ELECTROPHYSIOLOGY OF ARRHYTHMIAS

Second Edition

ELECTROPHYSIOLOGY OF ARRHYTHMIAS

Second Edition

Reginald T. Ho, MD, FACC, FHRS

Professor of Medicine
Department of Cardiology
Electrophysiology Service
Thomas Jefferson University Hospital
Philadelphia, Pennsylvania

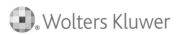. Wolters Kluwer

Philadelphia • Baltimore • New York • London
Buenos Aires • Hong Kong • Sydney • Tokyo

Senior Acquisitions Editor: Sharon Zinner
Development Editor: Ashley Fischer
Editorial Coordinator: Emily Buccieri
Editorial Assistant: Nicole Dunn
Production Project Manager: David Saltzberg
Design Coordinator: Holly Reid McLaughlin
Manufacturing Coordinator: Beth Welsh
Prepress Vendor: Absolute Service, Inc.

2nd edition

Library of Congress Cataloging-in-Publication Data

Names: Ho, Reginald T., author.
Title: Electrophysiology of arrhythmias / Reginald T. Ho.
Description: Second edition. | Philadelphia : Wolters Kluwer, [2020] |
   Includes bibliographical references and index.
Identifiers: LCCN 2019019636 | ISBN 9781975101107
Subjects: | MESH: Arrhythmias, Cardiac—diagnosis | Arrhythmias,
   Cardiac—surgery | Catheter Ablation | Electrophysiological Phenomena
Classification: LCC RC685.A65 | NLM WG 330 | DDC 616.1/28—dc23 LC record available at https://lccn.loc.gov/2019019636

This book is dedicated to my family, especially to my wife, Maromi, and sons, Ethan and Jeremy, whose love, enduring patience, and encouragement made this book possible, and to my parents who have always been a source of love and inspiration to me.

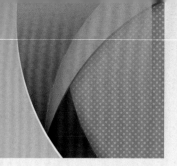

Preface

Since the first catheter recording of the human His bundle in 1960 and ablation in 1981, intracardiac electrophysiology has been the cornerstone of arrhythmia diagnosis and ablation. The ability to record electrical activity within the heart and observe its behavior to electrical stimulation has yielded valuable insights into the mechanisms and pathogenesis of arrhythmias. As a field where interpreting activation patterns, electrogram morphologies, and responses to pacing maneuvers are essential, electrophysiology is better understood through demonstration rather than description. This book is therefore purposefully designed to provide an understanding of arrhythmia diagnosis and ablation by using a comprehensive collection of intracardiac recordings; color-coded electro-anatomic maps; and fluoroscopy, intracardiac echocardiography (ICE),

and cardiac CT/MRI images detailing the "life" of each arrhythmia in the electrophysiology laboratory: induction, termination, transition zones, diagnostic pacing maneuvers, classic presentations, unique manifestations, mapping techniques, and target site criteria for successful ablation. Recordings were selected to emphasize physiology and illustrate important principles. Short but practical discussions systematically explain diagnostic and ablation criteria while providing a conceptual framework that puts each recording into context. It is hoped that through this library of quality recordings, the reader not only understands but also enjoys the electrophysiology of arrhythmias.

REGINALD T. HO, MD, FACC, FHRS

Contents

Bradycardias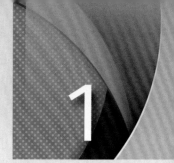

Introduction

The electrophysiologic (EP) study provides a means to assess sino-atrial node (SAN) function and the integrity of the atrio-ventricular node (AVN)–His-Purkinje axis.

The purpose of this chapter is to:
1. Discuss EP techniques to evaluate SAN, AVN, and His-Purkinje function.
2. Localize the site of atrio-ventricular (AV) block by 12-lead electrocardiogram (ECG) and His bundle recordings.
3. Differentiate physiologic from pathologic pacing-induced infrahisian block.
4. Recognize unusual manifestations of AV block in the His-Purkinje system.

SINUS NODE FUNCTION

The SAN, a crescent-shaped, subepicardial structure located along the lateral terminal groove at the junction of the right atrium and superior vena cava, is the site of impulse formation in the heart and densely innervated with cholinergic and adrenergic nerve fibers. The perinodal zone surrounding the SAN connects sinus nodal to right atrial cells. Sinus node function is an interplay of three variables: 1) sinus node automaticity, 2) perinodal conduction, and 3) autonomic tone. EP testing of the sinus node includes evaluation of its automaticity (sinus node recovery times or SNRTs), perinodal conduction (sino-atrial conduction times or SACTs), and the degree of autonomic control on the sinus node (intrinsic heart rate [IHR] and carotid sinus massage [CSM]).

SINUS NODE RECOVERY TIME

SNRTs measure spontaneous recovery of the sinus node after overdrive suppression. Rapid pacing is delivered from the high right atrium (HRA) near the SAN at different cycle lengths (CLs) (e.g., 600 ms, 500 ms, and 400 ms) for 30 sec. At each pacing CL, the recovery interval or uncorrected SNRT (interval from last pacing stimulus to first spontaneous sinus electrogram at the HRA catheter) is measured (normal <1400 ms).[1] The uncorrected SNRT is a function of 1) retrograde perinodal conduction, 2) sinus node automaticity (and, therefore, sinus CL), and 3) antegrade perinodal conduction. The corrected SNRT accounts for the sinus CL by subtracting it from the recovery interval (corrected SNRT = recovery interval − sinus CL; normal <550 ms).[1] The pacing CL and SNRT demonstrate

an inverse relationship until a point where shorter pacing CLs cause paradoxical shortening of the SNRT because of pacing-induced entrance block into the perinodal zone. The peak pacing CL is the shortest pacing CL resulting in the longest SNRT and is longer for patients with SAN dysfunction. Secondary pauses after pacing termination are sinus intervals that are longer than the SNRT.[2] The total recovery time is the amount of time after pacing that is required for the sinus rate to return to baseline (normal <5 sec or 4–6 beats). While abnormal SNRTs are specific for SAN dysfunction, variable penetration of pacing stimuli into the perinodal zone affects its sensitivity. Atropine can either shorten SNRTs by improving SAN automaticity or paradoxically increase SNRTs by improving perinodal conduction.[3] The clinical equivalent of abnormal SNRTs are prolonged post-conversion pauses following abrupt termination of atrial tachyarrhythmias (Fig. 1-1).

SINO-ATRIAL CONDUCTION TIME

SACTs measure perinodal conduction after the SAN has been reset (but not suppressed) by pacing.[4,5] With the Narula method, burst pacing is delivered just slightly faster (≤10 bpm) than the sinus rate. With the Strauss technique, single atrial extrastimuli scan sinus rhythm during diastole. Extrastimuli fall into one of four zones: 1) collision (compensation), 2) resetting, 3) interpolation, and 4) reentry, but only extrastimuli falling into the zone of resetting are analyzed. With either method, the return interval (time from the last stimulus to the first spontaneous sinus electrogram at the HRA catheter) is measured and is the summation of the retrograde conduction time from pacing site to SAN + sinus CL + antegrade conduction time from SAN to pacing site.

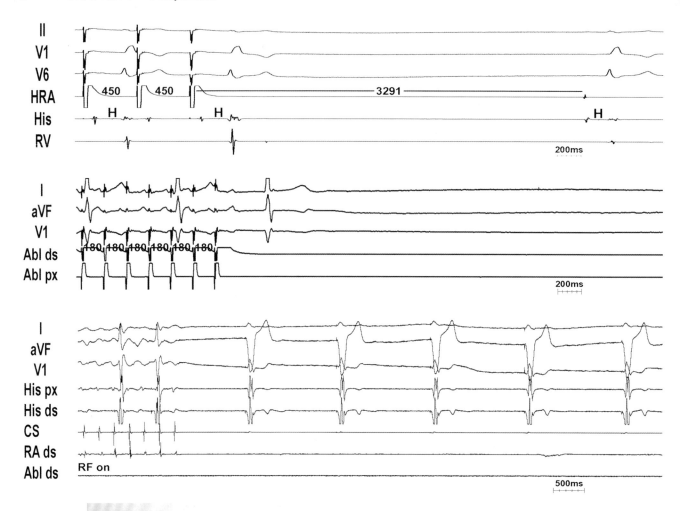

FIGURE 1-1 Manifestations of sinus node dysfunction. Prolonged SNRT (*top*). Sinus arrest following termination of atrial flutter by antitachycardia pacing (*middle*) and radiofrequency ablation (*bottom*).

Assuming that conduction times to and from the SAN are equal, the SACT = (return interval − sinus CL) / 2 (normal: 45–125 ms).[1] Poor or absent perinodal conduction causes prolonged SACT, the clinical equivalent of which is sino-atrial exit block (**Fig. 1-2**).

INTRINSIC HEART RATE

The IHR is a measure of sinus node automaticity when devoid of autonomic control. Autonomic blockade is achieved by propranolol (0.2 mg/kg at 1 mg/min) (sympathetic block) followed 10 min later by atropine (0.04 mg/kg over 2 min) (cholinergic block).[6,7] After autonomic blockade, the sinus rate is measured and compared to the predicted IHR (predicted IHR = 118.1 − [0.57 × age]).[8] An IHR that is less than the predicted IHR demonstrates intrinsic SAN disease. An IHR that is equal to the predicted IHR demonstrates lack of intrinsic SAN disease and implicates exaggerated autonomic tone for SAN dysfunction.

CAROTID SINUS MASSAGE

Carotid sinus hypersensitivity causes an exaggerated autonomic reflex in response to carotid sinus baroreceptor stimulation (**Fig. 1-3**).[9,10] It is associated with older age and organic heart disease. Gentle pressure on the carotid sinus (massage, stiff neck collars, tight neckties) triggers activation of baroreceptors located in the carotid bulb. Afferent nerve fibers travel from the baroreceptors via the glossopharyngeal nerve to the nucleus tractus solitarius (vasodepressor medullary region of the brain). The efferent limb of the reflex arc is the vagus nerve whose terminals richly innervate the SAN and AVN causing sinus pauses and/or AV block. Cardioinhibitory and vasodepressor responses are defined as ventricular asystole >3 sec and >50 mm Hg drop in systolic blood pressure, respectively.[9,11] Because cholinergic fibers innervate both the SAN and AVN, the combination of sinus slowing and PR prolongation before AV block suggests hypervagotonia (vagotonic AV block).

AVN–HIS-PURKINJE AXIS

The surface ECG PR interval is the summation of three sequential intracardiac intervals: PA + AH + HV, abnormalities of which can cause PR prolongation (first-degree AV block). The PA interval (onset of earliest surface P wave or intracardiac atrial activation to onset of the atrial electrogram on the His bundle catheter) represents the right atrial or internodal

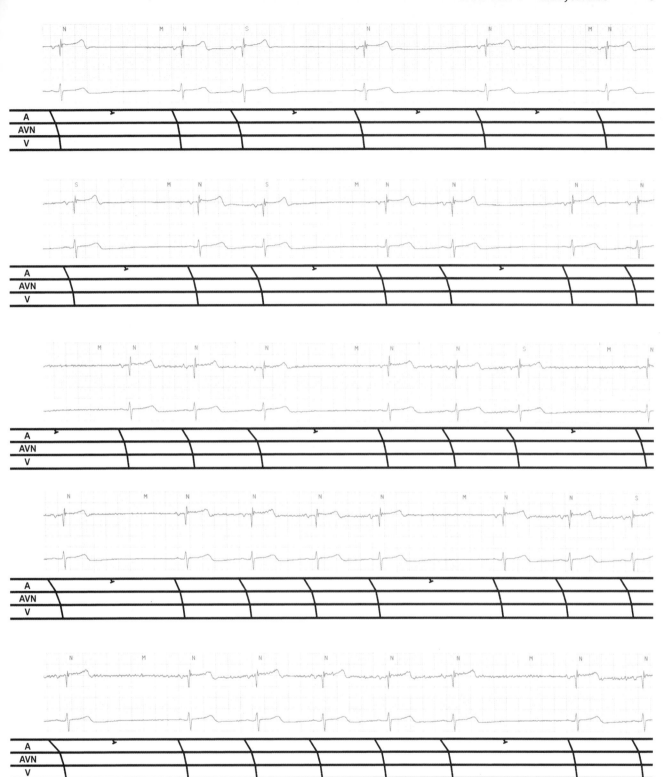

FIGURE 1-2 Sino-atrial exit block with conduction ratios ranging from 6:5 Wenckebach to 2:1.

(SAN to AVN) conduction time (normal: 20–60 ms).[12] The AH (atrio-His) interval (onset of the atrial electrogram on the His bundle catheter to onset of the His bundle potential) reflects the conduction time across the AVN (normal: 50–120 ms). The HV (His-ventricular) interval (onset of the His bundle potential to earliest surface [QRS complex] or intracardiac ventricular activation) represents the conduction time over the His-Purkinje system (normal: 35–55 ms).[12,13] The width of the His bundle electrogram, itself, represents the conduction time over the His bundle (normal: 15–25 ms).

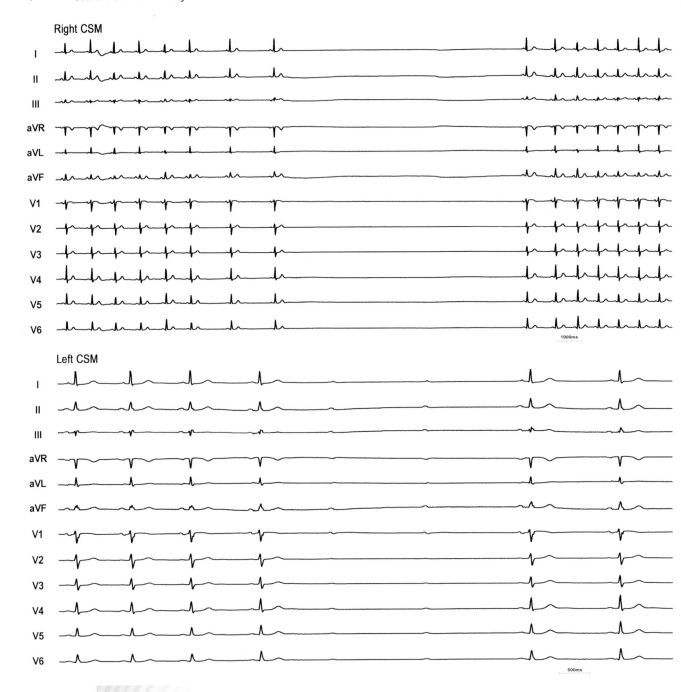

FIGURE 1-3 Carotid sinus hypersensitivity. Right CSM induces sinus slowing followed by 10.2 sec of sinus arrest. Left CSM triggers concomitant sinus slowing and 4.4 sec of AV block.

AVN FUNCTION

Programmed atrial extrastimulation and decremental atrial pacing assess antegrade AVN refractory periods and Wenckebach CLs, respectively.

AVN REFRACTORY PERIODS

During programmed atrial extrastimulation, single extrastimuli (A_2) are delivered with progressively shorter (10 ms) coupling intervals after a pacing drive train (A_1). At coupling intervals beyond the relative refractory period (RRP), the AH interval remains constant ($A_1H_1 = A_2H_2$). When the coupling interval reaches the AVN RRP, the AH interval prolongs because of decremental conduction over the AVN. The longest A_1A_2 interval causing $A_2H_2 > A_1H_1$ defines the AVN RRP. At a critically short coupling interval, the AVN effective refractory period (ERP) is reached and conduction blocks in the AVN. The longest A_1A_2 interval causing block in the AVN (A_2 without H_2) defines the AVN ERP. The shortest H_1H_2 interval for a given A_1A_2 interval defines the AVN functional refractory period (FRP) (AVN function curves plot A_1A_2 versus A_2H_2 or A_1A_2 versus H_1H_2).

WENCKEBACH CYCLE LENGTH

Rapid atrial pacing with progressively shorter CLs causes steady prolongation of the AH interval because of decremental AVN conduction. The point at which block occurs in the AVN defines its Wenckebach CL.

HIS-PURKINJE FUNCTION

Rapid atrial pacing tests the integrity of the His-Purkinje system and its ability to maintain 1:1 conduction.

PHYSIOLOGIC VERSUS PATHOLOGIC BLOCK

Pacing-induced infrahisian block can either be 1) physiologic (functional) or 2) pathologic.[14] Physiologic pacing-induced infrahisian block results from functional refractoriness in healthy His-Purkinje tissue often triggered by long–short sequences at the onset of rapid atrial pacing (normal His-Purkinje ERP ≤450 ms) (**Fig. 1-4**).[15] Because His-Purkinje refractory periods are directly related to sinus CL, abrupt onset rapid pacing during slow sinus rates facilitates physiologic infrahisian block. In contrast, pathologic pacing-induced intra- and infrahisian block

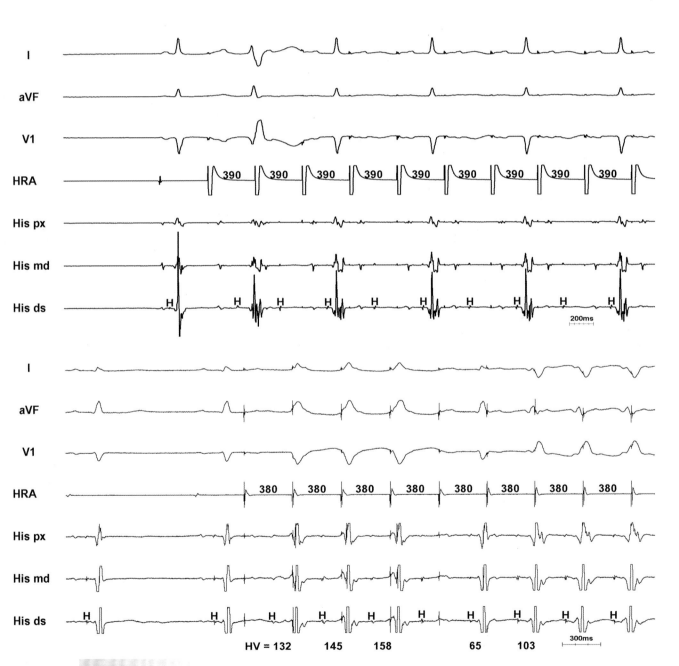

FIGURE 1-4 Physiologic pacing-induced infrahisian block. Baseline QRS complexes are normal. Abrupt onset rapid atrial pacing exposes the His-Purkinje system to long–short sequences that induce functional aberration, HV prolongation, and infrahisian AV block.

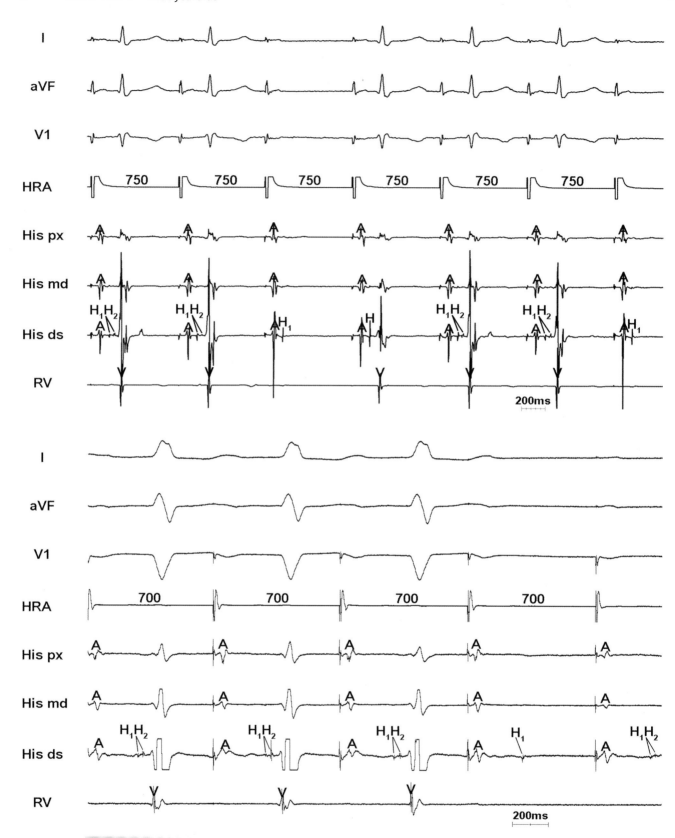

FIGURE 1-5 Pathologic pacing-induced intrahisian block. Split His bundle potentials (H₁H₂) are recorded during conduction. Slow atrial pacing induces block within the His bundle. Note that in the top tracing, the split His bundle electrogram becomes a large single potential after the pause due to recovery of His bundle conduction.

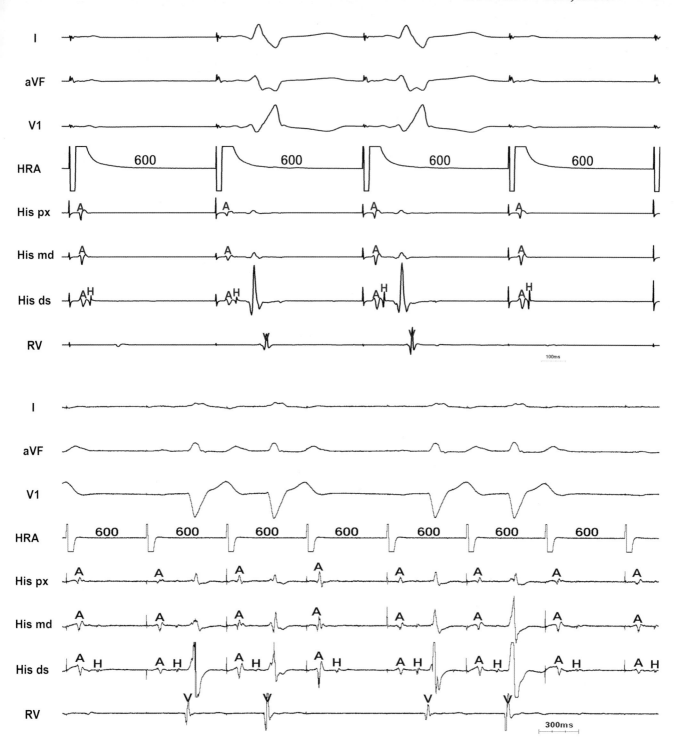

FIGURE 1-6 Pathologic pacing-induced infrahisian block. Slow atrial pacing induces block below the His bundle in the setting of RBBB (*top*) and LBBB (*bottom*).

results from abnormal refractoriness in diseased His-Purkinje tissue and observed during incremental or longer pacing CLs (>450 ms) (**Figs. 1-5 and 1-6**).[15]

ATROPINE OR ISOPROTERENOL

Adrenergic and cholinergic innervation of the AVN but not His-Purkinje system allows autonomic manipulation of the conduction system to identify the site of block. The AVN protects the His-Purkinje system from rapid atrial rates, and the evaluation of His-Purkinje system function is limited by the AVN FRP. Shortening AVN refractoriness by atropine or isoproterenol allows more atrial inputs to reach the His-Purkinje system. While atropine and isoproterenol improve intranodal AV block, it paradoxically worsens AV block in the His-Purkinje system (**Fig. 1-7**).[16] Conversely, while CSM increases vagal tone

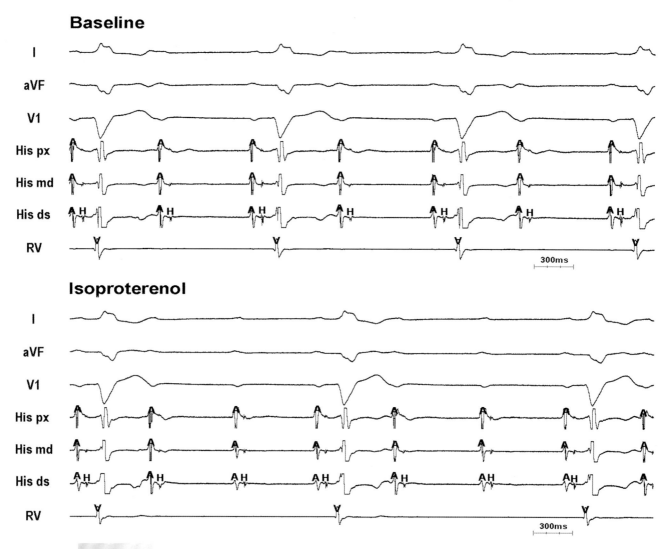

FIGURE 1-7 Paradoxical worsening of AV block by isoproterenol. *Top*: At a sinus rate of 86 bpm, 2:1 block in the setting of LBBB occurs below the His bundle resulting in a ventricular rate of 43 bpm. The HV interval measures 81 ms. *Bottom*: Sinus acceleration to 100 bpm on isoproterenol worsens the conduction ratio to 3:1 and paradoxically slows the ventricular rate to 33 bpm.

and worsens intranodal AV block, it slows the sinus rate and can improve AV block in the His-Purkinje system.

PROCAINAMIDE

Procainamide slows His-Purkinje conduction by blocking Na channels and delaying the upstroke (phase 0) of its action potential. It can, therefore, be a provocative test of His-Purkinje function.[17] While procainamide normally increases HV intervals by 15–20%, the following responses are abnormal: 1) HV increase by 100%, 2) HV >100 ms, 3) spontaneous second- and third-degree infrahisian block, and 4) pathologic pacing-induced infrahisian block not observed at baseline.[15]

LOCALIZING THE SITE OF AV BLOCK

AV block can occur at one of three sites along the AVN–His-Purkinje axis: AVN (intranodal), His bundle (intrahisian),

and bundle branches (infrahisian). The level of block is important prognostically because it determines the adequacy of subsidiary escape pacemakers. Junctional escape rhythms associated with intranodal AV block are faster and more reliable than ventricular escape rhythms.

12-LEAD ECG

The ECG clues providing a presumptive localization of the site of AV block are the 1) PR interval, 2) QRS width, 3) pattern of AV block, and 4) morphology of escape complexes. During AV block, long conducted PR intervals (>300 ms) and narrow QRS complexes favor block in the AVN, while normal or mildly prolonged PR intervals with bundle branch block (BBB) suggest block below the His bundle. The presence of normal or mildly prolonged PR intervals and narrow QRS complexes raises the possibility of block within the His bundle (**Figs. 1-8 and 1-9**). Escape QRS complexes that are identical to conducted QRS

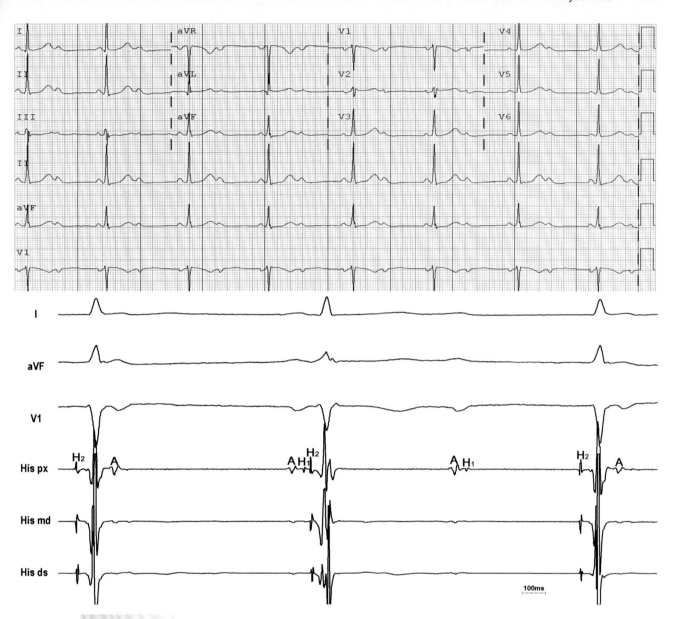

FIGURE 1-8 2:1 intrahisian AV block. Conducted PR intervals are normal and QRS complex are narrow suggesting block within the His bundle and confirmed by His bundle recordings: split His bundle potentials during conduction followed by H_1 block and H_2 preceding narrow escape complexes. Note that the sinus beat after escape complexes block in the AVN due to functional refractoriness caused by retrograde penetration of distal His bundle escape complexes into the AVN. Note also the slight difference in morphology between conducted and escape QRS complexes.

complex originate above the bifurcation of the His bundle and localize block to either the AVN or His bundle. While the AVN exhibits decremental conduction, His-Purkinje conduction is typically "all or none." Therefore, second-degree AV block (Mobitz type I or Wenckebach) suggests block in the AVN, particularly if the difference between the first and last PR interval of a Wenckebach sequence is large and the QRS complex is narrow. Rarely, however, diseased His-Purkinje tissue can exhibit decremental conduction, but the increment in PR interval before block is generally smaller. A Wenckebach pattern with only small increments in the PR interval and a narrow QRS complex suggests intrahisian Wenckebach (Fig. 1-9). A Wenckebach pattern in the setting of BBB especially when prolongation of

the PR interval is accompanied by changes in QRS morphology indicates infrahisian Wenckebach because bundle branch conduction contributes to formation of both the PR interval and QRS complex (Figs. 1-10 and 1-11). In contrast, second-degree AV block (Mobitz type II) indicates block in the His-Purkinje system. While Mobitz type II block typically occurs in the setting of BBB, the presence of a narrow QRS complex indicates block within the His bundle (Fig. 1-9).

HIS BUNDLE RECORDINGS

The presence of a His bundle electrogram localizes the site of AV block.

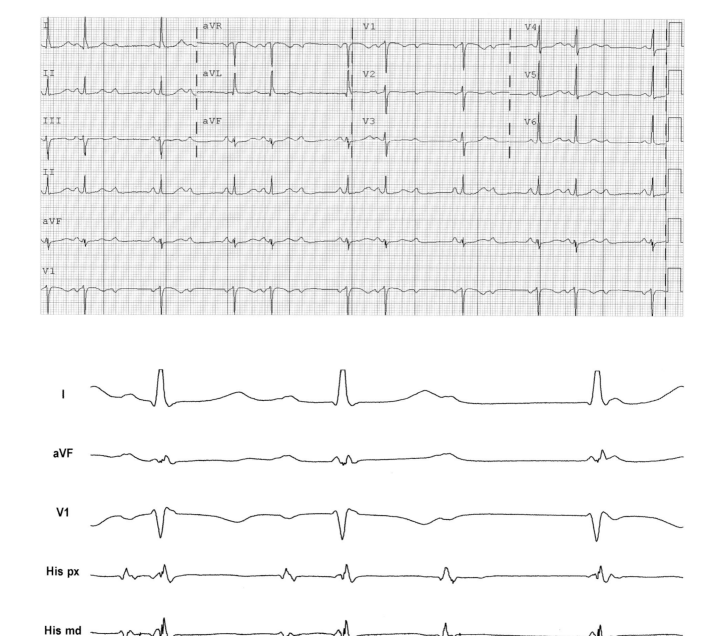

FIGURE 1-9 Mobitz type I and type II intrahisian blocks. The 12-lead ECG shows 3:2 Mobtiz Type 2 and 2:1 AV block in the setting of a normal PR and narrow QRS complex. Intracardiac recordings show 3:2 intrahisian Wenckebach (Mobitz type I). The sharp, single His bundle potential splits (H_1H_2 = 93 ms) during PR prolongation followed by block after H_1. H_2 precedes the junctional escape complex. Note that splitting causes diminution of the His bundle electrogram because of slow conduction.

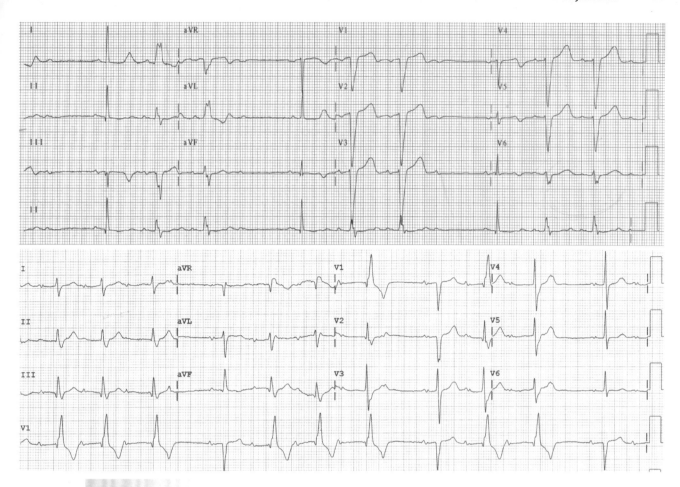

FIGURE 1-10 Unusual pattern of Mobitz type I infrahisian AV block in the setting of LBBB (*top*) and RBBB (*bottom*). After AV block, PR intervals shorten and QRS complexes narrow due to recovery of His-Purkinje conduction. Subsequent PR intervals lengthen and QRS complexes aberrate due to exposure of the diseased His-Purkinje system to a long–short sequence until AV block occurs. Increase in the PR interval accompanied by widening of the QRS complex indicates that the site of conduction delay and block is below the His bundle.

Intranodal Block

The characteristic feature of intranodal AV block is absence of His bundle activation following block. Second-degree AV block (Mobitz Type 1 or Wenckebach) shows progressive AH prolongation preceding block, while third-degree AV block with a junctional escape rhythm demonstrates complete failure of AVN conduction with His bundle activation linked to the junctional escape rhythm (**Fig. 1-12**).

Intrahisian Block

The characteristic feature of intrahisian AV block is a fractionated or split (H_1H_2) His bundle electrogram during conduction but failure of conduction between the two His bundle potentials during block.[18–20] Second-degree AV block (Mobitz Type 1 or Wenckebach) shows progressive prolongation of the H_1H_2 interval preceding block, while second-degree AV block (Mobitz Type II) is characterized by fixed H_1H_2 intervals preceding block (**Fig. 1-13**).[21] Third-degree AV block with a junctional (distal His bundle) escape rhythm shows complete failure of

His bundle conduction so that the two His bundle potentials are dissociated from each other (H_1 linked to the atrium and H_2 linked to the escape rhythm) (**Fig. 1-14**).

Infrahisian Block

The characteristic feature of infrahisian AV block is activation of the His bundle without conduction to the ventricle. Second-degree AV block (Mobitz Type 1 or Wenckebach) demonstrates progressive HV prolongation preceding block, while second-degree AV block (Mobitz Type II) shows constant HV intervals before block (**Figs. 1-15 to 1-18**). Third-degree AV block with a ventricular escape rhythm shows complete failure of conduction below the His bundle so that the His bundle and ventricle are dissociated from each other, the former being linked to the atrium (**Figs. 1-19 to 1-21**). Rarely, ventricular complexes can be narrower than the conducted BBB if the ventricular complex arises from the septum resulting in rapid engagement of the His-Purkinje system and simultaneous right and left ventricular activation (**Fig. 1-17**).[22]

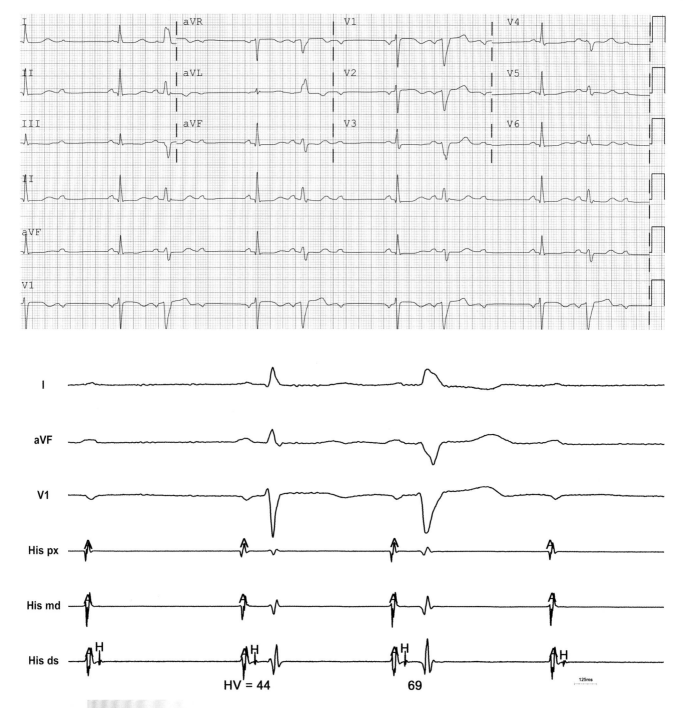

FIGURE 1-11 Unusual pattern of 3:2 Mobitz type I infrahisian AV block in the setting of LBBB. A normal PR interval and narrow QRS complex start each Wenckebach cycle. Exposure of the diseased His-Purkinje system to a long–short sequence from previous AV block causes HV prolongation and LBBB until infrahisian AV block occurs. The pause allows recovery of His-Purkinje conduction with subsequent normalization of the PR interval and QRS complex. Slight increase in the PR interval accompanied by widening of the QRS complex implicates the His-Purkinje system as the site of conduction delay and block.

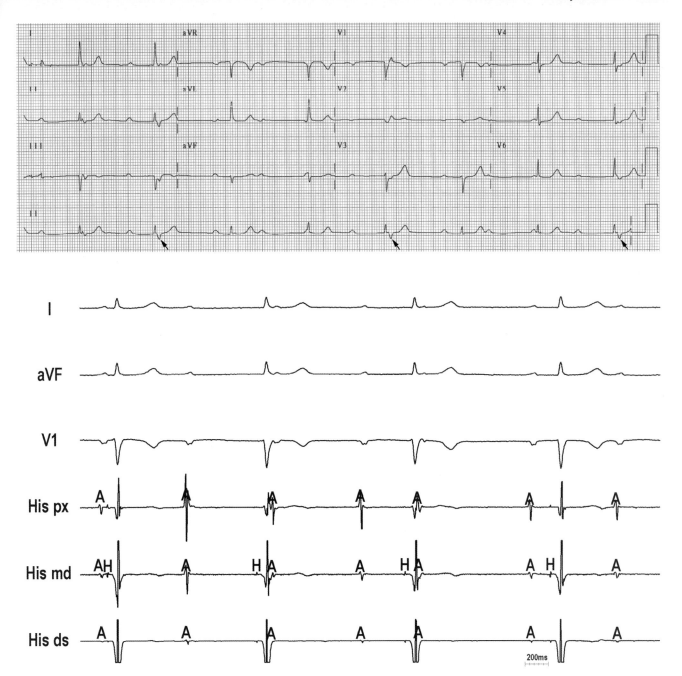

FIGURE 1-12 Complete intranodal AV block. The rhythm is sinus with complete AV block and junctional escape rhythm. Escape complexes falling into a window during late atrial diastole (when the atrium and AVN are not refractory but before the next sinus beat) conduct retrogradely over the AVN causing retrograde P waves (*arrows*). His bundle recordings show that the site of block is at the level of the AVN with His bundle potentials linked to escape complexes. (Retrograde AVN conduction during intranodal AV block is uncommon and more common with His-Purkinje block. Another possibility is intrahisian block but that a His bundle potential following the atrial electrogram is not visible.)

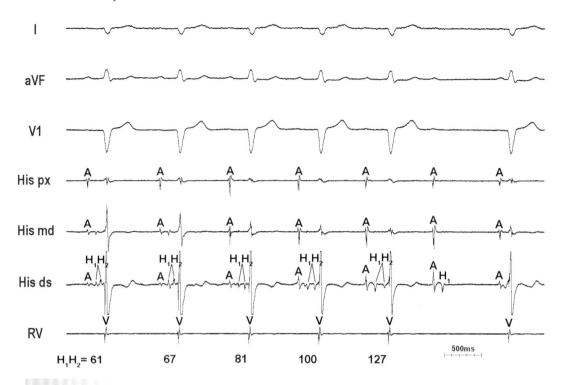

FIGURE 1-13 Intrahisian Wenckebach. During sinus rhythm, PR intervals progressively prolong in the setting of a narrow QRS complex preceding AV block. Note that the total increment between the first and last conducted PR interval is small. His bundle recordings show progressive splitting of His potentials (H_1H_2) followed by block within the His bundle and a distal His bundle escape complex.

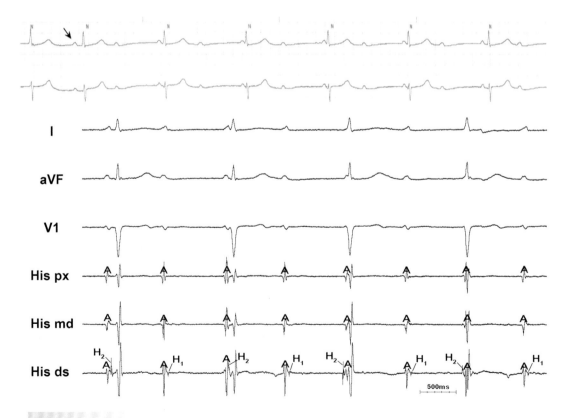

FIGURE 1-14 Complete intrahisian AV block. Telemetry strip (leads II and V1) demonstrates sinus rhythm with third-degree AV block and a narrow QRS complex escape rhythm except for a single P wave (*arrow*) that conducts to the ventricle with a normal PR interval. His bundle recordings reveal that the site of block is within the His bundle with dissociated His bundle potentials: H_1 linked to the atrium; H_2 linked to the ventricle.

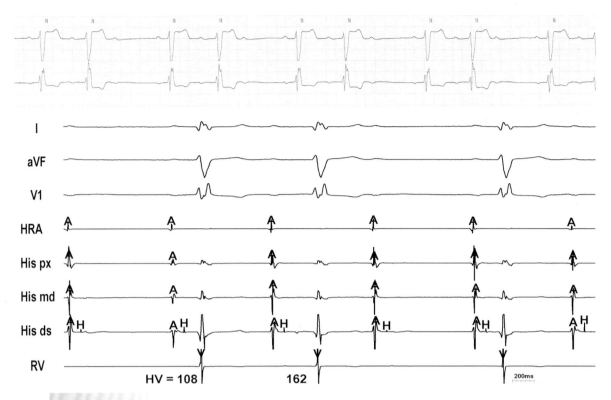

FIGURE 1-15 Infrahisian Wenckebach with RBBB. Telemetry strip (leads II and V1) shows sinus rhythm with Mobitz type I (Wenckebach) AV block in the setting of RBBB/LAFB. His bundle recordings show marked HV prolongation preceding infrahisian block. In the setting of RBBB/LAFB, Wenckebach occurs over the diseased left posterior fascicle.

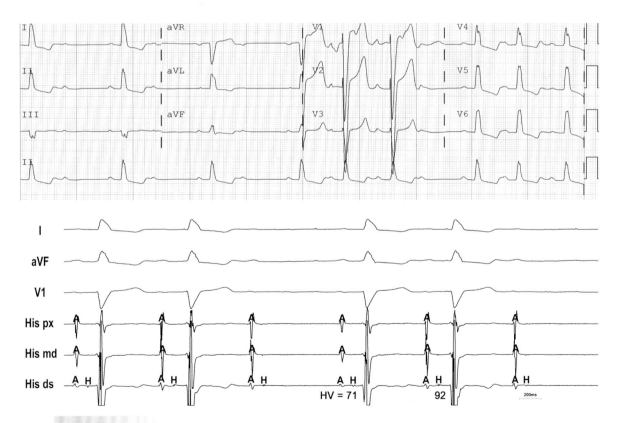

FIGURE 1-16 Infrahisian Wenckebach with LBBB. The 12-lead ECG shows sinus rhythm with Mobitz type I (Wenckebach) AV block in the setting of LBBB. His bundle recordings show prolongation of the HV interval preceding infrahisian block due to Wenckebach conduction over the right bundle.

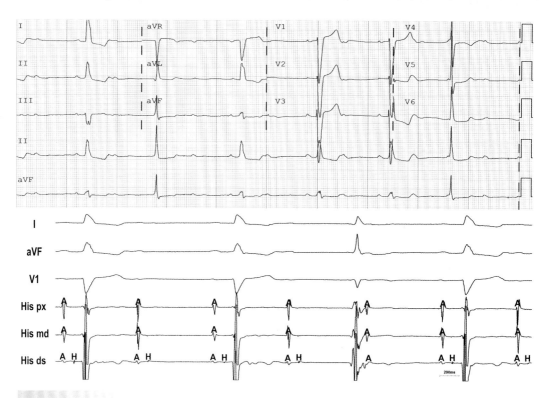

FIGURE 1-17 2:1 infrahisian AV block with LBBB and septal PVCs. The 12-lead ECG shows sinus rhythm with 2:1 AV block in the setting of LBBB. His bundle recordings show block below the His bundle. Note that the PVCs are paradoxically narrower than conducted LBBB QRS complexes because they arise from the anteroseptum (early ventricular activation on the His bundle channel) resulting in rapid penetration of the His-Purkinje system and simultaneous right ventricle (RV)/ left ventricle (LV) activation.

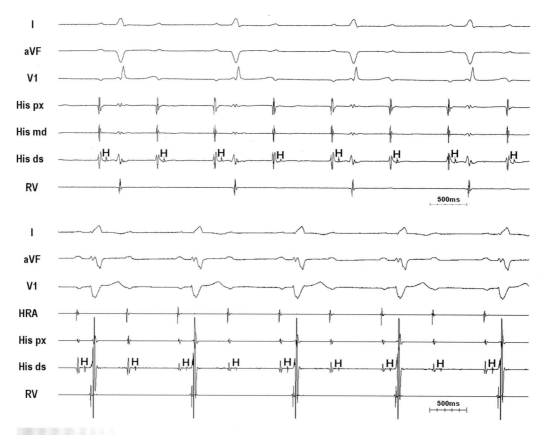

FIGURE 1-18 2:1 infrahisian AV in the setting of RBBB/LAFB (*top*) and LBBB (*bottom*). The HV interval of conducted QRS complexes measures 125 and 75 ms, respectively.

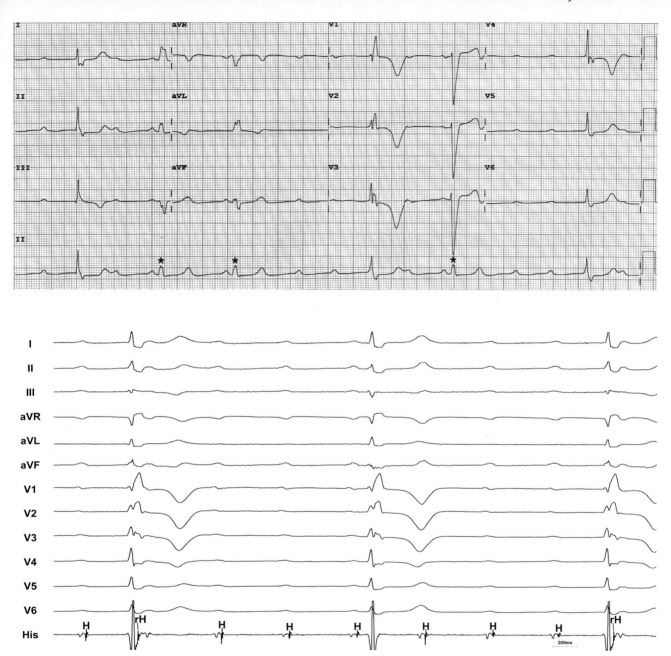

FIGURE 1-19 Advanced infrahisian AV block in the setting of LBBB. The 12-lead ECG shows sinus rhythm with high-grade AV block and intermittent AV conduction with normal PR interval and LBBB (*asterisks*). Escape complexes have RBBB morphology (left ventricular origin). His bundle recordings demonstrate block below the His bundle. Note that ventricular escape complexes are followed by retrograde activation of the His bundle (rH), which causes functional refractoriness in the AVN. Subsequent P waves, therefore, block in the AVN.

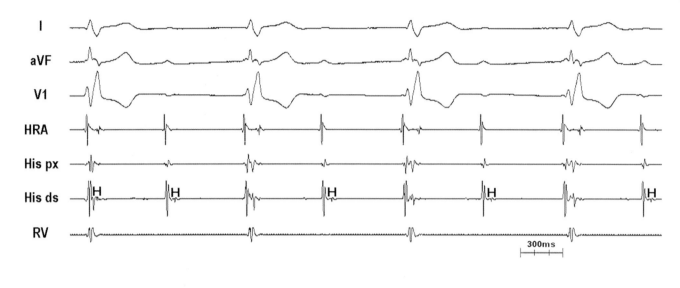

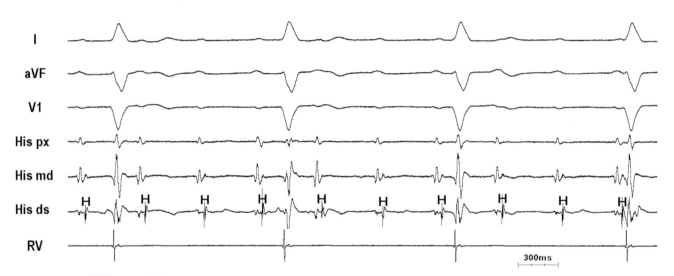

FIGURE 1-20 Complete infrahisian AV block with RBBB (*top*) and LBBB (*bottom*) morphology escape rhythms.

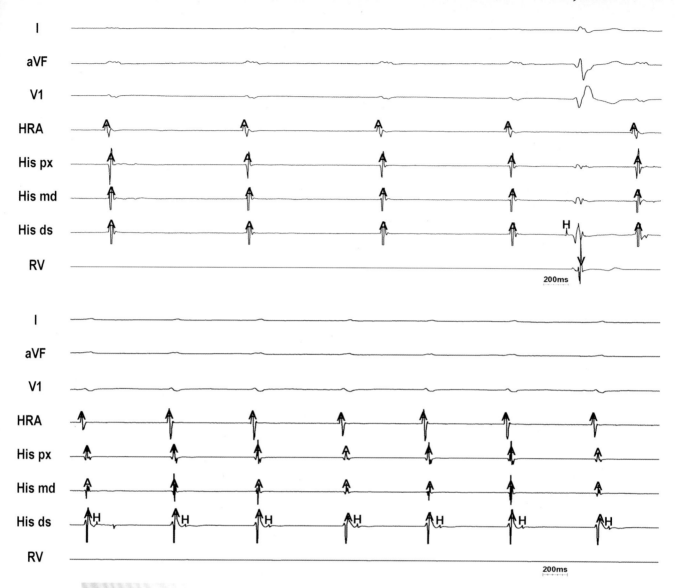

FIGURE 1-21 Asystole due to intranodal (*top*) and infrahisian (*bottom*) AV block. The single RBBB/LAFB QRS complex on the top tracing is either a conducted complex preceded by a long AH interval or a junctional escape.

UNUSUAL ELECTROPHYSIOLOGIC PHENOMENA

PAROXYSMAL AV BLOCK

Paroxysmal AV block (PAVB) is an abrupt form of high-grade AV block that can be bradycardia dependent, tachycardia dependent, or rate independent.[23] Bradycardia-dependent PAVB (also called phase IV AV block) results from spontaneous diastolic depolarizations in diseased His-Purkinje tissue.[24–27] Classically, it is triggered by premature impulses (e.g., atrial premature complex (APCs), premature ventricular complex (PVCs), junctional premature complex (JPCs)) that conceal into diseased His-Purkinje tissue exposing it to a longer diastolic interval (pause) than the sinus CL (**Figs. 1-22 to 1-25**). It can also be triggered paradoxically by a malfunctioning pacemaker (**Fig. 1-26**).[28] Resumption of conduction often manifests a predictable temporal relationship

to escape complexes resulting from various potential mechanisms (summation, supernormality, Wedensky facilitation). Tachycardia-dependent PAVB occurs during acceleration of the atrial rate causing repetitive concealed conduction into diseased His-Purkinje tissue and exacerbated by post-repolarization refractoriness. Acceleration of the sinus rate and lack of PR prolongation preceding high-grade AV block differentiate PAVB from vagotonic AV block. Some cases of PAVB occur spontaneously without any perceptible changes in atrial rate (rate independent).

BILATERAL BBB

The ECG manifestations of bilateral BBB include 1) alternating right bundle branch block (RBBB)/left bundle branch block (LBBB), 2) RBBB with alternating hemiblock (left anterior fascicular block [LAFB]/left posterior fascicular block [LPFB]), and 3) masquerading (or masked) BBB (**Figs. 1-27 to 1-32**).[29–33]

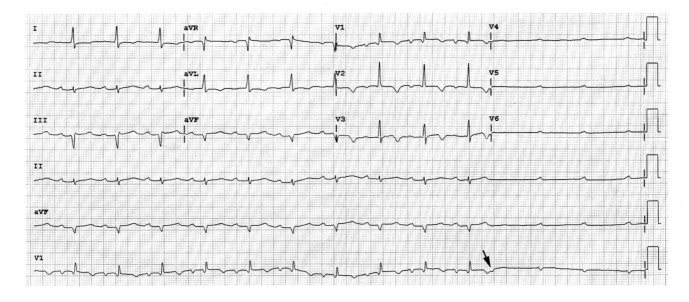

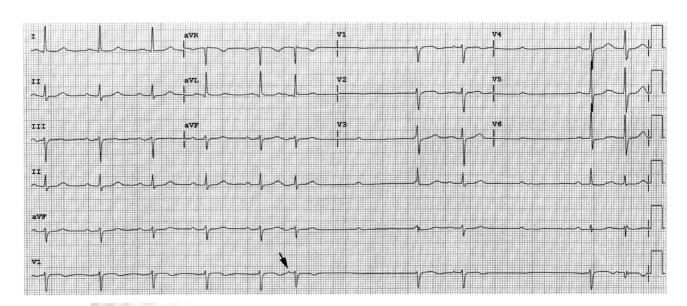

FIGURE 1-22 PAVB triggered by APCs (*arrows*). PR intervals are only mildly prolonged, and QRS complexes are narrow.

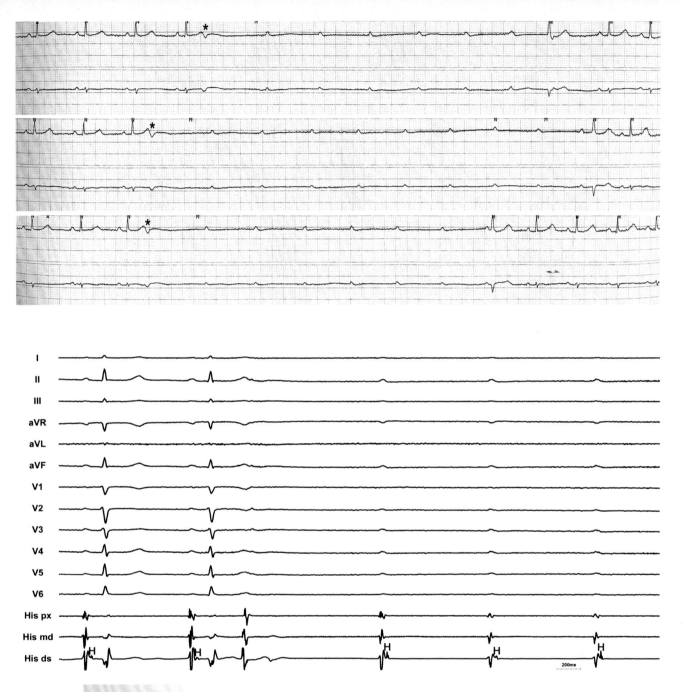

FIGURE 1-23 PAVB triggered repetitively by APCs (*asterisks*). Block is subnodal: distal His bundle (beyond the His bundle recording site) or simultaneously in both bundle branches.

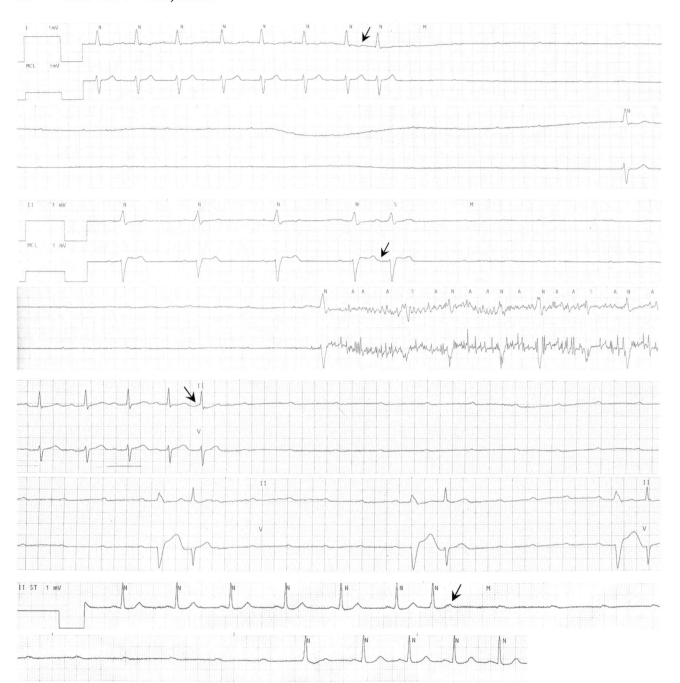

FIGURE 1-24 PAVB triggered by APCs (*first and second panels*) and JPCs (*third and fourth panels*). *First and second panels*: APCs (*arrows*) reset the sinus timetable causing a noncompensatory pause and provoking bradycardia-dependent AV block. Note the muscle artifact during convulsive syncope in the second episode. *Third and fourth panels*: JPCs coincide with or precede sinus complexes (*arrows*) and do not reset the sinus timetable, exposing the His-Purkinje system to a compensatory pause and provoking bradycardia-dependent AV block. In the third episode, phase IV LBBB accompanies intermittent resumption of AV conduction.

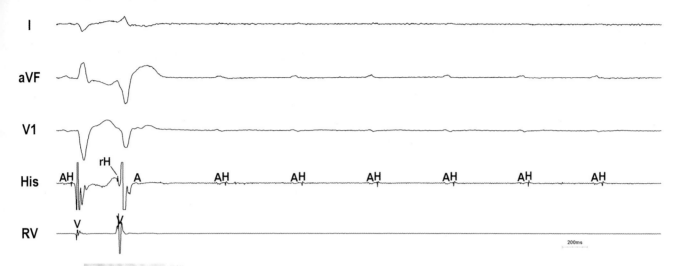

FIGURE 1-25 PAVB triggered by a PVC. During LBBB, a spontaneous PVC from the right ventricle (RV) apex retrogradely activates the His bundle (rH) causing one beat of intranodal AV block. Premature activation of the His-Purkinje system and subsequent exposure of the right bundle to a compensatory pause induces high-grade phase IV AV block.

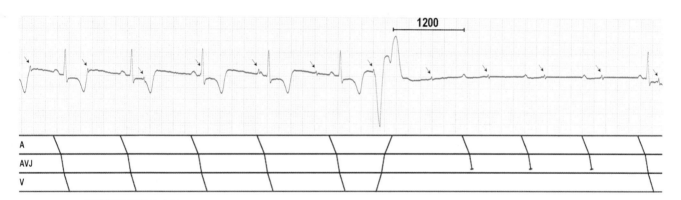

FIGURE 1-26 PAVB triggered paradoxically by a pacemaker. Pacing stimuli (*arrows*) fail to sense and capture the ventricle except for a single stimulus occurring shortly after the T wave and falling into the supernormal period of ventricular excitability. Premature ventricular capture results in retrograde conduction to the atrium, exposing the His-Purkinje system to a noncompensatory pause (1200 ms) and triggering phase IV AV block.

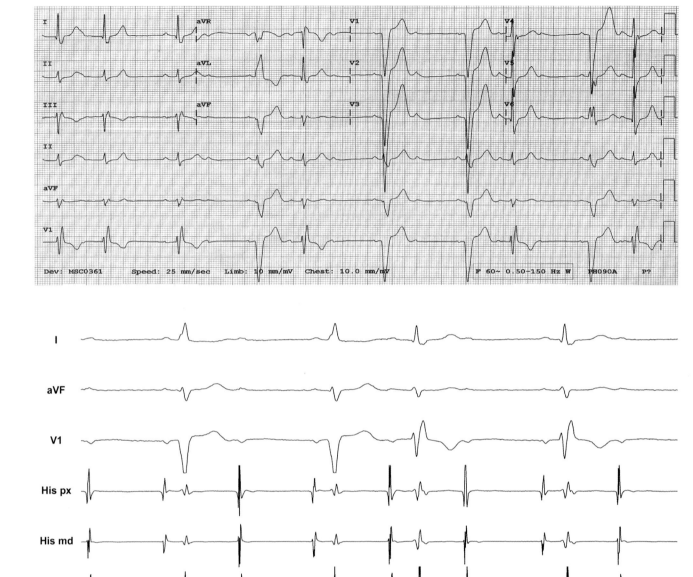

FIGURE 1-27 Bilateral BBB (alternating RBBB/LBBB). The 12-lead ECG shows sinus rhythm with both RBBB and LBBB conducted QRS complexes interspersed among AV block. His bundle recordings show that changes in the PR (HV) interval accompany changes in BBB with AV block below the His bundle.

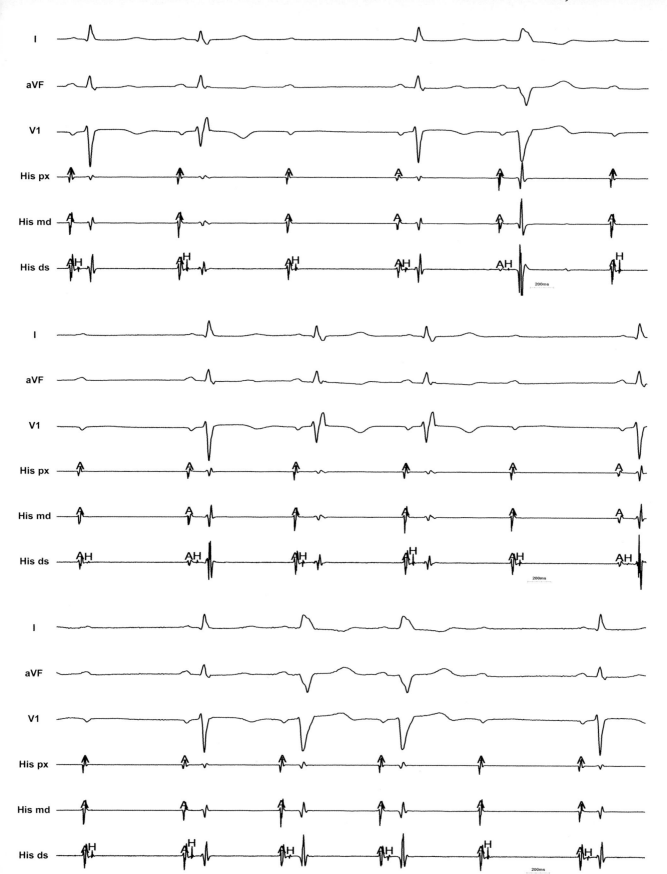

FIGURE 1-28 Bilateral BBB (alternating RBBB/LBBB). Episodes of infrahisian AV block are followed by narrow QRS complexes because the pause allows recovery of His-Purkinje conduction. Subsequent exposure of diseased His-Purkinje tissue to long–short sequences causes both RBBB and LBBB preceding AV block.

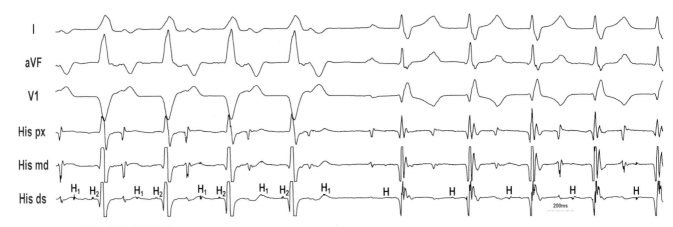

FIGURE 1-29 Bilateral BBB (alternating LBBB/RBBB). On the left half of the tracing, split His bundle potentials (H_1H_2 = 142 ms) precede LBBB QRS complexes. A single episode of AV block within the His bundle is followed by a pause that allows partial recovery of His-Purkinje conduction. Subsequent single His bundle potentials precede RBBB QRS complexes after a prolonged HV interval (HV = 134 ms).

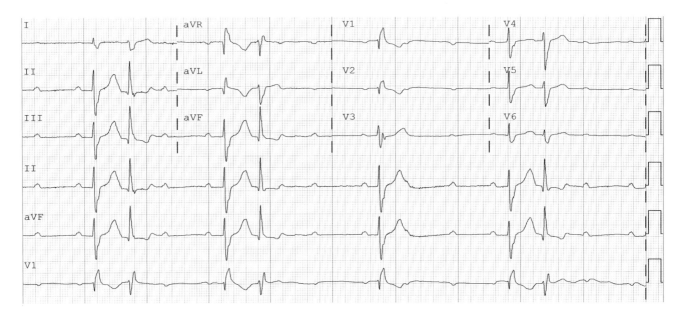

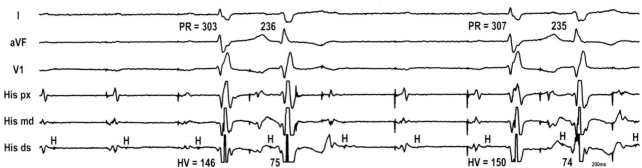

FIGURE 1-30 Bilateral BBB (RBBB with alternating LAFB/LPFB). The 12-lead ECG shows sinus rhythm with RBBB and alternating hemiblock among periods of AV block. His bundle recordings show block below the His bundle. The PR (and HV) interval of each second conducted QRS complex (RBBB/LPFB) paradoxically shortens because of conduction during the supernormal period of the left anterior fascicle.

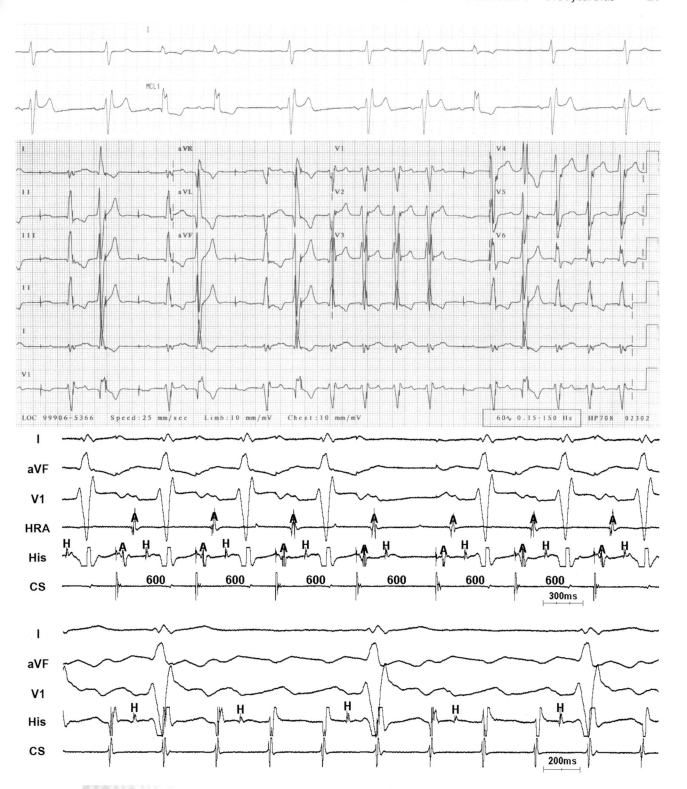

FIGURE 1-31 Bilateral BBB (RBBB with alternating LAFB/LPFB). Telemetry strips (leads I and V1) show sinus arrhythmia with faster rates associated with longer PR intervals and RBBB/LAFB and slower rates associated with shorter PR intervals and RBBB/LPFB. Both atrial pacing and atrial flutter cause pathologic infrahisian AV block. Note that the switch in hemiblock pattern causes a change in RBBB morphology due to activation from a different part of the left ventricle.

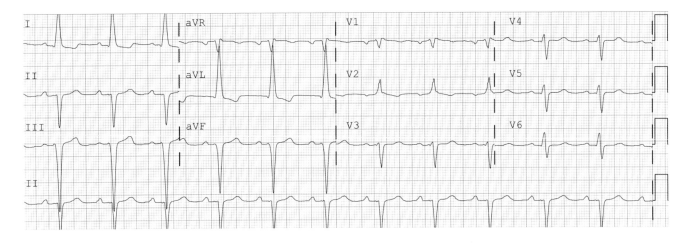

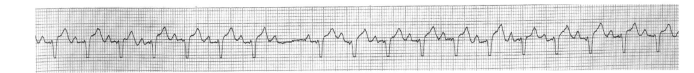

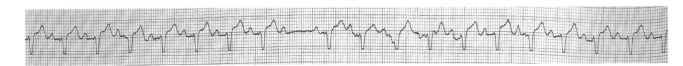

FIGURE 1-32 Masked BBB with AV block. Lead V1 shows an rSr′ pattern (RBBB), while lead I has a prominent R with no s wave (LBBB). The frontal QRS axis is leftward. Telemetry shows Mobitz type II AV block. Masked BBB is a form of bilateral BBB.

Masked BBB is a RBBB pattern in lead V1 (precordial lead) but an LBBB pattern in lead I (limb lead [absence of an s wave]) (Fig. 1-32).[34,35] Bilateral BBB is associated with a high risk of AV block below the His bundle.

SUPERNORMALITY

Supernormality is a brief period at the end of recovery during which an otherwise subthreshold impulse unexpectedly demonstrates conduction or excitation.[32,36–39] It is observed in diseased His-Purkinje tissue during infrahisian AV block when critically timed sinus impulses falling into the supernormal window of the His-Purkinje system demonstrate unexpected conduction to the ventricle (Figs. 1-30 and 1-33; see also Fig. 22-9). It explains unusual 3:2, 4:2, and 5:2 conduction ratios during high-grade infrahisian AV block (Figs. 1-34 and 1-35).[40]

FATIGUE PHENOMENA

Retrograde penetration and overdrive suppression of diseased His-Purkinje tissue by rapid ventricular pacing can induce transient high-grade or complete AV block upon pacing cessation (Fig. 1-36). The degree of fatigue in the His-Purkinje system is directly related to the rate and duration of pacing.[41]

INFRAHISIAN AV BLOCK DURING ATRIAL FIBRILLATION/FLUTTER

Typically, atrial fibrillation and flutter conceal antegradely into the AVN. Uncommonly, AV block occurs below the His bundle in the setting of severe His-Purkinje disease (Figs. 1-31, 1-37, and 1-38; see also Fig. 22-5).

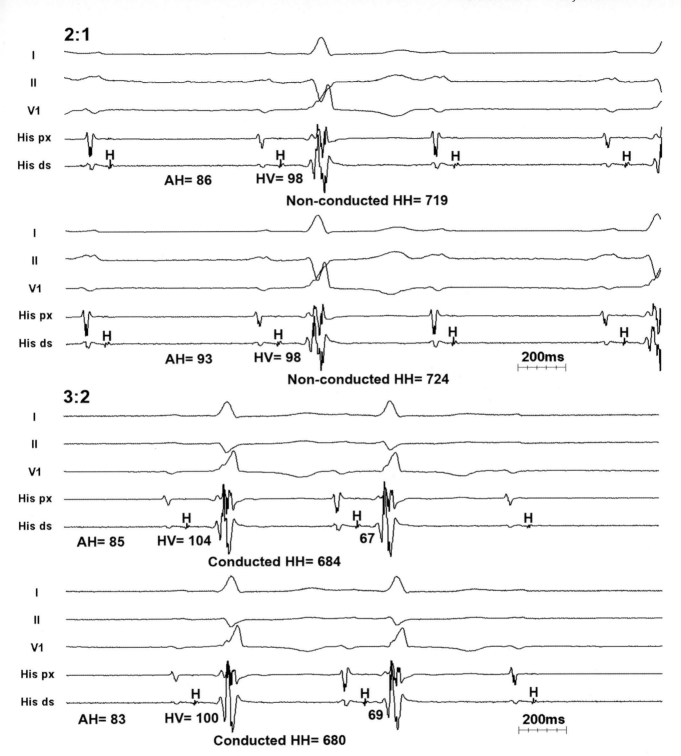

FIGURE 1-33 Infrahisian AV block with supernormality. Slight acceleration of the sinus rates causes transition from 2:1 to 3:2 conduction in the setting of RBBB/LAFB. During 3:2 conduction, the second conducted P wave falls into the supernormal period of the left posterior fascicle (LPF). Conduction over the LPF is not only "better than expected" but also "faster than expected" resulting in paradoxical shortening of the HV interval. Consecutive activation of the LPF narrows and shifts its supernormal period leftward causing the third P wave to fall outside the supernormal period and fail to conduct to the ventricle.

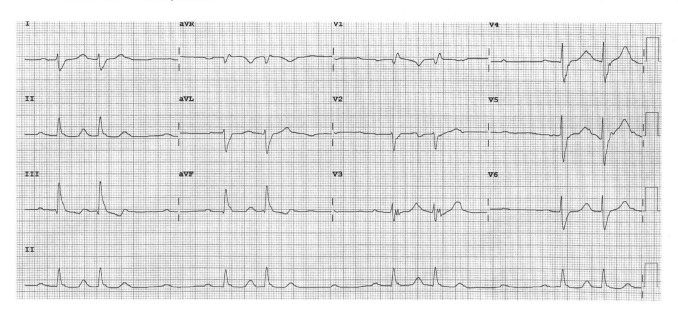

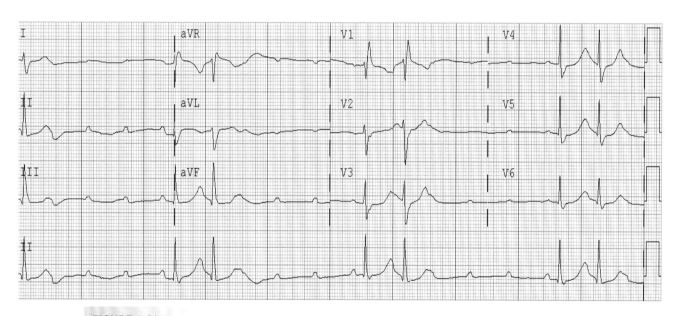

FIGURE 1-34 Unusual pattern of 4:2 and 5:2 AV block in the setting of RBBB/LPFB. The second conducted P wave of each cycle falls into the supernormal period of the left anterior fascicle resulting in unexpected conduction. The long preceding diastolic interval due to high-grade AV block causes a rightward shift and widening of the left anterior fascicle supernormal window. Following consecutive activation of the left anterior fascicle, its supernormal period narrows and shifts leftward so that the third P wave of each cycle falls outside the supernormal period and fails to conduct to the ventricle.

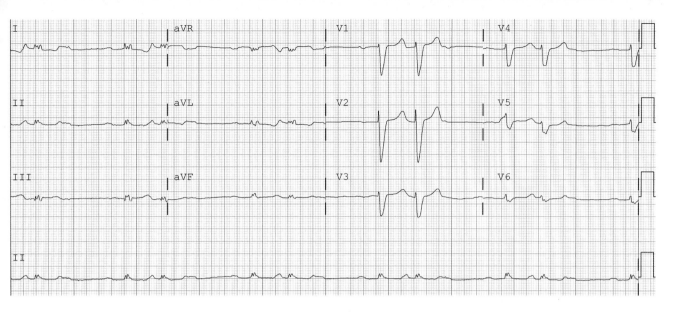

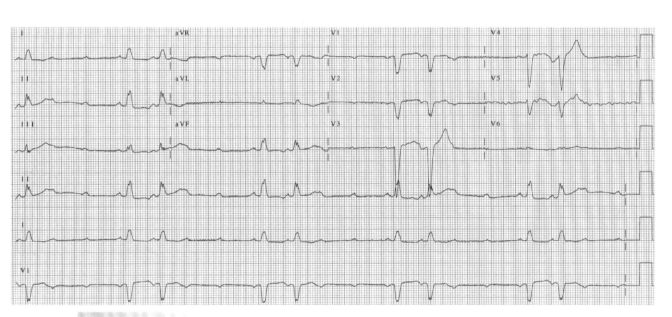

FIGURE 1-35 Unusual pattern of 3:2 and 4:2 AV block in the setting of LBBB. The second conducted P wave of each cycle falls into the supernormal period of the right bundle resulting in unexpected conduction. The long preceding diastolic interval due to high-grade AV block causes a rightward shift and widening of the right bundle supernormal window. Following consecutive activation of the right bundle, its supernormal period narrows and shifts leftward so that the third P wave of each cycle falls outside the supernormal period and fails to conduct to the ventricle. Note that in the top ECG, the second PR interval is paradoxically shorter than the first as supernormal conduction over the right bundle results not only in "better than expected" but also in "faster than expected" conduction.

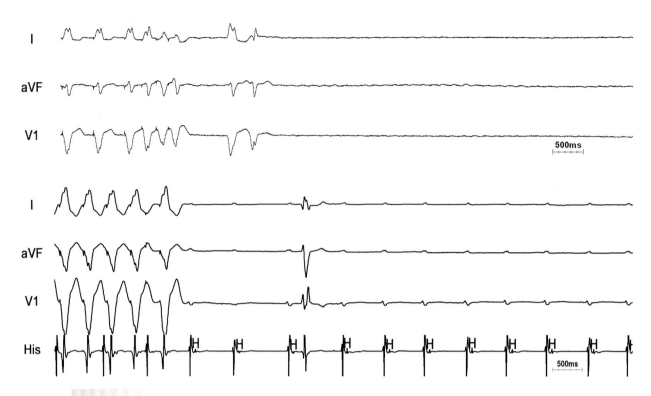

FIGURE 1-36 Fatigue phenomena. *Top*: During atrial fibrillation with LBBB, programmed ventricular stimulation using triple extrastimulation retrogradely penetrates the diseased right bundle causing fatigue and ventricular asystole. *Bottom*: During sinus rhythm with RBBB/LAFB, programmed ventricular stimulation using double extrastimulation penetrates the diseased left posterior fascicle causing fatigue and prolonged infrahisian AV block.

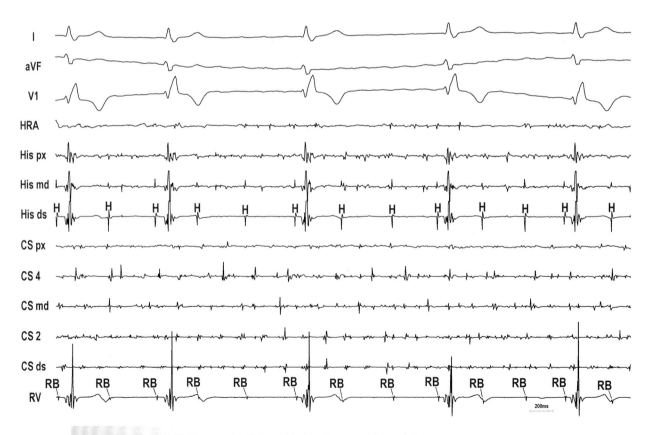

FIGURE 1-37 Atrial fibrillation with infrahisian block in the setting of RBBB/LAFB.

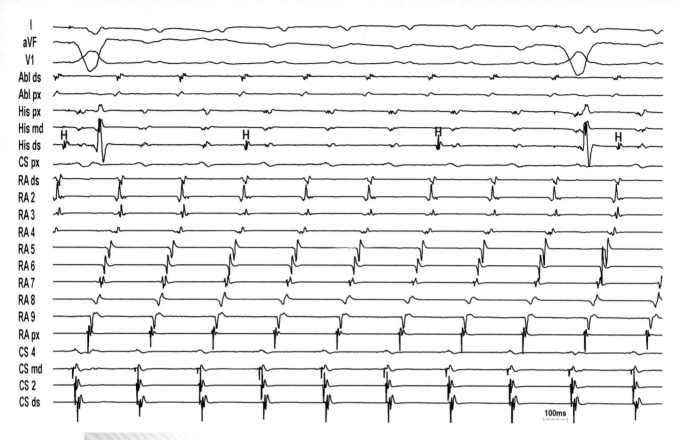

FIGURE 1-38 Counterclockwise CTI-dependent atrial flutter with complete infrahisian block and ventricular paced rhythm.

PSEUDO AV BLOCK

Pseudo AV block refers to functional or physiologic episodes of AV block (commonly in the AVN) resulting from concealed conduction that can mimic pathologic AV block.

Nonpropagated His Bundle Extrasystoles

Nonpropagated (concealed) His bundle extrasystoles are a rare cause of intermittent AV block (**Fig. 1-39**).[42,43] His bundle discharges typically manifest on the surface ECG because they conduct retrogradely to the atrium and/or antegradely to the ventricle. Nonpropagated discharges, however, neither conduct retrogradely nor antegradely and are hidden (hence, the term "concealed") on the ECG. Critically-timed concealed His bundle extrasystoles can retrogradely penetrate the AVN and render it refractory so that the subsequent sinus impulse fails to conduct to the ventricle (pseudo AV block).

Nodo-Fascicular/Ventricular Accessory Pathways

Nodo-fascicular (or ventricular) accessory pathways (NFAPs) are another rare cause of pseudo AV block. In the presence of a concealed NFAP, conduction can occur antegradely over the AVN–His-Purkinje axis and retrogradely over the NFAP. When this occurs repetitively, orthodromic reentrant tachycardia develops. When this occurs once, the AVN is rendered physiologically refractory so that the subsequent sinus beat fails to conduct to the ventricle (pseudo AV block).[44]

Self-Perpetuating Cycle of Intranodal AV Block and Phase IV BBB

Deceleration in heart rate can trigger phase IV BBB in diseased His-Purkinje tissue (bradycardia-dependent BBB). After BBB, retrograde transeptal conduction from "unblocked" to "blocked" bundle with subsequent retrograde activation of the His bundle and concealment into the AVN produces functional intranodal AV block. Deceleration in the heart rate due to intranodal AV block reinduces phase IV BBB, thereby perpetuating a self-repeating, continuous cycle of intranodal AV block and phase IV BBB (**Fig. 1-40**).[45]

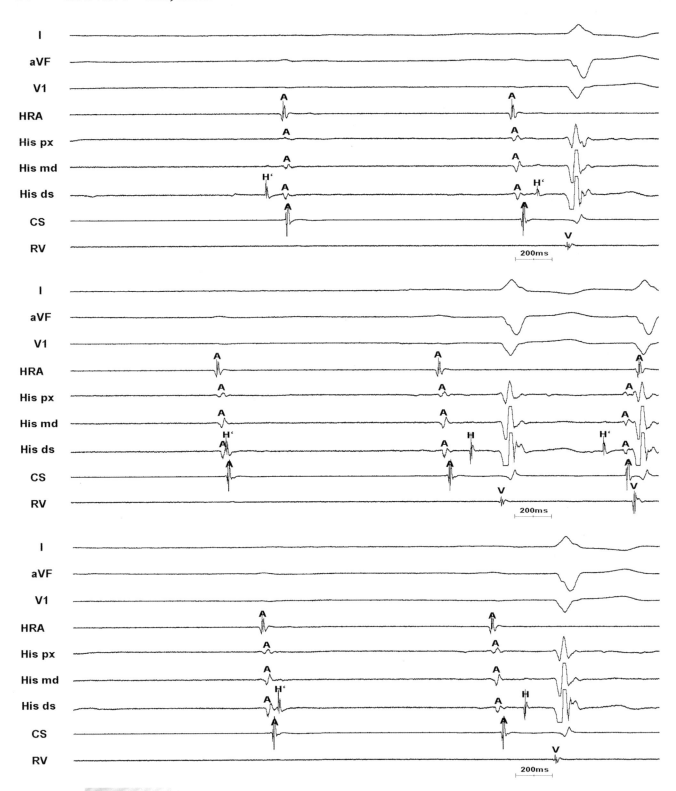

FIGURE 1-39 Pseudo AV block (nonpropagated His bundle discharges). Concealed His bundle extrasystoles (H′) precede (*top*), coincide with (*middle*), and follow (*bottom*) sinus P waves. Each extrasystole renders the AVN functionally refractory causing AV block (pseudo AV block). Manifest His bundle extrasystoles are also present and conduct only to the ventricle (*top*) and both atrium and ventricle (*middle*). The AH and HV intervals of sinus-conducted LBBB QRS complexes measure 150 and 161 ms, respectively.

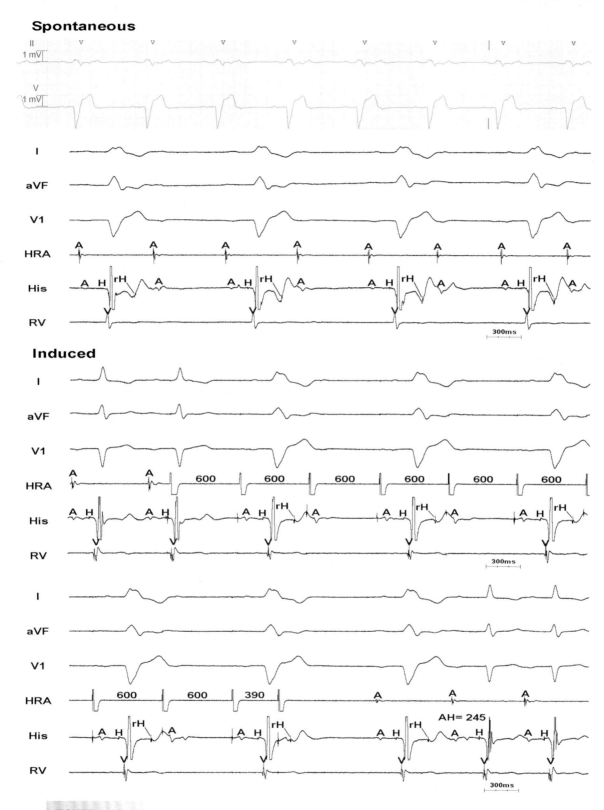

FIGURE 1-40 Self-perpetuating cycle of 2:1 intranodal AV block and phase IV LBBB. Telemetry and His bundle recording show spontaneous 2:1 intranodal AV block with LBBB. Retrograde activation of the His bundle (rH) follows LBBB. Induction: The first pacing stimulus captures the atrium and fails to conduct over the AVN exposing the His-Purkinje system to a long diastolic interval. The second pacing stimulus conducts over the AVN but because of bradycardia-dependent LBBB must travel over right bundle; crosses the septum; and retrogradely activates the left bundle, His bundle, and AVN. The third pacing stimulus falls into the ERP of the recently depolarized AVN resulting in functional AV block, which again induces phase IV LBBB. This self-perpetuating cycle continues until pacing stops. LBBB and rH accompany the first return sinus beat. The second sinus beat, however, falls into the RRP of the AVN (AH = 245 ms), conducts to the ventricle, and breaks the cycle.

REFERENCES

1. Josephson ME. Sinus node function. In: Josephson ME, ed. Clinical Cardiac Electrophysiology: Techniques and Interpretations. 2nd ed. Philadelphia, PA: Lea & Febiger, 1993:71–95.

2. Benditt DG, Strauss HC, Scheinman MM, Behar VS, Wallace AG. Analysis of secondary pauses following termination of rapid atrial pacing in man. Circulation 1976;54:436–441.

3. Reiffel JA, Bigger JT, Giardina EV. "Paradoxical" prolongation of sinus nodal recovery time after atropine in the sick sinus syndrome. Am J Cardiol 1975;36:98–104.

4. Narula OS, Shantha N, Vasquez M, Towne WD, Linhart JW. A new method for measurement of sinoatrial conduction time. Circulation 1978;58:706–714.

5. Strauss HC, Saroff AL, Bigger JT, Giardinia EV. Premature atrial stimulation as a key to the understanding of sinoatrial conduction in man. Presentation of data and critical review of the literature. Circulation 1973;47:86–93.

6. Jose AD. Effect of combined sympathetic and parasympathetic blockade on heart rate and cardiac function in man. Am J Cardiol 1966;18:476–478.

7. Jose AD, Taylor RR. Autonomic blockade by propranolol and atropine to study intrinsic myocardial function in man. J Clin Invest 1969;48:2019–2031.

8. Jose AD, Collison D. The normal range and determinants of the intrinsic heart rate in man. Cardiovasc Res 1970;4:160–167.

9. Huang S, Ezri MD, Hauser RG, Denes P. Carotid sinus hypersensitivity in patients with unexplained syncope: clinical, electrophysiologic and long-term follow-up observations. Am Heart J 1988;116:989–996.

10. Heron JR, Anderson EG, Noble IM. Cardiac abnormalities associated with carotid sinus syndrome. Lancet 1965;2:214–216.

11. Weiss S, Baker JP. The carotid sinus reflex in health and disease. Its role in the causation of fainting and convulsions. Medicine 1933;12:297–354.

12. Zaim B, Zaim S, Garan H. Invasive cardiac electrophysiology studies in assessment and management of cardiac arrhythmias. In: Podrid PJ, Kowey PR, eds. Cardiac Arrhythmia: Mechanisms, Diagnosis, and Management. Baltimore, MD: Williams & Wilkins, 1995:258–279.

13. Kupersmith J, Krongrad E, Waldo A. Conduction intervals and conduction velocity in the human cardiac system: studies during open-heart surgery. Circulation 1973;47:776–785.

14. Dhingra RC, Wyndham C, Bauernfeind R, et al. Significance of block distal to the His bundle induced by atrial pacing in patients with chronic bifascicular block. Circulation 1979;60:1455–1464.

15. Josephson ME. Clinical Cardiac Electrophysiology: Techniques and Interpretations. 2nd ed. Philadelphia, PA: Lea & Febiger, 1993:117–149.

16. Akhtar M, Damato AN, Carcacta AR, Batsford WP, Josephson ME, Lau SH. Electrophysiologic effects of atropine on atrioventricular conduction studied by His bundle electrogram. Am J Cardiol 1974;33:333–343.

17. Tonkin AM, Heddle WF, Tornos P. Intermittent atrioventricular block: procainamide administration as a provocative test. Aust NZ J Med 1978;8:594–602.

18. Bharati S, Lev M, Wu D, Denes P, Dhingra R, Rosen KM. Pathophysiologic correlations in two cases of split His bundle potentials. Circulation 1974;49:615–623.

19. Amat-y-Leon F, Dhingra R, Denes P, et al. The clinical spectrum of chronic His bundle block. Chest 1976;70:747–754.

20. Gupta PK, Lichstein E, Chadda KD. Chronic His bundle block: clinical, electrocardiographic, electrophysiological, and follow-up studies in 16 patients. Br Heart J 1976;38:1343–1349.

21. Pasquié JL, Grolleau R. Intrahisian block with Wenckebach phenomenon. Heart Rhythm 2004;1:368.

22. Kenia A, Ho RT, Pavri BB. Narrowing with prematurity—what is the mechanism? Pacing Clin Electrophysiol 2014;37:1404–1407.

23. El-Sherif N, Jalife J. Paroxysmal atrioventricular block: are phase 3 and phase 4 block mechanisms or misnomers? Heart Rhythm 2009;6:1514–1521.

24. Sachs A, Traynor R. Paroxysmal complete auriculo-ventricular heart block. Am Heart J 1933;9:267–271.

25. Rosenbaum MB, Elizari MV, Levi RJ, Nau GJ. Paroxysmal atrioventricular block related to hypopolarization and spontaneous diastolic depolarization. Chest 1973;63:678–688.

26. Coumel P, Fabiato A, Waynberger M, Motte G, Salma R, Bouvrain Y. Bradycardia-dependent atrio-ventricular block. Report of two cases of A-V block elicited by premature beat. J Electrocardiology 1971;4:168–177.

27. Castellanos A, Khuddus SA, Sommer LS, Sung RJ, Myerburg RJ. His bundle recordings in bradycardia-dependent AV block induced by premature beats. British Heart J 1975;37:570–575.

28. Mallya R, Pavri BB, Greenspon AJ, Ho RT. Recurrent paroxysmal atrioventricular block triggered paradoxically by a pacemaker. Heart Rhythm 2005;2:185–187.

29. Wu D, Denes P, Dhingra RC, et al. Electrophysiological and clinical observations in patients with alternating bundle branch block. Circulation 1976;53:456–464.

30. Rosenbaum MB, Elizari MV, Lázzari JO, Halpern MS, Nau GJ. Bilateral bundle branch block: its recognition and significance. Cardiovasc Clin 1971;2:151–179.

31. Ho RT, Stopper M, Koka A. Alternating bundle branch block. Pacing Clin Electrophysiol 2012;35:223–226.

32. Ho RT. An uncommon manifestation of atrio-ventricular block: what is the mechanism? Pacing Clin Electrophysiol 2014;37:900–903.

33. Ho RT, DeCaro M. Atrio-ventricular block from metastatic lung cancer to the aortic root. Europace 2017;19:946.

34. Unger PN, Lesser ME, Kugel VH, Lev M. The concept of masquerading bundle-branch block. An electrocardiographic-pathologic correlation. Circulation 1958;17:397–409.

35. Richman JL, Wolff L. Left bundle branch block masquerading as right bundle branch block. Am Heart J 1954;47:383–393.

36. Adrian ED, Lucas K. On the summation of propagated disturbances in nerve and muscle. J Physiol 1912;44:68–124.

37. Lewis T, Master AM. Supernormal recovery phase, illustrated by two clinical cases of heart-block. Heart 1924;11:371–387.

38. Massumi RA, Amsterdam EZ, Mason DT. Phenomenon of supernormality in the human heart. Circulation 1972;46:264–275.

39. Ho RT, Rhim ES, Pavri BB, Greenspon AJ. An unusual pattern of atrioventricular block. J Cardiovasc Electrophysiol 2007;18:1000–1002.

40. Satullo G, Donato A, Busà G, Grassi R. 4:2 Atrioventricular block: what is the mechanism? J Cardiovasc Electrophysiology 2003;14:1252–1253.

41. Wald RW, Waxman MB. Depression of distal AV conduction following ventricular pacing. Pacing Clin Electrophysiol 1981;4:84–91.

42. Rosen KM, Rahimtoola SH, Gunnar RM. Pseudo A-V block secondary to premature nonpropagated His bundle depolarizations. Documentation by His bundle electrocardiography. Circulation 1970;42:367–373.

43. Ho RT, Tecce M. Atrioventricular block: what is the mechanism? Heart Rhythm 2006;3:488–489.

44. Tuohy S, Saliba W, Pai M, Tchou P. Catheter ablation as a treatment of atrioventricular block. Heart Rhythm 2018;15:90–96.

45. Fedgchin B, Pavri BB, Greenspon AJ, Ho RT. A unique self-perpetuating cycle of intranodal atrio-ventricular block and phase IV LBBB in a patient with bundle branch reentrant tachycardia. Heart Rhythm 2004;1:493–496.

Mechanisms of Tachycardia

2

Introduction

The three mechanisms responsible for tachycardia are 1) reentry, 2) enhanced automaticity, and 3) triggered activity. Electrocardiographic presentations of tachycardia are mechanism specific including its initiation, termination, and response to pacing maneuvers. Understanding tachycardia mechanisms are important for developing specific mapping strategies for ablation.

The purpose of this chapter is to:
1. Discuss different mechanisms and clinical presentations of tachycardia.
2. Discuss mapping strategies for ablation based on tachycardia mechanism.

MECHANISMS

REENTRY

The mechanism responsible for the majority of pathologic tachycardias is reentry. These tachycardias include atrial fibrillation, atrial flutter, intraatrial reentrant tachycardia, atrio-ventricular nodal reentrant tachycardia (AVNRT), accessory pathway–mediated reentrant tachycardias (ortho- and antidromic reentrant tachycardia), sinus node reentrant tachycardia (SNRT), bundle branch reentrant tachycardia (BBRT), idiopathic left ventricular tachycardia (VT), and scar-related VT.

Circuit

A simplified reentrant circuit is composed of two longitudinally dissociated but complementary pathways (α and β) linked to form a functional circuit (**Fig. 2-1**).[1] The α pathway has slow conduction and short refractoriness, while the β pathway has rapid conduction and long refractoriness. The conduction and refractory properties of each pathway must complement the other so that conduction times over one pathway exceeds the refractory period of its counterpart. The depolarizing wavefront, therefore, always encounters excitable tissue to perpetuate reentrant excitation. An exit site allows the depolarizing wavefront to leave the circuit and activate the rest of the heart. The revolution time around the circuit equals the tachycardia cycle length (TCL). Tissue refractory periods are dynamic and show restitution or cycle length dependency (hyperbolic relationship between action potential [AP] duration and preceding diastolic interval) contributing to dispersion of refractoriness (particularly at the steep portion of the restitution curve) that facilitates reentry.

Two basic models of reentry depict circus movement around either a 1) fixed anatomic obstacle or 2) functional area of block.[2,3] During anatomical reentry, the circuit length is fixed and exceeds the tachycardia wavelength (λ = conduction velocity $\times$ refractory period). The difference between the circuit length and λ is the excitable gap. The excitable gap allows premature stimulation to penetrate the circuit and reset or entrain tachycardia. Antiarrhythmic drugs that prolong refractoriness (K channel blockers) increase the tachycardia λ, narrow the excitable gap, and terminate or prevent tachycardias by increasing the λ beyond the circuit length.[4] Antiarrhythmic drugs that slow conduction velocity (Na channel blockers) decrease conduction velocity and promote conduction block, particularly at fast rates (use dependence) causing tachycardia termination. However, reducing the λ can also cause tachycardia to become incessant. Because the circuit length is fixed in anatomical reentry, the TCL (revolution time around the circuit) is inversely related to conduction velocity. By contrast, functional reentry is the smallest circuit ("leading circle") around a central area (core) of refractoriness created by the convergence of multiple centripetal wavelets. The head of the excitatory wavefront is continuously biting its tail of refractoriness, and therefore, a fully excitable gap is absent. In functional reentry, the TCL is proportional to the tissue refractory period (not conduction velocity).

Variations of the reentrant model include 1) spiral wave reentry, 2) phase 2 reentry, and 3) reflection.[5,6] In the spiral wave theory, wave curvature and conduction velocity are inversely related. Spiral waves rotate around a central inexcitable rotor core where wave curvature is greatest, conduction velocity is slowest, and therefore propagation fails. The more distal parts of

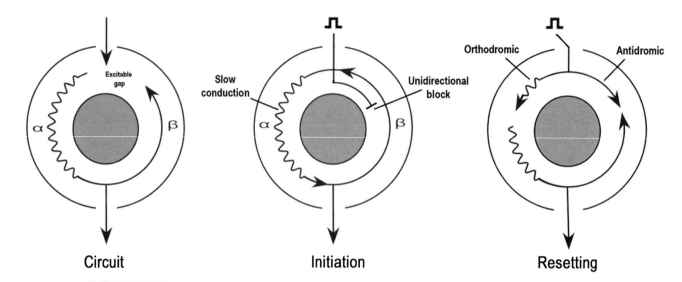

FIGURE 2-1 Diagram illustrating a functional circuit (*left*), criteria for reentrant initiation (*middle*), and resetting (*right*). The depicted circuit has separate entrance and exit sites. The α pathway exhibits slow conduction and short refractoriness, while its β counterpart demonstrates fast conduction and long refractoriness. The excitable gap is a zone of nonrefractory tissue between the head of the depolarizing wavefront and tail of refractoriness. Initiation of reentry requires a 1) functional circuit, 2) unidirectional block (β limb), and 3) slow conduction (α limb). A premature impulse falling into the tachycardia window (difference in refractory periods between the two limbs) fails to conduct over the β pathway (unidirectional block) and conducts exclusively over the α pathway (slow conduction). Sufficient delay over the α pathway allows the β pathway time to recover excitability and initiate reentry. During resetting, a premature impulse penetrates the excitable gap and generates an orthodromic and antidromic wavefront. The antidromic wavefront collides with tachycardia, while its orthodromic counterpart advances the circuit.

the spiral wave have less curvature and faster conduction. Stationary (anchored) and drifting spiral waves have been implicated in monomorphic and polymorphic VT, respectively. Spiral waves that encounter inexcitable tissue can break up and form daughter waves whose multiplicity is responsible for fibrillation. Phase 2 reentry is the presumptive mechanism underlying ventricular fibrillation (VF) in the Brugada syndrome. Compared to the endocardial AP, the normal epicardial AP shows a "spike and dome" configuration. The spike or epicardial notch (phase 1) results from the outward K current, I_{to}, while the dome (phase 2) results from inward ICa. Brugada syndrome results in an exaggerated spike (prominent I_{to} in the RV epicardium) and loss of the AP dome resulting in a transmural (epicardium–endocardium) gradient of repolarization that gives rise to the prominent J waves and ST segment elevation in ECG lead V1). Propagation of the dome (inward ICa) to nearby sites having loss of the dome causes local reentry (hence, termed phase 2 reentry) within the epicardium generating tightly coupled extrasystoles that trigger VF in the milieu of a transmural repolarization gradient. Reflection (reflected reentry) is the to and fro propagation of an impulse over a functionally inexcitable pathway and might contribute to ischemic ventricular extrasystoles.

Initiation

Three criteria necessary for initiation of reentry are 1) unidirectional block, 2) slow conduction, and a 3) functional circuit (Fig. 2-1).[5–7] Absolute and post-repolarization refractoriness are factors that can contribute to unidirectional block facilitating reentry. Relative refractoriness and anisotropy (differences in

conduction velocity related to fiber orientation) are factors contributing to slow conduction. Premature impulses (hence, the rationale behind programmed extrastimulation) are effective triggers of reentry by exposing differences in refractory periods between two longitudinally dissociated pathways. Premature impulses that fall into the tachycardia window (defined as the difference in refractory periods between the α and β pathways) fail to conduct over the β pathway with its longer refractory period (unidirectional block) and conduct exclusively over the α pathway (slow conduction), thereby fulfilling two requirements for reentry. Sufficient delay over the α pathway allows the β pathway time to recover excitability and initiate the first beat of reentry (functional circuit).

Reentrant initiation shows abrupt onset with an inverse relationship between the coupling interval of the initiating complex and the first beat of tachycardia due to slow conduction within the circuit. Induction is facilitated by rapid pacing (causing conduction slowing) especially with stimulation close to the tachycardia circuit.

Resetting and Entrainment

The existence of an excitable gap allows reentrant tachycardias to be reset or entrained. During resetting, a critically timed extrastimulus penetrates the excitable gap giving rise to two activation wavefronts: orthodromic and antidromic (Fig. 2-1). The orthodromic wavefront advances and resets the tachycardia, while its antidromic counterpart collides with the tachycardia wavefront. The resetting zone (difference between the longest and shortest coupled extrastimuli that reset tachycardia) defines the excitable gap. The ability of a premature impulse to reset tachycardia is dependent on the 1) size of the excitable gap, 2) distance between the pacing site and circuit, and 3) electrophysiologic properties (e.g., conduction velocity) of the intervening tissue. A macroreentrant circuit can be reset with fusion (resetting + fusion = macroreentry). Although automatic tachycardias can be reset, they cannot be reset with fusion. Entrainment is continuous resetting of tachycardia by overdrive pacing without tachycardia termination. Entrainment (as determined by presence of any four criteria of transient entrainment) establishes existence of an excitable gap and is specific for a reentrant mechanism.

Criteria of Transient Entrainment

The four criteria of transient entrainment are 1) constant ECG fusion (except for the last entrained beat, which is unfused and occurs at the pacing cycle length [PCL]), 2) progressive ECG fusion, 3) tachycardia termination associated with localized conduction block to a site activated orthodromically by tachycardia followed by activation of that site from a different direction and with a shorter conduction time, and 4) progressive electrogram (EGM) fusion.[8-14] While it is not always possible to demonstrate these four criteria, the presence of any one of them indicates a reentrant mechanism. The presence of constant and progressive ECG fusion implies that the circuit has separate entrance and exit sites (not to be confused with the entrance and exit sites of the critical isthmus or zone of slow conduction within the circuit). During transient entrainment, pacing stimuli collide with tachycardia outside the circuit (resulting in ECG fusion) while penetrating the circuit within its excitable gap to produce orthodromic and antidromic wavefronts. The antidromic wavefront of the first pacing stimulus (n) collides with tachycardia. Its orthodromic counterpart advances it. Pacing accelerates tachycardia to the pacing rate with each orthodromic (n) wavefront colliding with the subsequent antidromic (n + 1) wavefront. Upon pacing cessation, the last orthodromic wavefront has no antidromic wavefront with which to collide producing an orthodromically activated (unfused) complex occurring at the PCL. Transient entrainment at a fixed PCL causes a stable collision site between orthodromic (n) and antidromic (n + 1) wavefronts (constant ECG [and intracardiac] fusion) (**Figs. 2-2 to 2-4**). Accelerating the pacing rate shifts the collision site farther from the pacing site so that more of the ECG complex is paced (progressive ECG fusion) and more EGM sites are antidromically captured by pacing (progressive EGM fusion) (**Figs. 2-5 to 2-10**). Interruption of tachycardia is associated with localized conduction block to a site orthodromically activated

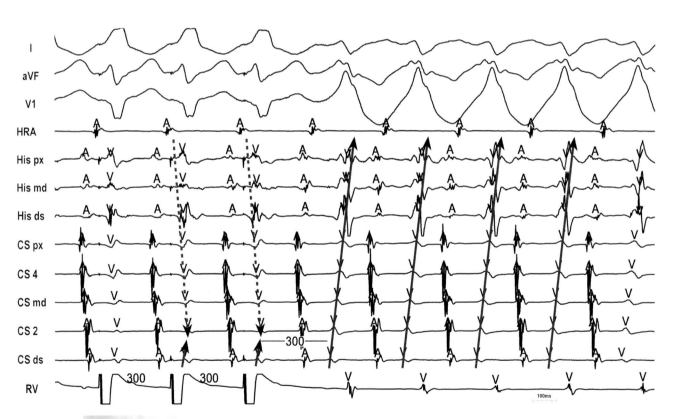

FIGURE 2-2 Constant ECG fusion during antidromic tachycardia (first criteria of transient entrainment). Entrainment from the RV results in constant QRS fusion (fixed collision [CS 2–CS ds] between paced RV antidromic wavefronts [*dashed arrows*] and orthodromic LV wavefronts [*solid arrows*] from an antegradely conducting left free wall accessory pathway). The last entrained ventricular complex occurs at the PCL (last entrained ventricular EGM on CS ds is orthodromically captured at 300 ms) and is unfused. Note that the morphology of orthodromically (CS ds) but not antidromically (CS px–CS 2) captured ventricular EGM is identical to tachycardia.

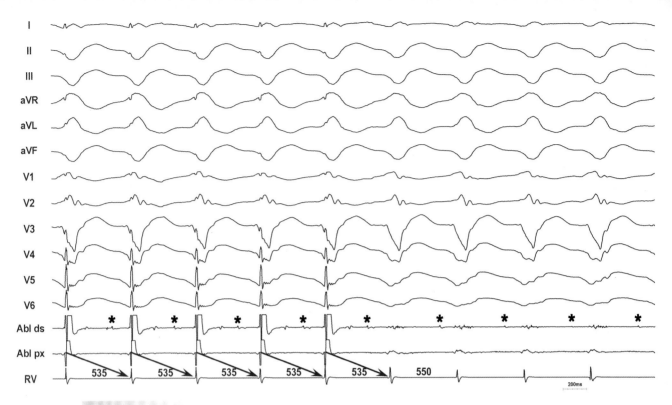

FIGURE 2-3 Constant ECG fusion during scar-mediated VT (first criteria of transient entrainment). Entrainment from the LV (Abl ds) results in constant QRS fusion. The last entrained ventricular complex accompanied by orthodromic capture of the RV EGM occurs at the PCL (535 ms) and is unfused. Note the low amplitude diastolic potentials (*asterisks*) recorded on the ablation catheter, which are not directly captured during entrainment, are accelerated to the PCL and are, therefore, "far-field."

by tachycardia followed by activation of that site from a different direction and with a shorter conduction time from the pacing stimulus. Transient entrainment from within the circuit (e.g., entrainment with concealed fusion during VT mapping—all pure tachycardia QRS complexes) or from outside the circuit having a single entrance and exit site to the chamber paced (e.g., concealed entrainment of AVNRT from the ventricle—all pure paced QRS complexes) causes orthodromic and antidromic collision exclusively within the circuit and, therefore, absence of paced ECG fusion (hence, the term "concealed").[15–17]

Termination

Spontaneous termination of reentrant tachycardias is generally abrupt. Termination can follow any single pacing stimulus that penetrates its excitable gap, collides with tachycardia antidromically, and fails to conduct orthodromically.

ENHANCED AUTOMATICITY

A second mechanism responsible for tachycardia is enhanced or abnormal automaticity. It is responsible for inappropriate sinus tachycardia and automatic atrial and junctional tachycardias. Automaticity arises from tissue with spontaneous phase 4 (diastolic) depolarizations of its transmembrane potential that reach threshold value to trigger an AP. Enhanced automaticity occurs when the 1) starting diastolic transmembrane potential is higher (more

positive), 2) threshold value for depolarization is lower (more negative), or 3) slope of the diastolic depolarization curve is steeper.

Initiation

The characteristic feature of automatic initiation is gradual acceleration in rate (warm-up).[18] Automatic tachycardias are generally not inducible by electrical stimulation, and induction is facilitated by catecholamine provocation (e.g., isoproterenol).[19]

Resetting and Overdrive Suppression

An appropriately-timed extrastimulus delivered during diastole can penetrate the region of abnormal automaticity and reset tachycardia but without fusion. In contrast to reentrant tachycardias, automatic tachycardias cannot be entrained. Rapid pacing causes variable ECG fusion or overdrive suppression of tachycardia.

Termination

Automatic tachycardias characteristically show gradual deceleration of rate (cool down) and are generally not interrupted by electrical stimulation.

TRIGGERED ACTIVITY

A third mechanism of tachycardia is triggered activity resulting from afterdepolarizations. Afterdepolarizations are oscillations in the transmembrane potential that attend (early afterdepolarizations [EADs]) or follow (delayed afterdepolarizations [DADs])

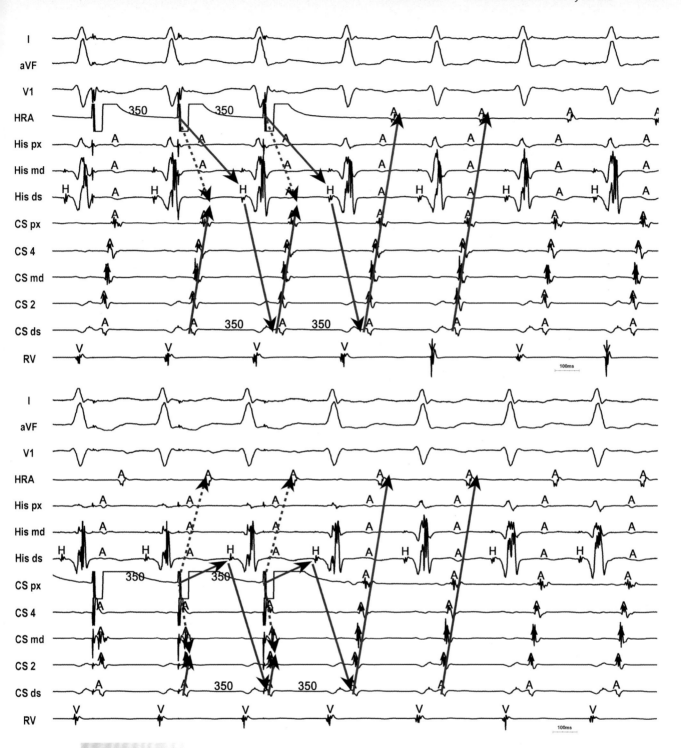

FIGURE 2-4 Constant EGM fusion during ORT (first criteria of transient entrainment). *Top:* Entrainment from the high right atrium (HRA) results in constant atrial fusion (fixed collision [His ds–CS px] between paced right atrial antidromic wavefronts [*dashed arrows*] and orthodromic left atrial wavefronts [*solid arrows*] from a retrogradely conducting left free wall accessory pathway). The last entrained atrial complex occurs at the PCL (last entrained atrial EGMs on CS ds to px are orthodromically captured at 350 ms) and is unfused. *Bottom:* Entrainment from the proximal CS results in constant atrial fusion with collision between antidromic (*dashed arrows*) and orthodromic wavefronts (*solid arrows*) at CS md–CS 2. The last entrained atrial complex occurs at the PCL (last entrained atrial EGMs on CS ds–CS 2 are orthodromically captured at 350 ms) and is unfused.

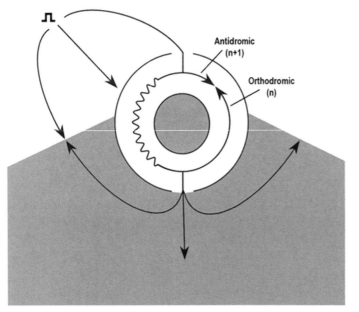
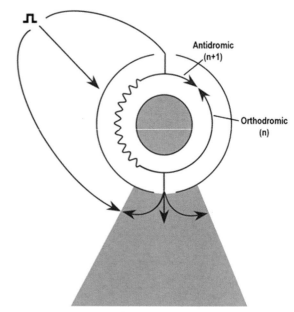

Longer PCL

Shorter PCL

FIGURE 2-5 Diagram illustrating entrainment with constant and progressive ECG fusion. (Circuit with anatomically separate entrance and exit sites within the chamber of interest.) Within the circuit, pacing stimuli enter the entrance site, penetrate its excitable gap, and continuously reset tachycardia with fixed collision between orthodromic (*n*) and antidromic (*n* + 1) wavefronts. Outside the circuit, fixed collision point between paced and tachycardia wavefronts produces constant ECG fusion. At faster pacing rates, the collision point shifts farther from the pacing site (progressive fusion). Shaded areas represent area activated by tachycardia.

the AP. Depolarizing afterpotentials that reach threshold can result in repetitive excitation called triggered activity. Triggered activity has been implicated as a mechanism for torsade de pointes initiation (EADs), digitalis-induced tachyarrhythmias (DADs), and cAMP-mediated right ventricular outflow tract (RVOT) tachycardia (**Figs. 2-11 and 2-12**).[20–23]

Initiation

Triggered activity can be induced by programmed extrastimulation and rapid pacing. In contrast to reentry, however, it manifests a direct relationship between the coupling interval of the initiating premature impulse (or pacing rate) and the first beat of tachycardia (or tachycardia rate).

Overdrive Acceleration

Rapid pacing can cause overdrive acceleration of tachycardia.

Termination

Similar to reentry, termination of triggered activity can be abrupt and result from rapid pacing or a premature extrastimulus.

MAPPING

The site for ablation of reentrant tachycardias is often the critical isthmus of slow conduction or a narrow limb necessary for reentry that can be successfully targeted with a catheter: 1) slow pathway of the atrio-ventricular node (AVNRT), 2) accessory pathway (orthodromic atrio-ventricular tachycardia [ORT]), 3) cavo-tricuspid isthmus (CTI) (CTI-dependent atrial flutter),

4) diseased bundle branch or fascicle (BBRT or interfascicular reentrant tachycardia), or 5) protected isthmus of slow conduction (scar-related atrial tachycardia [AT] or VT). Entrainment mapping is a technique employed to identify this critical region of slow conduction and has been used for AVNRT but generally for macroreentrant tachycardias (atrial flutter and scar-related AT and VT).[23–31] The target site for focal tachycardias (abnormal automaticity, triggered activity, or microreentry) is the site of earliest activation within the chamber of interest, which can be identified by activation mapping.[24–32] Besides activation mapping, focal AT can also be mapped using the post-pacing interval (PPI).[33] A third mechanism, localized reentry has been described for AT arising after ablation of atrial fibrillation and has features of both focal origin (centrifugal activation from a small area <2 cm²) and macroreentry (>75% of cycle length recordable).[34]

ENTRAINMENT MAPPING

Entrainment mapping identifies whether or not a specific pacing site is an integral part of the reentrant circuit. For macroreentrant tachycardia, activation mapping should be coupled with entrainment mapping. When entraining a critical portion of the circuit, a small region "upstream" to the pacing site is antidromically captured. With the last pacing stimulus, the region "downstream" to the pacing site is orthodromically captured to the PCL, but the EGM at the pacing site returns at the TCL because the orthodromic wavefront completes one

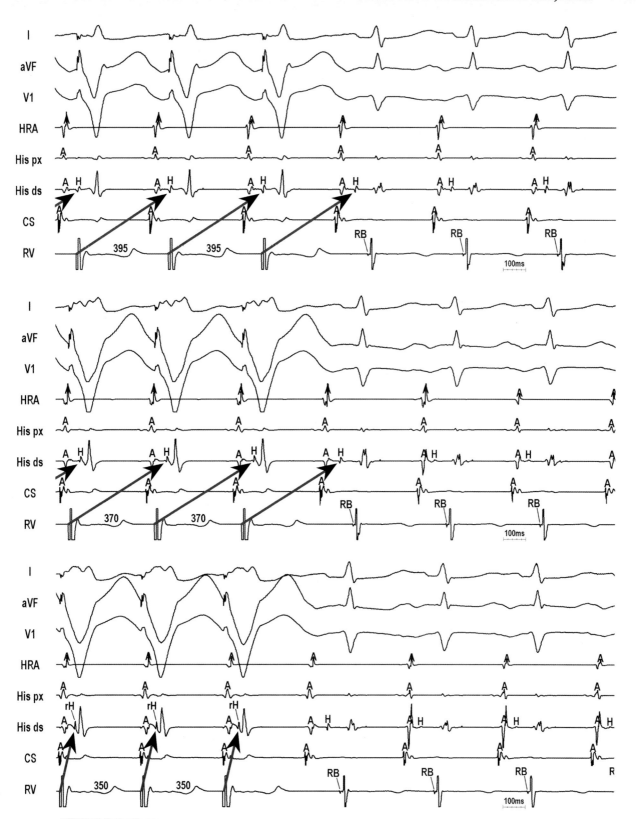

FIGURE 2-6 Constant and progressive ECG and EGM fusion during permanent form of junctional reciprocating tachycardia (PJRT) (first, second, and fourth criteria of transient entrainment). During PJRT, entrainment is performed from the RV apex with acceleration of the atrium to the pacing rate and constant QRS fusion at each PCL. At PCL of 395 and 370 ms, the His bundle is orthodromically captured and QRS complexes at the faster pacing rate are more fully paced (progressive ECG fusion). At PCL of 350 ms, the His bundle is antidromically captured and QRS complexes are maximally paced (progressive EGM and ECG fusion). Note that the morphology of orthodromically but not antidromically captured His bundle EGMs is identical to tachycardia.

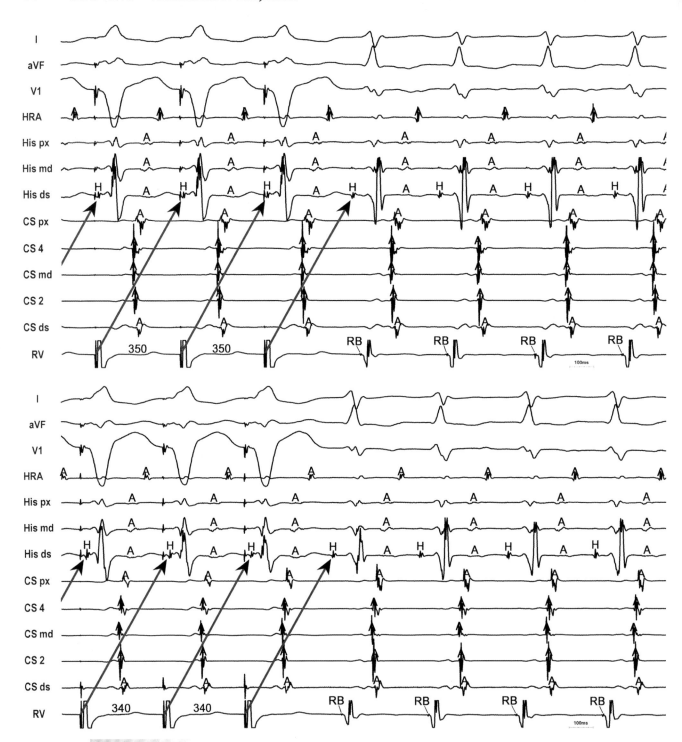

FIGURE 2-7 Progressive ECG fusion during ORT (second criteria of transient entrainment). *Top*: Entrainment from the RV apex at 350 ms results in orthodromic capture of the His bundle and constant QRS fusion. *Bottom*: A 10 ms shorter PCL (340 ms) still results in orthodromic capture of the His bundle, but QRS complexes are more fully paced. The last entrained QRS complex in each case occurs at the PCL (last entrained His bundle is orthodromically captured at 350 and 340 ms, respectively) and is unfused. Note that the morphology of orthodromically captured His bundle EGMs is identical to tachycardia.

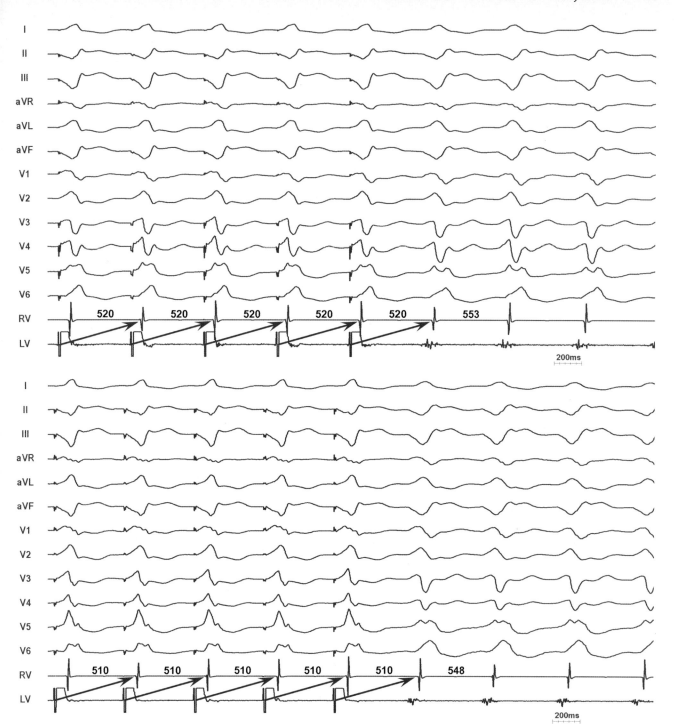

FIGURE 2-8 Progressive ECG fusion during scar-mediated VT (second criteria of transient entrainment). *Top:* Entrainment from the LV results in constant QRS fusion. *Bottom:* A 10 ms shorter PCL results in more fully paced QRS complexes. In both instances, the last entrained ventricular complexes accompanied by orthodromic capture of the RV EGMs occur at the PCL (520 and 510 ms, respectively) and are unfused.

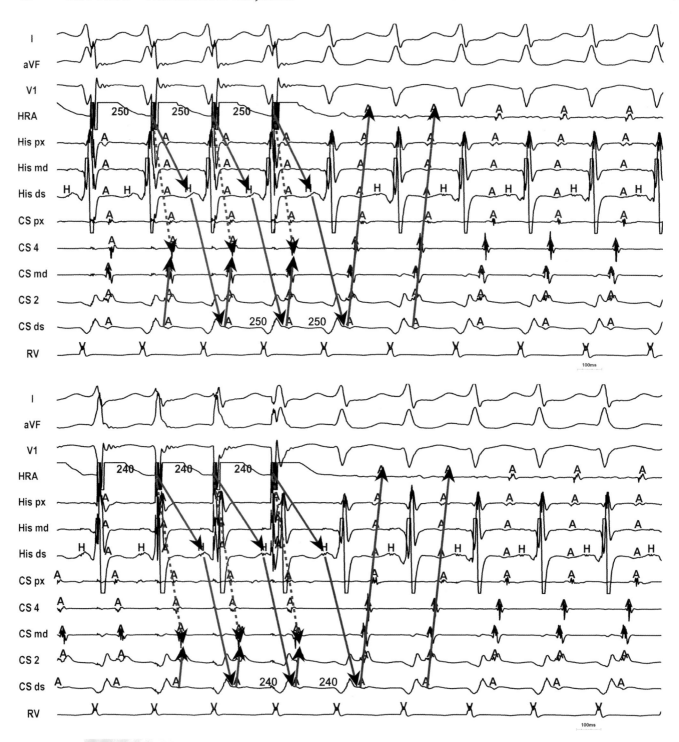

FIGURE 2-9 Progressive EGM fusion during ORT (fourth criteria of transient entrainment). *Top:* Entrainment from the high right atrium (HRA) at 250 ms results in constant atrial fusion with fixed collision (CS 4–CS md) between paced antidromic (*dashed arrows*) and orthodromic (*solid arrows*) wavefronts from a retrogradely conducting left free wall AP. The last entrained atrial complex occurs at the PCL (last entrained atrial EGMs on CS ds–CS md are orthodromically captured at 250 ms) and is unfused. *Bottom:* A 10 ms shorter PCL (240 ms) shifts the collision point farther from the HRA to between CS md and CS 2. The last entrained atrial complex occurs at the PCL (last entrained atrial EGMs on CS ds–CS 2 are orthodromically captured at 240 ms) and is unfused. Note that the morphology of orthodromically but not antidromically captured atrial EGMs is identical to tachycardia.

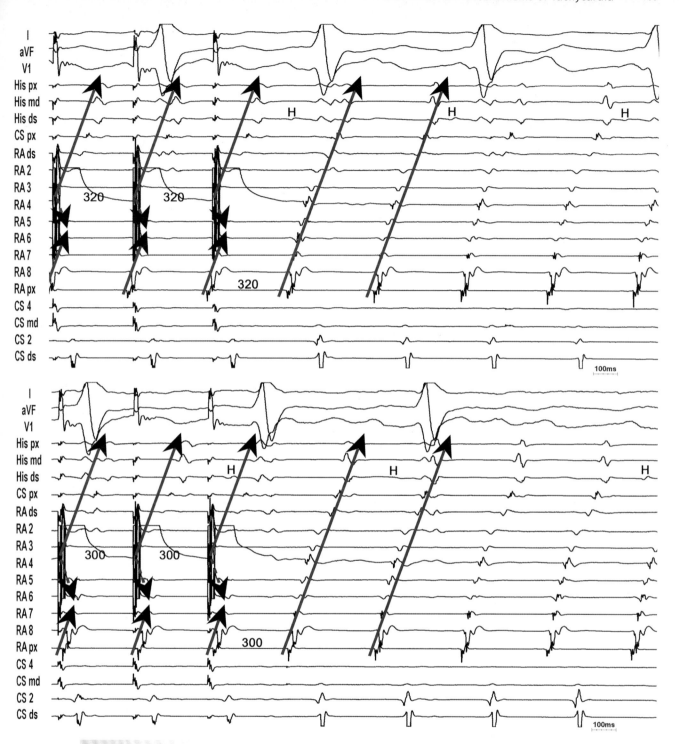

FIGURE 2-10 Progressive EGM fusion during atrial flutter (fourth criteria of transient entrainment). *Top*: Entrainment from the CTI at 320 ms during counterclockwise CTI-dependent atrial flutter results in fixed collision (RA 5–RA 6) between orthodromic (*n*) (*solid arrows*) and antidromic (*n* + 1) (*dashed arrows*) wavefronts upstream from the pacing site. *Bottom*: A 20 ms shorter PCL shifts the collision point more upstream and away from the pacing site (RA 6–RA 7). In each instance, the last entrained atrial complexes occur at the PCL (orthodromically captured atrial EGMs downstream to pacing site [RA 4] to collision point RA 6 [PCL 320 ms] and RA 7 [PCL 300 ms]) and are unfused. Note that the morphology of ortho-dromically captured EGMs is identical to tachycardia.

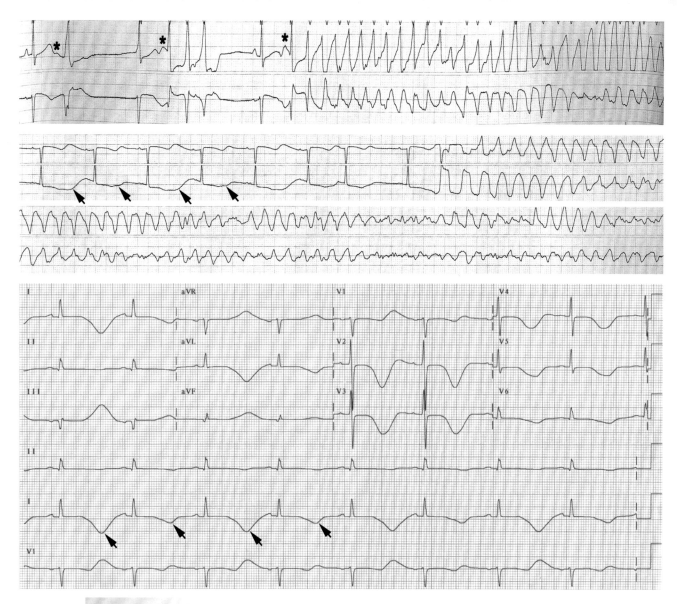

FIGURE 2-11 Torsade de pointes. Pause-dependent polymorphic VT preceded by U wave cascade (*asterisks*) and T wave alternans (*arrows*). U waves might represent EADs. Larger, more arrhythmogenic U waves reaching threshold potential trigger repetitive PVCs (triggered activity), which in the milieu of dispersion of refractoriness (long QT) initiate reentrant polymorphic VT.

full revolution around the circuit. The length of the PPI is, therefore, directly related to proximity of reentrant circuit. Sites integral to the circuit show PPI that is equal to TCL. In contrast, bystander sites show a PPI that is greater than TCL and equals the TCL plus conduction time to and from the circuit. During entrainment mapping, pacing from protected sites within the circuit (e.g., isthmus of slow conduction) activates the heart through its exit site so that paced and tachycardia complexes are identical (entrainment with concealed fusion). Collision between orthodromic and antidromic wavefronts occurs within the circuit and is undetectable on the surface ECG. Entrainment from nonprotected sites (e.g., remote bystander) produces paced complexes that are different from tachycardia (entrainment with manifest fusion).

First Criteria of Transient Entrainment versus Entrainment Mapping

The difference between the first criteria of transient entrainment and entrainment mapping might lead to confusion. During transient entrainment with constant ECG fusion, the last entrained complex is unfused and occurs at the PCL. It indicates a reentrant circuit with anatomically separate entrance and exit sites within the chamber of interest (different from the entrance and exit sites of the critical isthmus). Constant collision between paced and tachycardia wavefronts occurs outside the circuit (resulting in ECG fusion) and between paced orthodromic (n) and antidromic (n + 1) wavefronts within the circuit (allowing entrainment). The last paced orthodromic wavefront has no antidromic wavefront with which to collide resulting in an unfused

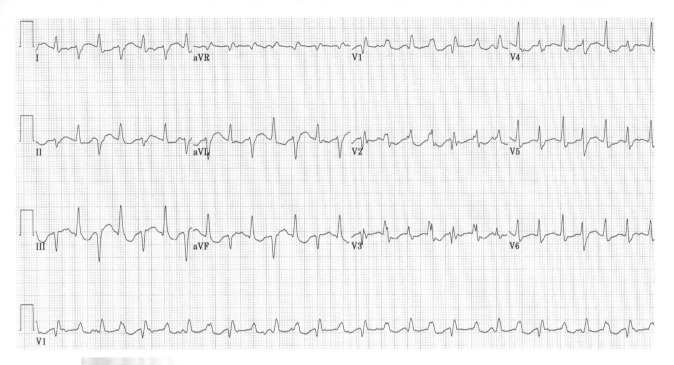

FIGURE 2-12 Bidirectional VT (digitalis toxicity). Bidirectional VT is due to DAD in the distal His-Purkinje system caused by calcium overload from digitalis toxicity. Elevated heart rates from DADs and triggered activity in the left anterior fascicle induce DADs and triggered activity in the left posterior fascicle and vice versa, resulting in ventricular ectopy arising from two alternating His-Purkinje sites ("ping pong" model).

complex (which along with orthodromically captured intracardiac sites downstream to the pacing site) occurring at the PCL. Because pacing occurs outside the circuit for ECG fusion to occur, the return interval on the pacing catheter (PPI) is long. Transient entrainment is used to show that a tachycardia mechanism is reentrant, but demonstrating the first criteria is not always possible if the entrance and exit sites within the chamber of interest are the same (e.g., AVNRT). In contrast, entrainment mapping is used to identify the critical isthmus of slow conduction of the reentrant circuit. Pacing within the critical portions of the circuit results in concealed (entrance, central, exit sites) or manifest (outer loop sites) fusion, and the return interval on the pacing catheter occurs at the TCL. Pacing outside the circuit (remote bystander site) results in manifest fusion and a PPI that is greater than TCL. Demonstrating the first criteria of transient entrainment during entrainment mapping of VT is uncommon and identifies a specific VT circuit with separate entrance and exit sites (Figs. 2-3 and 2-8).[35]

ACTIVATION MAPPING

In contrast to macroreentrant tachycardias where electrical activity within the circuit spans the entire TCL, focal tachycardias arise from a discrete "point source" that spreads radially from this site. The target site of ablation for focal tachycardias is, therefore, the earliest site of activation (presystolic EGM) referenced to the P wave (for AT), QRS complex (for VT), or an intracardiac reference point involving the chamber of interest.[36–38] A color-coded three-dimensional electro-anatomic activation map can differentiate focal versus macroreentrant mechanisms (Fig. 2-13). However, a focal tachycardia can produce a

Focal

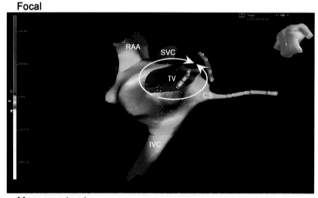

Macroreentrant

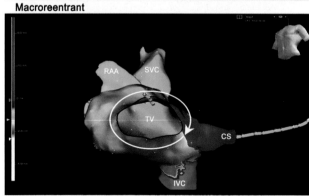

FIGURE 2-13 Electro-anatomic activation map of a focal (*top*) and macroreentrant (*bottom*) tachycardia. *Top*: atrial tachycardia. Note the centrifugal spread of activation from the site of origin (*white*) around the tricuspid annulus. *Bottom*: Clockwise CTI-dependent atrial flutter. Note the early (*white*) meets late (*purple*) activation pattern.

macroreentrant pattern if the point source is adjacent to a line of block (pseudo-macroreentrant) (see Fig. 6-18). Conversely, a macroreentrant circuit can generate a focal pattern at the endocardial breakthrough site of an epicardial structure critical to the circuit (e.g., macroreentrant LA vein of Marshall tachycardia).

REFERENCES

1. Moe GK, Preston JB, Burlington H. Physiologic evidence for a dual A-V transmission system. Circ Res 1956;4:357–375.
2. Mines GR. On dynamic equilibrium in the heart. J Physiol 1913;46:349–383.
3. Allessie M, Bonke F, Schopman F. Circus movement in rabbit atrial muscle as a mechanism of tachycardia. Circ Res 1977;41:9–18.
4. Task Force on the Working Group of Arrhythmias of the European Society of Cardiology. The Sicilian Gambit. A new approach to the classification of antiarrhythmic drugs based on their actions on arrhythmogenic mechanism. Circulation 1991;84:1831–1851.
5. Antzelevitch C. Basic mechanisms of reentrant arrhythmias. Curr Opin Cardiol 2001;16:1–7.
6. Spector P. Principles of cardiac electric propagation and their implications for re-entrant arrhythmias. Circ Arrhythm Electrophysiol 2013;6:655–661.
7. Coumel P. Junctional reciprocating tachycardias. The permanent and paroxysmal forms of A-V nodal reciprocating tachycardias. J Electrocardiol 1975;8:79–90.
8. Waldo AL, Maclean WA, Karp RB, Kouchoukos NT, James TN. Entrainment and interruption of atrial flutter with atrial pacing: studies in man following open heart surgery. Circulation 1977;56:737–745.
9. MacLean WA, Plumb VJ, Waldo AL. Transient entrainment and interruption of ventricular tachycardia. Pacing Clin Electrophysiol 1981;4:358–366.
10. Waldo AL, Henthorn RW, Plumb VJ, MacLean WAH. Demonstration of the mechanism of transient entrainment and interruption of ventricular tachycardia with rapid atrial pacing. J Am Coll Cardiol 1984;3:422–430.
11. Okumura K, Olshansky B, Henthorn RW, Epstein AE, Plumb VJ, Waldo AL. Demonstration of the presence of slow conduction during sustained ventricular tachycardia in man: use of transient entrainment of the tachycardia. Circulation 1987;75:369–378.
12. Waldo AL, Plumb VJ, Arciniegas JA, et al. Transient entrainment and interruption of the atrioventricular bypass pathway type of paroxysmal atrial tachycardia. A model for understanding and identifying reentrant arrhythmias. Circulation 1983;67:73–83.
13. Ormaetxe JM, Almendral J, Arenal A, et al. Ventricular fusion during resetting and entrainment of orthodromic supraventricular tachycardia involving septal accessory pathways. Implications for the differential diagnosis with atrioventricular nodal reentry. Circulation 1993;88:2623–2631.
14. Saoudi N, Anselme F, Poty H, Cribier A, Castellanos A. Entrainment of supraventricular tachycardias: a review. Pacing Clin Electrophysiol 1998;21:2105–2125.
15. Okumura K, Henthorn RW, Epstein AE, Plumb VJ, Waldo AL. Further observations on transient entrainment: importance of pacing site and properties of the components of the reentry circuit. Circulation 1985;72:1293–1307.
16. Almendral J. Resetting and entrainment of reentrant arrhythmias: part II: informative content and practical use of these responses. Pacing Clin Electrophysiol 2013;36:641–661.
17. Almendral J, Caulier-Cisterna R, Rojo-Álvarez JL. Resetting and entrainment of reentrant arrhythmias: part I: concepts, recognition, and protocol for evaluation: surface ECG versus intracardiac recordings. Pacing Clin Electrophysiol 2013;36:508–532.
18. Goldreyer BN, Gallagher JJ, Damato AN. The electrophysiologic demonstration of atrial ectopic tachycardia in man. Am Heart J 1973;85:205–215.
19. Lerman BB, Stein KM, Markowitz SM, Mittal S, Slotwiner DJ. Ventricular tachycardia in patients with structurally normal hearts. In: Zipes DP, Jalife J, eds. Cardiac Electrophysiology: From Cell to Bedside. 3rd ed. Philadelphia, PA: WB Saunders, 2000:640–656.
20. Cranefield P. Action potentials, afterpotentials, and arrhythmias. Circ Res 1977;41:415–423.
21. Surawicz B. Brief history of cardiac arrhythmias since the end of the nineteenth century: part II. J Cardiovasc Electrophysiol 2004;15:101–111.
22. Baher AA, Uy M, Xie F, Garfinkel A, Qu Z, Weiss JN. Bidirectional ventricular tachycardia: ping pong in the His-Purkinje system. Heart Rhythm 2011;8:599–605.
23. Lerman BB, Belardinelli L, West GA, Berne RM, DiMarco JP. Adenosine-sensitive ventricular tachycardia: evidence suggesting cyclic AMP-mediated triggered activity. Circulation 1986;74:270–280.
24. Haines DE, Nath S, DiMarco JP, Lobban JH. Entrainment mapping in patients with sustained atrioventricular nodal reentrant tachycardia: insights into the sites of conduction slowing in the slow atrioventricular nodal pathway. Am J Cardiol 1997;80:883–888.
25. Feld GK, Fleck RP, Chen P, et al. Radiofrequency catheter ablation for the treatment of human type 1 atrial flutter. Identification of a critical zone in the reentrant circuit by endocardial mapping techniques. Circulation 1992;86:1233–1240.
26. Olgin JE, Kalman JM, Fitzpatrick AP, Lesh MD. Role of right atrial endocardial structures as barriers to conduction during human type I atrial flutter. Activation and entrainment mapping guided by intracardiac echocardiography. Circulation 1995;92:1839–1848.
27. Kalman JM, Olgin JE, Saxon LA, Fisher WG, Lee RJ, Lesh MD. Activation and entrainment mapping defines the tricuspid annulus as the anterior barrier in typical atrial flutter. Circulation 1996;94:398–406.
28. Kalman JM, VanHare GF, Olgin JE, Saxon LA, Stark SI, Lesh MD. Ablation of "incisional" reentrant atrial tachycardia complicating surgery for congenital heart disease. Use of entrainment to define a critical isthmus of conduction. Circulation 1996;93:502–512.
29. Triedman JK, Saul JP, Weindling SN, Walsh EP. Radiofrequency ablation of intra-atrial reentrant tachycardia after surgical palliation of congenital heart disease. Circulation 1995;91:707–714.
30. Chen S, Chiang C, Yang C, et al. Radiofrequency catheter ablation of sustained intra-atrial reentrant tachycardia in adult patients. Identification of electrophysiological characteristics and endocardial mapping techniques. Circulation 1993;88:578–587.
31. Morady F, Frank R, Kou WH, et al. Identification and catheter ablation of a zone of slow conduction in the reentrant circuit of ventricular tachycardia in humans. J Am Coll Cardiol 1988;11:775–782.
32. Stevenson WG, Khan H, Sager P, et al. Identification of reentry circuit sites during catheter mapping and radiofrequency ablation of ventricular tachycardia late after myocardial infarction. Circulation 1993;88:1647–1670.
33. Mohamed U, Skanes AC, Gula LJ, et al. A novel pacing maneuver to localize focal atrial tachycardia. J Cardiovasc Electrophysiol 2007;18:1–6.
34. Jaïs P, Matsuo S, Knecht S, et al. A deductive mapping strategy for atrial tachycardia following atrial fibrillation ablation: importance of localized reentry. J Cardiovasc Electrophysiol 2009;20:480–491.
35. Almendral JM, Gottlieb CD, Rosenthal ME, et al. Entrainment of ventricular tachycardia: explanation for surface electrocardiographic phenomena by analysis of electrograms recorded within the tachycardia circuit. Circulation 1988;77:569–580.
36. Stevenson WG, Nademanee K, Weiss JN, Wiener I. Treatment of catecholamine-sensitive right ventricular tachycardia by endocardial catheter ablation. J Am Coll Cardiol 1990;16:752–755.
37. Klein LS, Shih H, Hackett FK, Zipes DP, Miles WM. Radiofrequency catheter ablation of ventricular tachycardia in patients without structural heart disease. Circulation 1992;85:1666–1674.
38. Coggins DL, Lee RJ, Sweeney J, et al. Radiofrequency catheter ablation as a cure for idiopathic tachycardia of both right and left ventricular origin. J Am Coll Cardiol 1994;23:1333–1341.

Intracardiac Echocardiography

3

Introduction

Intracardiac echocardiography (ICE) provides an invaluable tool during invasive electrophysiologic procedures by providing an important link between anatomy and electrophysiology, particularly when integrated with an electro-anatomic map. It serves several functions including 1) identifying critical structures involved in arrhythmogenesis, 2) visualizing the fossa ovalis for transeptal access, and 3) monitoring radiofrequency lesions and ablation complications (e.g., pericardial effusion, thrombus formation).

The purpose of this chapter is to:

1. Provide an understanding of different ICE views relative to transducer position and beam orientation within the heart.
2. Provide techniques to image important structures involved in arrhythmogenesis.

TYPES OF ICE CATHETERS

Two basic types of ICE catheters are 1) radial ICE and 2) phased-array ICE.[1–5] Radial ICE (9–12 MHz) uses a single, rotating (1800 rpm) crystal element mounted to the end of a nonsteerable catheter providing a 360-degree field of view *perpendicular* to the long axis of the shaft. It lacks Doppler capabilities and far-field resolution (penetration depth of <5 cm), limiting visualization of left heart structures from the right atrium (RA). Phased-array ICE (5.5–10 MHz) uses a 64-element transducer mounted longitudinally to a steerable (4-way articulation) catheter, providing a 90-degree ultrasound (US) sector *parallel* to the long axis of the shaft. It possesses Doppler capabilities and, because of its lower frequency, has greater tissue penetration (12 cm), allowing visualization of the left heart from the RA. Because of its greater capabilities for complex left heart ablations, this discussion primarily involves use of phased-array ICE with standard imaging from the right heart (RA/right ventricle [RV]), although imaging from the left atrium (LA), coronary sinus (CS), and pericardial space has also been described.[2,3]

ICE VIEWS

HOME VIEW

The characteristic neutral or home view provides a starting reference plane for orientation (Fig. 3-1). The ICE catheter is positioned in the mid-RA parallel to the spine with the US beam directed anteriorly toward the tricuspid valve (TV). The home view images the anterior RA, septal TV, longitudinal RV and outflow tract, aortic valve (noncoronary cusp [NCC] and right coronary cusp [RCC]), and proximal aortic root. The catheter tip during ablation of the posteroseptum (e.g., slow pathway), midseptum (e.g., accessory pathway [AP]), anteroseptum (e.g., His bundle), and cusp tachycardias (e.g., NCC atrial tachycardia [AT]) can be visualized in this view (**see Figs. 8-2, 8-3, 13-6 to 13-8, and 16-5**). A posterior location of the ICE transducer in the RA with slight clockwise torque from the home view intersects the aortic valve (NCC and left coronary cusp [LCC]) and left ventricle (LV) longitudinally. Because of the apical displacement of the TV relative to the mitral valve (MV), the location where the RA and LV intersect ("atrio-ventricular [AV] septum") can be seen (**Fig. 3-2**).

LEFT ATRIUM

Further clockwise torque of the ICE catheter from the home view images the structures of the LA in the following order: 1) MV/left atrial appendage (LAA)/proximal CS, 2) left-sided pulmonary veins (longitudinal view), 3) posterior LA/esophagus, and 4) right-sided pulmonary veins (cross-sectional view) (**Figs. 3-3 to 3-6**).[6–8] The catheter for ablation of mitral annular-related tachycardias (e.g., AP) can be imaged in the MV view (**see Figs. 12-2 to 12-4 and 12-11 to 12-16**). This view also images the anterior portion of the fossa ovalis for more

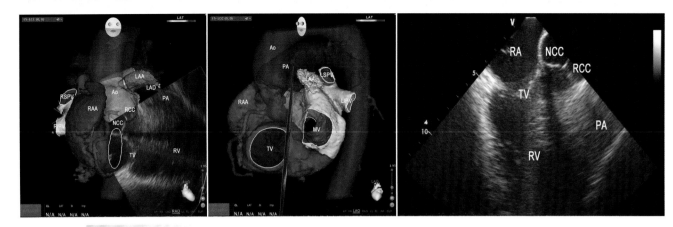

FIGURE 3-1 Home view. The US transducer is in the mid-RA with an anterior beam rotation.

anterior transeptal puncture sites (e.g., cryoablation).[9] With-drawal of the ICE catheter inferiorly visualizes the CS in cross section and the catheter during ablation of CS-related tachycar-dias (e.g., AP, AT) (Fig. 3-7; see also Fig. 13-10).

Additional views of the LAA can be obtained from the 1) RA (posterior tilt)/anterobasal RV (level with short axis view of the aortic valve), 2) RV beneath the pulmonic valve (anterior tilt; given the close proximity between the pulmonary artery [PA] and LAA), 3) from the LA (via a transeptal sheath), and 4) from within the CS (Figs. 3-8 and 3-9).[3,6] With the short axis view of the aortic valve, the Coumadin ridge between the LAA and left superior pulmonary vein (LSPV) (an important structure during LSPV isolation) is seen.

Clockwise torque of the ICE catheter from the MV view di-rects the US beam posterior to the LAA and views the left inferior pulmonary vein (LIPV), LSPV, and intervening carina longitu-dinally. This view images radiofrequency ablation and circum-ferential mapping catheters and cryoballoon seating at the vein antrum during pulmonary vein isolation (see Figs. 15-4, 15-16,

and 15-17). Color or pulsed-wave Doppler over the pulmonary veins can assess for pulmonary vein stenosis (increased flow velocity with an ostial gradient) or ostial leaks during cryobal-loon veno-occlusion. This view also images the posterior fossa ovalis for more posterior transeptal puncture sites (e.g., LAA occlusion).

Clockwise torque from the left pulmonary vein (LPV) view images the posterior LA, esophagus, and descending aorta and provides an understanding of the proximity of the esophagus to the pulmonary veins during atrial fibrillation ablation.

Clockwise torque from the posterior LA view visualizes the right inferior pulmonary vein (RIPV), right superior pulmonary vein (RSPV), intervening carina in cross section, and right pul-monary artery (see Figs. 15-10 and 15-19). Further posterior rotation with the ICE catheter near the interatrial septum helps to achieve a longitudinal view of the right pulmonary veins. Imaging the RSPV might require advancement of the ICE cath-eter superiorly toward the superior vena cava (SVC) given the close proximity between the SVC and RSPV.

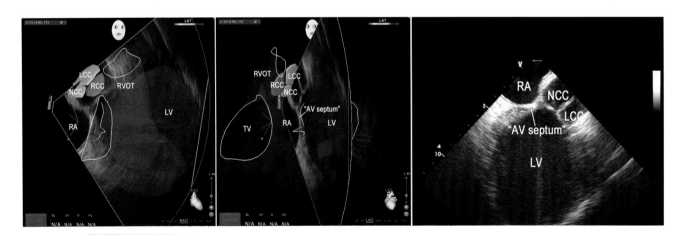

FIGURE 3-2 "AV septum." The US transducer is in the mid-RA with its beam directed leftward (clockwise torque) from the home view cutting through the aortic valve (NCC and LCC) and LV. The interface between the RA and LV ("AV septum") is seen.

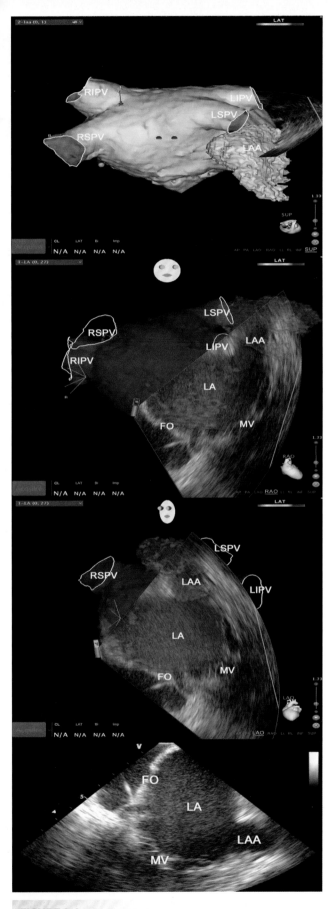

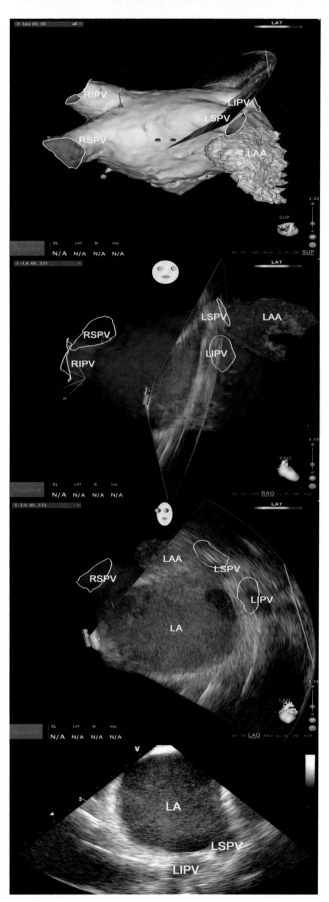

FIGURE 3-3 MV and LAA view.

FIGURE 3-4 Left-sided pulmonary vein view. The LSPV and LIPV are imaged longitudinally ("pant legs").

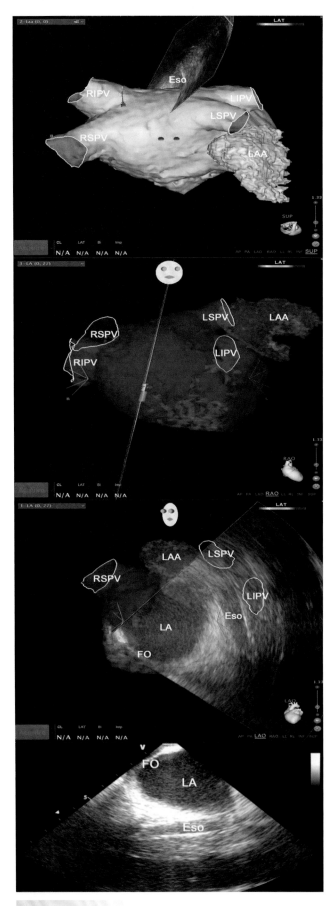

FIGURE 3-5 Esophageal view.

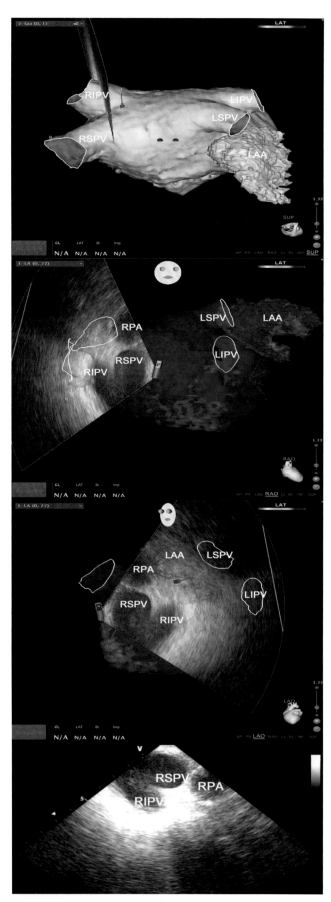

FIGURE 3-6 Right-sided pulmonary vein view. The RSPV and RIPV are imaged cross-sectionally ("owl eyes").

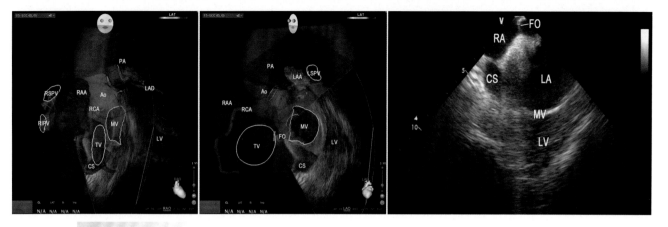

FIGURE 3-7 CS. The US transducer is in the inferior RA and directed leftward to visualize the CS (cross-sectional view) and MV.

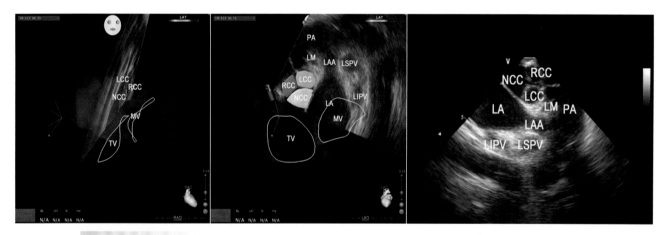

FIGURE 3-8 LAA (from the RA with posterior tilt). Note the proximity among the LAA, left main coronary artery, and PA. The Coumadin ridge between the LAA and LSPV can be seen in this view.

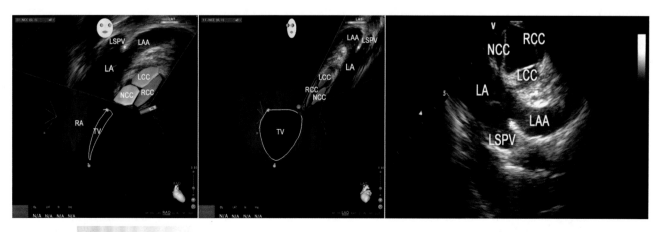

FIGURE 3-9 LAA (from the anterobasal RV). The Coumadin ridge (*asterisk*) between the LAA and LSPV is prominent.

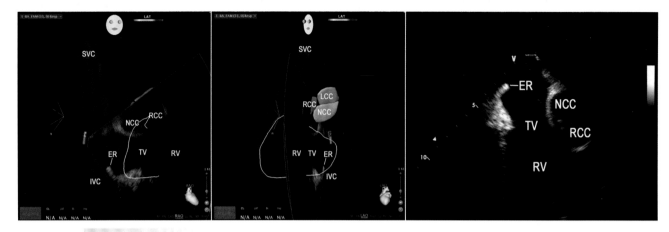

FIGURE 3-10 CTI. A prominent eustachian ridge (ER) takes off 90 degrees from the posterior end of a short CTI.

RIGHT ATRIUM

From the home view, counterclockwise torque of the ICE catheter scans the TV from septal to lateral margin. Anterior tilt directs the US beam inferiorly imaging the cavo-tricuspid isthmus (CTI) and anatomical structures (e.g., eustachian ridge, pouches) that can make CTI ablation difficult (Fig. 3-10; see also Fig. 14-19).[10] Counterclockwise torque of the ICE catheter views the lateral tricuspid annulus and right atrial appendage (RAA) (Fig. 3-11). Further counterclockwise torque images the crista terminalis along the anterolateral RA border—the superior extension of which is the sinus node (Fig. 3-12). Both structures can be the target site of ablation for crista tachycardias and sinus node modification, respectively.[11]

RIGHT VENTRICLE

While portions of the RV can be imaged from the RA, the moderator band (septomarginal trabeculae) and anterior papillary muscle are best viewed by advancing the ICE catheter across the TV (anterior tilt). Counterclockwise torque from a septal view images the RV and moderator band as it crosses the RV cavity from septum to lateral margin (Fig. 3-13). The moderator band can be a source of RV ectopy—particularly short-coupled premature ventricular contractions that trigger ventricular fibrillation (see Figs. 19-31 and 19-32). While the home view visualizes the right ventricular outflow tract (RVOT), additional views of the RVOT can be obtained by advancing the ICE catheter into the RV and clocking the catheter so that the US beam points superiorly to image the RVOT/PV and PA longitudinally.

LEFT VENTRICLE

The basal LV can be imaged from the RA, but the best images of the LV are obtained from the RV. From the home view, the ICE catheter is tilted anteriorly and advanced into the RV. Clockwise torque beneath the aortic valve images the LV from apex to base in the following orders: 1) LV septum/apex; 2) posteromedial papillary (PMP) muscle; 3) anterolateral papillary (ALP) muscle; 4) MV/aorto-mitral continuity; 5) aortic (cross-sectional view) and pulmonary valves; and 6) aortic valves, aorta, and pulmonary artery (longitudinal view) (Figs. 3-14 to 3-18). The papillary muscle and chordal attachments to the MV are imaged from a mid-LV oblique view. The papillary

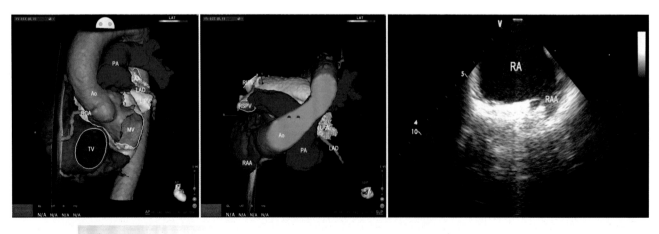

FIGURE 3-11 RAA. The US transducer is in the mid-RA and directed rightward (counterclockwise torque) from the home view.

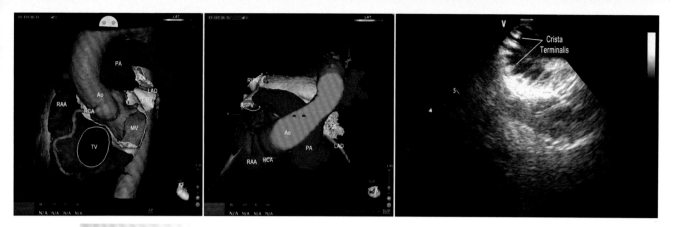

FIGURE 3-12 Crista terminalis. Further counterclockwise torque from the RAA images the crista terminalis, which is characterized by its "shaggy" appearance due to pectinate muscles.

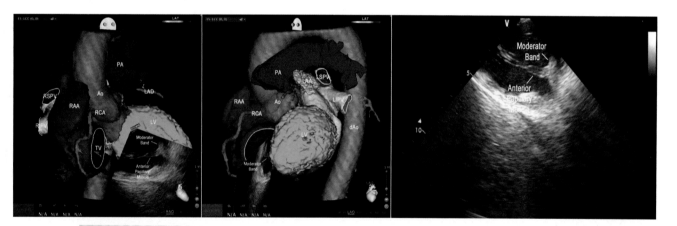

FIGURE 3-13 Moderator band. The US transducer is in the RV with its beam directed inferiorly (anterior tilt) to image the moderator band–anterior papillary muscle complex.

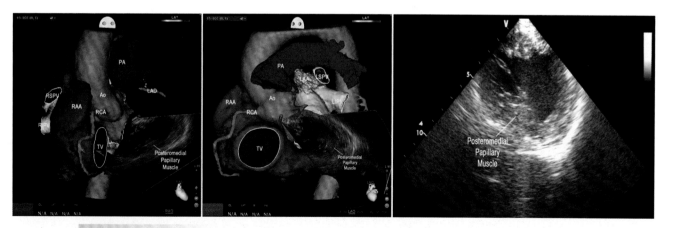

FIGURE 3-14 PMP muscle. The US transducer is in the RV with clockwise torque to direct its beam toward the LV cavity and image the PMP muscle.

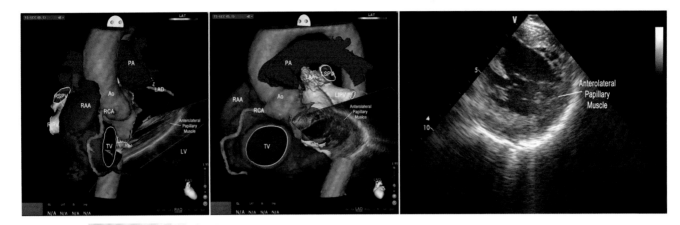

FIGURE 3-15 ALP muscle. Clockwise torque of the US transducer from the PMP muscle directs the beam onto the ALP muscle.

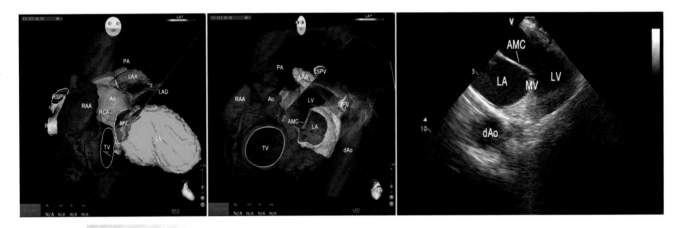

FIGURE 3-16 Aorto-mitral continuity (AMC). Clockwise torque from the papillary muscles images the AMC and LV outflow tract.

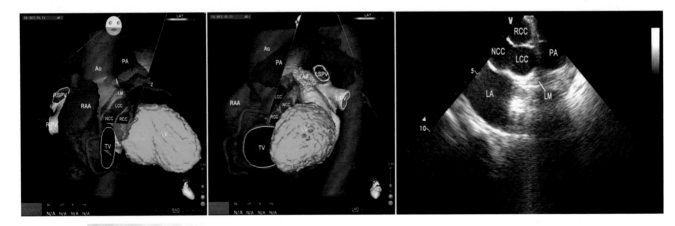

FIGURE 3-17 Aortic valve (cross-sectional view). The left main coronary artery can be imaged from this view.

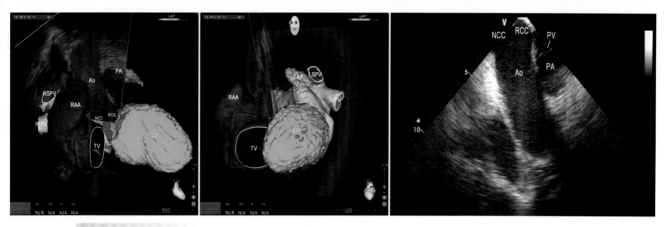

FIGURE 3-18 Aortic valve (longitudinal view). The ascending aorta (Ao) and pulmonary artery are also imaged in long axis.

muscles are another common source of ventricular ectopy (see Figs. 19-22 to 19-24). Identifying LV scar (akinetic areas with increased echogenicity) and aneurysms (dyskinetic areas) facilitates substrate mapping during ventricular tachycardia ablation (see Figs. 20-3, 20-22, and 20-23). Ventricular ectopy can also originate from the outflow tracts, especially the anteroseptum of the RVOT beneath the pulmonary valve, pulmonary artery, RCC, LCC, and the aorto-mitral continuity (see Figs. 19-6 to 19-10, 19-11 to 19-14, 19-16, 19-17, and 19-19 to 19-21). With ablation within the aortic cusps, ICE can view the proximity of the coronary arteries to the ablation catheter. The aortic cusps can be visualized from the 1) home view, 2) RA (cross-sectional view of aortic valve), 3) RV (cross-sectional view of aortic valve), and 4) RV (longitudinal view of aortic valve). While visualizing all three leaflets of the pulmonary

valve is difficult with transthoracic and transesophageal echocardiography because of its anterior location, a unique trileaflet cross-sectional view of the pulmonary valve can be obtained by positioning the ICE transducer in the RAA and directing the beam leftward toward the neighboring pulmonary artery (Fig. 3-19).

ICE MONITORING

ICE provides real-time monitoring of ablation lesions and complications. During radiofrequency ablation, ICE can show the location and stability of electrode/tissue contact, radiofrequency-induced changes in tissue character (increased echogenicity, swelling, crater formation), and ablation complications

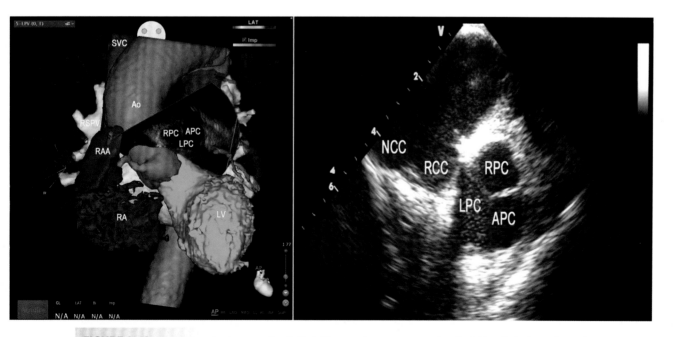

FIGURE 3-19 Pulmonary valve (cross-sectional view). The transducer is positioned in the RAA with the beam directed leftward toward the nearby pulmonary artery to visualize the right, left, and anterior pulmonary cusps.

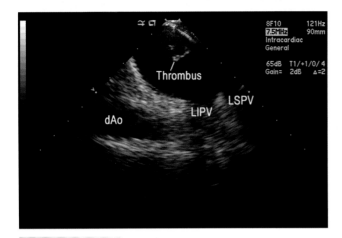

FIGURE 3-20 Mobile thrombus is attached to the ablation catheter in the LA.

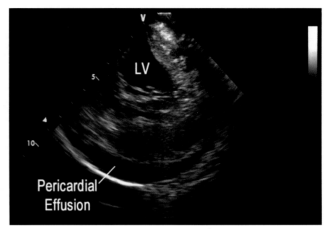

FIGURE 3-21 Echolucent pericardial effusion around the LV.

(thrombus formation, shower of accelerated microbubble formation [indicative of tissue overheating], and pericardial effusions) (**Figs. 3-20 and 3-21**).

REFERENCES

1. Kim SS, Hijazi ZM, Lang RM, Knight BP. The use of intracardiac echocardiography and other intracardiac imaging tools to guide noncoronary cardiac interventions. J Am Coll Cardiol 2009;53:2217–2228.
2. Hijazi ZM, Shivkumar K, Sahn DJ. Intracardiac echocardiography during interventional and electrophysiological cardiac catheterization. Circulation 2009;119:587–596.
3. Banchs JE, Patel P, Naccarelli GV, Gonzalez MD. Intracardiac echocardiography in complex cardiac catheter ablation procedures. J Interv Card Electrophysiol 2010;28:167–184.
4. Ali S, George LK, Das P, Koshy SK. Intracardiac echocardiography: clinical utility and application. Echocardiography 2011;28:582–590.
5. Bruce CJ, Friedman PA. Intracardiac echocardiography. Eur J Echocardiogr 2001;2:234–244.
6. Ruisi CP, Brysiewicz N, Asnes JD, et al. Use of intracardiac echocardiography during atrial fibrillation ablation. Pacing Clin Electrophysiol 2013;36:781–788.
7. Dello Russo A, Russo E, Fassini G, et al. Role of intracardiac echocardiography in atrial fibrillation ablation. J Atr Fibrillation 2013;5:786.
8. Ren JF, Marchlinski FE. Utility of intracardiac echocardiography in left heart ablation for tachyarrhythmias. Echocardiography 2007;24:533–540.
9. Merchant FM, Delurgio DB. Site-specific transseptal cardiac catheterization guided by intracardiac echocardiography for emerging electrophysiology applications. J Innov Card Rhythm Manage 2013;4:1415–1427.
10. Bencsik G. Novel strategies in the ablation of typical atrial flutter: role of intracardiac echocardiography. Curr Cardiol Rev 2015;11:127–133.
11. Nagarakanti R, Saksena S. Three-dimensional mapping and intracardiac echocardiography in the treatment of sinoatrial nodal tachycardias. J Interv Card Electrophysiol 2016;46:55–61.

Transeptal Catheterization

4

Introduction

Transeptal catheterization was originally developed to access the left atrium directly for left-sided hemodynamic measurements.[1–5] It has become a mainstay technique of electrophysiologist to provide access for different left atrial (e.g., pulmonary vein isolation) and ventricular (e.g., ventricular tachycardia ablation) procedures and can be performed safely using both tactile and visual clues.

The purpose of this chapter is to:

1. Discuss the anatomy of the interatrial septum and fossa ovalis.
2. Describe different techniques and troubleshooting tips for transeptal catheterization.

FOSSA OVALIS

The primary target site for transeptal catheterization is the thinnest portion of the interatrial septum—the fossa ovalis (a shallow, thumbprint-sized oval depression in the middle of the interatrial septum) (**Fig. 4-1**). An alternative transeptal access site is the foramen ovale—a slit-like recess superior to the fossa ovalis between the septum primum and secundum. Crossing the foramen ovale superior to the fossa ovalis, however, could make catheter manipulation toward inferior left atrial targets more difficult.

EMBRYOLOGY/ANATOMY

The primitive atrium is divided into right and left atria by two septae: the thin, membrane-like septum primum and the thicker septum secundum. The septum primum grows caudally from the roof of the atrium to fuse with the endocardial cushions and close the foramen primum. Coalescing perforations and resorption of the cranial portion of the septum primum creates the foramen secundum. The septum secundum then grows caudally from the roof of the atrium to the right of the septum primum and closes the foramen secundum. The slit-like recess that forms between the two septae tucked behind the thick inferior muscular rim of the septum secundum is the foramen ovale, which is incompletely fused in 25% (patent foramen ovale).[6] The fossa ovalis is a central depression in the right face of the septum primum inferior to the foramen ovale and in situ lying obliquely off the coronal plane (**Fig. 4-2**). It is bounded superiorly by the thick septum secundum (superior limbus)—the most caudal portion of which is the "limbic ledge."[7]

Critical structures surrounding the fossa ovalis include the aortic root/mound (anterior and superior), coronary sinus (CS) (anterior and inferior), and posterior right atrium. The posterior atrium is created by an infolding of the right and left atrial tissue between layers of epicardial fat where transeptal puncture would initially be epicardial before entering the left atrium. Late tamponade can occur once the sheath is removed from the left atrium.

TRANSEPTAL CATHETERIZATION

EQUIPMENT

The basic equipment for transeptal catheterization are the 1) transeptal needle (TN), 2) transeptal dilator (TD) and sheath (TS), 3) arterial (not venous) pressure tubing connected to a pressure transducer, and 4) anticoagulation.[8] The classic manual Brockenbrough TN has a 135-degree curve to directly engage the fossa ovalis and an inner lumen with an end hole for contrast/saline injection, pressure transduction, and insertion of a 0.014-inch wire. An arrow at the base of the TN points in the direction of the TN curve. A 0.0315-inch SafeSept™ needle (Pressure Products) needle can also be used alone or in conjunction with the Brockenbrough TN to puncture the fossa ovalis.[9] It assumes an atraumatic J-tip when it enters the left atrium allowing it to be positioned in a left pulmonary vein for support of the TD/TS assembly. An alternative to manual (forceful) transeptal puncture with the Brockenbrough TN is a dedicated

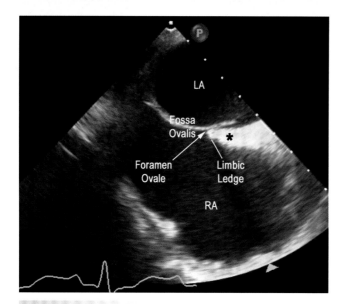

FIGURE 4-1 Anatomy of the fossa ovalis (TEE). Note the thick muscular septum secundum (*asterisk*) that forms the "limbic ledge" with the thin septum primum.

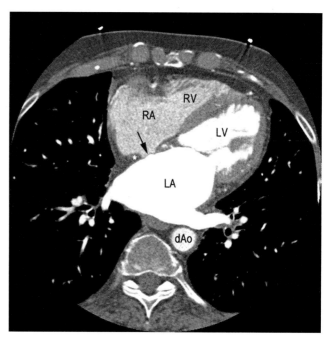

FIGURE 4-2 Anatomy of the fossa ovalis (CT). The fossa ovalis lies obliquely off the coronal plane and is therefore accessed by a TN pointed between 4 and 5 o'clock in the horizontal plane (*arrow*). Note the prominent "limbic ledge" from the thick muscular septum secundum (*asterisk*) to thin septum primum.

NRG™ radiofrequency TN (Baylis Medical) that contains an inner lumen but side holes that allow for fluid injection/pressure transduction but not delivery of an inner 0.014-inch wire.[10] Radiofrequency energy can also be applied to the Brockenbrough TN through an electrocautery pen or ablation catheter.[11–13]

The TS comes in various lengths and curves depending on the intended application. Curves can be steerable or fixed (short curves to target the posterior pulmonary veins and long curves to reach the anterior mitral annulus and left ventricle). The side arm of the TS lies in the same plane and generally points in the direction of the TS curve. A mark on the hub of the TD indicates the direction of the TD curve. When assembling the TD/TS, the side arm of the TS should line up with the mark of the TD hub so that the curves of the TD/TS unit are aligned with each other.

AVOIDING CRITICAL STRUCTURES

Because critical structures neighboring the fossa ovalis are fluoroscopically invisible, it is important to understand their location in order to avoid inadvertent puncture.[14–16] The aortic root anterior to the fossa ovalis can be marked by a pigtail catheter placed in the noncoronary cusp (NCC) of the aortic valve or a properly positioned His bundle catheter because the His bundle penetrates the membranous septum beneath the commissure of the NCC and right coronary cusp (RCC). A deflectable catheter within the CS inferior to the fossa ovalis outlines its course along the left atrio-ventricular groove.

PULL-DOWN TECHNIQUE

Rather than a direct approach, the most common transeptal technique is the pull-down or drag approach that takes

advantage not only of the coaxial relationship of the superior vena cava (SVC), interatrial septum, and inferior vena cava but also the movement of the TN over specific landmarks giving the operator an understanding of the TN tip location relative to the fossa ovalis.[7] The initial setup requires that the TN/TD/TS assembly is meticulously flushed with heparinized saline. Over a 0.032-inch guidewire, the TD/TS is advanced to the SVC (level of the carina). The TN is advanced into the TD/TS unit so that the TN tip is just within (but not beyond) the tip of the TD under high magnification fluoroscopy (a packaged stylet can also be used with the Brockenbrough TN to guide delivery of the TN into the TD/TS and avoid puncturing the wall of the TD/TS assembly). Once the TN tip is just within the tip of the TD, it is important to keep the distance between the hubs of the TN/TD fixed to avoid the advancement of the TN out of the TD. The arrow of the TN should be aligned with the side arm of the TS and hub mark of the TD so that the curves of all three (TN/TD/TS) are aligned and not fighting each other.[14] Using the arrow of the TD, the assembly is then rotated so that the TN tip points posteromedially (4–5 o'clock) when looking down the barrel of the needle (horizontal plane) and in the same direction as the intracardiac echocardiography (ICE) beam visualizing the fossa ovalis.[14] Clockwise and counterclockwise torque directs the needle more posteriorly (toward the posterior atrial wall) and anteriorly (toward the aortic root), respectively.

Pull-down

With the TN tip pointed posteromedially (4–5 o'clock), the entire TN/TD/TS unit is slowly pulled down together from the SVC keeping the distance between hubs of the TN and TD fixed. During the pull-down, three tactile and visible clues ("bumps" or "jumps") occur at the level of the 1) aortic knob, 2) SVC–RA junction, and 3) limbic ledge.[3,7,14–16] In particular, the "jump" off the limbic ledge as the assembly falls off the thick muscular septum secundum into the depression of the fossa ovalis is most prominent. Once the TN/TD/TS assembly snags the fossa ovalis, gentle forward pressure further tents the fossa ovalis (not uncommonly, this simple forward pressure can puncture the septum without a TN because the fossa ovalis can be very thin [sometimes nearly transparent] or the assembly crosses a probe patent foramen ovale more superiorly).[17,18]

Tenting

Before deployment of the TN out of the TD, it is crucial to verify that the TN has engaged the fossa ovalis and not any other structure by demonstrating tenting of the fossa ovalis. Fluoroscopically, the TN is posterior to the His bundle (aortic root) and aligned nearly parallel to the CS catheter (RAO) and toward the left atrium (LAO) (**Fig. 4-3**).[19,20] By tactile sensation, the TN can be felt moving with the beating heart. Tenting can be confirmed by 1) ICE (or transesophageal echocardiography [TEE]) or 2) dye staining of the interatrial septum (end-hole TNs) (**Figs. 4-3 to 4-6**).[21] In particular, ICE identifies the point of maximal tenting on the fossa ovalis and the trajectory of the TN toward the left atrium.

The Puncture

Once tenting is confirmed, forward pressure of the TN out of the TD is used to puncture the septum. Successful puncture of the fossa ovalis is often associated with a tactile "pop" or "give" and visual loss of tenting on ICE (**Figs. 4-4 to 4-6**). Alternatively, transeptal puncture can also be achieved using a powered TN with radiofrequency energy (**Fig. 4-7**).

TD/TS Deployment

Before deployment of the TD/TS across the interatrial septum, it is crucial to verify that the TN tip is in the left atrium. Confirmation of left atrial access can be confirmed by 1) bubbles in the left atrium with saline injection under ICE imaging, 2) swirl of contrast in the left atrium under fluoroscopy, 3) SafeSept or 0.014-inch guidewire inserted through the TN and positioned in a left pulmonary vein, 4) left atrial (not aortic) pressure waveforms with pressure transduction, 5) arterial oxygen saturation (although this does not exclude aortic puncture), and 6) electro-anatomic localization of the TN in the left atrium (**Figs. 4-4, 4-5, and 4-7 to 4-10**). Because of the different viscosities between contrast and saline, contrast affects pressure waveforms and therefore should be thoroughly flushed from the TN. The TN can be located on the electro-anatomic mapping system but requires a special adapter that turns the metal TN tip into an electrode,

and visualization requires that the TN tip is outside the TD/TS assembly.

Once left atrial access is confirmed, the TN is kept fixed and the TD/TS is advanced over the TN into the left atrium under LAO fluoroscopy to a point where the TS crosses the septum but the TD does not reach the left atrial free wall to avoid free wall puncture (**Fig. 4-11**). At this point, the TD/TN is kept fixed and the TS is advanced over the TD into the left atrium. Once the TS is in the left atrium, both the TN and TD are removed slowly from the TS (rapid removal of the TN/TD can create negative pressure within the TS [Venturi effect], introduce air into the TS, and cause air emboli). The TS is then meticulously de-aired, flushed, and connected to fluid-filled arterial tubing and the pressure transducer.

PUNCTURE TYPES

Double Transeptal Puncture

Certain applications (e.g., pulmonary vein isolation) might require a second transeptal puncture. The second TN/TD/TS assembly is pulled down in fashion similar to the first assembly. The RAO/LAO fluoroscopic location of the first TS provides a visual reference to the fossa ovalis for a second puncture site (e.g., slightly inferiorly), but acoustic interference from the first TS might limit ICE images (**Fig. 4-12**). An alternative to double transeptal puncture is the one-puncture, double transeptal catheterization technique.[22] After initial puncture, a 0.032-inch guidewire is inserted into the TD/TS unit and positioned in a left pulmonary vein for support. Back and forth movement of the TD/TS across the septum dilates the puncture site. In one form of this technique, the TD/TS is then pulled back into the right atrium. An ablation catheter is then advanced across the dilated puncture site into the left atrium, curved anteriorly and inferiorly toward the mitral valve (MV), and pulled down to stretch the puncture site. The TD/TS assembly is then re-advanced over the guidewire back into the left atrium. In another form of this technique, the TD is removed after dilating the puncture site. Two 0.032-inch guidewires are then advanced through the TS into the left pulmonary veins providing double left atrial access. The TS is then removed and two TD/TS sheaths are advanced separately over each wire into the left atrium. This technique, however, can be associated with a higher risk of femoral vein bleeding and a residual atrial septal defect.

Site-Selective Transeptal Puncture

Certain applications might require a more anterior (plane directed toward the MV/left atrial appendage [LAA]) or posterior (plane directed toward the left pulmonary veins) puncture site, particularly when using bulky sheaths with large turning radii (**Figs. 4-13 and 4-14**).[23,24] Cryoablation of the posterior pulmonary veins (particularly, right inferior pulmonary vein) might require a more anterior-inferior puncture site, while LAA occlusion (e.g., Watchman) of the anteriorly and superiorly situated left appendage is easier with a posterior-inferior puncture site.

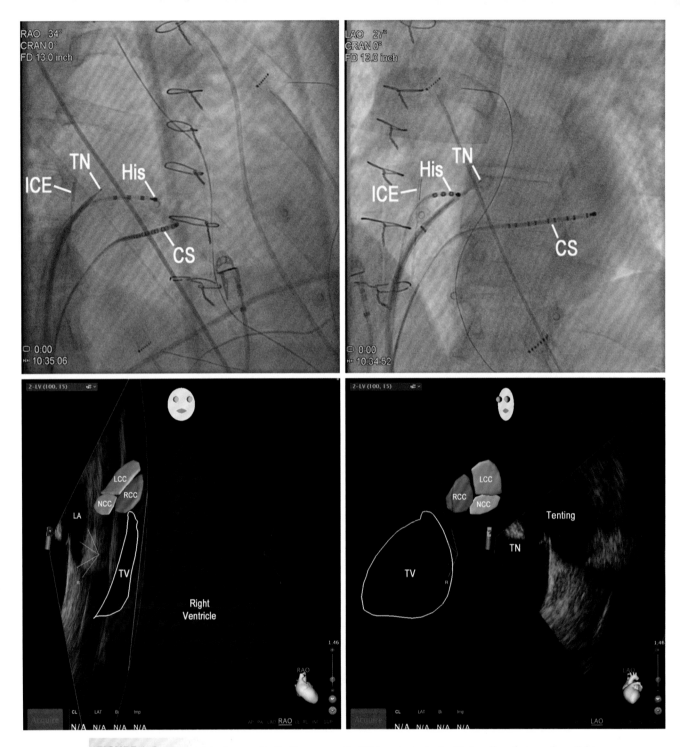

FIGURE 4-3 Tenting of the fossa ovalis. On fluoroscopy, the TN is posterior to the His bundle catheter and parallel to the CS catheter. Tenting into the left atrium is seen on ICE. Note the location of the fossa ovalis relative to the aortic valve.

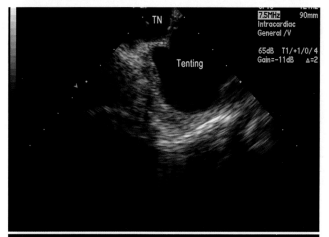

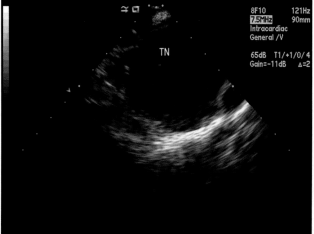

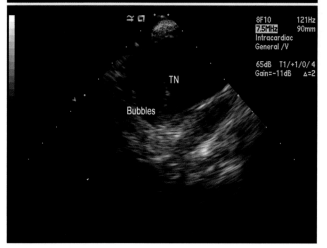

FIGURE 4-4 Transeptal puncture. Tenting of the fossa ovalis is seen on ICE. Successful puncture is confirmed by the loss of tenting and visualizing the tip of the TN and bubbles in the left atrium.

TROUBLESHOOTING

FIRST PASS FAILURE

During the pull-down, the TN/TD/TS assembly might bypass the fossa ovalis either because the assembly was not aligned with the fossa ovalis (too posterior or anterior) or the TN curve had insufficient reach to the fossa ovalis (e.g., right atrial enlargement). With the assembly inferior to the fossa ovalis, the TN is removed and replaced by a 0.032-inch guidewire, which is then re-advanced back to the SVC, and the process is repeated. A second pull-down is done with a different rotational axis of the TN (more posterior [toward 5 o'clock] or anterior [toward 4 o'clock]) and/or larger TN curve (e.g., manually curved or BRK-1 [107 degrees]). An alternative to repeated guidewire and needle exchanges is the anterior staircase technique, which takes advantage of the anterior free space in the right atrium. With the TN within the TD/TS, the assembly is rotated so that the TN arrow and curve points anteriorly (12 o'clock). The whole assembly is then slowly advanced to the SVC with back-and-forth rotation of the curve between 10 o'clock (counterclockwise rotation) and 2 o'clock (clockwise rotation) to prevent snagging of the assembly in the right atrium.[25]

DIFFERENT SEPTA

Certain interatrial septum can make transeptal puncture challenging and difficult. A floppy, aneurysmal septum can stretch the fossa ovalis during tenting so that the point of maximal tenting is close to the left atrial free wall (**Fig. 4-15**). A "give" of the septum and lunging of the TN forward can puncture the left atrial free wall. Radiofrequency energy or use of the SafeSept needle allows puncture of the septum without the need for excessive force applied to the TN. Conversely, a thick, fibrotic septum (e.g., repeated transeptal procedures) can be difficult to puncture with a TN or deploy a TD/TS. Radiofrequency energy can also be used to puncture the septum. Sheath deployment might require dilation and/or using a TD/TS unit with a smooth transition and without a significant step-up between TD and TS. Some surgically repaired septal patches (pericardial or Dacron but generally not resistant Gore-Tex) can be punctured.[14] Interatrial septal occluding devices can also be directly punctured, although an alternative is puncturing the native septum surrounding the rim of the prosthetic device.[26]

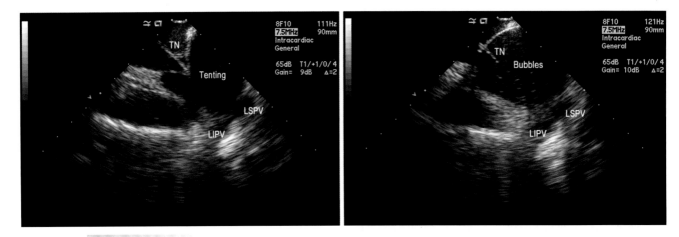

FIGURE 4-5 Transeptal puncture. Tenting of the fossa ovalis is seen on ICE. Successful puncture is confirmed by the loss of tenting and identifying the tip of the TN and bubbles in the left atrium. Transeptal crossing in the direction of the left-sided pulmonary veins identifies a more posterior puncture site.

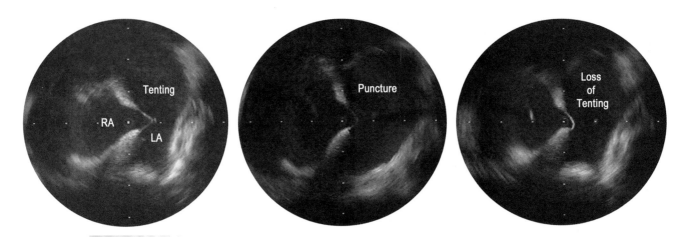

FIGURE 4-6 Transeptal puncture. Tenting of the fossa ovalis is seen on radial ICE.

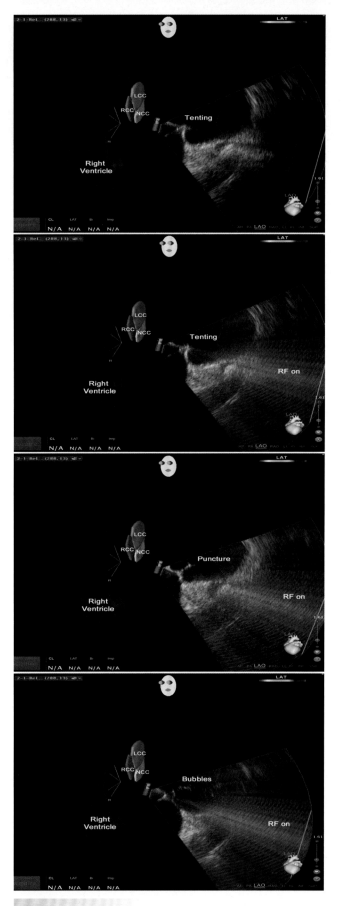

FIGURE 4-7 Transeptal puncture using radiofrequency energy.

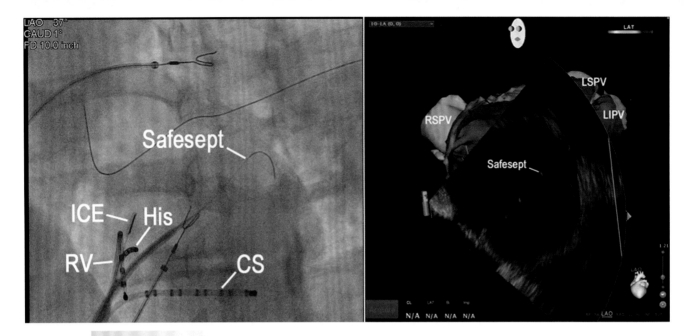

FIGURE 4-8 Transeptal puncture using a SafeSept wire. Confirmation of left atrial access is confirmed by visualizing the 0.0315-inch SafeSept wire in the left atrium on fluoroscopy and ICE.

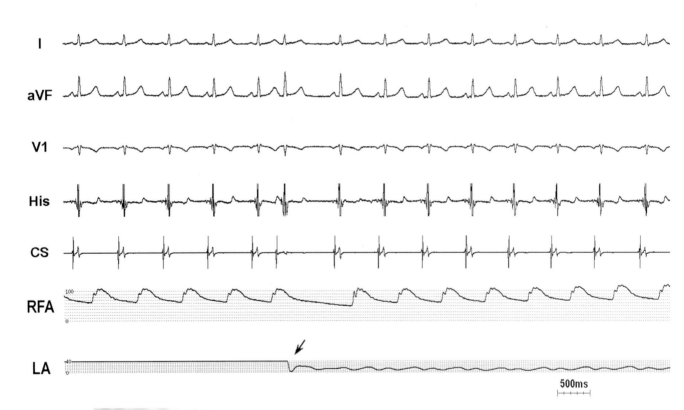

FIGURE 4-9 Left atrium pressure waveform. Left atrial access is confirmed by recording a left atrial hemodynamic waveform. The waveform is dampened while the needle is against the septum. Successful puncture (*arrow*) causes an APC followed by a left atrial pressure recording.

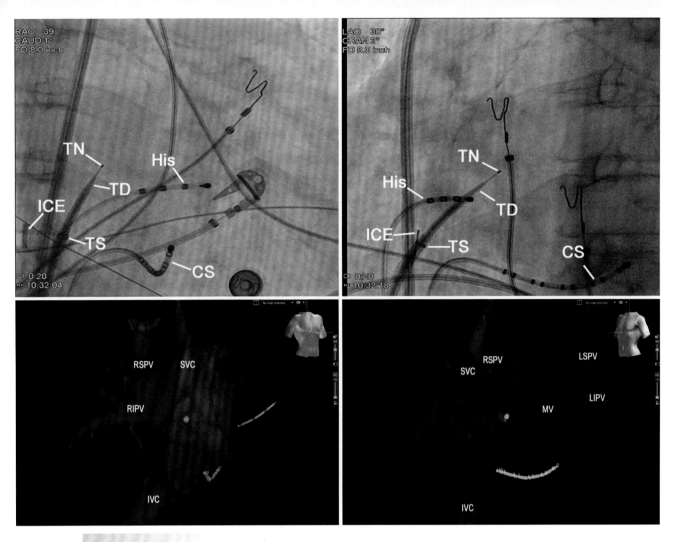

FIGURE 4-10 Electro-anatomic localization of the TN. On fluoroscopy, the TN is posterior to the His bundle and nearly parallel to the CS catheter. Left atrial access is confirmed by visualizing the TN tip (*green dot*) in the left atrium on the three-dimensional electro-anatomic map.

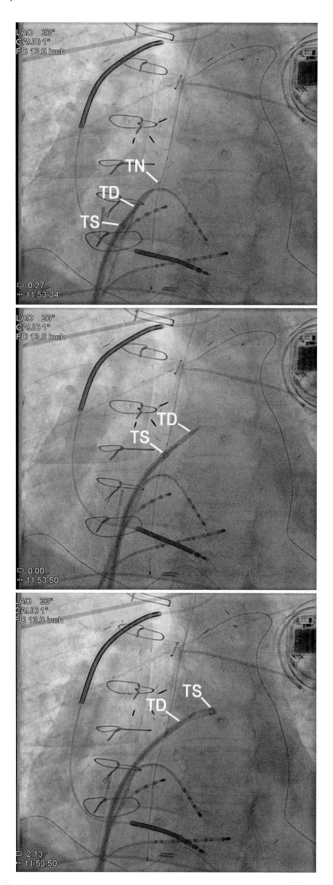

FIGURE 4-11 TS deployment. *Top*: The TN has punctured the fossa ovalis. *Middle*: The TN is kept fixed, and the TD/TS assembly is advanced over the TN into the left atrium until the TS has just crossed the septum. *Bottom*: The TN/TD is then kept fixed, and the TS sheath is advanced over the TD into the left atrium.

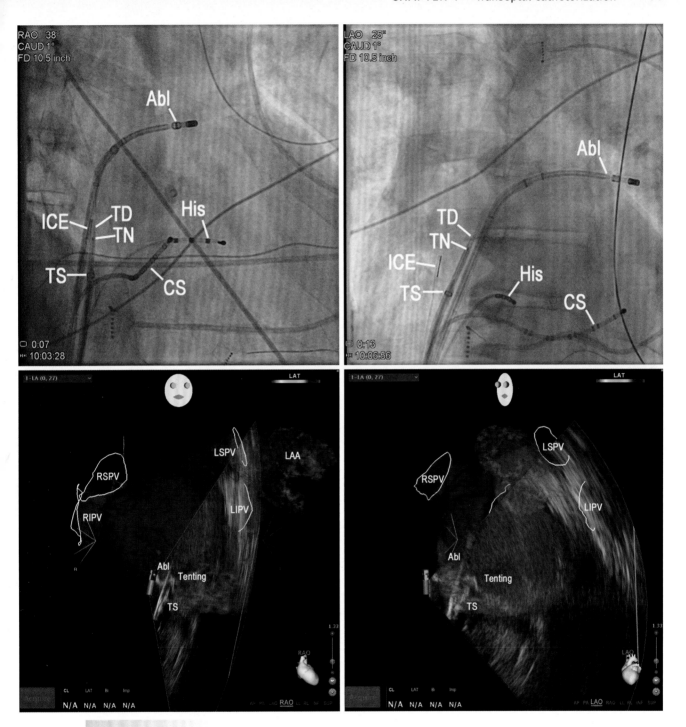

FIGURE 4-12 Double transeptal puncture. On fluoroscopy, the ablation catheter from the first transeptal puncture provides a reference landmark to the location of the fossa ovalis. ICE imaging shows tenting of the fossa ovalis inferior to the ablation catheter where the second transeptal puncture was made.

Posterior Puncture

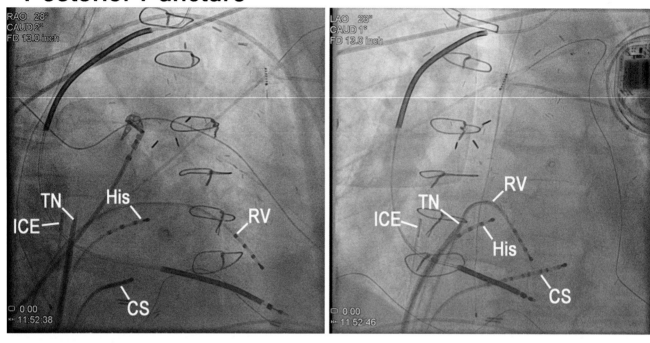

Anterior Puncture

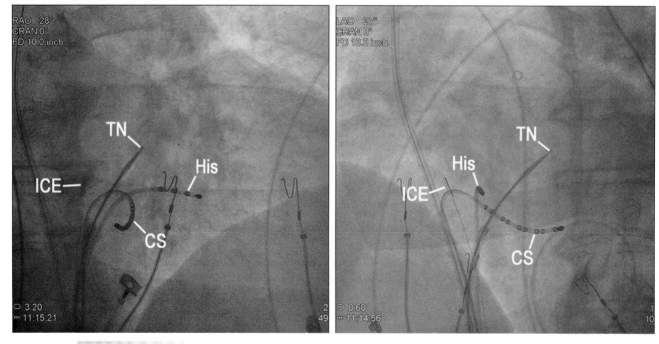

FIGURE 4-13 Site-selective transeptal puncture. *Top*: With a posterior puncture, RAO fluoroscopy shows the TN pointed away from the His bundle and CS and closer to the spine ("vertical or straight" appearing). *Bottom*: With an anterior puncture, RAO fluoroscopy shows the TN pointed closer to the His bundle and CS and farther from the spine ("curved" appearing).

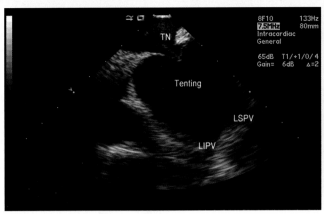

Posterior Puncture

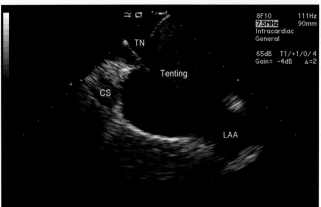

Anterior Puncture

FIGURE 4-14 Site-selective transeptal puncture. *Left:* posterior puncture with the ICE plane directed toward the LIPV/LSPV. *Right:* anterior puncture with the ICE plane directed toward the MV/LAA. The puncture is also inferior on the fossa ovalis for atrial fibrillation cryoablation.

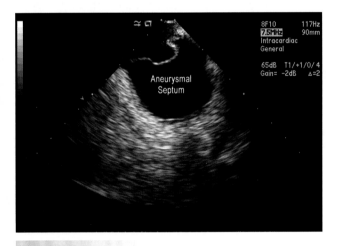

FIGURE 4-15 Aneurysmal ("floppy") septum. Tenting could stretch the septum close to the left atrial free wall risking puncture if the septum suddenly "gives" and the TN lunges toward the free wall. In this situation, a radiofrequency needle or SafeSept wire might be beneficial.

REFERENCES

1. Ross J Jr. Transeptal left heart catheterization: a new method of left atrial puncture. Ann Surg 1959;149:395–401.
2. Ross J Jr, Braunwald E, Morrow AG. Transseptal left atrial puncture; new technique for the measurement of left atrial pressure in man. Am J Cardiol 1959;3:653–655.
3. Ross J Jr. Considerations regarding the technique for transseptal left heart catheterization. Circulation 1966;34:391–399.
4. Brockenbrough EC, Braunwald E, Ross J Jr. Transseptal left heart catheterization. A review of 450 studies and description of an improved technic. Circulation 1962;225:15–21.
5. Ross J Jr. Transseptal left heart catheterization: a 50-year odyssey. J Am Coll Cardiol 2008;51:2107–2115.
6. Hara H, Virmani R, Ladich E, et al. Patent foramen ovale: current pathology, pathophysiology, and clinical status. J Am Coll Cardiol 2005;46: 1768–1776.
7. Bloomfield DA, Sinclair-Smith BC. The limbic ledge. A landmark for transseptal left heart catheterization. Circulation 1965;331:103–107.
8. Mullins CE. Transseptal left heart catheterization: experience with a new technique in 520 pediatric and adult patients. Pediatr Cardiol 1983;4: 239–245.
9. de Asmundis C, Chierchia GB, Sarkozy A, et al. Novel trans-septal approach using a Safe Sept J-shaped guidewire in difficult left atrial access during atrial fibrillation ablation. Europace 2009;11:657–659.
10. Winkle RA, Mead RH, Engel G, Patrawala RA. The use of a radiofrequency needle improves the safety and efficacy of transseptal puncture for atrial fibrillation ablation. Heart Rhythm 2011;8:1411–1415.
11. Bidart C, Vaseghi M, Cesario DA, et al. Radiofrequency current delivery via transseptal needle to facilitate septal puncture. Heart Rhythm 2007;4: 1573–1576.
12. Knecht S, Jais P, Nault I, et al. Radiofrequency puncture of the fossa ovalis for resistant transseptal access. Circ Arrhythm Electrophysiol 2008;1:169–174.
13. McWilliams MJ, Tchou P. The use of a standard radiofrequency energy delivery system to facilitate transseptal puncture. J Cardiovasc Electrophysiol 2009;20:238–240.
14. Tzeis S, Andrikopoulos G, Deisenhofer I, Ho SY, Theodorakis G. Transseptal catheterization: considerations and caveats. Pacing Clin Electrophysiol 2010;33:231–242.
15. Earley MJ. How to perform a transseptal puncture. Heart 2009;95:85–92.
16. Gard J, Swale M, Asirvatham SJ. Transseptal access for the electrophysiologist: anatomic considerations to enhance safety and efficacy. J Innov Cardiac Rhythm Manage 2011;2:332–338.
17. Gorlin R, Krasnow N, Levine HJ, Neill WA, Wagman RJ, Messer JV. A modification of the technic of transseptal left heart catheterization. Am J Cardiol 1961;7:580.
18. Aldridge HE. Transseptal left heart catheterization without needle puncture of the interatrial septum. Am J Cardiol 1964;13:239–243.
19. Cheng A, Calkins H. A conservative approach to performing transseptal punctures without the use of intracardiac echocardiography: stepwise approach with real-time video clips. J Cardiovasc Electrophysiol 2007; 18:686–689.
20. Croft CH, Lipscomb K. Modified technique of transseptal left heart catheterization. J Am Coll Cardiol 1985;5:904–910.
21. Daoud EG, Kalbfleisch SJ, Hummel JD. Intracardiac echocardiography to guide transseptal left heart catheterization for radiofrequency catheter ablation. J Cardiovasc Electrophysiol 1999;10:358–363.
22. Yamada T, McElderry HT, Epstein AE, Plumb VJ, Kay GN. One-puncture, double-transseptal catheterization manoeuvre in the catheter ablation of atrial fibrillation. Europace 2007;9:487–489.
23. Bazaz R, Schwartzman D. Site-selective atrial septal puncture. J Cardiovasc Electrophysiol 2003;14:196–199.
24. Merchant FM, Delurgio DB. Site-specific transseptal cardiac catheterization guided by intracardiac echocardiography for emerging electrophysiology applications. J Innov Cardiac Rhythm Manage 2013;4:1415–1427.
25. Shaw TR. Anterior staircase manoeuvre for atrial transseptal puncture. Br Heart J 1994;71:297–301.
26. Santangeli P, Di Biase L, Burkhardt JD, et al. Transseptal access and atrial fibrillation ablation guided by intracardiac echocardiography in patients with atrial septal closure devices. Heart Rhythm 2011;8:1669–1675.

5 Narrow Complex Tachycardias

Introduction

The three major causes of a paroxysmal supraventricular tachycardia (SVT) are 1) atrio-ventricular nodal reentrant tachycardia (AVNRT ~80%), 2) orthodromic reciprocating tachycardia (ORT ~15%), and 3) atrial tachycardia (AT ~5%). Least common are junctional tachycardias (JT) (more commonly seen in pediatric populations or postoperatively after cardiac surgery). Clinically, ORT presents at a younger age than AVNRT.[1] Rapid regular pulsations in the neck (frog sign) is characteristic of AVNRT (due to right atrial contraction against a closed tricuspid valve).[2] Electrophysiologically, diagnosis of a narrow complex tachycardia (NCT) is established by systematic evaluation of its 1) 12-lead ECG and electrophysiologic features, 2) zones of transition, and 3) response to pacing and vagal maneuvers.[3] Particularly important is evaluation of the P-wave morphology and intracardiac pattern of atrial activation, atrio-ventricular (AV) relationship, and the effect of bundle branch block (BBB) on tachycardia. Transition zones are regions of spontaneous or induced changes in tachycardia (initiation, termination, oscillations in cycle length) that provide valuable clues about the tachycardia mechanism. Lastly, perturbations in tachycardia induced by pacing or vagal maneuvers (adenosine, carotid sinus massage) also provide important information about diagnosis.

The purpose of this chapter is to:

1. Diagnose NCT by systematic evaluation of its 12-lead ECG, electrophysiologic features, and transition zones.
2. Understand specific pacing maneuvers differentiating 1) ORT versus AVNRT, 2) AT versus AVNRT/ORT, and 3) AVNRT versus JT.

ELECTROPHYSIOLOGIC FEATURES

12-LEAD ECG

Presumptive diagnosis of an NCT can often be established by inspection of the 12-lead ECG.[4] The most important clue is derived from the P-wave morphology, which is often seen as a high-frequency deflection (in contrast to the low-frequency T wave) distorting the terminal portion of the QRS complex or ST segment. A sinus rhythm ECG is invaluable in establishing a template of the baseline QRS complex and ST segment for comparison.

RP Interval

NCTs are categorized by the length of its RP interval (onset of QRS complex to onset of P wave) into short and long RP tachycardias. Short RP tachycardias (RP < PR) include typical (slow–fast) AVNRT, ORT, AT with PR prolongation, and JT with retrograde fast pathway (FP) conduction. During typical (slow–fast) AVNRT, simultaneous activation of the atrium and ventricle produces a very short RP interval (<70 ms) ("A on V" tachycardia) with P waves buried within the QRS complex or distorting its terminal portion (pseudo S waves in II, III, aVF; pseudo r′ wave in V1) (see Fig. 7-13).[5,6] Sequential activation from ventricle to atrium during ORT imposes a mandatory finite VA interval during tachycardia (≥70 ms; ≥50 ms for pediatric populations) so that P waves are generally buried within the ST segment.[6,7] Therefore, a NCT with an RP interval <70 ms essentially excludes ORT. Long RP tachycardias (RP > PR) include atypical (fast–slow) AVNRT, ORT using a slowly conducting, decremental accessory pathway (AP) (permanent form of junctional reciprocating tachycardia [PJRT] or nodo-fascicular reentrant tachycardia [NFRT]), and AT (see Chapter 6). A mid-RP tachycardia with P waves buried exactly between QRS complexes (RP = PR) should raise suspicion of typical AVNRT with 2:1 block in the lower common final pathway (LCFP) (Fig. 5-1). NCTs without identifiable P waves

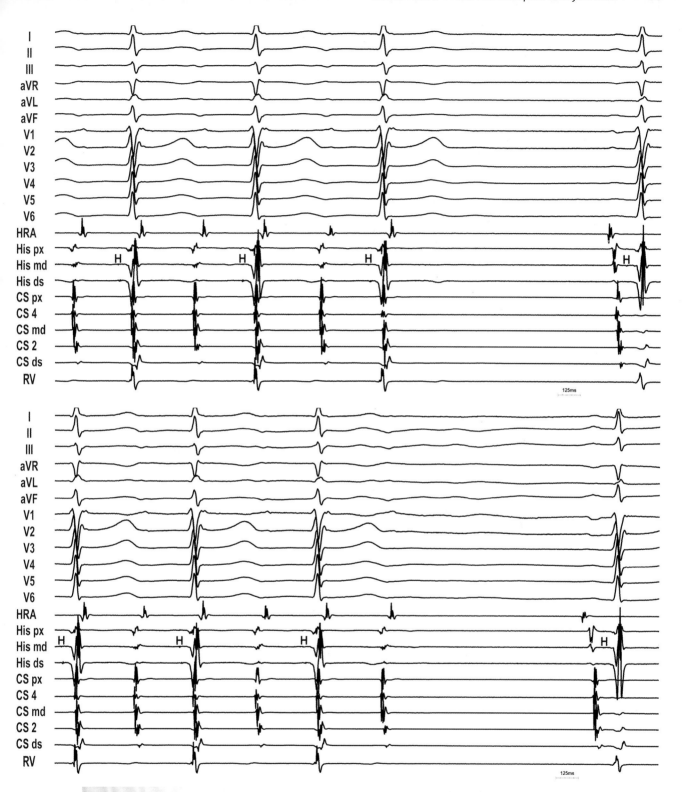

FIGURE 5-1 Typical (slow–fast) AVNRT with 2:1 block in the distal AV node (LCFP). Tachycardia terminates with block in the SP during two different cycles of LCFP conduction/block. Alternate P waves (narrow, superiorly directed) are buried exactly in mid-diastole.

include typical AVNRT (P waves buried within QRS complexes) and atrial flutter with 2:1 AV conduction (flutter waves buried within QRS complexes and T waves) especially when the ventricular rate is ~150 bpm.

P-Wave Morphology

The site of atrial origin during tachycardia determines its P-wave morphology. P waves originating from the septum tend to be narrower than those from the free wall. In general, low septal origin (AVNRT, ORT using a septal AP, septal AT) have a superior (inverted in leads II, III, aVF) and midline (aVR P [+] ~ aVL P [+]) axis. Left atrial origin (ORT using a left-sided AP, left AT, AVNRT with left atrio-nodal inputs) has an anterior (V1 P [+]) and rightward (aVR P [+], aVL P [−]) axis. Right atrial origin (ORT using a right-sided AP, right AT) have a posterior (V1 P [−]) and leftward (aVR P [−], aVL P [+]) axis. P waves with an inferior axis (upright in leads II, III, aVF) are generally due to AT, although ORT using an anteroseptal AP can produce positive P waves inferiorly.[8]

QRS Alternans

QRS alternans is the beat-to-beat variation in R-wave amplitude (≥1 mm) during stable tachycardia. While some evidence suggests that QRS alternans favors ORT with slower rates (<180 bpm), it is likely a rate-related phenomenon and not specific for a particular tachycardia mechanism.[4,9,10]

NCT Rate

Because of the large overlap in rates of different NCT, a specific rate criterion is generally not helpful for discrimination. However, a ventricular rate of 150 bpm suggests the possibility of atrial flutter with 2:1 AV conduction. An extremely rapid ("ultrafast") SVT (>250 bpm) should raise suspicion of atrial flutter with 1:1 AV conduction.

ELECTROPHYSIOLOGIC STUDY

Definitive diagnosis of a NCT is established in the electrophysiology laboratory by systematically analyzing its electrophysiologic features, zones of transition, and response to specific pacing maneuvers (Table 5-1).

VA Interval

The VA interval (onset of QRS complex to earliest site of atrial activation) is the intracardiac equivalent of the RP interval. A VA <70 ms (<50 ms in pediatric populations) excludes ORT.[6,7]

Atrial Activation Pattern

Atrial activation patterns dictate P-wave morphology and are either concentric (midline) or eccentric.[11–13] Concentric patterns show earliest activation along the interatrial septum near the coronary sinus ostium (posteroseptum) or His bundle region (anteroseptum). NCTs with earliest activation at the anteroseptum include typical AVNRT, ORT using an anteroseptal AP, AT arising near the His bundle (e.g., noncoronary cusp), and JT with retrograde conduction over the FP. NCT with earliest activation at the posteroseptum include atypical AVNRT; ORT using a posteroseptal AP; AT arising near the coronary sinus

TABLE 5-1 Distinguishing features of the three major NCTs

	AVNRT	ORT	AT
VA < 70	Common (typical AVNRT)	No	Uncommon (long PR ≈ TCL)
AV block	Uncommon	No	Common
BBB	No effect	↑ VA (and generally TCL) with BBB ipsilateral to AP	No effect
Spontaneous termination with AV block	Yes	Yes	No
Pre- or postexcitation/ termination by His refractory VPDs	No (unless bystander NF AP present)	Yes	No
"AV or AAV" response	"AV"	"AV"	"AAV"
PPI − TCL	>115	≤115	—
cPPI	≥110	<110	—
ΔHA	>0	<0	—
ΔVA	>85	≤85	—
ΔAH	>40	<20	<10

Abbreviations: $\Delta AH = AH_{(A\ pacing\ at\ TCL)} - AH_{(SVT)}$; $\Delta HA = HA_{(entrainment)} - HA_{(SVT)}$; $\Delta VA = St\text{-}A_{(entrainment)} - VA_{(SVT)}$; *NF, nodo-fascicular.*

ostium; and theoretically, JT with retrograde conduction over the slow pathway (SP). Eccentric patterns show earliest activation away from the septum and generally argue against retrograde AV nodal conduction except with left atrio-nodal inputs. NCTs with left eccentric atrial activation include ORT using a left-sided AP, left AT, and uncommonly AVNRT with left atrio-nodal inputs.[14] NCT with right eccentric atrial activation includes ORT using a right-sided AP and right AT. Because both the typical (AV) AP and the AV node are annular structures, an NCT with early activation from a nonannular site is most likely an AT.

AV Relationship

ORT is the only NCT that incorporates the ventricle as an integral part of its reentrant circuit, and therefore, a NCT with AV block excludes ORT. AV block, on the other hand, is possible but uncommon during AVNRT and common during AT. AVNRT with LCFP block is generally a transient phenomenon precipitated by abrupt changes (long–short sequence) in cycle length (particularly at SVT initiation) (Fig. 5-1).[15,16] A NCT with sustained and varying degrees of AV block is likely AT. During 1:1 AV association, changes in AH intervals that precede and predict VV and subsequent AA intervals indicate an AV node–dependent tachycardia (AVNRT or ORT) and argue against AT. Constant AA intervals despite changes in AH and VV intervals demonstrate AV node independence (AT).

In contrast to NCT with AV block, NCT with AV dissociation is rare and includes 1) AVNRT with upper common final pathway (UCFP) block, 2) JT with JA block, 3) ORT using a nodo-fascicular/nodo-ventricular AP with nodo-atrial block, and 4) intrahisian reentry with His-atrial block (see below).[17,18] While ORT using an AV AP obligates a 1:1 AV relationship, ORT using a nodo-fascicular/ventricular AP does not and can show AV dissociation (but not AV block).

Bundle Branch Block

ORT is the only NCT that incorporates the His-Purkinje system as an integral part of its reentrant circuit and specifically uses the bundle branch and Purkinje fibers ipsilateral to the AP to form the shortest functional circuit sustaining reentry. Block in the bundle branch ipsilateral to the AP forces antegrade conduction over the contralateral bundle enlarging the circuit with transeptal conduction.[19–22] The addition of transeptal conduction time to the tachycardia increases its 1) VA interval and, generally, 2) cycle length (Coumel's sign) (Figs. 5-2 and 5-3). VA intervals increase by >35 ms for free wall AP and <25 ms for septal AP.[20]

Therefore, cycle length deceleration with BBB (or conversely, cycle length acceleration with loss of BBB) indicates that the His-Purkinje system is an integral part of the circuit and establishes a diagnosis of ORT using an AP ipsilateral to the blocked bundle. By contrast, failure of cycle length deceleration with BBB is not specific for a tachycardia mechanism and even does not exclude ORT using an AP ipsilateral to BBB. The increase in VA interval can be compensated by an equivalent shortening of the AV interval, generally due to a decrease in the AH interval (see Figs. 10-5 and 10-6).

ZONES OF TRANSITION

INITIATION

Spontaneous

Important clues to tachycardia diagnosis during spontaneous initiation include its 1) mode of onset and 2) initiating complexes. Gradual onset (warm-up phenomenon) occurs with automatic tachycardias (e.g., automatic AT). Abrupt onset is observed with triggered activity and reentry (e.g., AVNRT, ORT). NCTs whose initial P wave is identical to tachycardia P waves include automatic AT (where an ectopic focus drives all tachycardia P waves) and PJRT (which occurs spontaneously during sinus rhythm without the need for atrial prematurity).

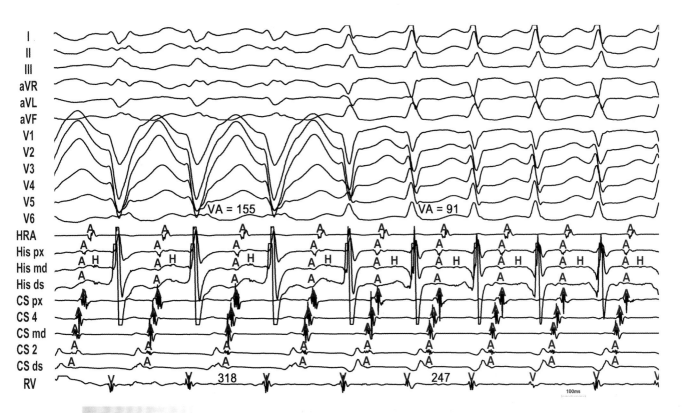

FIGURE 5-2 Coumel's sign (ORT using a left free wall AP). Atrial activation is left eccentric (earliest at CS ds). Loss of left bundle branch block (LBBB) causes a 64 ms and 71 ms shortening of the VA interval and TCL, respectively, indicating that the His-Purkinje system is an integral part of the tachycardia circuit.

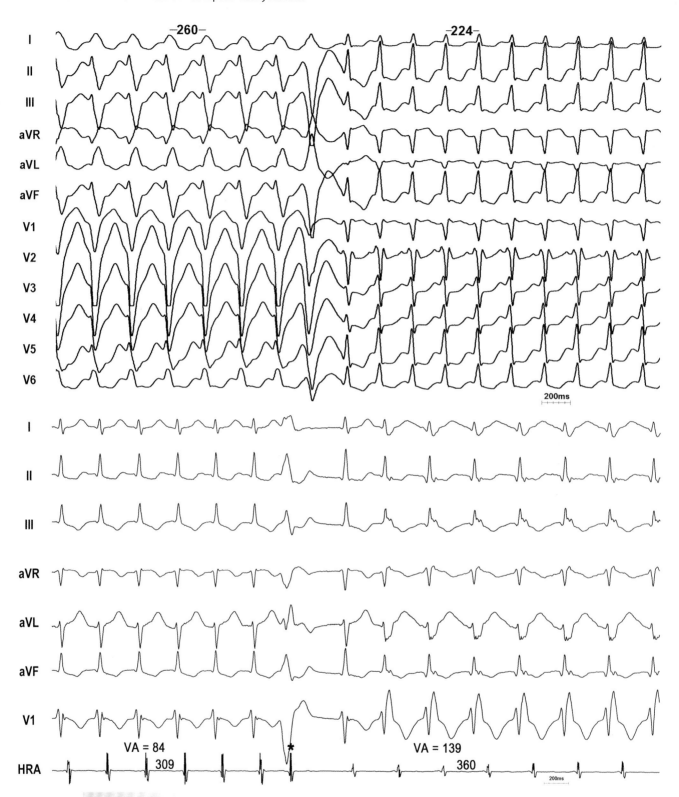

FIGURE 5-3 Coumel's sign. *Top*: During ORT using a left free wall AP, a spontaneous premature ventricular contraction (PVC) breaks the transeptal link that perpetuates LBBB causing acceleration of tachycardia and demonstrating tachycardia dependence on the His-Purkinje system. *Bottom*: During ORT using a right free wall AP, a late-coupled PVC advances the atrium (*asterisk*) indicating the presence of an AP. Tachycardia is reset with delay in the AV node exposing the His-Purkinje system to a long–short sequence that induces phase 3 RBBB and subsequent prolongation of both the VA interval (55 ms) and TCL (51 ms).

NCTs triggered by an atrial premature depolarization (APD) (initial P wave ≠ tachycardia P waves) include AVNRT, ORT, and triggered and reentrant AT. NCT initiated by a ventricular premature depolarization (VPD) (particularly, late-coupled VPDs) favors ORT because the ventricle is an integral part of the circuit. Rarely, NCT can be induced upon termination of atrial fibrillation (**Fig. 5-4**).

Induced

Programmed atrial extrastimulation facilitates induction of reentrant tachycardias by providing triggers that fall into the tachycardia window (difference in refractory periods between the two limbs of the reentrant circuit). The premature impulse fails to conduct over the β limb with longer refractoriness (unidirectional block) and conducts with sufficient delay

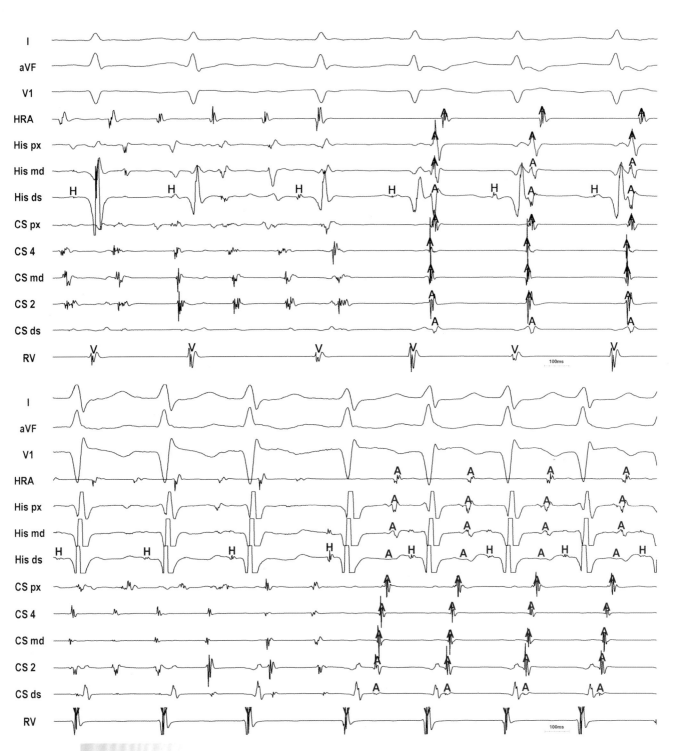

FIGURE 5-4 Spontaneous termination of atrial fibrillation to AVNRT (*top*) and ORT (*bottom*) using a left free wall AP.

(slow conduction) over its counterpart α limb allowing sufficient time to recover excitability and initiate reentry. Induction of intra-atrial reentrant tachycardia, AVNRT, and ORT requires a critical degree of slow conduction within the atrium, the AV node, and along the AV node–His-Purkinje axis, respectively.[23] The critical AH interval for typical AVNRT is achieved by switch from FP to SP conduction (see Figs. 7-32 and 7-33). The critical AV interval for ORT can occur within the AV node, His bundle, and/or bundle branches (particularly BBB ipsilateral to the AP) (see Figs. 10-8 to 10-10). While programmed ventricular extrastimulation can induce both AVNRT and ORT, atypical AVNRT is more easily induced from the ventricle than its typical counterpart. A feature characteristic of ORT using a left-sided AP is induction following typical bundle branch reentrant (BBR) complexes (Fig. 5-5). Single, typical BBR complexes cross the lower interventricular septum, fail to conduct over the AV node due to retrograde left bundle (LB) refractoriness (unidirectional block), and reach the AP with sufficient VA delay (transeptal conduction) to initiate tachycardia.

When single-site atrial and ventricular extrastimulation fail to induce tachycardia, several techniques might facilitate induction: 1) stimulation from different sites (site-dependent induction), 2) extrastimulation following different drive cycles or during sinus rhythm (simulating clinical APD or VPDs), 3) double atrial extrastimulation, and 4) drug provocation (isoproterenol or atropine).

TERMINATION

Spontaneous

Important clues during spontaneous termination of tachycardia include the 1) mode of termination and 2) terminating complexes. Gradual deceleration preceding termination (cool-down period) suggests an automatic tachycardia (e.g., automatic AT), while sudden termination occurs with triggered and reentrant mechanisms. Spontaneous termination with AV block (tachycardia termination with a P wave) demonstrates tachycardia dependence on the AV node (AVNRT, ORT) and excludes AT (Figs. 5-6 and 5-7). Tachycardia termination by a VPD that fails to reach the atrium (VA block) also excludes AT (Figs. 5-8 and 5-9). Electrocardiographically, VA block is suggested by early return of a sinus beat (less than the sinus cycle length) following the VPD. Termination of tachycardia by a late-coupled VPD (≥85% of tachycardia cycle length [TCL]) favors diagnosis of ORT.

Induced

Late-coupled VPDs delivered when the His bundle has been antegradely depolarized ("committed") by tachycardia are "His refractory" and do not affect AVNRT (unless a nodo-fascicular/nodo-ventricular AP is present) or AT (unless an AV AP with its atrial insertion site at the AT site of origin is present). Tachycardia termination by His refractory VPD that fails to reach the atrium (VA block) excludes pure AVNRT and AT and strongly favors a diagnosis of ORT (Fig. 5-10). Tachycardia

termination by early-coupled (non–His refractory) VPD that fails to reach the atrium (VA block) excludes AT (Figs. 5-8 and 5-9).

PACING MANEUVERS FROM THE VENTRICLE (INVERSE RULE)

Critical to the diagnosis of NCT is identifying the retrograde limb of tachycardia: AV node (AVNRT), AP (ORT), none (AT). Therefore, NCT diagnosis is best established by pacing maneuvers from the ventricle (inverse rule).

DURING NSR (AV NODE VERSUS AP)

Ventricular pacing identifies if VA conduction is absent and when present, its pattern of retrograde atrial activation. Complete absence of VA conduction (even on isoproterenol) suggests AT and excludes ORT. Rarely, retrograde VA conduction can be absent during AVNRT with retrograde LCFP block. In the presence of VA conduction, retrograde atrial activation that is identical to atrial activation during tachycardia argues against AT (unless AT arises near the retrogradely conducting structure). Concentric atrial activation earliest at the anteroseptum (His bundle region) indicates retrograde conduction over the FP or an anteroseptal AP, while earliest at the posteroseptum (coronary sinus ostium) indicates retrograde conduction over the SP or a posteroseptal AP. Left eccentric atrial activation results from a left-sided AP or less commonly left-sided inputs to the AV node, while right eccentric atrial activation indicates the presence of a right-sided AP.

The hallmark of retrograde AV nodal conduction is midline, decremental (rate-dependent), adenosine-sensitive conduction, which is linked to retrograde activation of the His bundle. In contrast, typical (AV) AP shows nondecremental (rate-independent) or minimally decremental adenosine-insensitive conduction independent of retrograde His bundle activation.[24,25] The FP, however, can show only minimal decrement before block. Certain APs in the posteroseptal region can also manifest slow, decremental, adenosine-sensitive conduction (PJRT) mimicking retrograde conduction over the SP. Given the overlap of these findings, 1) ventricular extrastimulation, 2) differential RV, and 3) parahisian pacing are three useful maneuvers to differentiate AV nodal from AP conduction—each separately determining whether or not retrograde atrial activation depends on preceding His bundle activation.

Ventricular Extrastimulation (Retrograde RBBB)

Programmed ventricular extrastimulation with tightly coupled extrastimuli can induce a "VH jump" when retrograde right bundle (RB) refractoriness (retrograde right bundle branch block [RBBB]) is reached (particularly at long drive cycles when RB effective refractory period [ERP] is greater than RV ERP). During the VH jump, retrograde RBBB forces retrograde activation to cross the interventricular septum and conduct retrogradely over

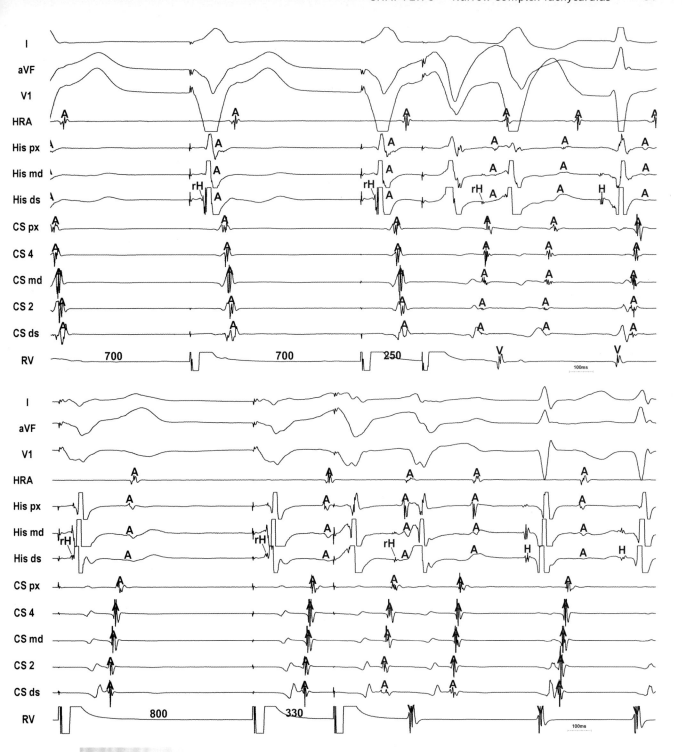

FIGURE 5-5 Induction of left-sided ORT by single BBR beats. *Top*: During the drive train, retrograde atrial activation is concentric and occurs over the FP. A single ventricular extrastimulus induces a "VH jump" exposing a left free wall AP (eccentric atrial activation earliest at CS ds that precedes retrograde His bundle activation) and producing a BBR beat. The BBR beat crosses the septum, fails to conduct retrogradely over the LB (unidirectional block), and conducts over the AP to initiate ORT. *Bottom*: During the drive train, retrograde atrial activation is eccentric over a left free wall AP (earliest at CS ds). A single ventricular extrastimulus induces a "VH jump" confirming an AP (retrograde atrial preceding His bundle activation) and producing a BBR beat which initiates ORT. Both retrograde concealment into the AV node after the VH jump and repetitive antegrade activation of the atrium over the AP cause the first AH to be greater than the second AH at ORT onset.

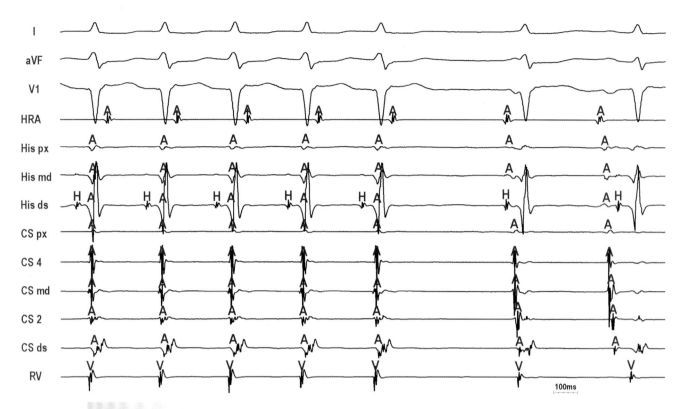

FIGURE 5-6 Spontaneous termination of NCT with AV block (typical AVNRT). Simultaneous AV activation ("A on V" tachycardia) excludes ORT. Spontaneous termination with intranodal AV block excludes AT.

the LB to activate the His bundle. Taking advantage of the VH jump allows determination of whether retrograde atrial activation is associated (AV node) or dissociated (AP) from the His bundle.[26] With retrograde AV node conduction, the increase in VH interval is accompanied by an equivalent (fully excitable AV node) or longer (relative refractory AV node) increase in VA interval (HA is unchanged or longer) (**Fig. 5-11**). With retrograde AP conduction, the increase in the VH interval is accompanied by no change in the VA interval (nondecremental AP) (HA becomes shorter or paradoxically negative). A negative HA interval (retrograde atrial activation preceding retrograde His bundle activation) shows that atrial activation is not linked to retrograde activation of the His bundle and identifies the presence of an extranodal AP (**Figs. 5-12 to 5-14**).

Differential RV Pacing

Differential RV pacing takes advantage of the site dependency of retrograde atrial activation, which differs between the AV node and AP.[27,28] The VA interval is directly related to the proximity of the RV pacing site to the entrance site of the retrogradely conducting structure. Because retrograde conduction over the AV node is linked to the His bundle, the VA interval at the RV apex (near the RB terminus) is shorter than at the base (**Fig. 5-15**). In contrast, the VA interval for AP at the RV base (near its ventricular insertion site) is shorter than at the apex (**Figs. 5-15 and 5-16**).

Parahisian Pacing

Parahisian pacing takes advantage of the ability to directly capture the His-Purkinje system and therefore determines whether retrograde atrial activation is dependent on capture of the His bundle/RB (AV node) or myocardium (AP).[29] High-output pacing is delivered near the His bundle at the RV anterobasal septum directly capturing the His bundle/RB complex and myocardium (His/RV capture). The stimulation strength is lowered until His bundle/RB capture is lost and stimulation only captures the RV (RV-only capture). Loss of direct His bundle/RB capture delays activation of the His bundle by forcing the depolarizing wavefront to travel from the basal pacing site to the terminus of the RB (RV base → apex) and then retrogradely over the RB back to the His bundle (RV apex → base). With retrograde conduction over the AV node, loss of His bundle capture causes 1) prolongation of the stimulus-A (St-A) interval at the expense of the stimulus-H (St-H) interval (demonstrating dependency of retrograde atrial activation on His bundle activation), 2) no change in the HA interval, and 3) no change in the atrial activation pattern (AV node response) (**Figs. 5-17 and 5-18**). With retrograde conduction over an AP, loss of His bundle capture causes 1) no change in the St-A interval (demonstrating dependency of retrograde atrial activation on myocardial not His bundle activation), 2) shortening or reversal of the HA interval, and 3) no change in the atrial activation pattern (AP response) (**Figs. 5-17 and 5-18**). With retrograde

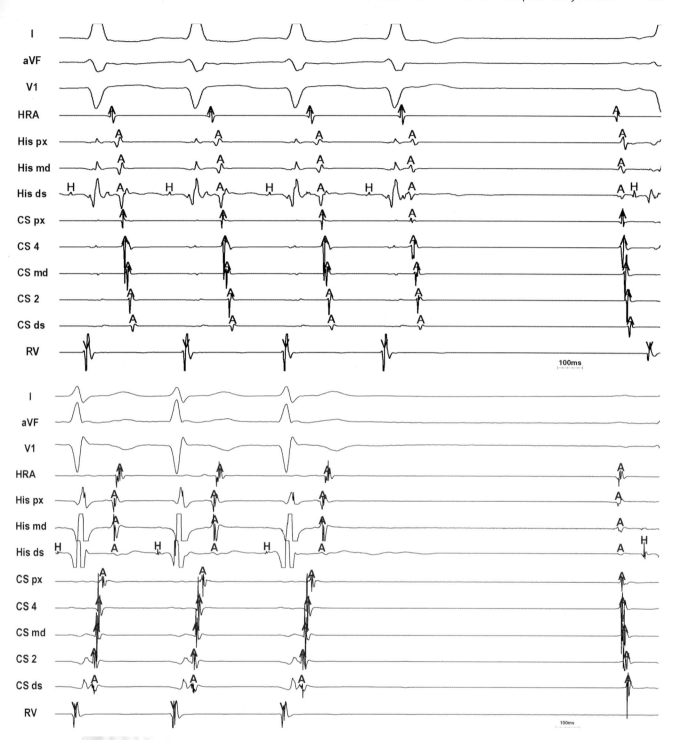

FIGURE 5-7 Spontaneous termination of NCT with AV block. *Top*: ORT using a right free wall AP. *Bottom*: ORT using a left free wall AP. Eccentric atrial activation excludes AVNRT (except AVNRT with eccentric left atrio-nodal inputs). Spontaneous termination with AV block excludes AT.

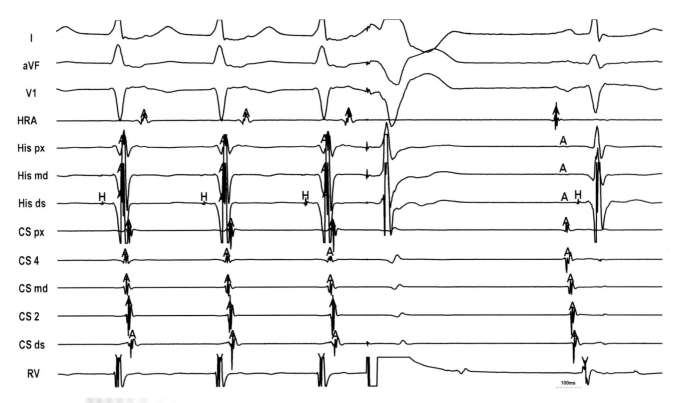

FIGURE 5-8 Termination of NCT by early-coupled VPD with VA block (typical AVNRT). Simultaneous AV activation ("A on V" tachycardia) excludes ORT. Termination by a VPD with VA block excludes AT.

fusion over both the AV node and an AP, loss of His bundle capture shows a possible increase in St-A intervals (depending on the relative conduction times over the AV node and AP) but a change in the retrograde atrial activation pattern (Fig. 5-19). Because a finite amount of time (generally ≥35 ms) is required for the pacing stimulus that only captures the right ventricle to retrogradely activate the His bundle, small increases (<35 ms) in St-A interval with loss of His bundle capture should raise suspicion for presence of an AP. The addition of pure His bundle pacing (selective His only capture) can identify other APs not identified by parahisian pacing alone.[30]

Pitfalls of parahisian pacing include 1) FP preempting AP conduction, 2) atrial capture, 3) LB capture, 4) retrograde RBBB, and 5) nodo-fascicular APs.[31–33] Parahisian pacing (or any pacing maneuver during sinus rhythm) identifies the structure conducting retrogradely during sinus rhythm, which is not necessarily the same structure operative during tachycardia. In the presence of two retrogradely conducting structures (FP and AP), FP conduction can preempt AP conduction even with loss of His bundle capture falsely excluding the presence of an AP. Therefore, it is important that the retrograde atrial activation during parahisian pacing is identical to that during tachycardia. With a proximal parahisian pacing site, the capture threshold for the atrium might be lower than for the His bundle/RB and ventricle resulting in atrial capture during both His/RV and RV-only capture. The "St-A" interval, therefore, does not change

with loss of His bundle capture resulting in false diagnosis of an AP. Very short St-A intervals—St-A (CS px) <60 ms, St-A (high right atrium [HRA]) <70 ms—indicate direct atrial capture (Fig. 5-20).[32] With a left-sided AP, the St-A time with His/RV capture might be paradoxically shorter than during RV-only capture (AV node response). Despite a longer distance, rapid conduction over the His-Purkinje system to the AP might result in a shorter conduction time than slower muscle-to-muscle activation from RV base to AP, particularly for a left free wall location where differences between His-Purkinje and myocardial conduction are exaggerated. Additionally, high-output pacing with a large virtual electrode that captures the His/RB might also capture the LB (fibers within the His bundle destined for the LB), resulting in even faster conduction times. A left eccentric atrial activation pattern alone should raise suspicion of the presence of an AP (although rare eccentric left atrio-nodal inputs are possible). In order to determine if retrograde conduction occurs over the AV node, parahisian pacing requires that retrograde conduction occurs over the His bundle following direct His/RB capture distally. The presence of retrograde block proximal to the pacing site (retrograde RBBB) can confound the use of this maneuver. Lastly, an AV node response can be seen with a nodo-fascicular AP because retrograde conduction is dependent on His/RB capture. Conversely, a nodo-ventricular AP causes an AP response because retrograde conduction is dependent on myocardial capture (see Chapters 6 and 11).[34]

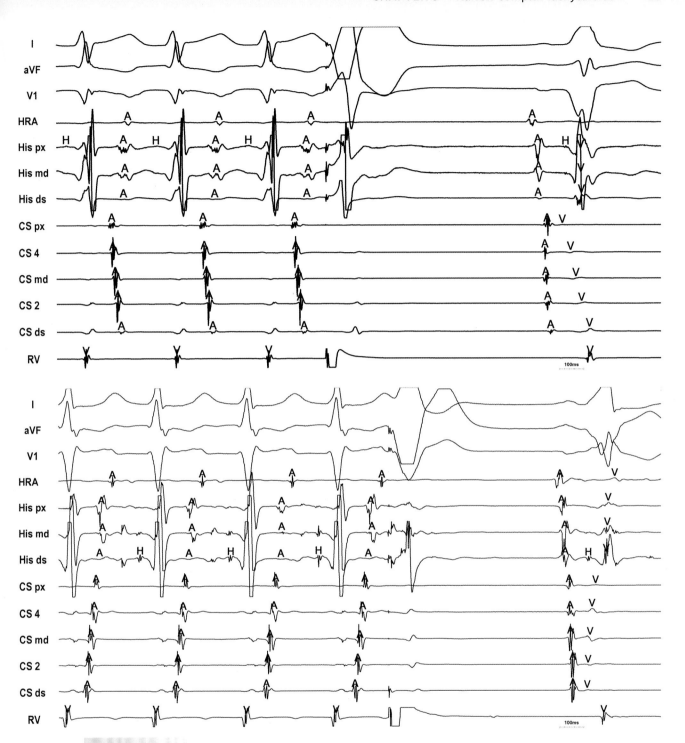

FIGURE 5-9 Termination of NCT by early-coupled VPD with VA block (ORT using a manifest right posteroseptal [*top*] and left free wall [*bottom*] AP). Termination by an early-coupled VPD with VA block excludes AT. The earliest site of atrial activation during ORT matches the earliest site of ventricular activation during preexcited sinus rhythm.

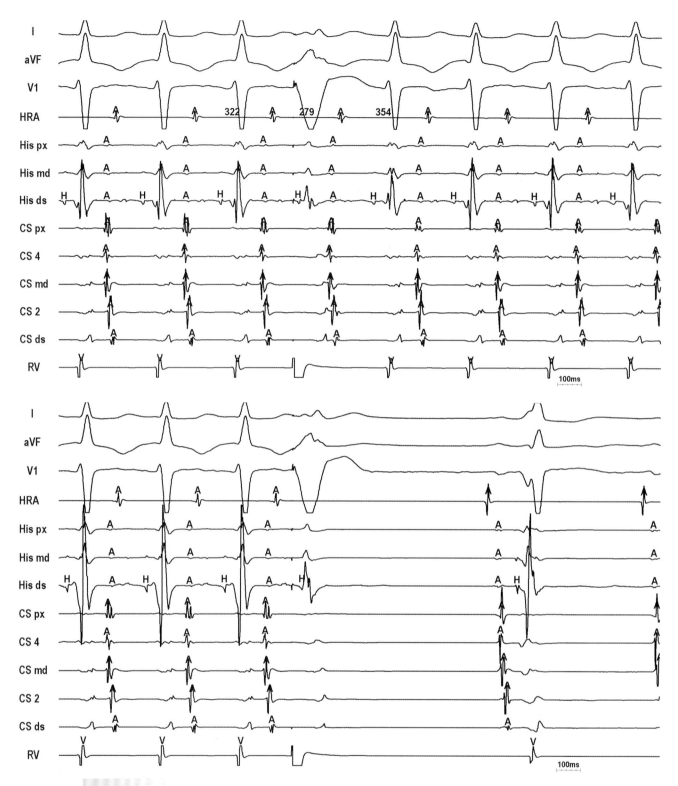

FIGURE 5-10 Resetting (*top*) and termination (*bottom*) of NCT by His refractory VPD (ORT using a posteroseptal AP). *Top*: A His refractory VPD advances the atrium by 43 ms. *Bottom*: A His refractory VPD terminates tachycardia with VA block. Both positive responses are proof of the presence of an AP.

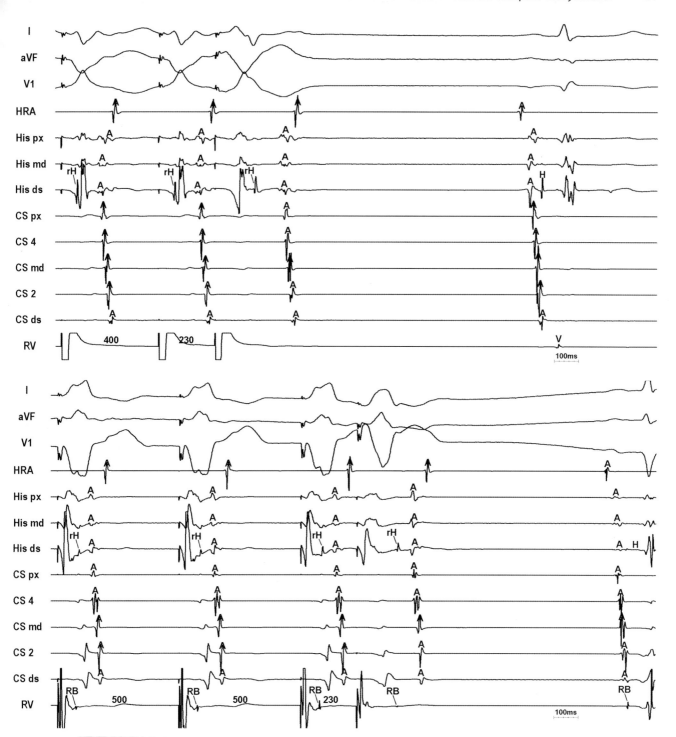

FIGURE 5-11 Ventricular extrastimulation with retrograde RBBB (AV node). During the drive train, retrograde atrial activation is concentric (earliest at His bundle region). The extrastimulus encounters retrograde RB refractoriness inducing a "VH jump." The increase in VH interval is accompanied by an equivalent increase in the VA interval (constant HA) indicating that retrograde atrial activation is linked to the His bundle and therefore occurs over the FP of the AV node. Note that retrograde His bundle potentials precede local ventricular electrograms during RV apical pacing (*top*) but follow them during RV basal (*bottom*) pacing.

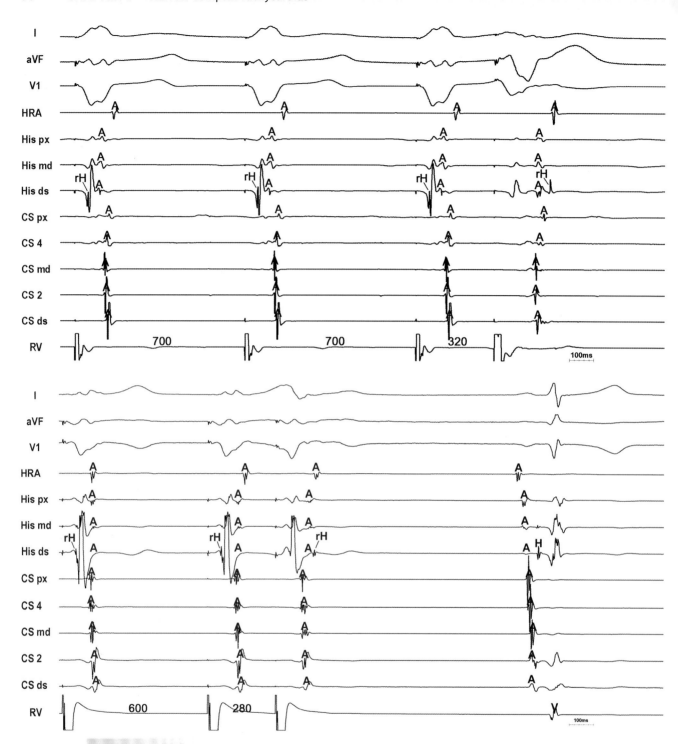

FIGURE 5-12 Ventricular extrastimulation with retrograde RBBB (FP and AP). During the drive train, retrograde atrial activation is concentric (earliest at the His bundle region). The extrastimulus encounters retrograde RB refractoriness inducing a "VH jump" and a change in atrial activation (earliest at CS md [*top*] and CS px [*bottom*]). The new retrograde atrial activation patterns precede retrograde activation of the His bundle indicating the presence of an AP. During the drive train, retrograde atrial activation represents fusion over the FP and AP.

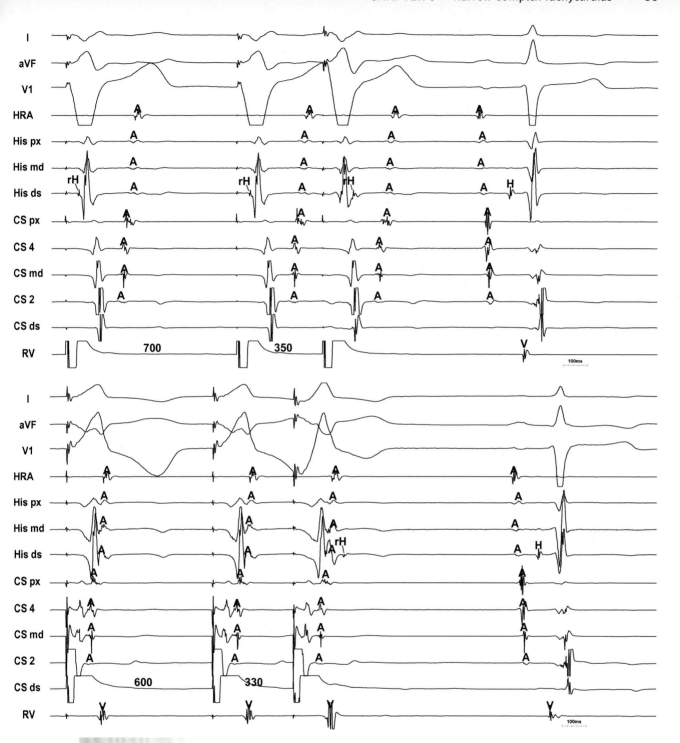

FIGURE 5-13 Ventricular extrastimulation with retrograde RBBB and LBBB (AP). During the drive train, retrograde atrial activation is eccentric (earliest at CS 2) suggestive of a left free wall AP. *Top*: With RV apical pacing, the extrastimulus encounters retrograde RB refractoriness inducing a "VH jump" (over the LB). Despite increase in VH interval, however, the VA interval remains unchanged (shorter HA), indicating that retrograde atrial activation is not linked to the His bundle and confirming the presence of an AP. *Bottom*: With left ventricular basal pacing (CS ds in ventricular branch of the coronary sinus), the extrastimulus encounters retrograde LB refractoriness inducing a "VH jump" (over the RB). Retrograde atrial activation precedes His bundle activation again confirming the presence of an AP.

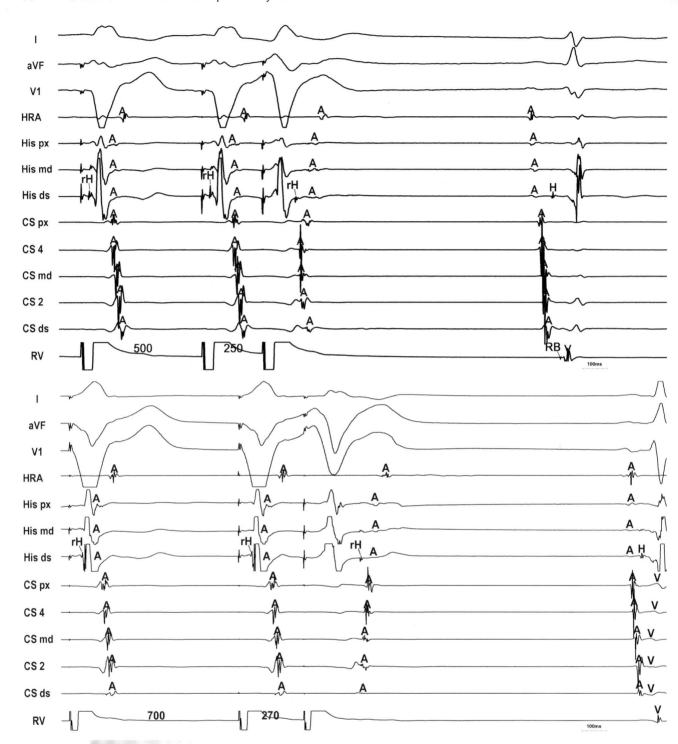

FIGURE 5-14 Ventricular extrastimulation with retrograde RBBB (FP and AP). During the drive train, retrograde atrial activation is concentric (earliest at the His bundle region). The extrastimulus encounters retrograde RB refractoriness inducing a "VH jump" and a change in atrial activation (earliest at CS md [*top*] and CS ds [*bottom*]). The new retrograde atrial activation patterns are nearly simultaneous with retrograde activation of the His bundle indicating the presence of an AP. During the drive train, retrograde atrial activation represents conduction over the FP. In the bottom tracing, minimal (inapparent) preexcitation is present with a short HV interval (29 ms) and earliest local ventricular activation at CS ds.

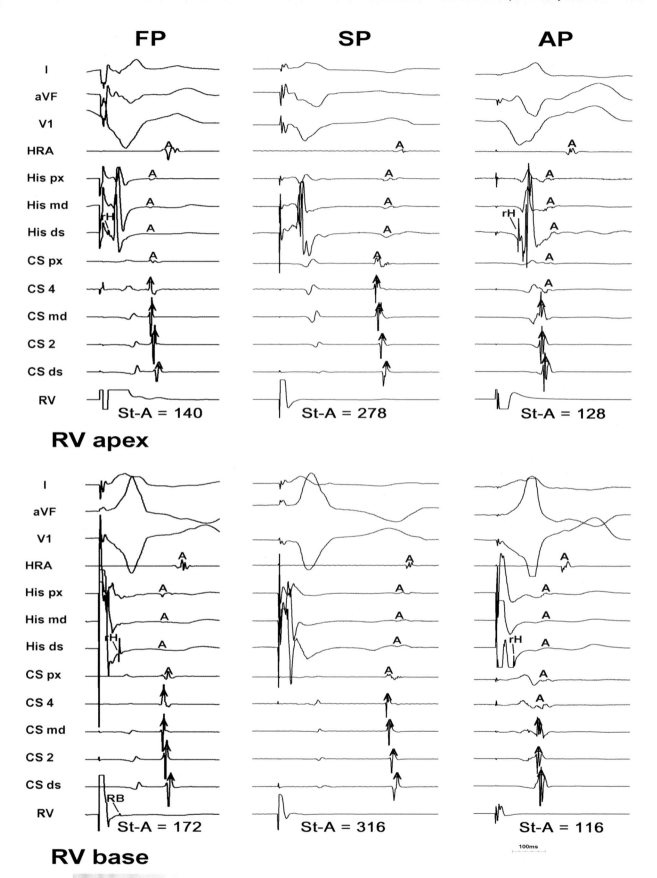

FIGURE 5-15 Differential RV pacing (FP, SP, and AP). RV apical pacing causes a shorter St-A interval than basal pacing with retrograde conduction over the AV node but the opposite over an AP. Note that retrograde activation of the His bundle (rH) precedes the local ventricular electrogram during RV apical pacing but follows it during RV basal pacing.

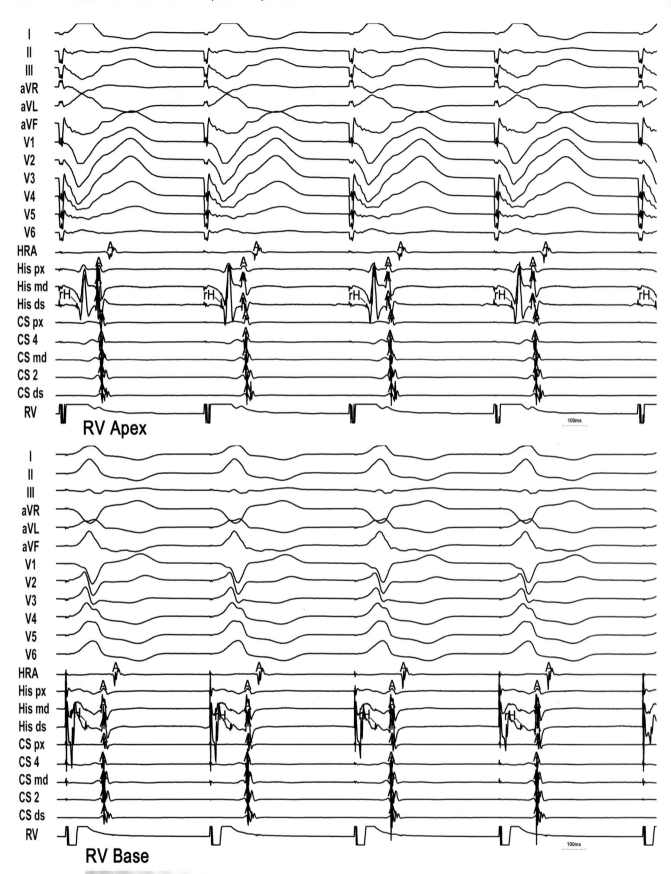

FIGURE 5-16 Differential RV pacing (FP and AP). During RV apical pacing, retrograde conduction is earliest at the His bundle region due to retrograde conduction over the FP. RV basal pacing causes delay over the FP unmasking the presence of a posteroseptal AP (earliest at CS 4). Note that retrograde activation of the His bundle (rH) precedes the local ventricular electrogram during RV apical pacing but follows it during RV basal pacing.

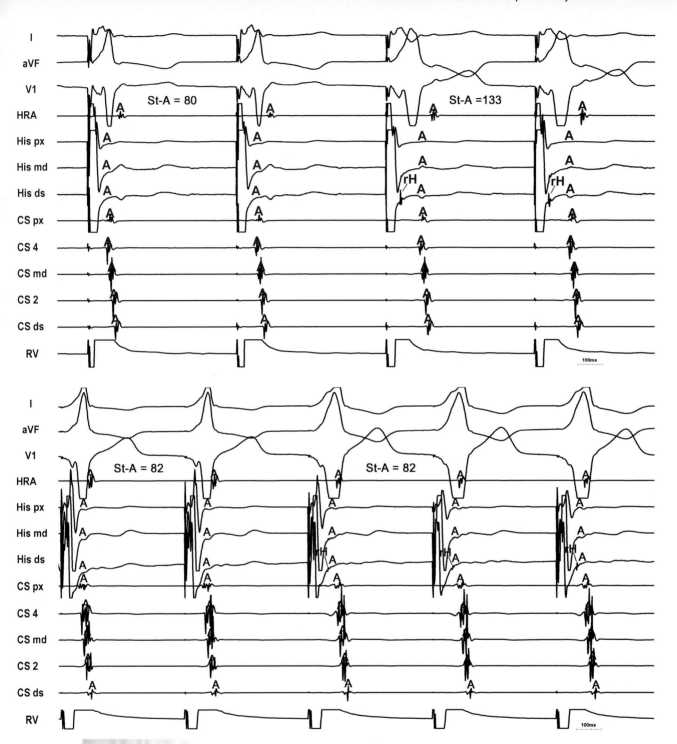

FIGURE 5-17 Parahisian pacing (*top*: FP; *bottom*: anteroseptal AP). Retrograde atrial activation is rapid and concentric (earliest at His bundle region). *Top*: Loss of His bundle capture results in the appearance of a retrograde His bundle potential and a 53 ms increase in the St-A interval demonstrating dependence of retrograde atrial activation on His bundle activation and indicating retrograde conduction over the FP. *Bottom*: Loss of His bundle capture results in appearance of a retrograde His bundle potential but no change in the St-A interval indicating that retrograde atrial activation is independent of His bundle activation and therefore occurs over an anteroseptal AP.

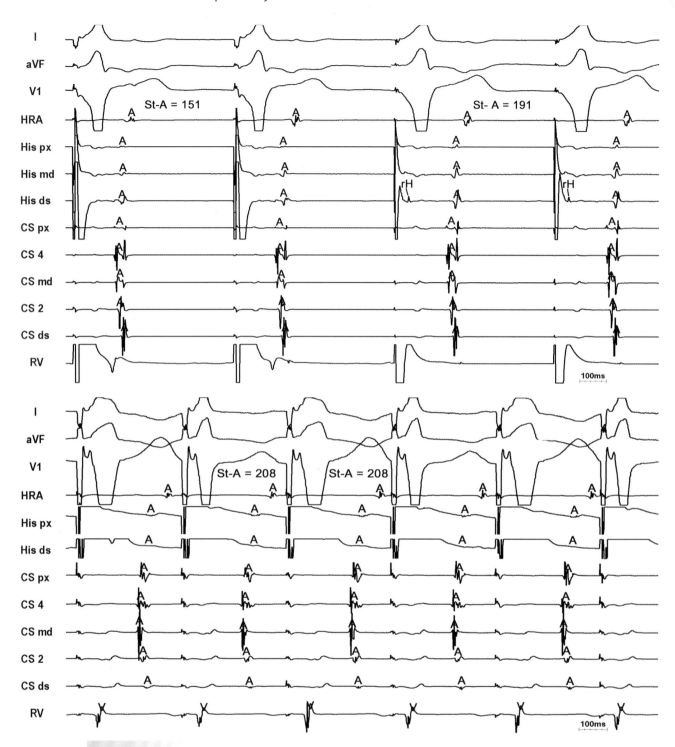

FIGURE 5-18 Parahisian pacing (*top*: SP; *bottom*: posteroseptal AP). Retrograde atrial activation is slow and concentric (earliest at CS os region). *Top*: Loss of His bundle capture results in the appearance of a retrograde His bundle potential and a 40 ms increase in the St-A interval demonstrating dependence of retrograde atrial activation on His bundle activation and indicating retrograde conduction over the SP. *Bottom*: Loss of His bundle capture causes no change in the St-A interval indicating that retrograde atrial activation is independent of His bundle activation and therefore occurs over a slowly conducting posteroseptal AP.

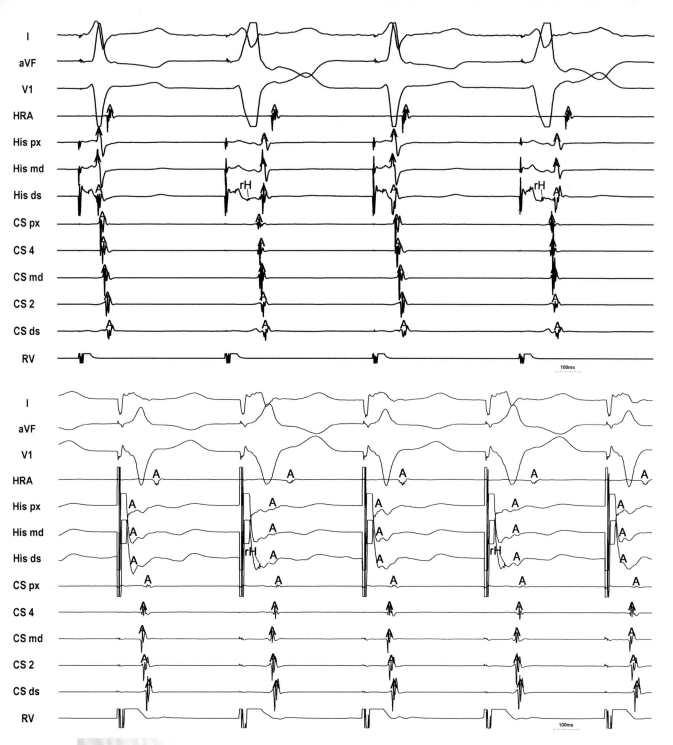

FIGURE 5-19 Parahisian pacing (FP and AP). With His bundle capture, retrograde atrial activation is rapid and concentric (earliest at His bundle region) occurring over the FP. Loss of His bundle capture results in the appearance of a retrograde His bundle potential and a change in the retrograde atrial activation pattern (now earliest at CS px [*top*] and CS md [*bottom*]) exposing the presence of an AP.

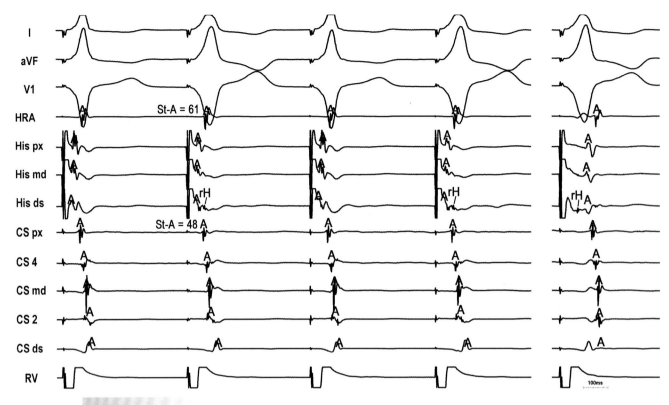

FIGURE 5-20 Parahisian pacing (atrial capture). Atrial activation is concentric (earliest at the His bundle region) with a short St-A time (31 ms at His, 48 ms at CS, 61 ms at HRA). Loss of His bundle capture results in the appearance of a retrograde His bundle potential after the atrium and no change in St-A intervals giving false diagnosis of an AP (pseudo AP response). The last panel shows the true St-A interval with loss of atrial capture and retrograde conduction over the FP.

A paradoxical parahisian response occurs when the St-A interval prolongs with His bundle capture. In this case, the transition from pure RV capture with late activation of the His bundle to direct His/RV capture shortens the HH interval, which by encroaching on the AV node ERP causes block and allows conduction of a slower alternate pathway (SP, slow AP).

The major limitation of ventricular extrastimulation, differential RV, and parahisian pacing is that they identify the retrogradely conducting structure during sinus rhythm, which is not necessarily the same structure responsible for tachycardia. This is particularly evident when FP preempts AP conduction and can be overcome by performing these same maneuvers during tachycardia: scanning VPDs, differential RV, and parahisian entrainment.[35–37] However, differential RV and parahisian entrainment can be difficult to perform because of frequent catheter ectopy, inability to capture the His bundle during tachycardia, and unwanted pacing-induced termination of tachycardia.

DURING NCT

Because the retrogradely conducting structure responsible for tachycardia may not be evident during sinus rhythm, pacing maneuvers during tachycardia more accurately establish the diagnosis. These pacing maneuvers include 1) scanning diastolic VPDs and 2) entrainment from the ventricle.

Diastolic VPDs

Single extrastimuli delivered from the RV during the diastolic period of tachycardia (diastolic scanning) can reset (preexcite/ postexcite) or terminate tachycardia. The ability of the extrastimulus to perturb tachycardia depends on the proximity of the pacing site (apex versus base) relative to the circuit (AVNRT versus ORT).[38]

Preexcitation Index

During diastolic scanning, the longest coupling interval that preexcites the atrium establishes the preexcitation index (PI).[39] The PI = TCL − longest coupling interval preexciting the atrium. The PI is dependent on the location of the RV pacing catheter (standardly positioned at the RV apex) relative to the tachycardia circuit. The PI for ORT using a septal AP is small (<45 ms) because the short distance between the RV pacing site and AP allows long-coupled VPDs to preexcite the atrium, while a left free wall AP has a PI >75 ms because short-coupled VPDs are required to penetrate the circuit and preexcite the atrium. Because of the large distance between the RV apex and AV node, the PI for AVNRT is ≥100 ms.

His Refractory VPD ("V on H" Maneuver)

A late-coupled VPD delivered when the His bundle has been antegradely depolarized ("committed") by tachycardia is termed "His refractory" and is important in determining the presence of an AP because it cannot conduct retrogradely to the atrium unless an AP is present.[40] Three signs that a VPD is His refractory are 1) delivery synchronous with an on-time His bundle electrogram ("His synchronous" or "V on H"), 2) delivery in the presence of a visible on-time His bundle electrogram but not necessarily His synchronous, and 3) paced QRS fusion. Three positive responses of a His refractory VPD during tachycardia that prove the presence of an AP (but not necessarily its participation in tachycardia) are 1) advancement (preexcitation) of the atrium, 2) delay (postexcitation) of the atrium, and 3) termination without reaching the atrium (VA block) (Fig. 5-10; see also Figs. 6-11 to 6-14). All three positive responses indicate the presence of an AP and exclude pure AVNRT and AT. While ORT is most likely, they do not necessarily prove it. (A His refractory VPD can reset or terminate AVNRT in the presence of a bystander nodo-fascicular/nodo-ventricular pathway.) Postexcitation delay is observed with decrementally conducting APs (long RP tachycardias) (see Chapter 6).[34,41–43]

Non–His Refractory VPD

While a His refractory VPD that perturbs tachycardia is more useful than a non–His refractory VPD for diagnosis, important information can also be derived from these early-coupled VPDs. An early VPD that terminates tachycardia with VA block excludes AT. An early VPD that advances the atrium and resets tachycardia is essentially equivalent to single beat entrainment of tachycardia from the ventricle. In the presence of a visible retrograde His bundle potential, ΔHA ($HA_{[reset]} - HA_{[SVT]}$) > or < 0 differentiate AVNRT from ORT, respectively (or an early VPD that advances the atrium more than the His bundle indicates the presence of an AP).

Entrainment from the Ventricle

Ventricular overdrive pacing delivered at a cycle length shorter than the NCT cycle length can penetrate the excitable gap of the reentrant circuit and accelerate the atrium to the pacing cycle length without terminating tachycardia. During entrainment, the (n) orthodromic wavefront of each pacing stimulus collides with the ($n + 1$) antidromic wavefront within the circuit until pacing stops. While collision between orthodromic and antidromic wavefronts during AVNRT occurs in the AV node, collision during ORT can occur either above or below the His bundle. Antidromic capture of the His bundle (collision point above the His bundle) occurs at faster pacing rates with retrograde activation of the His bundle. Orthodromic capture of the His bundle (collision point below the His bundle) occurs at slower pacing rates allowing antegrade activation of the His bundle.[44,45] Right ventricular basal pacing (far from the RB terminus) facilitates orthodromic capture of the His bundle.[46]

Orthodromic Capture of the His Bundle

It is important to recognize orthodromic capture of the His bundle during entrainment of NCT from the ventricle because it is equivalent to continuous resetting of tachycardia by repetitive His refractory VPDs, indicates the presence of an AP, and establishes a likely diagnosis of ORT. (An alternative to ORT is the theoretical possibility of AVNRT with a bystander nodo-fascicular/nodo-ventricular AP that bypasses the His bundle and allows entrainment of AVNRT with orthodromic His

bundle capture.) Identifying the last His bundle electrogram accelerated to the pacing cycle length is critical to determining whether the His bundle is orthodromically or antidromically captured (Fig. 2-6). Orthodromic capture of the His bundle causes constant paced QRS fusion with the last orthodromically captured His bundle electrogram (same morphology as during tachycardia) occurring at the pacing cycle length (first criteria of transient entrainment) (Fig. 5-21).

Four Post-Entrainment Criteria

While identifying orthodromic capture of the His bundle during entrainment is useful, His bundle potentials are not always visible during pacing. The following observations following entrainment help establish tachycardia diagnosis: 1) "AV" or "AAV" response (AVNRT/ORT versus AT), 2) post-pacing interval (PPI)–TCL (AVNRT versus ORT), 3) ΔHA value (AVNRT versus ORT), and 4) ΔVA value (AVNRT versus ORT) (Figs. 5-21 and 5-22).[44,47–50]

"AV" or "AAV" Response

The response to entrainment from the ventricle is "AV" for both AVNRT and ORT (fulfilling the obligatory 1:1 AV relationship in the latter) and "AAV" for AT (Figs. 5-21 to 5-23).[47] An AV response is very specific for AVNRT/ORT and described only rarely for AT (a macroreentrant AT when the circuit time exceeds the AV node-His-Purkinje refractory period and recording is from an orthodromically captured atrial site).[51] An AAV response, however, is less specific for AT and can be seen with AVNRT/ORT in various settings (Table 5-2) (see also Figs. 6-12 to 6-14 and 6-16).[41,42,52–55]

Post-pacing Interval–Tachycardia Cycle Length

The PPI following entrainment of tachycardia from the ventricle reflects the distance between the pacing site (RV apex) and tachycardia circuit. The PPI–TCL for AVNRT is long (>115 ms) because of the large distance between the RV apex and AV node but is short (≤115 ms) for ORT because the ventricle is an integral part of its reentrant circuit.[48] A PPI − TCL ≤115 ms is very specific for ORT. However, a PPI − TCL >115 ms is less specific for AVNRT and can occur with ORT due to 1) retrograde decrement in the AP (PJRT) or 2) antegrade decrement in the AV node, particular with fast-pacing rates (see Figs. 6-14 and 10-27). Fast-pacing rates facilitate antidromic capture of the His bundle with retrograde penetration of the AV node rendering it relatively refractory or causing a switch from FP to SP upon pacing cessation.[44,56] This limitation can be overcome by pacing at a cycle length just below (10–20 ms) the TCL and/or correcting the PPI for the delay in the AV node (corrected PPI [cPPI] <110 ms: ORT; cPPI ≥110 ms: AVNRT).[57,58] Correcting the PPI for the delay in the AV node, however, does not correct a long PPI due to retrograde decrement in an AP (PJRT).[34]

ΔHA Value

The His bundle and atria are activated sequentially over the AV node during entrainment of AVNRT from the ventricle but simultaneously during tachycardia ($HA_{[entrainment]}$ > $HA_{[AVNRT]}$ or $\Delta HA = HA_{[entrainment]} - HA_{[AVNRT]}$ > 0). In contrast, they are activated in parallel over the His bundle and

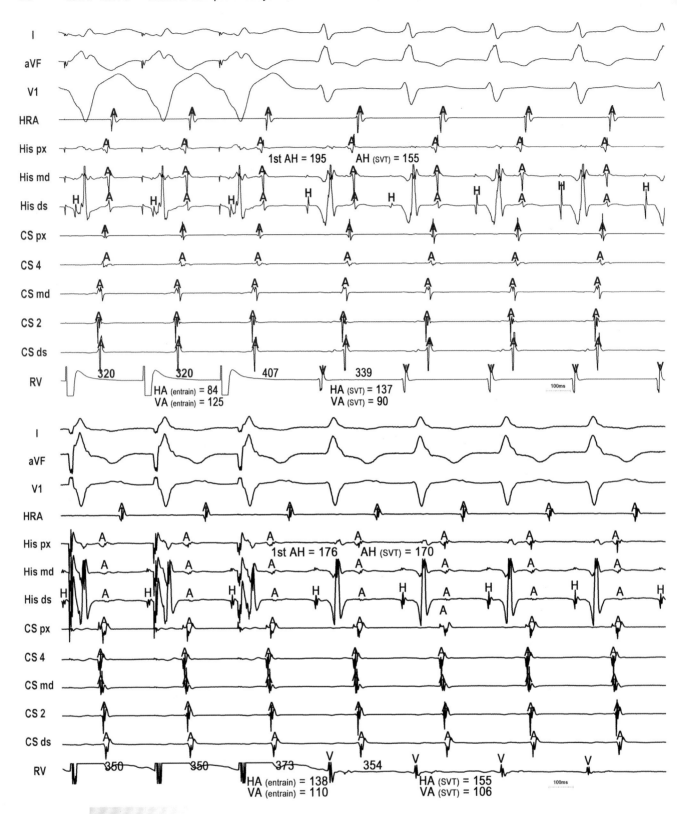

FIGURE 5-21 Entrainment of ORT with orthodromic capture of the His bundle. The response to entrainment is AVA excluding AT. *Top*: ORT using a left posterolateral AP. The PPI − TCL = 68 ms, cPPI = 28 ms, ΔHA = −53, ΔVA = 35. *Bottom*: ORT using a right posteroseptal AP. The PPI − TCL = 19 ms, cPPI = 13 ms, ΔHA = −17, ΔVA = 4 ms. In both cases, the His bundle is orthodromically captured, which alone indicates the presence of an AP. Note that the His bundle morphology during entrainment and tachycardia are identical.

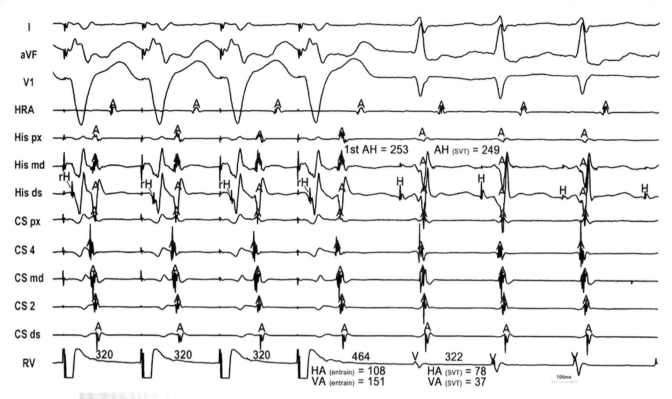

FIGURE 5-22 Entrainment of NCT from the ventricle (typical AVNRT). The response to entrainment is AVA (AHA) excluding AT. Atrial activation is concentric and simultaneous with the ventricle ("A on V" tachycardia) excluding ORT. The PPI − TCL = 142, cPPI = 138, ΔHA = 30, and ΔVA = 114.

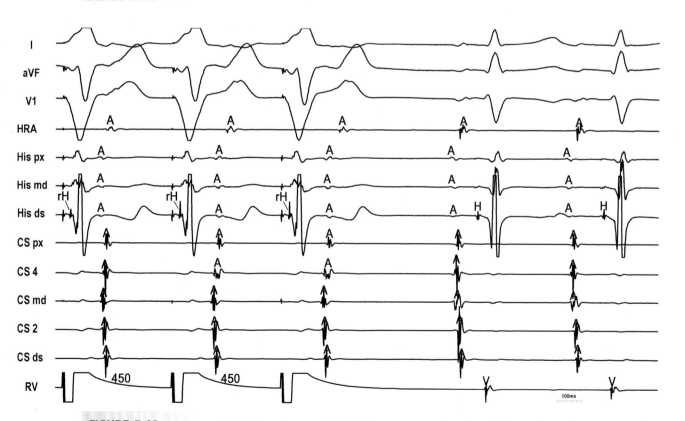

FIGURE 5-23 Entrainment of NCT from the ventricle (AT). The response to "entrainment" (ventricular overdrive pacing) is AAV. Note that atrial activation patterns during entrainment and tachycardia differ and the tachycardia P-wave morphology is inconsistent with AVNRT or ORT. AT arose from the noncoronary cusp of the aortic valve.

TABLE 5-2 AAV responses not due to AT

Diagnosis	Type	Atrial activation pattern (entrained versus tachycardia)	His bundle position	Explanation
Typical AVNRT	Pseudo AAV	Identical (FP)	AHA	HV > HA
Atypical AVNRT/PJRT	Pseudo AAV (classic)	Identical (SP or AP)	AAH	VA (entrained) > VV (PCL)
Atypical AVNRT/PJRT	True AAV	Different (FP versus SP or AP)	AAH	Dual retrograde response
Atypical AVNRT	Pseudo AAV	Identical (SP) unless dual retrograde response present	AHA (infrahisian block) AAH (suprahisian block)	LCFP block
Atypical AVNRT	Pseudo AAV	Identical (SP)	AAH	Long AH > TCL

Abbreviation: PCL, pacing cycle length.

AP during entrainment of ORT but sequentially during tachycardia ($HA_{[entrainment]} < HA_{[ORT]}$ or $\Delta HA = HA_{[entrainment]} - HA_{[ORT]} < 0$) (**Figs. 5-21 and 5-22**).[44,49]

ΔVA Value

When His bundle potentials are not visible during entrainment, an alternative measurement is the difference between the St-A during entrainment and the VA interval during tachycardia (ΔVA interval). A ΔVA interval (St-A − VA) > and ≤85 ms differentiates AVNRT and ORT, respectively (**Figs. 5-21 and 5-22**).[48]

The PPI–TCL, ΔHA, and ΔVA are indirect measurements of AVNRT/ORT circuit and prone to "artificially" large values because of decremental conduction inherent in the antegrade (and possibly retrograde limb) of the circuits. While short cutoff values are specific for ORT, long values are less specific for AVNRT. These measurements might also be useful during induction of SVT from the ventricle when tachycardia cannot be entrained.[59]

Onset of Ventricular Overdrive Pacing

When tachycardia cannot be entrained because of repeated pacing-induced termination, identifying when tachycardia is perturbed differentiates AVNRT from ORT. Resetting (advancement/delay) of the atrium or termination (with VA block) within the transition zone (progressive paced QRS fusion) or by one fully paced QRS complex indicates a diagnosis of ORT (**Figs. 5-24 and 5-25**).[60,61] (Ventricular paced complexes within the transition zone are fused and therefore His refractory.)

PACING MANEUVERS FROM THE ATRIUM

While pacing maneuvers in the ventricle are more useful for diagnosis of NCT, pacing maneuvers in the atrium also play an important role.

ΔAH VALUE

During AVNRT, the AH interval is a pseudo-interval reflecting simultaneous activation of the atrium retrogradely and His bundle antegradely over the AV node. During ORT and AT, the AH interval is a true interval representing sequential activation of the atrium/AV node/His bundle and similar to the AH interval during atrial pacing at the TCL (or entrainment). Therefore, ΔAH ($AH_{[pacing @ TCL]} - AH_{[SVT]}$) differentiates AVNRT (>40 ms) from ORT (<20 ms) and AT (<10 ms).[62]

VA LINKING (AT VERSUS AVNRT/ORT)

In contrast to AT, both AVNRT and ORT use a fixed retrogradely conducting structure (AVN and AP, respectively). VA intervals one beat after atrial overdrive pacing are therefore similar ("linked") to tachycardia (conventional method), pacing at different rates (decremental pacing), or from different atrial sites (differential pacing) ($\Delta VA < 10$ ms). In contrast, $\Delta VA > 10$ ms for AT because the VA is not a true conduction interval but a value dependent on the AT return interval at the pacing site (which, itself, depends on the proximity of the pacing site to the AT site of origin) and AV nodal conduction time to the ventricle (**Figs. 5-26 and 5-27**).[6,63–65]

AVNRT VERSUS JT

Two commonly employed methods to differentiate AVNRT from JT are 1) atrial overdrive pacing and 2) atrial extrastimulation.[66–68] The response to atrial overdrive pacing is "AHA" for AVNRT and "AHH" for JT (**Figs. 5-28 to 5-30**). While an AHA response is very specific for AVNRT, AHH responses are less specific for JT and can be seen with AVNRT: 1) pseudo AHH response when AH (SP conduction) > AA (atrial pacing cycle length) and 2) true AHH due to dual antegrade response upon pacing cessation (either atrial overdrive pacing stopped and restarted AVNRT followed by a dual antegrade response or AVNRT has a large excitable gap so that the collision point between [n] orthodromic and [n + 1] antidromic wavefronts occurs in the antegrade SP [not retrograde FP], resulting in a dual antegrade response upon pacing cessation).

During atrial extrastimulation, a late-coupled (His refractory) APD that resets (advances/delays) or terminates tachycardia with AV block excludes JT (**Figs. 5-31 and 5-32**). An early-coupled APD that resets tachycardia by conducting over

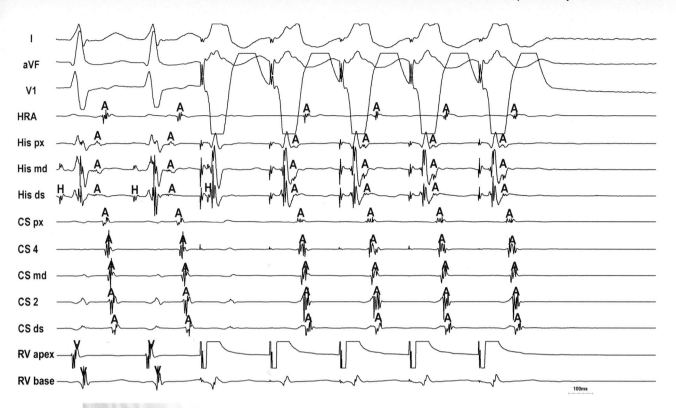

FIGURE 5-24 Onset of ventricular overdrive pacing during NCT (ORT using an anteroseptal AP). Atrial activation is concentric (earliest at His bundle region). The first paced complex is His refractory and terminates tachycardia with VA block indicating the presence of an AP.

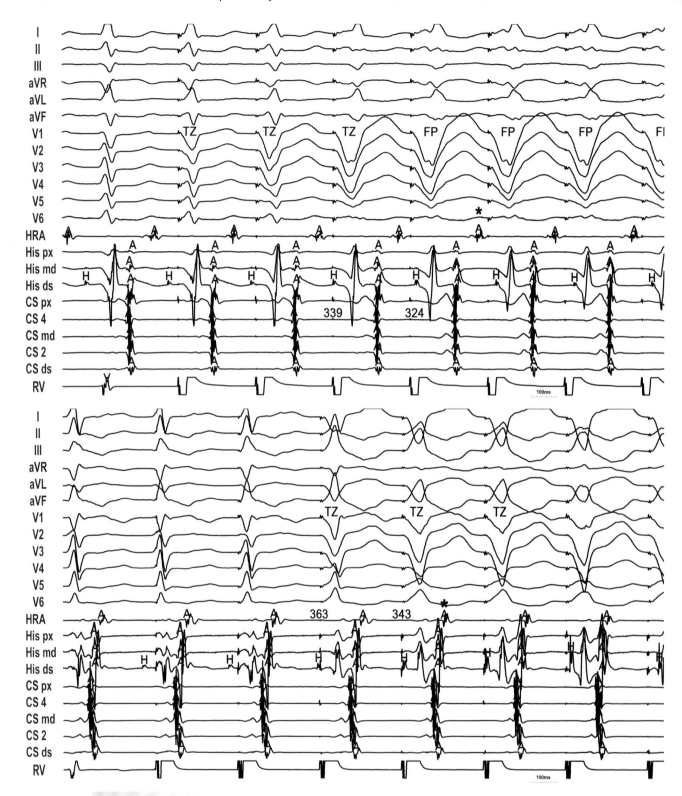

FIGURE 5-25 Onset of ventricular overdrive pacing during NCT. *Top*: ORT using a left posteroseptal AP. The first fully paced (FP) complex after the transition zone (TZ) remains His refractory and advances the atrium (*asterisk*) by 15 ms indicating the presence of an AP. *Bottom*: ORT using a left posteroseptal AP. A ventricular paced complex within the TZ (His refractory) advances the atrium (*asterisk*) by 20 ms indicating the presence of an AP.

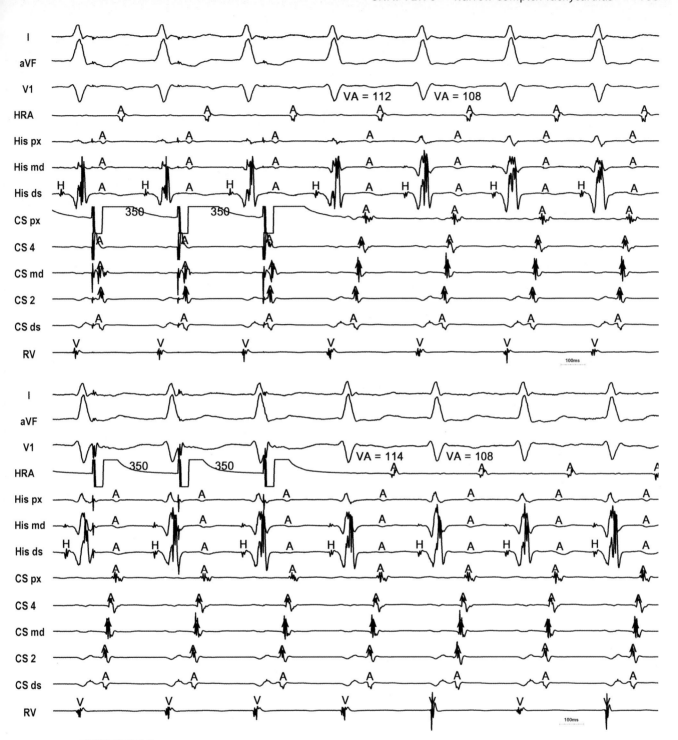

FIGURE 5-26 VA linking (ORT using a left free wall AP). Atrial overdrive pacing from CS px (*top*) and HRA (*bottom*) entrains ORT with constant atrial fusion (first criteria of transient entrainment). The ΔVA (1st VA [HRA] − 1st VA [CS px]) = 2 ms.

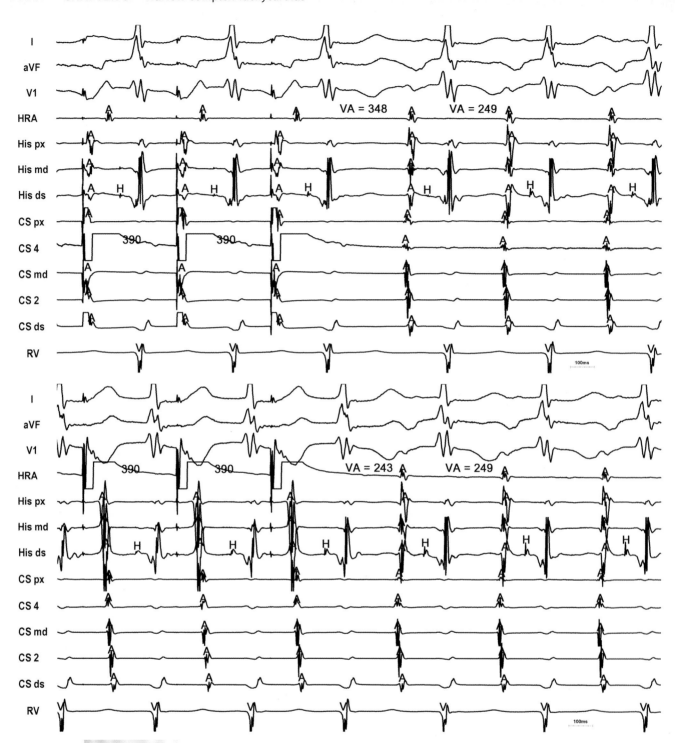

FIGURE 5-27 Absence of VA linking (AT). Atrial overdrive pacing from CS 4 (*top*) and HRA (*bottom*) accelerates the atrium to the pacing cycle length. The ΔVA (1st VA [CS 4] − 1st VA [HRA]) = 105 ms.

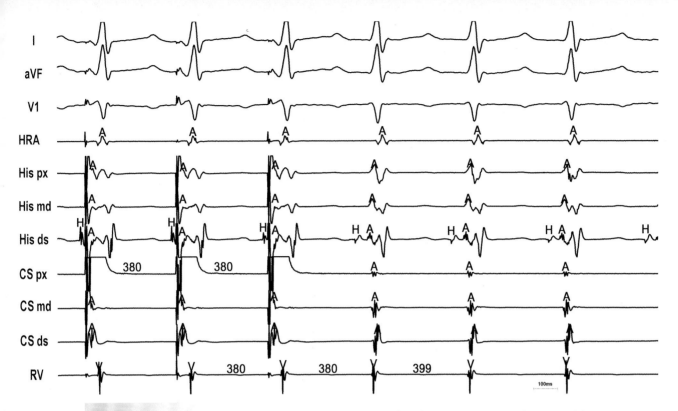

FIGURE 5-28 AHA response (typical AVNRT). Atrial overdrive pacing from the CS px entrains typical AVNRT and the response upon pacing cessation is "AHA."

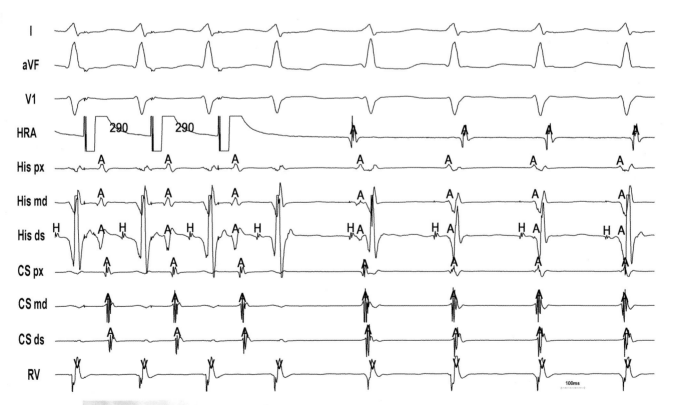

FIGURE 5-29 True AHH response (JT). Atrial overdrive pacing from the HRA yields a true "AHH" response upon pacing cessation indicating JT. An alternative possibility, however, is typical AVNRT with "double fire" (FP and SP) followed by resumption of tachycardia.

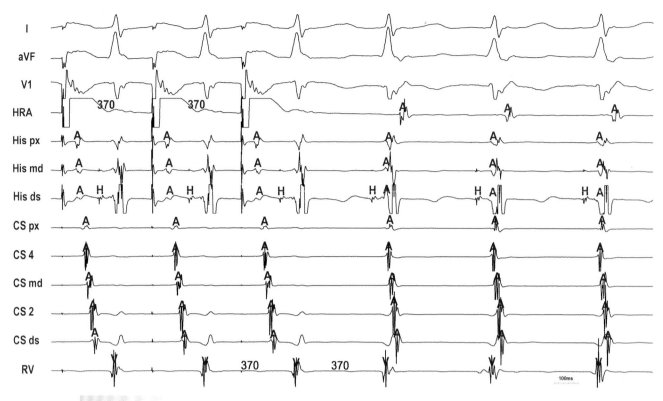

FIGURE 5-30 Pseudo AHH response (typical AVNRT). This is a true AHA response with an "AHH" pattern because of markedly prolonged conduction over the SP (the first and second H after pacing are driven by the penultimate and last pacing stimulus, respectively).

the FP without terminating it favors JT. (Another possibility, however, is an early-coupled APD that resets AVNRT followed by a dual antegrade response.)

VAGAL MANEUVERS

The AV node is an active participant in the reentrant circuit of AVNRT and ORT but not AT. Perpetuation of tachycardia despite vagally-induced AV block (adenosine or carotid sinus massage) is diagnostic of an AT. Adenosine-induced termination of NCT, however, is less specific and observed with AV node–dependent (AVNRT, ORT), SA node–dependent (sinus node reentrant tachycardia), and cyclic adenosine monophosphate (cAMP)-mediated (AT) tachycardias.[69,70]

UNUSUAL ELECTROPHYSIOLOGIC PHENOMENA

NCT WITH AV DISSOCIATION

The differential diagnosis of the rare NCT with AV dissociation is 1) AVNRT with UCFP block, 2) JT with JA block, 3) ORT using a nodo-fascicular/nodo-ventricular AP (NFRT) with nodo-atrial block, and 4) intrahisian reentry with HA block. Differentiating AVNRT from JT by the aforementioned atrial pacing maneuvers

can be difficult because of the failure of atrial pacing stimuli to affect tachycardia during AV dissociation. Other clues from transition zones (e.g., absence of dual AV node physiology at induction) might be required. NFRT with AV dissociation can be diagnosed by 1) His refractory VPDs that reset (advance/delay the next His bundle/ventricle but not necessarily the atrium because of AV dissociation) or terminate tachycardia or 2) short PPI following entrainment from the ventricle (see Figs. 11-11 and 11-12).[17,18,71,72] Intrahisian reentry due to longitudinal dissociation of the His bundle is characterized by split His bundle potentials.[73]

DUAL ANTEGRADE RESPONSE TACHYCARDIA

Another rare cause of NCT is dual antegrade response tachycardia (DART) where a single P wave generates two QRS complexes resulting from simultaneous conduction over the FP and SP of the AV node (Fig. 5-33).[74,75] This results in a bigeminal tachycardia where the ventricular rate is twice the sinus rate (and which might be mistaken for AV dissociation).

NARROW QRS VT

Not all NCTs are supraventricular in origin. Rarely, ventricular tachycardia (VT) can be associated with a narrow QRS complex (<120 ms), particularly in the setting of an inferior myocardial infarction or origin near the fascicles (Fig. 5-34).[76–78]

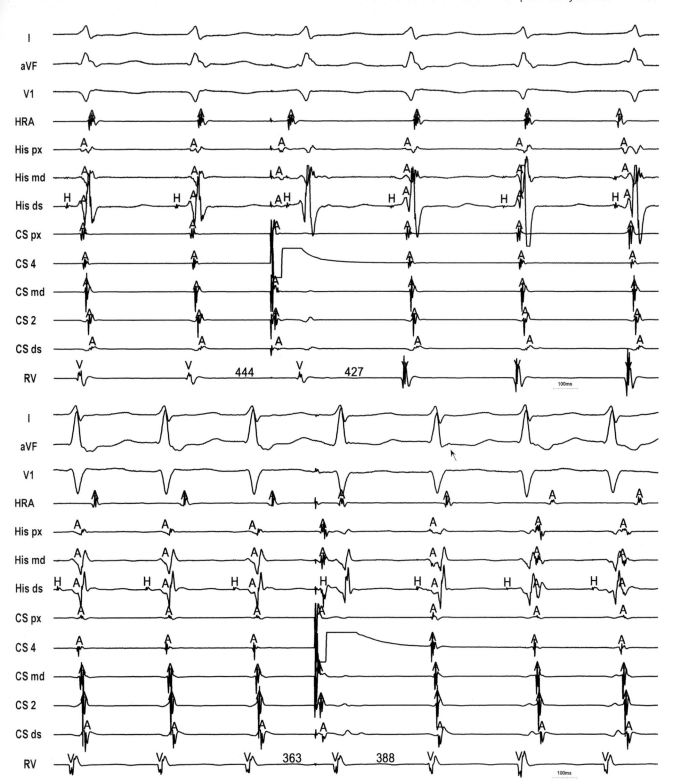

FIGURE 5-31 Resetting by His refractory APDs (typical AVNRT). His refractory APDs resets typical AVNRT by advancing (*top*) and delaying (*bottom*) the His bundle over the SP. These findings exclude JT. Resetting in the bottom tracing is confirmed by shift in retrograde P wave location from the end to the middle of the QRS complex (*arrow*).

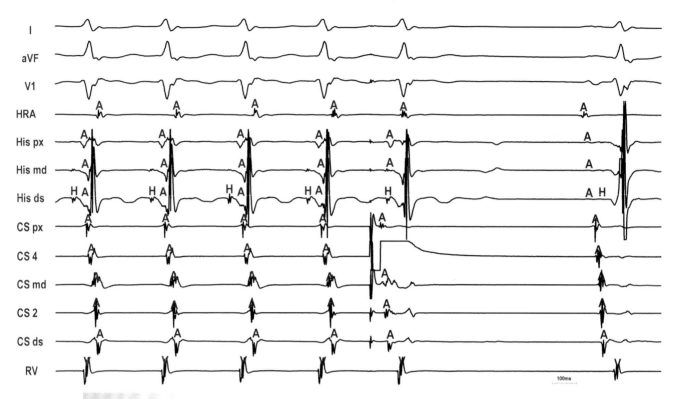

FIGURE 5-32 Termination by His refractory APDs (typical AVNRT). A His refractory APD terminates typical AVNRT by failing to conduct over the SP. Such a finding excludes JT.

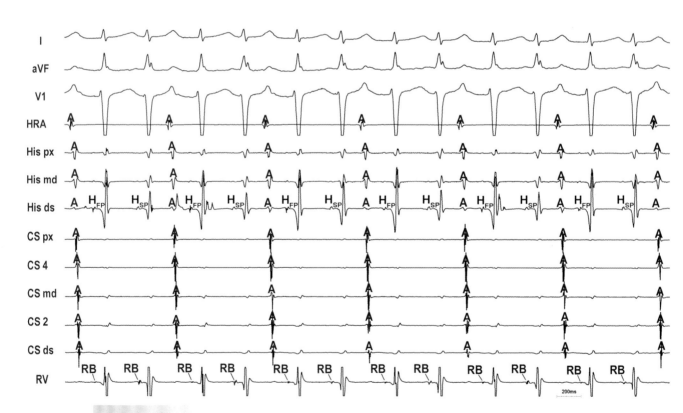

FIGURE 5-33 DART. Longitudinal dissociation of the AV node results in every sinus P wave generating two QRS complexes ("double fire") as conduction occurs simultaneously over FP and SP. Note that tachycardia is not regular but shows bigeminal (long–short) cycles.

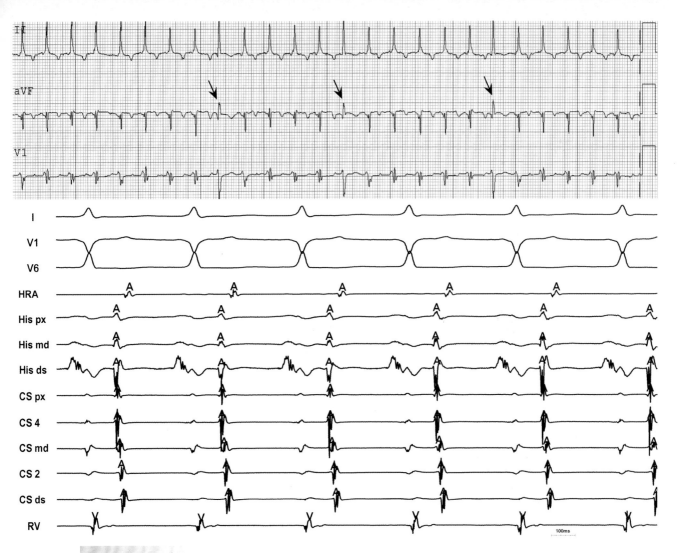

FIGURE 5-34 Narrow QRS complex VT. Retrograde Wenckebach over the AV node generates intermittent atypical AV nodal echoes (*arrows*) that reset VT with slight advancement. The ability of these capture beats to reset VT indicates close proximity of VT to the His-Purkinje system, thereby explaining its narrow QRS complex. Note that His bundle potentials do not precede QRS complexes.

REFERENCES

1. Goyal R, Zivin A, Souza J, et al. Comparison of the ages of tachycardia onset in patients with atrioventricular nodal reentrant tachycardia and accessory pathway-mediated tachycardia. Am Heart J 1996;132:765–767.

2. González-Torrecilla E, Almendral J, Arenal A, et al. Combined evaluation of bedside clinical variables and the electrocardiogram for the differential diagnosis of paroxysmal atrioventricular reciprocating tachycardias in patients without pre-excitation. J Am Coll Cardiol 2009;53:2353–2358.

3. Katritsis DG, Josephson ME. Differential diagnosis of regular, narrow-QRS tachycardia. Heart Rhythm 2015;12:1667–1676.

4. Kay GN, Pressley JC, Packer DL, Pritchett EL, German LD, Gilbert MR. Value of the 12-lead electrocardiogram in discriminating atrioventricular nodal reciprocating tachycardia from circus movement atrioventricular tachycardia utilizing a retrograde accessory pathway. Am J Cardiol 1987;59:296–300.

5. Benditt D, Pritchett E, Smith W, Gallagher J. Ventriculoatrial intervals: diagnostic use in paroxysmal supraventricular tachycardia. Ann Intern Med 1979;91:161–166.

6. Knight BP, Ebinger M, Oral H, et al. Diagnostic value of tachycardia features and pacing maneuvers during paroxysmal supraventricular tachycardia. J Am Coll Cardiol 2000;36:574–582.

7. Ceresnak SR, Doan LN, Motonaga KS, et al. 50 is the new 70: short ventriculoatrial times are common in children with atrioventricular reciprocating tachycardia. Heart Rhythm 2015;12:1541–1547.

8. Tai C, Chen S, Chiang C, Lee S, Chang M. Electrocardiographic and electrophysiologic characteristics of anteroseptal, midseptal, and para-Hisian accessory pathways. Implication for radiofrequency catheter ablation. Chest 1996;109:730–740.

9. Green M, Heddle B, Dassen W, et al. Value of QRS alteration in determining the site of origin of narrow QRS supraventricular tachycardia. Circulation 1983;68:368–373.

10. Morady F. Significance of QRS alternans during narrow QRS tachycardias. Pacing Clin Electrophysiol 1991;14:2193–2198.

11. Josephson M, Scharf D, Kastor J, Kitchen J. Atrial endocardial activation in man. Electrode catheter technique of endocardial mapping. Am J Cardiol 1977;39:972–981.

12. Wellens H, Durrer D. Patterns of ventriculo-atrial conduction in the Wolff-Parkinson-White syndrome. Circulation 1974;49:22–31.

13. Amat-y-Leon F, Dhingra R, Wu D, Denes P, Wyndham C, Rosen K. Catheter mapping of retrograde atrial activation. Observations during ventricular pacing and AV nodal re-entrant paroxysmal tachycardia. Br Heart J 1976;38:355–362.

14. Hwang C, Martin DJ, Goodman JS, et al. Atypical atrioventricular node reciprocating tachycardia masquerading as tachycardia using a left-sided accessory pathway. J Am Coll Cardiol 1997;30:218–225.

15. Wellens H, Wesdorp J, Düren D, Lie K. Second degree block during reciprocal atrioventricular nodal tachycardia. Circulation 1976;53:595–599.

16. Willems S, Shenasa M, Borggrefe M, et al. Atrioventricular nodal reentry tachycardia: electrophysiologic comparisons in patients with and without 2:1 infra-His block. Clin Cardiol 1993;16:883–888.

17. Lau EW. Infraatrial supraventricular tachycardias: mechanisms, diagnosis, and management. Pacing Clin Electrophysiol 2008;31:490–498.

18. Hamdan MH, Kalman JM, Lesh MD, et al. Narrow complex tachycardia with VA block: diagnostic and therapeutic implications. Pacing Clin Electrophysiol 1998;21:1196–1206.

19. Coumel P, Attuel P. Reciprocating tachycardia in overt and latent preexcitation. Influence of functional bundle branch block on the rate of the tachycardia. Eur J Cardiol 1974;1:423–436.

20. Kerr C, Gallagher J, German L. Changes in ventriculoatrial intervals with bundle branch block aberration during reciprocating tachycardia in patients with accessory atrioventricular pathways. Circulation 1982;66:196–201.

21. Pritchett E, Tonkin A, Dugan F, Wallace A, Gallagher J. Ventriculo-atrial conduction time during reciprocating tachycardia with intermittent bundle-branch block in Wolff-Parkinson-White syndrome. Br Heart J 1976;38:1058–1064.

22. Jazayeri M, Caceres J, Tchou P, Mahmud R, Denker S, Akhtar M. Electrophysiologic characteristics of sudden QRS axis deviation during orthodromic tachycardia. Role of functional fascicular block in localization of accessory pathway. J Clin Invest 1989;83:952–959.

23. Goldreyer B, Damato A. The essential role of atrioventricular conduction delay in the initiation of paroxysmal supraventricular tachycardia. Circulation 1971;43:679–687.

24. Rinne C, Sharma AD, Klein GJ, Yee R, Szabo T. Comparative effects of adenosine triphosphate on accessory pathway and atrioventricular nodal conduction. Am Heart J 1988;115:1042–1047.

25. Owada S, Iwasa A, Sasaki S, et al. "V-H-A pattern" as a criterion for the differential diagnosis of atypical AV nodal reentrant tachycardia from AV reciprocating tachycardia. Pacing Clin Electrophysiol 2005;28:667–674.

26. Kapa S, Henz B, Dib C, et al. Utilization of retrograde right bundle branch block to differentiate atrioventricular nodal from accessory pathway conduction. J Cardiovasc Electrophysiol 2009;20:751–758.

27. Martinez-Alday JD, Almendral J, Arenal A, et al. Identification of concealed posteroseptal Kent pathways by comparison of ventriculoatrial intervals from apical and posterobasal right ventricular sites. Circulation 1994;89:1060–1067.

28. Derval N, Skanes AC, Gula LJ, et al. Differential sequential septal pacing: a simple maneuver to differentiate nodal versus extranodal ventriculoatrial conduction. Heart Rhythm 2013;10:1785–1791.

29. Hirao K, Otomo K, Wang X, et al. Para-Hisian pacing. A new method for differentiating retrograde conduction over an accessory AV pathway from conduction over the AV node. Circulation 1996;94:1027–1035.

30. Takatsuki S, Mitamura H, Tanimoto K, et al. Clinical implications of "pure" Hisian pacing in addition to para-Hisian pacing for the diagnosis of supraventricular tachycardia. Heart Rhythm 2006;3:1412–1418.

31. Sheldon SH, Li H, Asirvatham SJ, McLeod CJ. Parahisian pacing: technique, utility, and pitfalls. J Interv Card Electrophysiol 2014;40:105–116.

32. Obeyesekere M, Leong-Sit P, Skanes A, et al. Determination of inadvertent atrial capture during para-Hisian pacing. Circ Arrhythm Electrophysiol 2011;4:510–514.

33. Kenia A, Ho RT, Pavri BB. An uncommon response to para-His pacing. J Cardiovasc Electrophysiol 2014;25:796–798.

34. Ho RT, Frisch DR, Pavri BB, Levi SA, Greenspon AJ. Electrophysiological features differentiating the atypical atrioventricular node-dependent long RP supraventricular tachycardias. Circ Arrhythm Electrophysiol 2013;6:597–605.

35. Segal OR, Gula LJ, Skanes AC, Krahn AD, Yee R, Klein GJ. Differential ventricular entrainment: a maneuver to differentiate AV node reentrant tachycardia from orthodromic reciprocating tachycardia. Heart Rhythm 2009;6:493–500.

36. Platonov M, Schroeder K, Veenhuyzen GD. Differential entrainment: beware from where you pace. Heart Rhythm 2007;4:1097–1099.

37. Reddy VY, Jongnarangsin K, Albert CM, et al. Para-Hisian entrainment: a novel pacing maneuver to differentiate orthodromic atrioventricular reentrant tachycardia from atrioventricular nodal reentrant tachycardia. J Cardiovasc Electrophysiol 2003;14:1321–1328.

38. Benditt D, Benson DW Jr, Dunnigan A, et al. Role of extrastimulus site and tachycardia cycle length in inducibility of atrial preexcitation by premature ventricular stimulation during reciprocating tachycardia. Am J Cardiol 1987;60:811–819.

39. Miles W, Yee R, Klein G, Zipes D, Prystowsky E. The preexcitation index: an aid in determining the mechanism of supraventricular tachycardia and localizing accessory pathways. Circulation 1986;74:493–500.

40. Zipes DP, De Joseph RL, Rothbaum DA. Unusual properties of accessory pathways. Circulation 1974;49:1200–1211.

41. Ho RT, Patel U, Weitz HH. Entrainment and resetting of a long RP tachycardia: which trumps which for diagnosis? Heart Rhythm 2010;7:714–715.

42. Ho RT, Fischman DL. Entrainment versus resetting of a long RP tachycardia: what is the diagnosis? Heart Rhythm 2012;9:312–314.

43. Bardy G, Packer D, German L, Coltorti F, Gallagher J. Paradoxical delay in accessory pathway conduction during long R-P' tachycardia after interpolated ventricular premature complexes. Am J Cardiol 1985;55:1223–1225.

44. Ho RT, Mark GE, Rhim ES, Pavri BB, Greenspon AJ. Differentiating atrioventricular nodal reentrant tachycardia from atrioventricular reentrant tachycardia by ΔHA values during entrainment from the ventricle. Heart Rhythm 2008;5:83–88.

45. Nagashima K, Kumar S, Stevenson WG, et al. Anterograde conduction to the His bundle during right ventricular overdrive pacing distinguishes septal pathway atrioventricular reentry from atypical atrioventricular nodal reentrant tachycardia. Heart Rhythm 2015;12:735–743.

46. Boyle PM, Veenhuyzen GD, Vigmond EJ. Fusion during entrainment of orthodromic reciprocating tachycardia is enhanced for basal pacing sites but diminished when pacing near Purkinje system end points. Heart Rhythm 2013;10:444–451.

47. Knight B, Zivin A, Souza J, et al. A technique for the rapid diagnosis of atrial tachycardia in the electrophysiology laboratory. J Am Coll Cardiol 1999;33:775–781.

48. Michaud GF, Tada H, Chough S, et al. Differentiation of atypical atrioventricular node re-entrant tachycardia from orthodromic reciprocating tachycardia using a septal accessory pathway by the response to ventricular pacing. J Am Coll Cardiol 2001;38:1163–1167.

49. Mark GE, Rhim ES, Pavri BB, Greenspon AJ, Ho RT. Differentiation of atrio-ventricular nodal reentrant tachycardia from orthodromic atrioventricular reentrant tachycardia by ΔhA intervals during entrainment from the ventricle. Heart Rhythm 2006;3:S321.

50. Miller JM, Rosenthal ME, Gottlieb CD, Vassallo JA, Josephson ME. Usefulness of the delta HA interval to accurately distinguish atrioventricular nodal reentry from orthodromic septal bypass tract tachycardias. Am J Cardiol 1991;68:1037–1044.

51. Jastrzebski M, Kukla P. The V-A-V response to ventricular entrainment during atrial tachycardia: what is the mechanism? J Cardiovasc Electrophysiol 2012;23:1266–1268.

52. Kaneko Y, Nakajima T, Irie T, Iizuka T, Tamura S, Kurabayashi M. Atrial and ventricular activation sequence after ventricular induction/entrainment pacing during fast-slow atrioventricular nodal reentrant tachycardia: new insight into the use of V-A-A-V for the differential diagnosis of supraventricular tachycardia. Heart Rhythm 2017;14:1615–1622.

53. Vijayaraman P, Lee BP, Kalahasty G, Wood MA, Ellenbogen KA. Reanalysis of the "pseudo A-A-V" response to ventricular entrainment of supraventricular tachycardia: importance of His-bundle timing. J Cardiovasc Electrophysiol 2006;17:25–28.

54. Vijayaraman P, Kok LC, Rhee B, Ellenbogen KA. Wide complex tachycardia: what is the mechanism? Heart Rhythm 2005;2:107–109.

55. Crawford TC, Morady F, Pelosi F Jr. A long R-P paroxysmal supraventricular tachycardia: what is the mechanism? Heart Rhythm 2007;4:1364–1365.

56. Michaud GF. Entrainment of a narrow QRS complex tachycardia from the right ventricular apex: what is the mechanism? Heart Rhythm 2005;2:559–560.

57. Michaud GF, Morady F. Letters to the editor. Heart Rhythm 2006;7:1114–1115.

58. González-Torrecilla E, Arenal A, Atienza F, et al. First postpacing interval after tachycardia entrainment with correction for atrioventricular node delay: a simple maneuver for differential diagnosis of atrioventricular nodal reentrant tachycardias versus orthodromic reciprocating tachycardias. Heart Rhythm 2006;3:674–679.

59. Obeyesekere M, Gula LJ, Modi S, et al. Tachycardia induction with ventricular extrastimuli differentiates atypical atrioventricular nodal reentrant tachycardia from orthodromic reciprocating tachycardia. Heart Rhythm 2012;9:335–341.

60. AlMahameed ST, Buxton AE, Michaud GF. New criteria during right ventricular pacing to determine the mechanism of supraventricular tachycardia. Circ Arrhythm Electrophysiol 2010;3:578–584.

61. Dandamudi G, Mokabberi R, Assal C, et al. A novel approach to differentiating orthodromic reciprocating tachycardia from atrioventricular nodal reentrant tachycardia. Heart Rhythm 2010;7:1326–1329.

62. Man KC, Niebauer M, Daoud E, et al. Comparison of atrial-His intervals during tachycardia and atrial pacing in patients with long RP tachycardia. J Cardiovasc Electrophysiol 1995;6:700–710.

63. Kadish AH, Morady F. The response of paroxysmal supraventricular tachycardia to overdrive atrial and ventricular pacing: can it help determine the tachycardia mechanism? J Cardiovasc Electrophysiol 1993;4:239–252.

64. Maruyama M, Kobayashi Y, Miyauchi Y, et al. The VA relationship after differential atrial overdrive pacing: a novel tool for the diagnosis of atrial tachycardia in the electrophysiologic laboratory. J Cardiovasc Electrophysiol 2007;18:1127–1133.

65. Sarkozy A, Richter S, Chierchia G, et al. A novel pacing manoeuvre to diagnose atrial tachycardia. Europace 2008;10:459–466.

66. Fan R, Tardos JG, Almasry I, Barbera S, Rashba EJ, Iwai S. Novel use of atrial overdrive pacing to rapidly differentiate junctional tachycardia from atrioventricular nodal reentrant tachycardia. Heart Rhythm 2011;8:840–844.

67. Padanilam BJ, Manfredi JA, Steinberg LA, Olson JA, Fogel RI, Prystowsky EN. Differentiating junctional tachycardia and atrioventricular node re-entry tachycardia based on response to atrial extrastimulus pacing. J Am Coll Cardiol 2008;52:1711–1717.

68. Roberts-Thomson KC, Seiler J, Steven D, et al. Short AV response to atrial extrastimuli during narrow complex tachycardia: what is the mechanism? J Cardiovasc Electrophysiol 2009;20:946–948.

69. DiMarco JP, Sellers TD, Berne RM, West GA, Belardinelli L. Adenosine: electrophysiologic effects and therapeutic use for terminating paroxysmal supraventricular tachycardia. Circulation 1983;68:1254–1263.

70. Camm AJ, Garratt CJ. Adenosine and supraventricular tachycardia. N Engl J Med 1991;325:1621–1629.
71. Ho RT. A narrow complex tachycardia with atrioventricular dissociation: what is the mechanism? Heart Rhythm 2017;14:1570–1573.
72. Roberts-Thomson KC, Seiler J, Raymond JM, Stevenson WG. Exercise induced tachycardia with atrioventricular dissociation: what is the mechanism? Heart Rhythm 2009;6:426–428.
73. Kusa S, Taniguchi H, Hachiya H, et al. Bundle branch reentrant ventricular tachycardia with wide and narrow QRS morphology. Circ Arrhythm Electrophysiol 2013;6:e87–e91.
74. Gaba D, Pavri BB, Greenspon AJ, Ho RT. Dual antegrade response tachycardia induced cardiomyopathy. Pacing Clin Electrophysiol 2004;27:533–536.
75. Wang N. Dual atrioventricular nodal nonreentrant tachycardia: a systematic review. Pacing Clin Electrophysiol 2011;34:1671–1681.
76. Sakamoto T, Fujiki A, Nakatani Y, Sakabe M, Mizumaki K, Inoue H. Narrow QRS ventricular tachycardia from the posterior mitral annulus without involvement of the His-Purkinje system in a patient with prior inferior myocardial infarction. Heart Vessels 2010;25:170–173.
77. Bogun F, Good E, Reich S, et al. Role of Purkinje fibers in post-infarction ventricular tachycardia. J Am Coll Cardiol 2006;48:2500–2507.
78. Talib AK, Nogami A, Nishiuchi S, et al. Verapamil-sensitive upper septal idiopathic left ventricular tachycardia: prevalence, mechanism, and electrophysiological characteristics. JACC Clin Electrophysiol 2015;1:369–380.

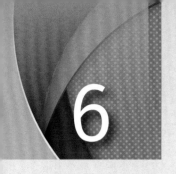

6 Long RP Tachycardias

Introduction

Long RP tachycardias are an unusual type of narrow complex tachycardia (NCT) that includes atrial tachycardia (AT) and four atrio-ventricular (AV) node–dependent tachycardias: 1) pure atypical (fast–slow) AV nodal reentrant tachycardia (AVNRT); 2) atypical AVNRT with a concealed, bystander nodo-fascicular (NF)/nodo-ventricular (NV) accessory pathway (AP) inserting into the slow pathway (SP) of the AV node (AVNRT–NF AP–SP); 3) orthodromic reciprocating tachycardia (ORT) using a concealed NF/NV AP inserting into the SP of the AV node (nodo-fascicular reentrant tachycardia [NFRT] AP–SP); and 4) ORT using a concealed, slowly conducting, decremental AV AP (also called the permanent form of junctional reciprocating tachycardia [PJRT]) (**Fig. 6-1**).[1] Because of their rarity, standard diagnostic criteria are lacking and often extrapolated from responses to conventional pacing maneuvers applied to the short RP tachycardia. These tachycardias, however, respond differently than their short RP counterparts to pacing maneuvers because of the decremental properties in the retrograde limb of their circuit.

The purpose of this chapter is to:
1. Discuss the electrophysiologic features of the four AV node–dependent long RP NCTs.
2. Discuss the delineation of the upper and lower limbs of each circuit by atrial and ventricular pacing maneuvers, respectively.
3. Discuss the target sites for successful ablation of each long RP tachycardia.

ELECTROPHYSIOLOGIC FEATURES

Because the retrograde limb of the AV node–dependent long RP tachycardia involves the SP (atypical AVNRT, NFRT AP–SP) or a slowly conducting decremental AP, which are often (but not always) posteroseptal in location (PJRT), atrial activation is generally midline and earliest along the posteroseptum (**Figs. 6-2 to 6-4**). Both the AV node and slowly conducting APs are adenosine-sensitive postulating that these decremental APs contain accessory AV nodal or depolarized atrial tissue.[2] While transition zone clues (spontaneous termination with AV block excluding AT, VA/tachycardia cycle length [TCL] prolongation with bundle branch block [BBB]) still apply to long RP tachycardias, such observations are less common than with their short RP counterpart (**Fig. 6-5**). Spontaneous termination commonly occurs in the retrograde limb (SP or slowly conducting AP), which is unhelpful for diagnosis. Additionally, BBB-induced VA/TCL changes are difficult to appreciate or even absent with long RP ORT because 1) tachycardia is

slower and less susceptible to aberration, 2) the septal location of most APs increases VA intervals only slightly (≤25 ms), and 3) any enlargement of the macroreentrant circuit by the addition of transeptal conduction is counterbalanced by faster conduction over the decremental AP, or conversely, reduction of the macroreentrant circuit by the loss of transeptal conduction (loss of BBB ipsilateral to the AP) is counterbalanced by slower conduction over the decremental AP (VA prolongation). Pacing maneuvers are therefore required to establish a more definitive diagnosis.

PACING MANEUVERS

For the AV node–dependent long RP tachycardias, pacing maneuvers from the ventricle during sinus rhythm (parahisian, differential RV pacing) are less useful than those during tachycardia (His refractory ventricular premature depolarizations [VPDs], entrainment) because 1) VA Wenckebach block might exist despite pacing at the slowest rate allowable by sinus rhythm, 2) fast pathway (FP) might preempt

Diagnosis	Atypical AVNRT	Atypical AVNRT + bystander NF	NFRT	PJRT

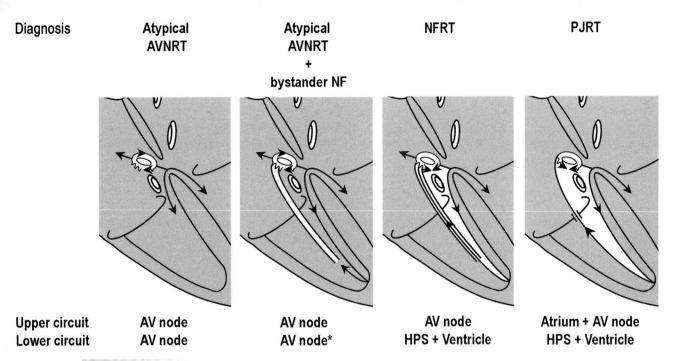

	Atypical AVNRT	Atypical AVNRT + bystander NF	NFRT	PJRT
Upper circuit	AV node	AV node	AV node	Atrium + AV node
Lower circuit	AV node	AV node*	HPS + Ventricle	HPS + Ventricle

FIGURE 6-1 The four AV node–dependent long RP tachycardias. The upper and lower limbs of the circuit are determined by pacing maneuvers in the atrium and ventricle, respectively. Asterisk denotes that NF/NV AP inserts into the SP.

slower SP or AP conduction and prevent identification of the slowly-conducting retrograde limb of the circuit responsible for tachycardia, and 3) reproducible tachycardia induction with onset of ventricular stimulation can interfere with pacing maneuvers.[3] Additionally, an "AV nodal response" during parahisian pacing can occur with a NF AP, while an "AV nodal response" during differential RV pacing can be seen with a long, insulated AV or NF/NV AP inserting closer to the RV apex than base (**Figs. 6-6 and 6-7**).[4,5]

His Refractory VPDs (Identifying Presence of a Decremental AP)

For long RP tachycardias, a positive response to His refractory VPDs is the single most useful maneuver to identify the existence of an AP.[1] With long RP tachycardias, positive responses include reproducible 1) termination with VA block, 2) resetting with advancement, and 3) resetting with delay—the latter occurring only in APs with significant decremental properties (**Figs. 6-8 to 6-14**).[6–13] A positive response, however, proves the presence of an AP but not necessarily its participation in the tachycardia mechanism (participant versus bystander).[8,9] It is possible for a His refractory VPD to terminate or reset atypical AVNRT in the presence of a concealed, bystander NF AP inserting into the SP (retrograde limb) of the AV node (**Figs. 6-12 and 6-13; see also Fig. 11-16**).[8–10] Such a VPD conducts over the NF AP–SP and penetrates the excitable gap in the SP ahead of the tachycardia wavefront, which had just crossed the lower turnaround point of the circuit. The paced antidromic wavefront collides with tachycardia, while its orthodromic wavefront finds absolute or relative distal SP refractoriness terminating or resetting tachycardia with delay, respectively.

His refractory VPDs that reset tachycardia with delay ("post-excitation") identify an AP with severe decremental properties (degree of AP delay > degree of VPD prematurity resulting in a more than fully compensatory pause) that can also generate long post-pacing intervals (PPIs) and pseudo AAV responses during entrainment from the ventricle, resulting in a potential misdiagnosis of AVNRT and AT, respectively (**Fig. 6-14**).[11,14] Additionally, it is important to deliver multiple VPDs because apparent absence of resetting following a single VPD (false negative) can occur if the degree of VPD prematurity is offset by an equal degree of AP delay (full compensation) (**Fig. 6-15**).

Entrainment

The different mechanisms of the AV node–dependent long RP tachycardias are complex. The lower limb of its circuit can involve the His-Purkinje system/ventricle (ORT: PJRT/NFRT) or not (AVNRT). The upper limb of its circuit can be confined to the AV node ("nodal tachycardias": AVNRT/NFRT) or not (PJRT).[1] Therefore, diagnosis requires separate pacing maneuvers in the atrium and ventricle to delineate the upper and lower limbs of the circuit, respectively (**Fig. 6-1**).

Entrainment from the Ventricle (Delineation of the Lower Circuit: Atypical ORT [PJRT/NFRT] Versus Atypical AVNRT)

In contrast to entrainment of short RP tachycardias from the ventricles, long RP tachycardias often demonstrate atypical responses (AAV patterns, long PPIs) because of the decremental properties of its retrograde limb (SP or AP). Additionally,

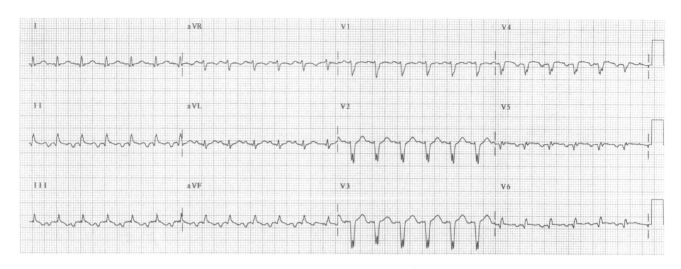

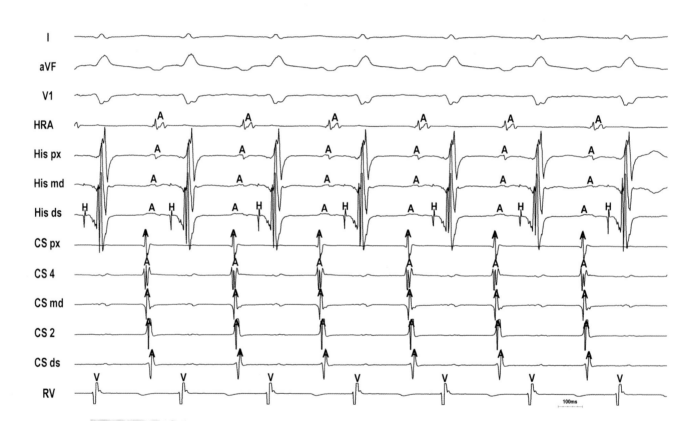

FIGURE 6-2 Atypical AVNRT. P waves are inverted inferiorly and slightly positive in V1. Atrial activation is midline (earliest along the posteroseptum).

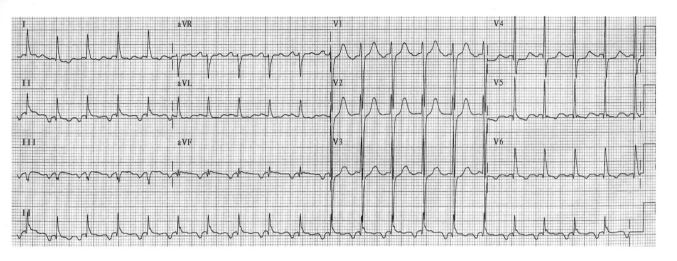

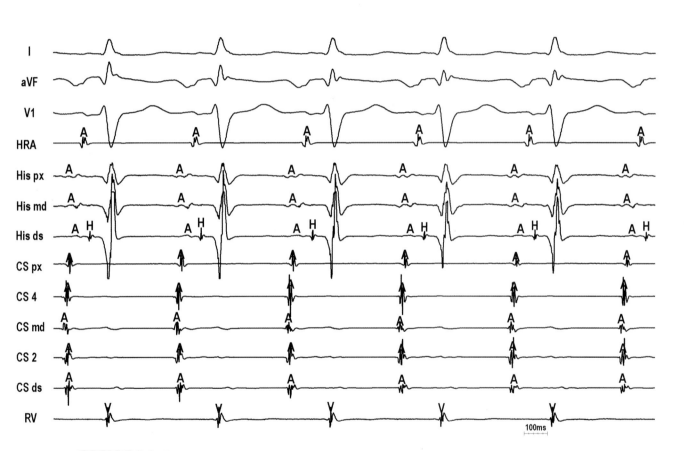

FIGURE 6-3 PJRT. P waves are inverted inferiorly and slightly negative in V1 (in contrast to the slight positivity in V1 of atypical AVNRT). Atrial activation is midline (nearly simultaneous between the antero- and posteroseptum).

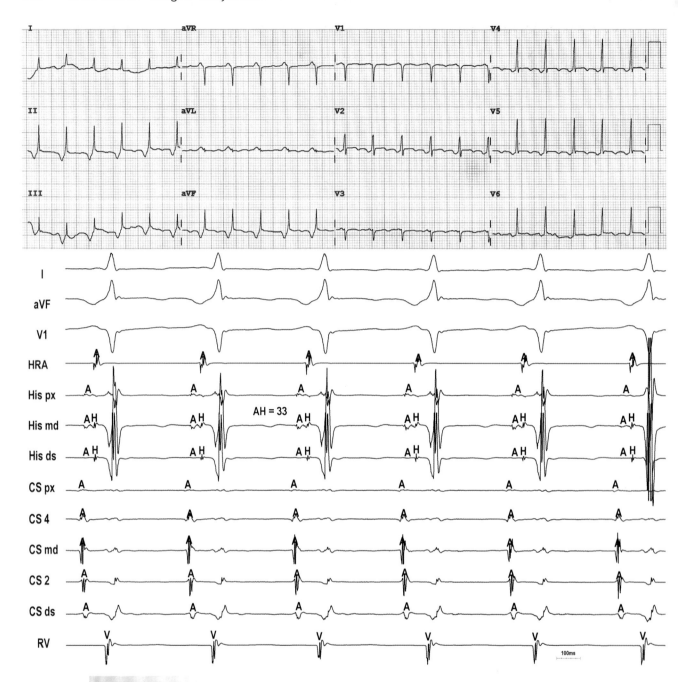

FIGURE 6-4 Atypical AVNRT with a concealed, bystander NF AP. P waves are inverted inferiorly and slightly positive in V1. The AH interval is very short (33 ms—the end of the atrial electrogram overlaps the His bundle potential) because it is actually a pseudo-interval that represents simultaneous activation of the atrium and His bundle (excludes PJRT). His refractory VPDs delayed the atrium proving the presence of an AP (Fig. 6-13).

oscillations in the cycle length and pacing-induced VA prolongation make interpretation of entrainment criteria difficult.

AAV Patterns

An AAV response is generally considered diagnostic of AT, but AAV patterns are common with AV node–dependent long RP tachycardias causing potential misdiagnosis of AT. The AAV pattern can either be a 1) pseudo AAV (true AV) response or 2) true AAV response resulting from retrograde "double fire"

(see Table 5-2) (Figs. 6-12 to 6-14 and 6-16).[8,9,11,15–19] Classic pseudo AAV responses are more common with atypical AVNRT than ORT because of its longer paced VA interval and occur when significant pacing-induced decrement over the SP or AP cause the paced VA interval to exceed the pacing cycle length (VV interval). In this case, the first atrial electrogram after entrainment is actually driven by the penultimate (second to last) pacing stimulus. Identifying the last entrained atrium after pacing demonstrates a true "AV" response and an

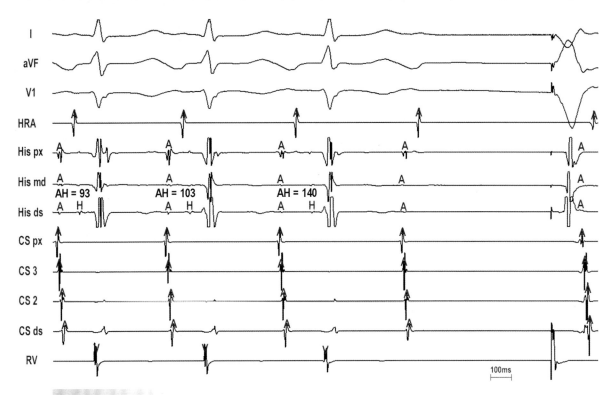

FIGURE 6-5 Spontaneous termination of atypical AVNRT with AV block. Antegrade FP Wenckebach causes tachycardia slowing and termination—indication that tachycardia is dependent on the AV node, thereby excluding AT. A paced ventricular complex conducts retrogradely over the FP (preempting the SP).

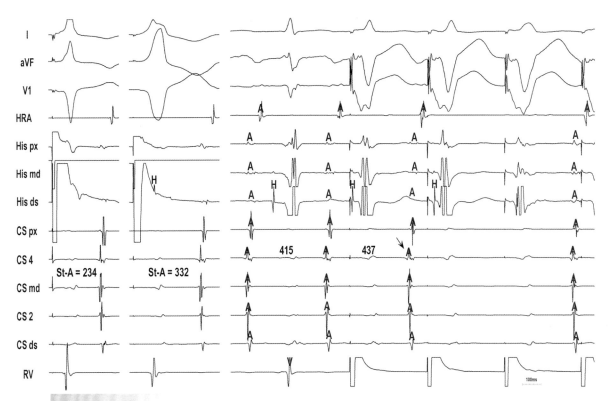

FIGURE 6-6 NFRT AP–SP. *Left*: Parahisian pacing elicits an "AV nodal response" excluding a slowly conducting AV AP (PJRT). Note that the atrial activation patterns during parahisian pacing and NFRT are identical. *Right*: Termination of NFRT AP–SP at onset of ventricular overdrive pacing. The first paced complex (His refractory) delays the atrium by 22 ms (*arrow*), while the second (also His refractory) terminates tachycardia with VA block—both proving the presence of an AP.

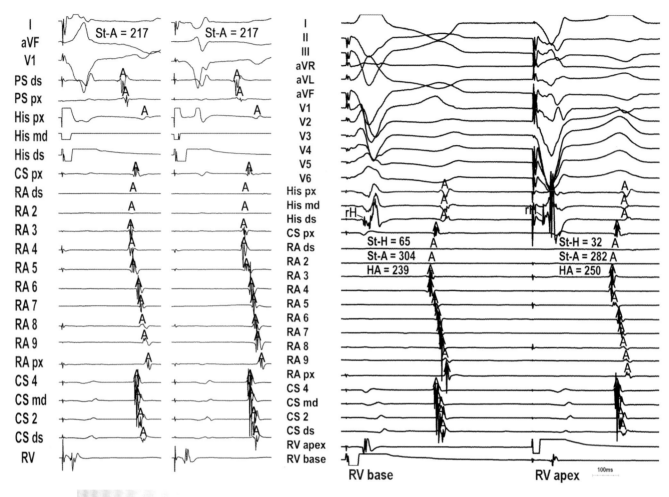

FIGURE 6-7 PJRT using a long, insulated AV AP. *Left*: Parahisian pacing elicits an "AP response." *Right*: Differential RV pacing, however, shows that the ventricular insertion site of the AP is closer to the RV apex than base. A similar finding could be seen with an NV AP inserting close to the RV apex but is excluded by demonstrating that the atrium is an integral part of the ORT circuit (**Fig. 6-22**). Note that RV basal pacing results in a longer St-H interval.

atrial activation pattern identical to tachycardia. Other rare causes of pseudo AAV responses during atypical AVNRT are seen when long AH intervals exceed the TCL or momentary lower common final pathway block develops upon cessation of pacing.[15,17,19] True AAV responses result from dual retrograde responses ("double fire") with simultaneous conduction over the FP and SP/slowly conducting AP. This is different from the true AAV response of AT where retrograde atrial activation over the AV node is followed by the first return beat of AT after pacing. In contrast to pseudo AAV responses, first and second atrial activation patterns with true AAV responses generally differ. One mechanism to explain dual retrograde responses during atypical AVNRT/ORT is the presence of a large excitable gap with collision between antidromic and orthodromic wavefronts in the SP or AP (orthodromic or retrograde limb) of the circuit. The last (*n*) paced antidromic wavefront conducts completely over the FP to the atrium (first A) while colliding with the previous (*n* − 1) orthodromic wavefront in the SP or AP. The last (*n*) paced orthodromic wavefront has no antidromic wavefront with which to collide, conducts slowly over the SP or AP to activate the atrium (second A) before conducting antegradely

over the FP to the His bundle/ventricle. An alternative mechanism is tachycardia termination and subsequent re-initiation. With onset of ventricular pacing, retrograde block occurs in the SP/AP effectively terminating tachycardia and conducts exclusively over the FP. When pacing stops, retrograde conduction occurs over both the FP and SP/AP, the latter re-initiating tachycardia with a dual retrograde response.

Long Post-pacing Intervals

Conventional NCT criteria (PPI–TCL, ΔVA, ΔHA) establish the lower portion of the circuit as macroreentrant involving the His-Purkinje system/ventricle (ORT: PJRT/NFRT) or not (AVNRT).[20,21] However, because of slow, decremental AP conduction, entrainment of atypical ORT can generate large PPI–TCL (>115 ms), ΔVA (>85 ms), and ΔHA (>0 ms) values causing misdiagnosis of AVNRT (**Fig. 6-14**).[1,11,22] A PPI–TCL cutoff value of 125 ms has been suggested to better discriminate atypical ORT from atypical AVNRT.[1] Furthermore, because decrement occurs retrogradely in the AP rather than antegradely in the AV node, correcting the PPI for the antegrade delay in the AV node (corrected PPI) is not helpful. In fact, the corrected PPI

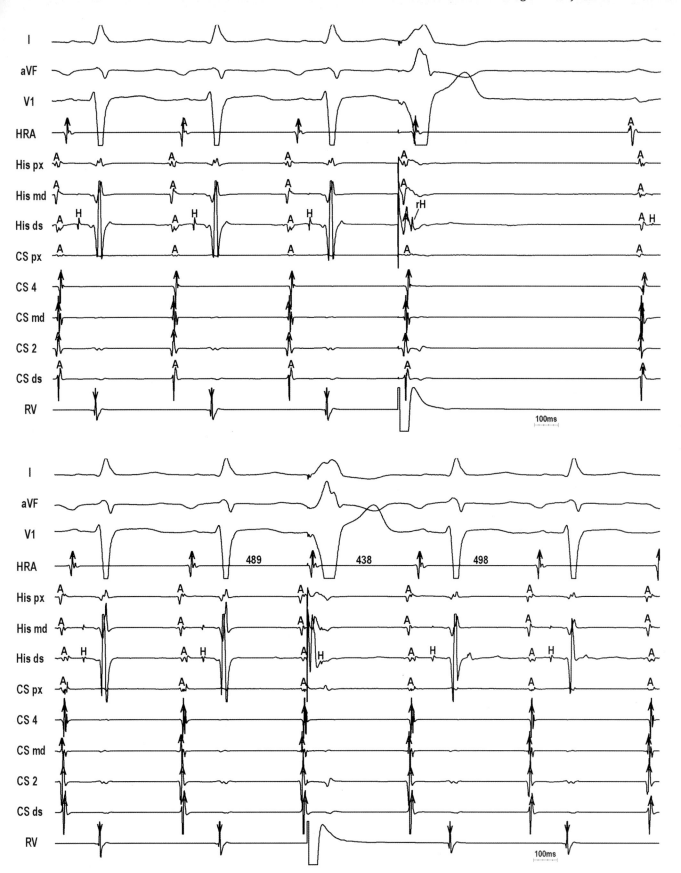

FIGURE 6-8 PJRT. *Top*: An early VPD terminates tachycardia with VA block excluding AT. *Bottom*: A His refractory VPD advances the atrium by 51 ms proving the presence of an AP. *Abbreviation*: rH, retrograde His bundle potential.

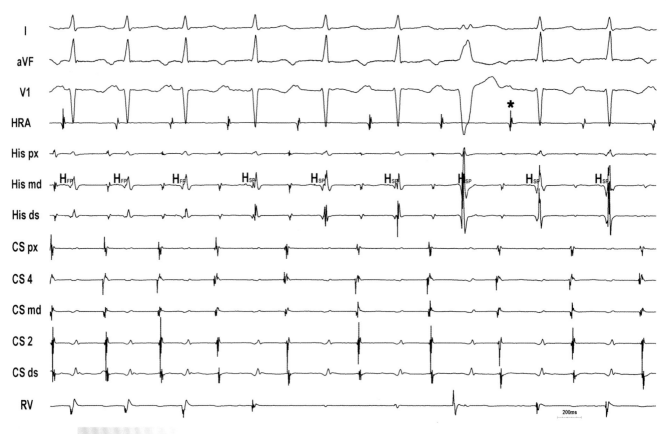

FIGURE 6-9 PJRT with dual AV node physiology. PJRT abruptly slows because of an antegrade shift from FP to SP, indicating dependence of tachycardia upon AV nodal conduction and excluding AT. A spontaneous His refractory VPD advances the atrium (*asterisk*) by 25 ms proving presence of an AP.

can be paradoxically longer than the PPI when very slow retrograde AP conduction allows the first post-pacing AH interval to shorten relative to tachycardia. While a short PPI (PPI − TCL ≤115 ms) is specific for atypical ORT, it is theoretically possible to have a short PPI during atypical AVNRT if a concealed, bystander NF AP is present. If the refractory period of the NF AP is sufficiently short to support 1:1 conduction during entrainment (but a dominant AVNRT circuit is faster than the putative NFRT circuit) and retrograde conduction over the NF AP is faster than over the His-Purkinje system, the pathway for entrainment of atypical AVNRT/NF AP and NFRT is the same and the single PPI return cycle might be misleadingly short.

Orthodromic Capture of the His Bundle
During entrainment from the ventricle, the presence of an AP allows the His bundle to be captured either antegradely (orthodromically) or retrogradely (antidromically)—the collision point between each orthodromic (*n*) and antidromic (*n* + 1) wavefronts being below or above the His bundle recording site, respectively. For AVNRT, the His bundle must be captured retrogradely in order for pacing stimuli to penetrate the tachycardia circuit within the AV node. Therefore, identifying His bundle potentials during pacing and determining whether or not they are orthodromically captured during entrainment (equivalent to delivery of His refractory VPDs) is a valuable clue demonstrating the presence of an AP (**Figs. 6-10 and 6-11**).[21]

Onset of Ventricular Overdrive Pacing
While the end of entrainment can provide important information regarding the mechanism of tachycardia (AV versus AAV response, PPI–TCL, ΔVA, ΔHA), additional clues can also be found at the beginning of ventricular overdrive pacing. During the transition zone, QRS complexes represent fusion between antegrade His-Purkinje activation from tachycardia and the paced activation wavefront (equivalent to variably timed His refractory VPDs). Therefore, any perturbation of tachycardia (advancement, delay, termination) within the transition zone or by one fully paced QRS complex indicates the presence of an AP and likely diagnosis of macroreentrant ORT (**Fig. 6-17**).[23,24]

Entrainment from the Atrium (Delineation of the Upper Circuit: Nodal Tachycardias [AVNRT/NFRT] Versus PJRT)
ΔAH Interval
Comparison of AH intervals during atrial entrainment can differentiate nodal tachycardia (AVNRT/NFRT) from PJRT.[7–9,25–27] The upper limb of the circuit for atypical AVNRT/NFRT ("nodal tachycardias") is confined to the AV node and its atrionodal inputs. The AH interval is a pseudo-interval reflecting simultaneous activation of the atrium retrogradely and FP/His bundle antegradely. Therefore, the AH interval of nodal tachycardias can be very short and paradoxically shorter than the AH interval during sinus rhythm (**Figs. 6-4, and 6-11 to 6-13**).

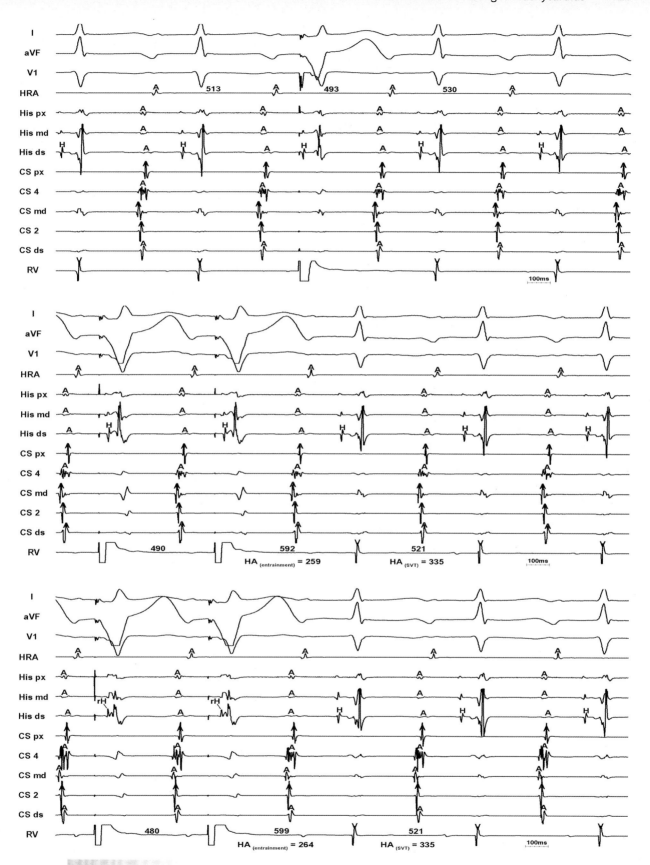

FIGURE 6-10 PJRT. *Top*: A His refractory VPD preexcites the atrium by 20 ms, indicating existence of an AP. *Middle*: Entrainment from the ventricle with orthodromic capture of the His bundle (constant QRS fusion) further confirming the presence of an AP. *Bottom*: Entrainment from the ventricle with antidromic capture of the His bundle at a shorter (10 ms) pacing cycle length (progressive QRS fusion). In both cases, the PPI − TCL <125 ms and ΔHA <0.

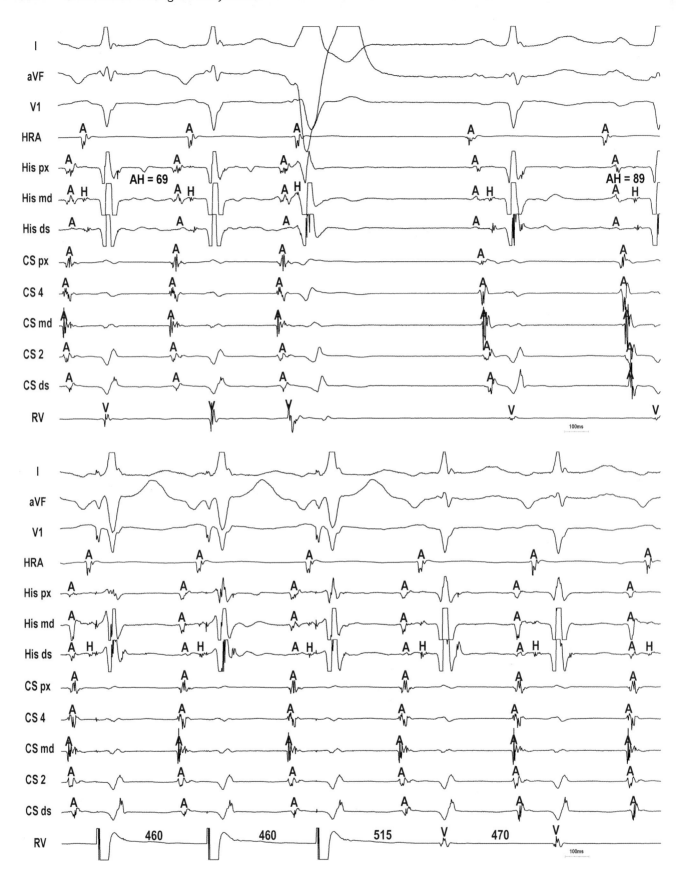

FIGURE 6-11 NFRT. *Top:* A His refractory VPD terminates tachycardia with VA block. Paradoxically, AH$_{(SVT)}$ < AH$_{(NSR)}$ excluding PJRT. *Bottom:* Entrainment from the ventricle with orthodromic capture of the His bundle. The PPI–TCL is short (45 ms) excluding long atypical AVNRT with a bystander NF AP.

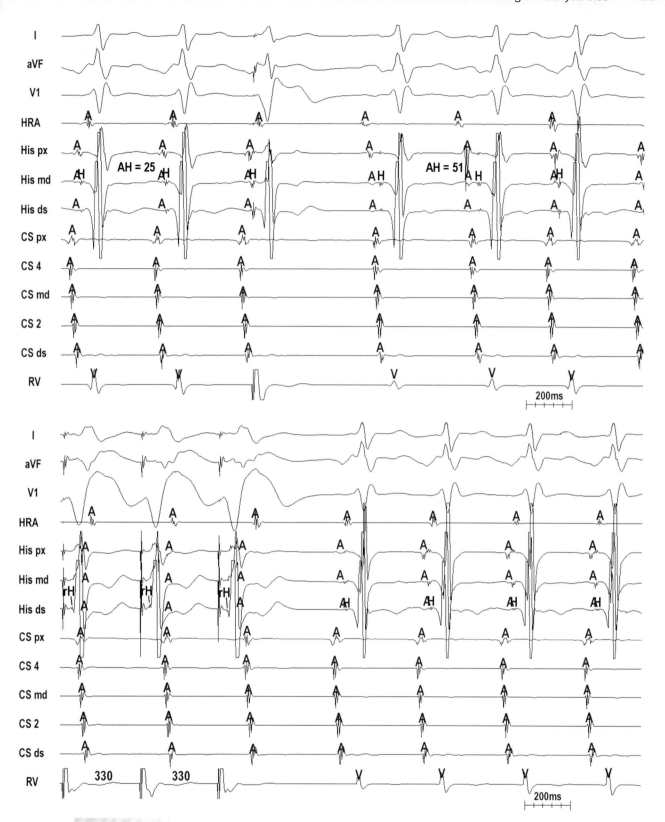

FIGURE 6-12 Atypical AVNRT with a bystander NF AP–SP. *Top*: A His refractory VPD momentarily terminates tachycardia with VA block before spontaneous resumption after two sinus beats. The $AH_{(SVT)}$ is extremely short (25 ms) and paradoxically shorter than $AH_{(NSR)}$ excluding PJRT. *Bottom*: Entrainment from the ventricle with antidromic capture of the His bundle and true AAV response (retrograde double fire). Ventricular paced complexes capture the His bundle retrogradely (rH) but do not entrain tachycardia until the last paced complex, indicating that the His bundle is not part of the circuit, thereby excluding NFRT. Pacing cessation results in retrograde conduction over the FP and NF AP–SP with a very long PPI (581 ms, PPI − TCL = 140 ms).

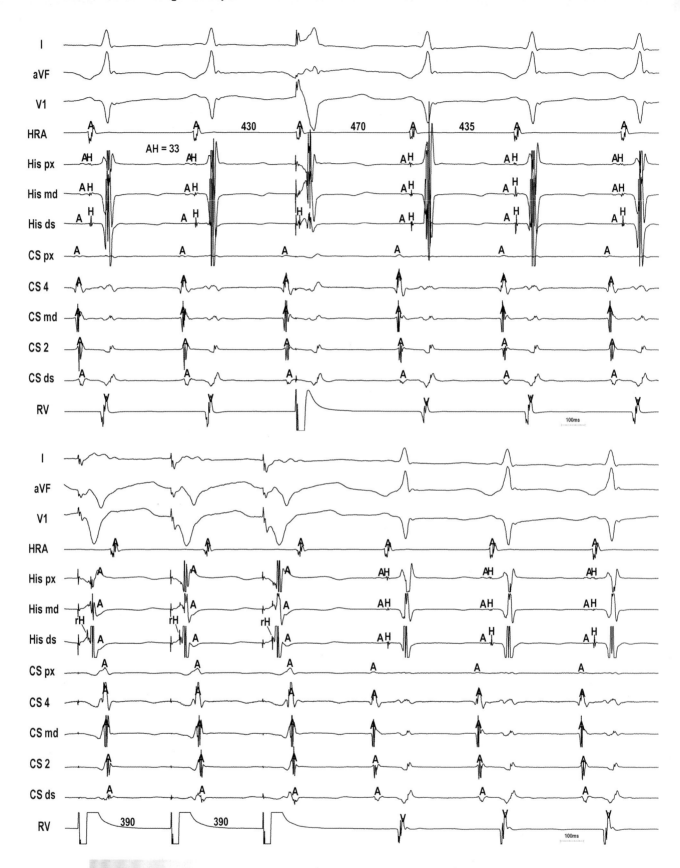

FIGURE 6-13 Atypical AVNRT with a bystander NF AP–SP. *Top*: A His refractory VPD delays the atrium by 40 ms. The AH(SVT) is very short (33 ms) excluding PJRT. *Bottom*: Entrainment from the ventricle with antidromic capture of the His bundle and a true AAV response (retrograde double fire). Pacing cessation results in retrograde conduction over the FP and NF AP–SP with a very long PPI (564 ms, PPI − TCL = 141 ms).

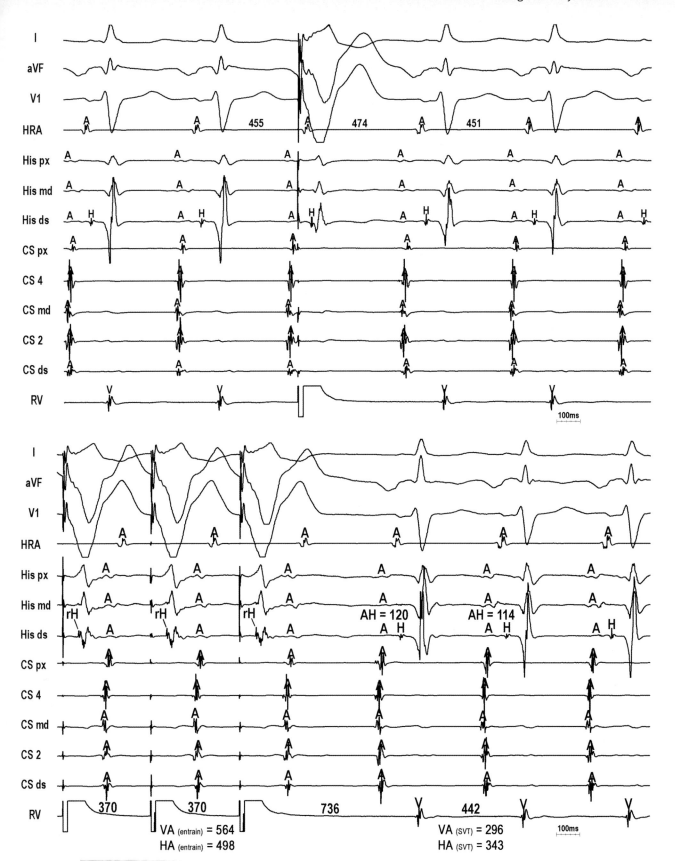

FIGURE 6-14 PJRT. *Top*: A His refractory VPD delays the atrium by 19 ms, indicating the presence of a decremental AP. *Bottom*: Entrainment from the ventricle with antidromic capture of the His bundle and a pseudo AAV response (true AV). Atrial activations during entrainment and tachycardia are identical. The PPI − TCL = 294 ms, corrected PPI (cPPI) = 288 ms, ΔVA = 268 ms, and ΔHA = 155 ms all yield a false diagnosis of atypical AVNRT.

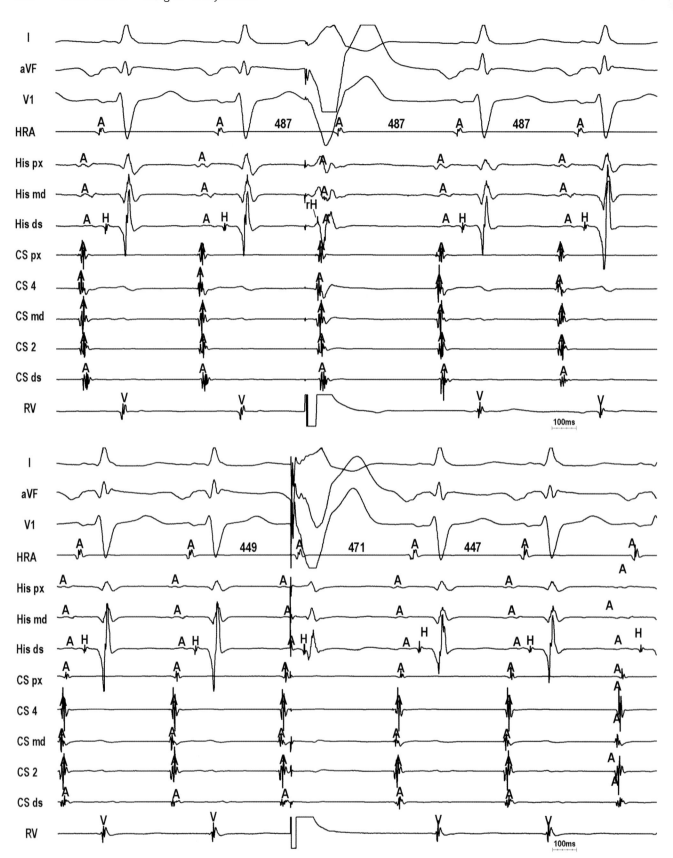

FIGURE 6-15 Apparent absence of resetting during PJRT. *Top*: An early-coupled VPD seemingly fails to reset tachycardia because the degree of VPD prematurity is offset by an equal degree of AP conduction delay (full compensation). *Bottom*: A late-coupled (His refractory) VPD resets tachycardia with delay (22 ms) confirming the presence of a decremental AP.

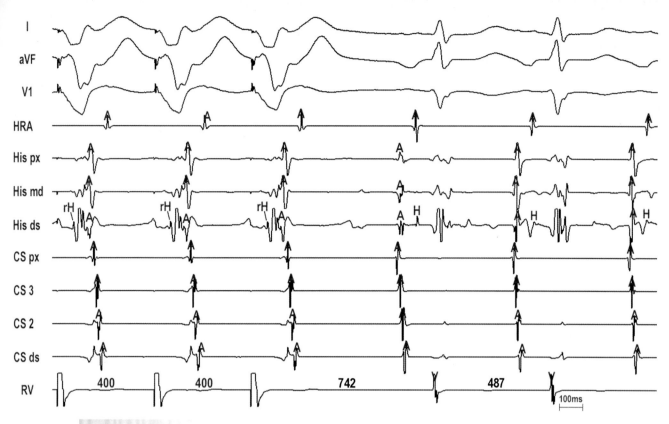

FIGURE 6-16 Atypical AVNRT with a true AAV response. During entrainment from the ventricle with antidromic capture of the His bundle, retrograde conduction occurs over the FP. Upon pacing cessation, retrograde conduction occurs over both the FP and SP (retrograde double fire), resulting in a true AAV response and very long PPI (742 ms, PPI − TCL = 255 ms).

In contrast, the upper limb of the circuit for PJRT involves both the atrium and AV node, and the AH interval is, therefore, a true interval reflecting sequential activation of the atrium/AV node/His bundle axis and similar to the AH interval during atrial entrainment. During entrainment of tachycardia from the atrium (or atrial pacing at the TCL), the ΔAH (AH$_{(entrainment)}$ − AH$_{(SVT)}$) criteria differentiates tachycardia circuits whose upper portion is completely intranodal (NFRT/atypical AVNRT) versus partially extranodal (PJRT).[1,27] The ΔAH is long (>40 ms) for AVNRT/NFRT but short (<20 ms) for PJRT. A major limitation of ΔAH criteria, however, is the sensitivity of the AV node to rapid fluctuations in autonomic tone so that comparison of AH intervals between tachycardia and pacing should be done close in time, allowing for minimal change in the autonomic state of the patient.

ABLATION

Because the ablation target depends on the mechanism of the AV node–dependent long RP tachycardia, it is critical to establish its exact diagnosis. Concealed, decremental AV APs (PJRT) can be localized by activation mapping either during ORT or constant ventricular pacing with most APs located along the posteroseptum near the coronary sinus ostium (Figs. 6-18 to 6-20). Mapping during ventricular pacing, however, can be more difficult than during ORT when 1) FP preempts AP

conduction, 2) retrograde block occurs over the AP despite the slowest ventricular pacing rate allowable by sinus rhythm, and 3) ORT is reproducibly initiated by ventricular stimulation. The concealed, NF/NV APs involved in long RP tachycardias (NFRT, atypical AVNRT-NF) seem to originate from the SP or left atrio-nodal input of the AV node.[4,7–9] The SP (or left atrio-nodal input) of the AV node can therefore be the target site of these APs as well as for atypical AVNRT using either standard SP ablation during sinus rhythm or activation mapping of the SP atrial exit site.[28] In contrast to SP ablation of typical (slow–fast) AVNRT, retrograde FP conduction may be absent for long RP tachycardias, making radiofrequency (RF) monitoring of junctional-atrio (JA) conduction difficult. A cautious piecemeal approach, accepting only slow junctional rhythms during RF delivery, and immediate discontinuation of RF energy with rapid junctional ectopy can allow for successful SP ablation without causing inadvertent AV block.

SUMMARY

For AV node–dependent long RP tachycardias, positive responses to His refractory VPDs (termination with VA block, resetting with advancement or delay) is the single best maneuver to identify the presence of an AP but does not necessarily prove its participation in the circuit. Establishing the exact mechanism

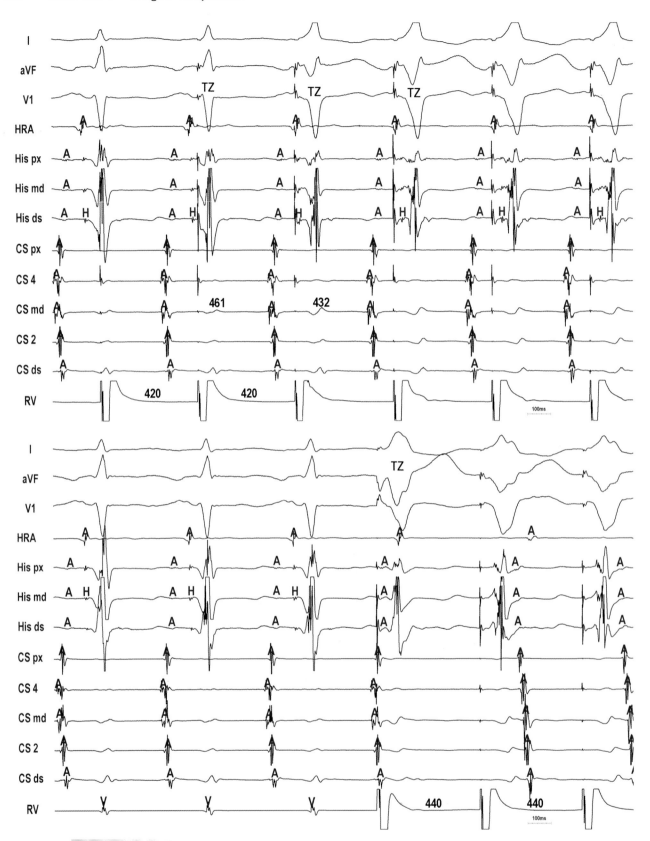

FIGURE 6-17 Advancement (*top*) and termination (*bottom*) of PJRT in the transition zone (TZ) during onset of ventricular overdrive pacing. *Top*: The third pacing stimulus is His refractory (unperturbed His bundle potential, QRS fusion) and advances the atrium by 29 ms, indicating the presence of an AP. *Bottom*: The first pacing stimulus is His refractory (QRS fusion) and terminates tachycardia with VA block—also identifying the presence of an AP. Subsequent paced complexes conduct over the FP of the AV node.

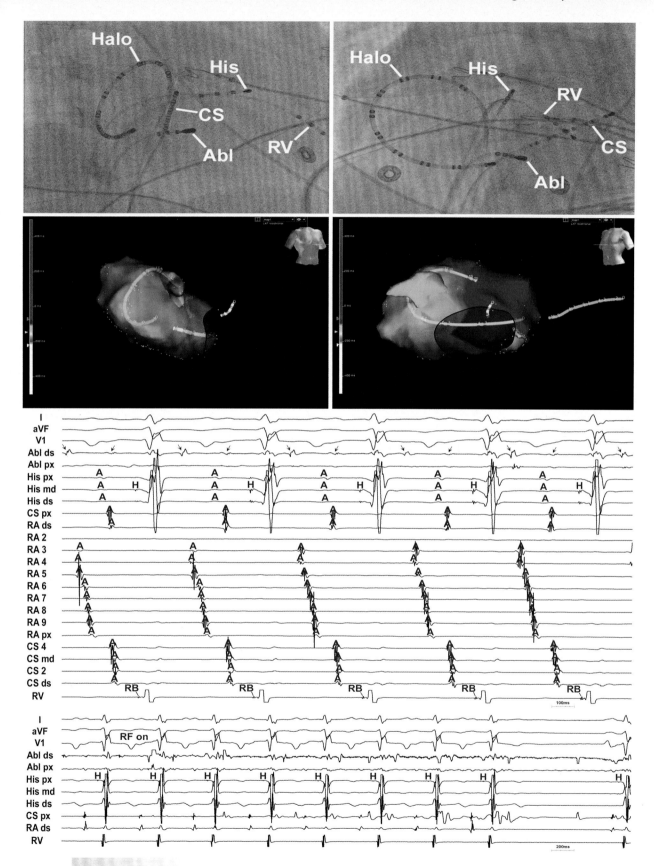

FIGURE 6-18 Ablation of PJRT. The ablation catheter is positioned along the right atrial posteroseptum where it records double potentials (*arrows*) across a functional line of counterclockwise cavo-tricuspid isthmus block during PJRT. Note the "early (*white*) meets late (*purple*)" along the posteroseptum with isochronal clustering between them. The first potential is very early (pre–P wave × 80 ms), where RF application terminated tachycardia in 2.9 sec.

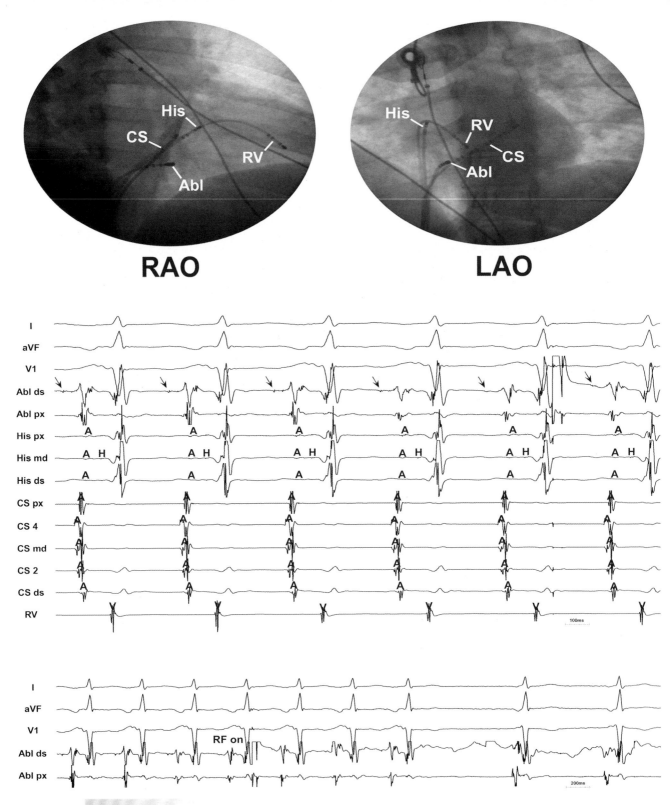

FIGURE 6-19 Ablation of PJRT. The ablation catheter is positioned along the right posteroseptum where it records high frequency potentials (*arrows*) preceding P wave onset × 77 ms. RF application terminated tachycardia in 1.3 sec.

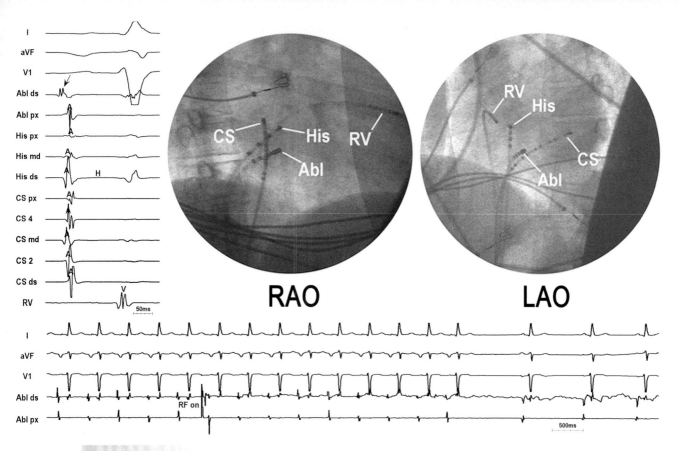

FIGURE 6-20 Ablation of PJRT. The ablation catheter is positioned along the right posteroseptum at the coronary sinus ostium where it records the earliest site of atrial activation during tachycardia (*arrow*, pre–P wave by 26 ms). Application of RF energy terminated tachycardia in 4.1 sec.

of a long RP tachycardia that demonstrates a positive response to His refractory VPDs requires additional pacing maneuvers in the atrium and ventricle to delineate the upper and lower limbs of its circuit, respectively (Table 6-1).[1]

UNUSUAL ELECTROPHYSIOLOGIC PHENOMENA

CYCLE LENGTH ALTERNANS

Cycle length alternans during a long RP tachycardia can result from alternating conduction over two different pathways in either the antegrade or retrograde limbs. During retrograde conduction, these two different pathways could be a longitudinally

dissociated SP/AP (or two distinct but closely spaced SPs/APs) with different conduction velocities/refractoriness that cause alternating short and long RP intervals with the same atrial activation pattern during atypical AVNRT or atypical ORT, respectively (**Fig. 6-21**; see also **Fig. 7-45**).

COUMEL'S LAW IN THE ATRIUM

Similar to the increase in VA interval with BBB ipsilateral to the AP during ORT, cavo-tricuspid or mitral isthmus block septal to a right- or left-sided AP, respectively, can increase the AV interval and generally the TCL (provided that the increase in AV interval is not equally counterbalanced by a decrease in the VA interval), demonstrating that the ipsilateral atrium is an integral part of the circuit (**Fig. 6-22**).[5] For long RP tachycardias,

---

TABLE 6-1 Criteria differentiating the three AV node–dependent long RP tachycardias terminated or reset by His refractory VPDs

Diagnosis	PJRT	NFRT	Atypical AVNRT + bystander NF AP
Upper circuit (ΔAH)	<20 ms	>40 ms or $AH_{(SVT)} < AH_{(NSR)}$	>40 ms or $AH_{(SVT)} < AH_{(NSR)}$
Lower circuit (PPI–TCL)	<125ms	<125 ms	>125 ms

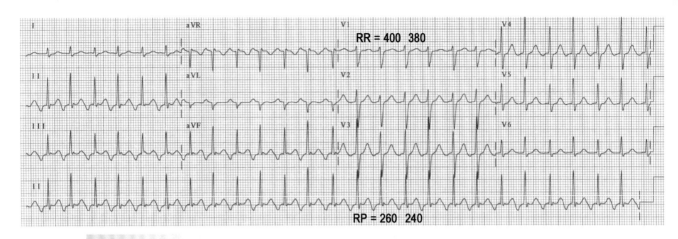

FIGURE 6-21 Long RP NCT with both cycle length and QRS alternans. The RP shortens and lengthens on a beat-to-beat basis causing cycle length alternans. QRS alternans is also present.

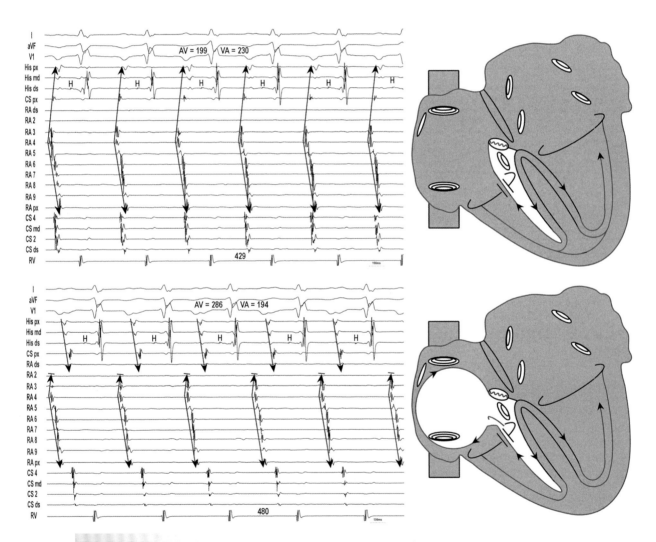

FIGURE 6-22 Coumel's law in the atrium. During PJRT, the earliest site of atrial activation is along the right posteroseptum (RA 4). *Top*: PJRT with counterclockwise (lateral to medial) cavo-tricuspid isthmus (CTI) conduction septal to the AP. *Bottom*: PJRT with functional counterclockwise (lateral to medial) CTI block septal to the AP. With CTI block, the RA free wall becomes incorporated into the circuit, increasing the intra-atrial (RA 4–His A) conduction time by 34 ms. An increase in the IACT along with a 53 ms increase in the AH interval converts the long RP tachycardia to a short RP tachycardia. The overall 87 ms increase in AV interval is partially compensated by a 36 ms decrease in the VA interval (because of the decremental properties of the AP), resulting in a net increase in TCL of 51 ms.

such a finding is unique to PJRT and excludes nodal tachycardias (atypical AVNRT, NFRT) where the atrium is not a part of the circuit.

REFERENCES

1. Ho RT, Frisch DR, Pavri BB, Levi SA, Greenspon AJ. Electrophysiological features differentiating the atypical atrioventricular node-dependent long RP supraventricular tachycardias. Circ Arrhythm Electrophysiol 2013;6:597–605.

2. Lerman BB, Greenberg M, Overholt ED, et al. Differential electrophysiologic properties of decremental retrograde pathways in long RP' tachycardia. Circulation 1987;76:21–31.

3. Ho RT. Diagnosis and ablation of long RP supraventricular tachycardias. Curr Treat Options Cardiovasc Med 2015;17:370.

4. Ho RT, Pavri BB. A long RP-interval tachycardia: what is the mechanism? Heart Rhythm 2013;10:456–458.

5. Ho RT, Yin A. Spontaneous conversion of a long RP to short RP tachycardia: what is the mechanism? Heart Rhythm 2014;11:522–525.

6. Rhim ES, Hillis MB, Mark GE, Ho RT. The ΔHA value during entrainment of a long RP tachycardia: another useful criterion for diagnosis of supraventricular tachycardia. J Cardiovasc Electrophysiol 2008;19:559–561.

7. Ho RT, Luebbert J. An unusual long RP tachycardia: what is the mechanism? Heart Rhythm 2012;9:1898–1901.

8. Ho RT, Levi SA. An atypical long RP tachycardia—what is the mechanism? Heart Rhythm 2013;10:1089–1090.

9. Ho RT, Fischman DL. Entrainment versus resetting of a long RP tachycardia: what is the diagnosis? Heart Rhythm 2012;9:312–314.

10. Bansal S, Berger RD, Spragg DD. An unusual long RP tachycardia: what is the mechanism? Heart Rhythm 2015;12:845–846.

11. Ho RT, Patel U, Weitz HH. Entrainment and resetting of a long RP tachycardia: which trumps which for diagnosis? Heart Rhythm 2010;7:714–715.

12. Bardy G, Packer D, German L, Coltorti F, Gallagher J. Paradoxical delay in accessory pathway conduction during long R-P' tachycardia after interpolated ventricular premature complexes. Am J Cardiol 1985;55:1223–1225.

13. Michaud GF, John R. Unusual response to a premature ventricular complex introduced during an episode of paroxysmal supraventricular tachycardia: what is the mechanism? Heart Rhythm 2009;6:279–280.

14. Divakara Menon S, Healey J, Nair G, et al. A case of long-RP tachycardia: what is the mechanism? J Cardiovasc Electrophysiol 2009;20:702–704.

15. Crawford TC, Morady F, Pelosi F Jr. A long R-P paroxysmal supraventricular tachycardia: what is the mechanism? Heart Rhythm 2007;4:1364–1365.

16. Yamabe H, Okumura K, Tabuchi T, Tsuchiya T, Yasue H. Double atrial responses to a single ventricular impulse in long RP' tachycardia. Pacing Clin Electrophysiol 1996;19:403–410.

17. Gauri AJ, Knight BP. Unusual response to ventricular pacing during a long RP tachycardia. J Cardiovasc Electrophysiol 2004;15:241–243.

18. Kaneko Y, Nakajima T, Irie T, Ota M, Iijima T, Kurabayashi M. V-A-A-V activation sequence at the onset of a long RP tachycardia: what is the mechanism? J Cardiovasc Electrophysiol 2015;26:101–103.

19. Kaneko Y, Nakajima T, Irie T, Iizuka T, Tamura S, Kurabayashi M. Atrial and ventricular activation sequence after ventricular induction/entrainment pacing during fast-slow atrioventricular nodal reentrant tachycardia: new insight into the use of V-A-A-V for the differential diagnosis of supraventricular tachycardia. Heart Rhythm 2017;14:1615–1622.

20. Michaud GF, Tada H, Chough S, et al. Differentiation of atypical atrioventricular node re-entrant tachycardia from orthodromic reciprocating tachycardia using a septal accessory pathway by the response to ventricular pacing. J Am Coll Cardiol 2001;38:1163–1167.

21. Ho RT, Mark GE, Rhim ES, Pavri BB, Greenspon AJ. Differentiating atrioventricular nodal reentrant tachycardia from atrioventricular reentrant tachycardia by ΔHA values during entrainment from the ventricle. Heart Rhythm 2008;5:83–88.

22. Bennett MT, Leong-Sit P, Gula LJ, et al. Entrainment for distinguishing atypical atrioventricular node reentrant tachycardia from atrioventricular reentrant tachycardia over septal accessory pathways with long-RP [corrected] tachycardia. Circ Arrhythm Electrophysiol 2011;4:506–509.

23. AlMahameed ST, Buxton AE, Michaud GF. New criteria during right ventricular pacing to determine the mechanism of supraventricular tachycardia. Circ Arrhythm Electrophysiol 2010;3:578–584.

24. Dandamudi G, Mokabberi R, Assal C, et al. A novel approach to differentiating orthodromic reciprocating tachycardia from atrioventricular nodal reentrant tachycardia. Heart Rhythm 2010;7:1326–1329.

25. Good E, Morady F. A long-RP supraventricular tachycardia: what is the mechanism? Heart Rhythm 2005;2:1387–1388.

26. Okabe T, Hummel JD, Kalbfleisch SJ. A long RP supraventricular tachycardia: what is the mechanism? Heart Rhythm 2017;14:462–464.

27. Man KC, Niebauer M, Daoud E, et al. Comparison of atrial-His intervals during tachycardia and atrial pacing in patients with long RP tachycardia. J Cardiovasc Electrophysiol 1995;6:700–710.

28. Jackman WM, Beckman KJ, McClelland JH, et al. Treatment of supraventricular tachycardia due to atrioventricular nodal reentry by radiofrequency catheter ablation of slow-pathway conduction. N Engl J Med 1992;327:313–318.

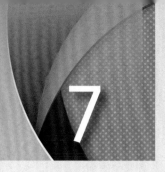

7 Atrio-ventricular Nodal Reentrant Tachycardia

> ## Introduction
> Atrio-ventricular nodal reentrant tachycardia (AVNRT) is the most common paroxysmal supraventricular tachycardia (SVT).

> ## The purpose of this chapter is to:
> 1. Discuss dual atrio-ventricular (AV) node physiology and its ECG manifestations.
> 2. Discuss the AVNRT circuit.
> 3. Describe the electrophysiologic features and transition zones of AVNRT.
> 4. Differentiate AVNRT from ORT/atrial tachycardia (AT).
> 5. Differentiate AVNRT from junctional tachycardia (JT).

DUAL AV NODE PHYSIOLOGY

Both the AV node and His bundle are located within the triangle of Koch, which is formed by the 1) septal leaflet of the tricuspid valve, 2) tendon of Todaro, and 3) coronary sinus (CS) ostium. The penetrating His bundle is located at the apex of the triangle. The compact AV node is a subendocardial structure in the right atrium located posterior and inferior to the His bundle along the interatrial septum. Dual AV node physiology (longitudinal dissociation of the AV node) refers to anatomically and functionally distinct inputs (or approaches) to the AV node: the slow pathway (SP, or right inferior extension) and fast pathway (FP, or superior extension).[1] The SP is located along the posteroseptal right atrium near the ostium of the CS and demonstrates slow conduction/short refractoriness (α limb). The FP is located along the anteroseptal right atrium superior to the His bundle and exhibits rapid conduction/long refractoriness (β limb). When the refractoriness of each pathway complements the conduction properties of the other, they can create the substrate for AVNRT. Left atrio-nodal connections (left inferior extensions) also exist and are generally found within 2 cm of the CS os.[2]

ECG MANIFESTATIONS OF DUAL AV NODE PHYSIOLOGY

12-Lead ECG manifestations of dual AV node physiology include 1) two distinct families of PR intervals for a given sinus rate, 2) PR alternans, 3) dual antegrade response tachycardia (DART, also called "double fire," "1:2" tachycardia, and paroxysmal non-reentrant tachycardia), and 4) AVNRT (**Figs. 7-1 to 7-11**).[3] Two families of PR intervals can occur spontaneously or be unmasked by critically timed atrial or ventricular premature depolarizations (VPDs) that conceal into a longitudinally dissociated AV node (sequential FP/SP conduction) (**Figs. 7-1 to 7-3**). Sustained conduction over the SP (or FP) is maintained by repetitive concealment from SP to FP (or vice versa), rendering the latter refractory with each subsequent sinus impulse.[4] A rare manifestation is PR alternans (alternating FP and SP conduction after each sinus complex) (**Figs. 7-4 and 7-5**).[5] PR alternans result from 2:1 block in the FP when the SP is capable of 1:1 conduction. SP conduction is only manifest when FP conduction is absent. Isolated or sustained dual antegrade responses result from simultaneous conduction over the FP and SP, generating two QRS complexes for each P wave—the latter potentially causing a tachycardia-mediated cardiomyopathy (simultaneous FP/SP conduction) (**Figs. 7-6 to 7-11**).[6–10] RR irregularity generated by 2:1 and 1:1 conduction can be mistaken for atrial fibrillation. Determinants of DART are 1) sufficient difference between SP and FP conduction times (generally, $AH_{SP} - AH_{FP} > 300$ ms), 2) $H_{SP}-H_{FP}$ interval is greater than the His-Purkinje effective refractory period (ERP), 3) absence of retrograde conduction over each AV nodal pathway following antegrade conduction over its counterpart, and 4) appropriate timing of sinus impulses relative to preceding AV nodal conduction (critical HA interval).[8,9] Dual antegrade responses often require $AH_{SP} > 400$ ms. The $H_{SP}-H_{FP}$ interval must exceed His-Purkinje refractoriness to allow consecutive activation of the His-Purkinje by a single sinus input. Aberration is common

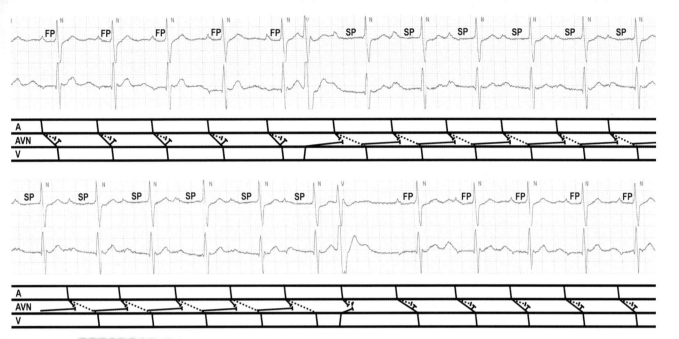

FIGURE 7-1 Dual AV node physiology (FP/SP alternans induced by PVCs). Sinus P waves conduct over the FP with mild PR prolongation (260 ms). An interpolated PVC conceals retrogradely into both the FP and SP. Because the FP has a longer refractory period, the subsequent P wave finds it refractory and conducts over the SP with a long PR interval (520 ms). Repetitive concealment from SP to FP ("linking") maintains SP conduction until another PVC. This second PVC again conceals into both the FP and SP rendering them refractory upon arrival of the next sinus impulse. The subsequent compensatory pause allows both pathways to recover, but FP then preempts SP conduction. Solid and dashed lines represent FP and SP conduction, respectively.

because of longitudinal dissociation within the His-Purkinje system (**Fig. 7-9**).

Dual Antegrade Response versus His Bundle Extrasystole

His bundle extrasystoles can mimic isolated dual antegrade responses. Similar to dual antegrade responses, His bundle extrasystoles can be associated with aberration due either to its prematurity relative to His-Purkinje refractoriness or site of origin within the His bundle (committed fibers in the His bundle destined for specific bundle branches). A short HV interval and retrograde His bundle activation sequence (His ds to px) suggest an extrasystole arising from the His bundle distal to the recording site (**Fig. 7-12**).[11] Antegrade His bundle activation, however, is not specific to a dual antegrade response and can occur with an extrasystole arising from the AV node or proximal His bundle. While the target ablation site for DART is the SP, ablation of His bundle extrasystoles carries a greater risk of AV block depending on its location along the AV node–His bundle axis.

ELECTROPHYSIOLOGIC STUDY

During programmed atrial extrastimulation, dual AV node physiology is defined by $\geq$50 ms increment in the AH interval ("AH jump" or discontinuity) for a 10 ms decrement in the A_1A_2 coupling interval.[12] An AH jump $\geq$50 ms arbitrarily differentiates physiologic decrement over the FP from SP conduction, and the A_1A_2 interval defines the antegrade FP ERP. During rapid atrial pacing, conduction over the SP is suggested when the PR interval

exceeds the atrial pacing cycle length (crossover phenomenon).[13] During programmed ventricular extrastimulation, retrograde dual AV node physiology is manifested by an increase in the VA interval accompanied by a switch from a midline atrial activation pattern earliest along the anteroseptum (FP) to the posteroseptum (SP).

ATRIO-VENTRICULAR NODAL REENTRANT TACHYCARDIA CIRCUIT

For typical (slow–fast) AVNRT, the antegrade and retrograde limbs of the circuit are the SP and FP, respectively, and reversed for its atypical counterpart (fast–slow AVNRT). The presence of variable AV nodal pathways (e.g., intermediate SP, "superior" SP, left atrio-nodal inputs), however, can produce other atypical AVNRTs (slow–slow, fast–slow with "superior" SP, and AVNRT with left atrio-nodal inputs mimicking ORT with a left-sided AP).[14–16] The conduction time over each pathway must exceed the refractory period of its counterpart to allow the depolarizing wavefront to constantly encounter excitable tissue. At the lower turnaround point of the circuit, the wavefront splits to activate the ventricle antegradely while simultaneously activating the atrium retrogradely (simultaneous ventriculo-atrial activation). At the upper turnaround point, the wavefront activates the atrium retrogradely while simultaneously activating the ventricle antegradely. The existence of an upper common final pathway (UCFP) separate from the atrium is controversial.[17,18] Occurrence of JA block during AVNRT supports the

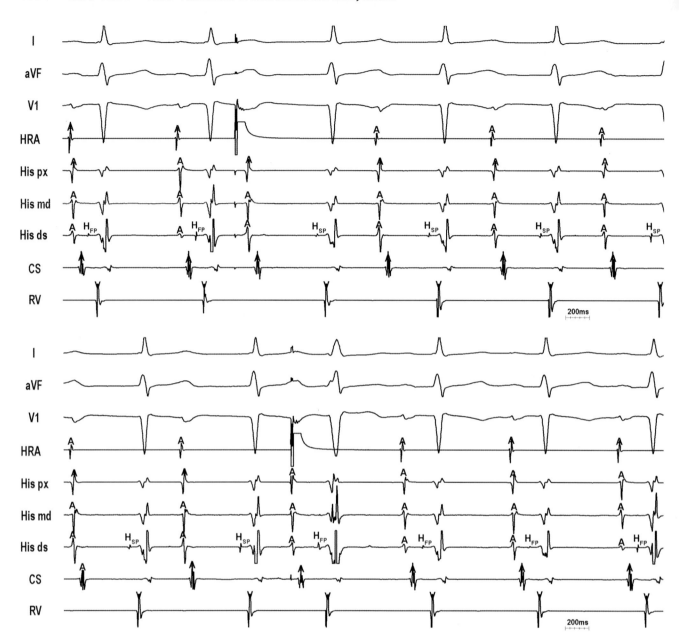

FIGURE 7-2 Dual AV node physiology (FP/SP alternans induced by APCs). Sinus impulses conduct over the FP. An APC is delivered, which encounters FP refractoriness and conducts over the SP. Repetitive concealment from SP to FP ("linking") maintains SP conduction. Spontaneous FP conduction resumes coincident with a pacing stimulus delivered during a sinus beat.

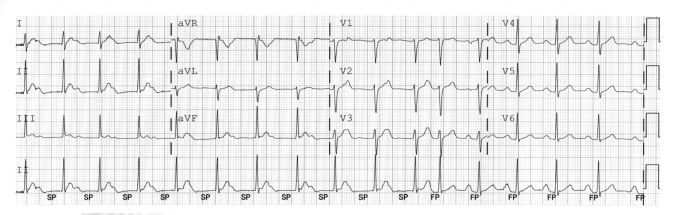

FIGURE 7-3 Dual AV node physiology. Spontaneous conversion from SP to FP conduction (sinus rhythm with two families of PR intervals).

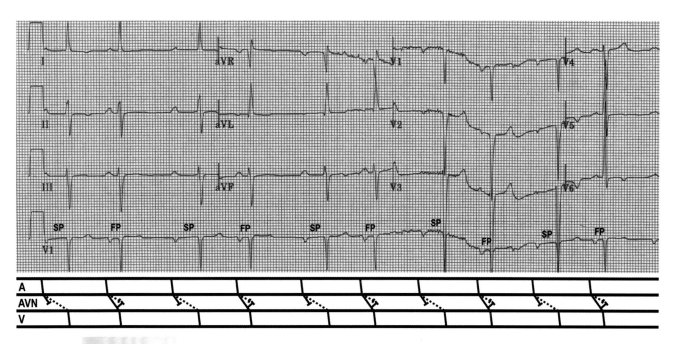

FIGURE 7-4 PR alternans. Alternating conduction over the FP and SP produces two sets of PR intervals (180 and 380 ms) changing on a beat-to-beat basis. Conduction over the SP becomes manifest only when FP conduction is absent. Solid and dashed lines represent FP and SP conduction, respectively.

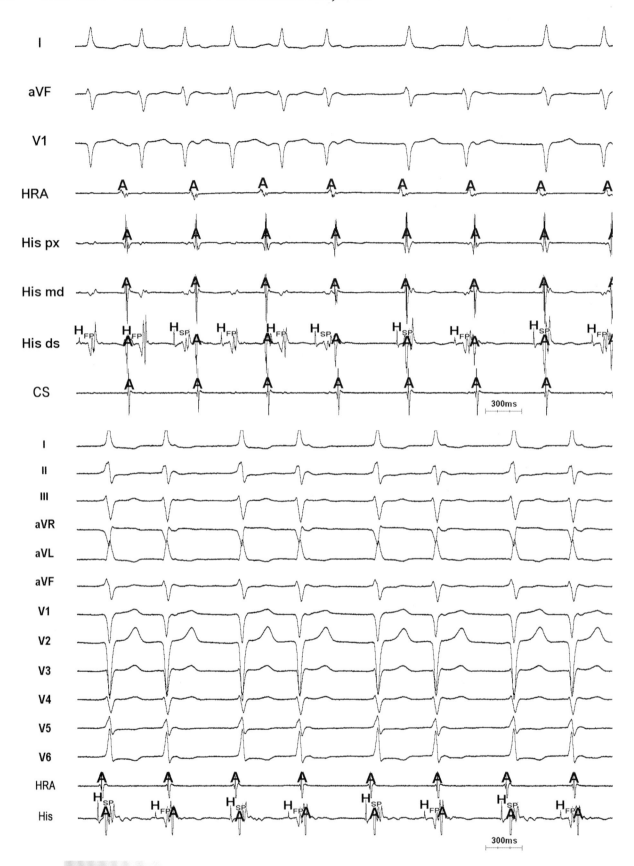

FIGURE 7-5 DART transitioning to PR alternans. During DART, retrograde concealment from SP into FP renders the FP relatively and absolutely refractory, abolishing the dual antegrade response after the second and fourth sinus beats, respectively. Isolated SP conduction after the fourth sinus beat is followed by alternating SP/FP conduction with prolonged AH_{FP} due to concealment from SP into FP ("linking") and relative FP refractoriness.

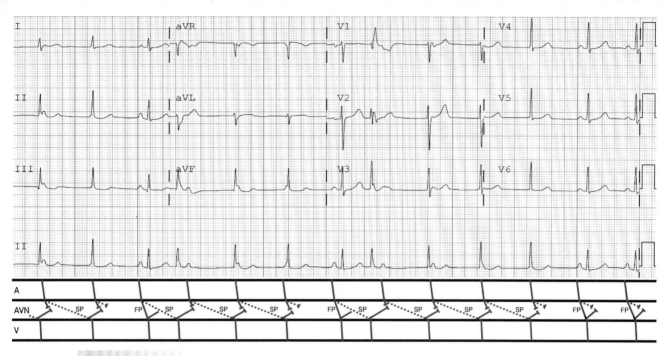

FIGURE 7-6 Intermittent dual antegrade responses followed by isolated SP Wenckebach conduction.

presence of a UCFP. A lower common final pathway (LCFP) is less controversial.[19–22] Wenckebach-type and 2:1 blocks above the His bundle recording site during AVNRT support a LCFP that involves the distal AV node/proximal His bundle.

ELECTROPHYSIOLOGIC FEATURES OF AVNRT

12-LEAD ECG

The 12-lead ECG of typical AVNRT is a 1) regular, narrow complex tachycardia; 2) short RP interval <70 ms; and a 3) midline, superior P-wave axis (**Figs. 7-13 and 7-14**).[23–25] Antegrade activation of the ventricle simultaneously with retrograde activation of FP and atrium results in a short RP interval <70 ms. Retrograde P waves are buried within or distort the terminal portion of the QRS complex causing pseudo S waves in the inferior leads and pseudo r′ in V1. Because atrial activation originates from the FP along the interatrial septum, P waves are narrow and have a midline, superior axis (negative in inferior leads, positive in aVR and aVL). Atypical AVNRT is a regular, narrow complex tachycardia with a long RP interval and a midline superior P-wave axis because retrograde conduction occurs over the SP (**Figs. 7-13 and 7-15**).

ELECTROPHYSIOLOGIC STUDY

The electrophysiologic features of typical AVNRT are 1) antegrade His bundle electrograms preceding QRS complexes, 2) VA interval <70 ms, and 3) earliest site of atrial activation at the FP (His bundle region) (**Fig. 7-14**).[23–25] The VA interval

is short (<70 ms) because activation of the ventricle is simultaneous with the atrium ("A on V" tachycardia). A negative VA interval occurs when the antegrade conduction time to the ventricle exceeds the retrograde conduction time to the atrium. Atrial activation is concentric and earliest at the His bundle region. Atypical AVNRT manifests a long VA interval and earliest site of atrial activation at the SP (CS os region) (**Fig. 7-15**). Variability of AV nodal pathways, however, can cause different types of AVNRT with midline or left eccentric atrial activation patterns occurring anywhere within the tachycardia cycle length (TCL).

AV Relationship

The existence of a LCFP and UCFP allows AVNRT to persist despite block to the ventricle and atrium, respectively. Therefore, AVNRT does not have an obligatory 1:1 AV relationship.[19,21,22] Physiologic block to the ventricle can occur either above or below the His bundle and is often a transient phenomenon induced by abrupt changes (long–short sequences) in cycle length (e.g., tachycardia initiation) (**Figs. 7-16 to 7-25**). An ECG clue to typical AVNRT with 2:1 LCFP block is the finding of a P wave (narrow, superior axis) buried exactly between two QRS complexes (mid-diastole). AVNRT with Wenckebach-type block above the His bundle suggests that the LCFP can involve the distal AV node (**Fig. 7-20**). AVNRT can also be induced despite pathologic AV block in the His-Purkinje system (**Figs. 7-26 and 7-27**).[26] Block to the atrium is less common and supports the existence of an UCFP (**Figs. 7-28 to 7-30**). Concealed AVNRT results from transient block in both UCFP and LCFP resulting in a pause, which is a multiple of the TCL.[27]

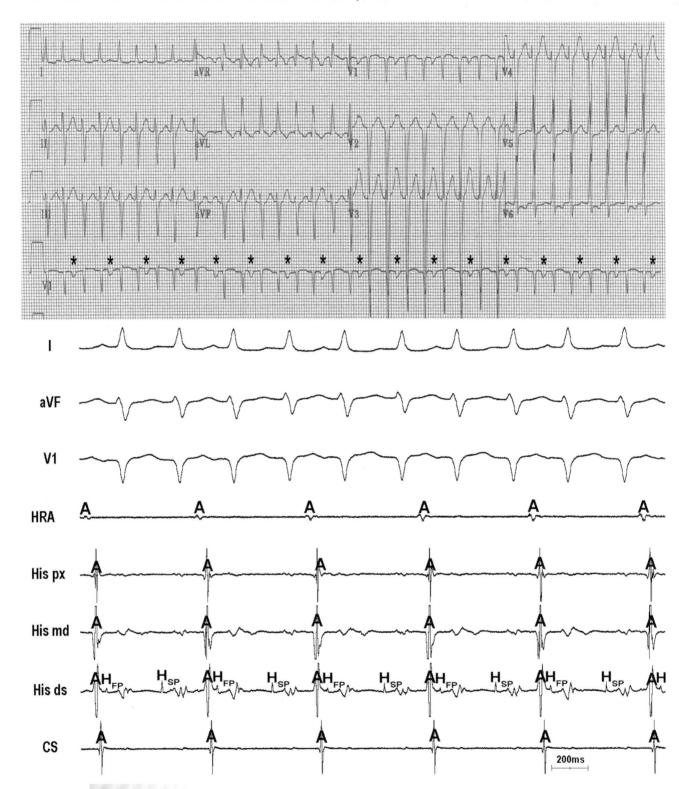

FIGURE 7-7 DART. Every P wave (*asterisks*) except the fourth conduct over the FP and SP producing two sets of PR intervals (160 and 460 ms). The fourth P wave is preceded by the shortest RP interval on the tracing, falls into the relative refractory period of the FP (due to preceding concealment from the SP), and conducts with delay over the FP (PR = 280 ms). Reduction in the difference between SP and FP conduction causes momentary loss of the dual antegrade response. His bundle recordings show each sinus impulse generating two His bundle potentials (AH_{FP} = 75 ms, AH_{SP} = 383 ms) and QRS complexes.

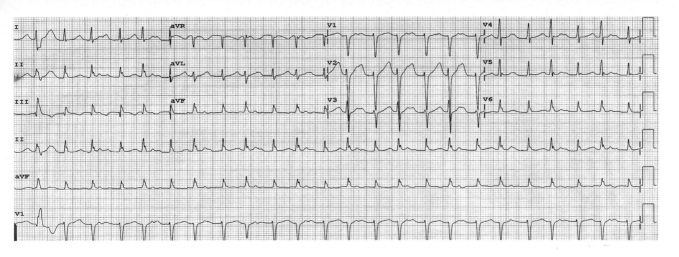

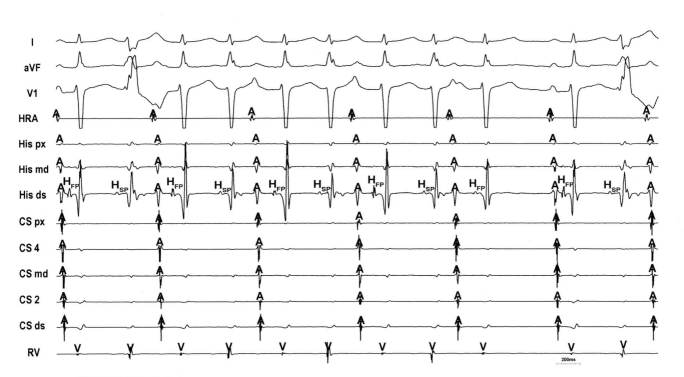

FIGURE 7-8 DART. P waves generate two His bundle potentials and QRS complexes resulting in a bigeminal tachycardia. Progressive decrease in the $H_{SP}A$ interval encroaches on FP refractoriness, resulting in prolongation of subsequent AH_{FP} intervals and eventual loss of the dual antegrade response. Resumption of the dual antegrade response is accompanied by a long–short sequence inducing RBBB aberration.

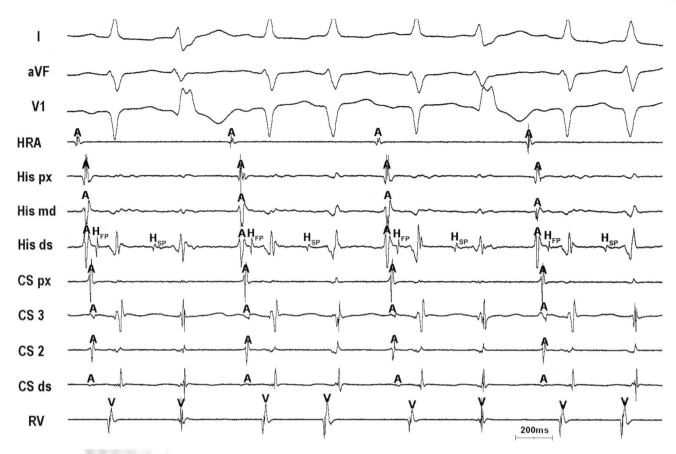

FIGURE 7-9 DART. Successive activations of the His bundle (H_{FP} + H_{SP}) encroach on His-Purkinje refractoriness causing HV prolongation and BBB. Alternating RBBB and LBBB is caused by retrograde concealed transeptal conduction from unblocked to blocked bundle, exposing each bundle branch to different alternating long–short sequences.

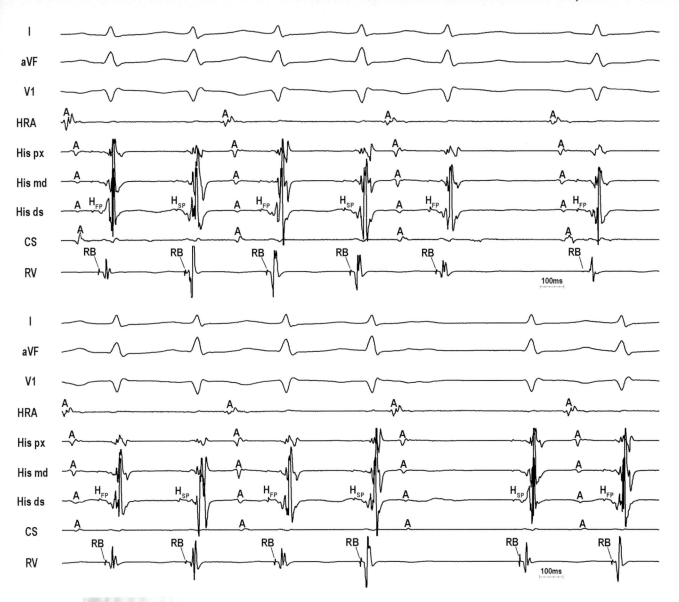

FIGURE 7-10 DART. Progressive decrease in the H$_{SP}$A interval encroaches on FP refractoriness resulting in prolongation of subsequent AH$_{FP}$ intervals. Sufficient conduction delay (*top*) or block (*bottom*) due to relative and absolute FP refractoriness causes momentary loss of the dual antegrade response. Note that the AH$_{SP}$ interval is longer with than without the dual antegrade response because of retrograde concealment from FP into SP.

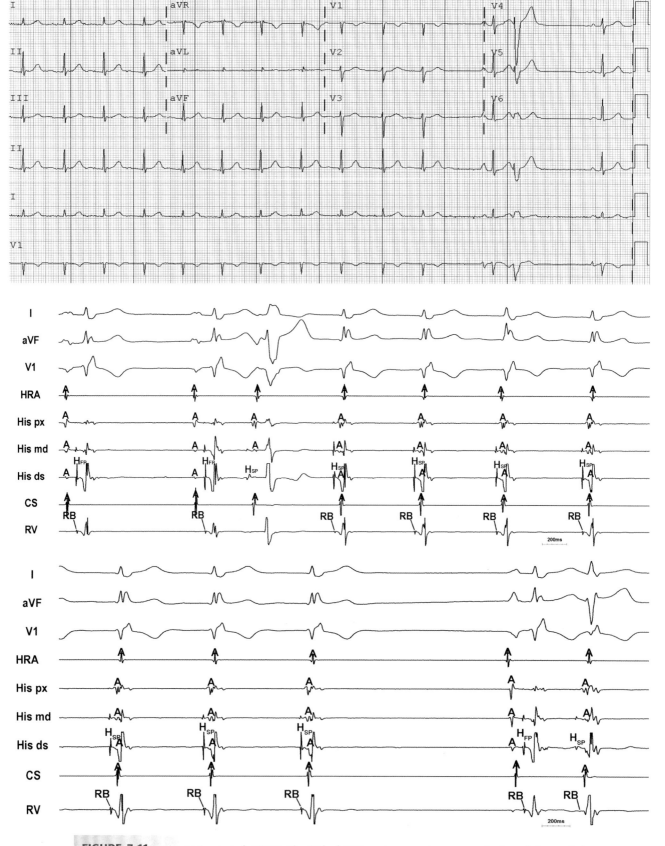

FIGURE 7-11 DAR initiating typical AVNRT. The 12-lead ECG captures spontaneous termination of slow typical AVNRT followed by a dual antegrade response. Intracardiac recordings show a sinus P wave conducting with a dual antegrade response followed by initiation of AVNRT. Long–short sequences cause LBBB aberration. Tachycardia terminates with AV block followed by another dual antegrade reeponse.

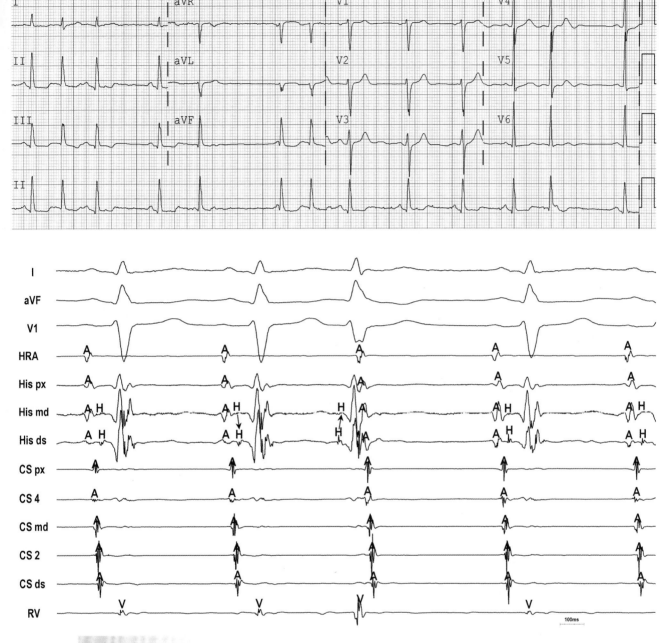

FIGURE 7-12 His bundle extrasystoles mimicking dual antegrade responses. Note the retrograde His bundle activation sequence (His ds to His md) preceding the extrasystoles.

Typical AVNRT

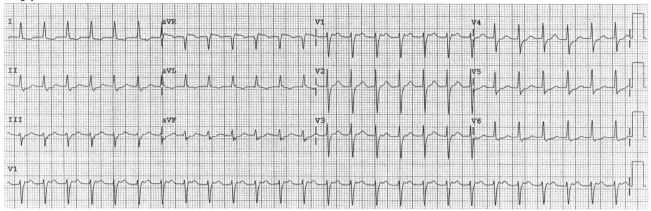

Atypical AVNRT

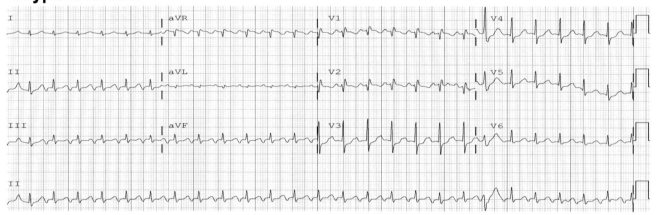

FIGURE 7-13 Typical and atypical AVNRT. During typical AVNRT, the RP interval is short and narrow retrograde P waves deform the end of the QRS complex causing terminal positivity in V1 (pseudo R′) and negativity inferiorly (pseudo S wave). During atypical AVNRT, the RP interval is long and retrograde P waves are also positive in V1 and negative inferiorly. A late-coupled PVC fails to affect tachycardia.

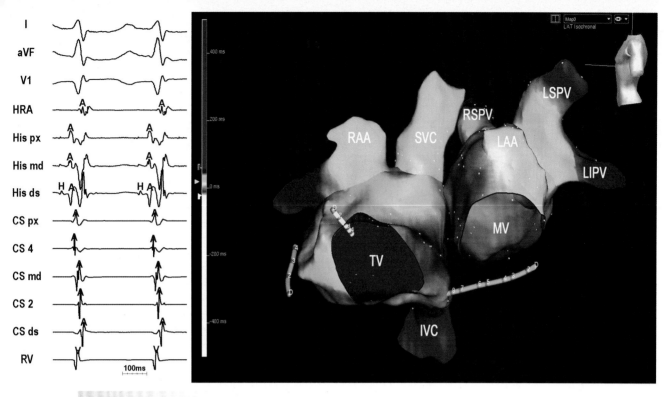

FIGURE 7-14 Typical AVNRT. The earliest site of atrial activation (*white*) is at the anteroseptum (His bundle region).

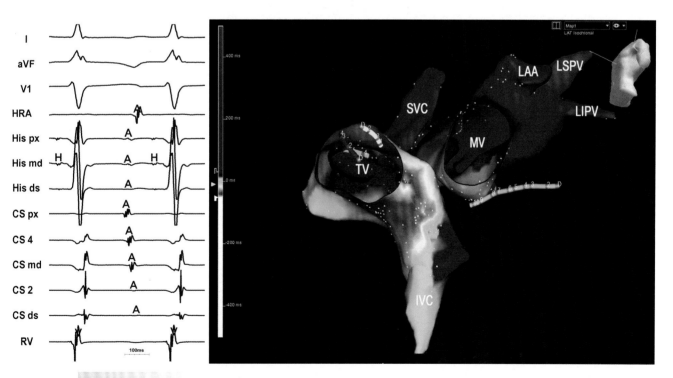

FIGURE 7-15 Atypical AVNRT. The earliest site of atrial activation (*white*) is at the posteroseptum (CS os region).

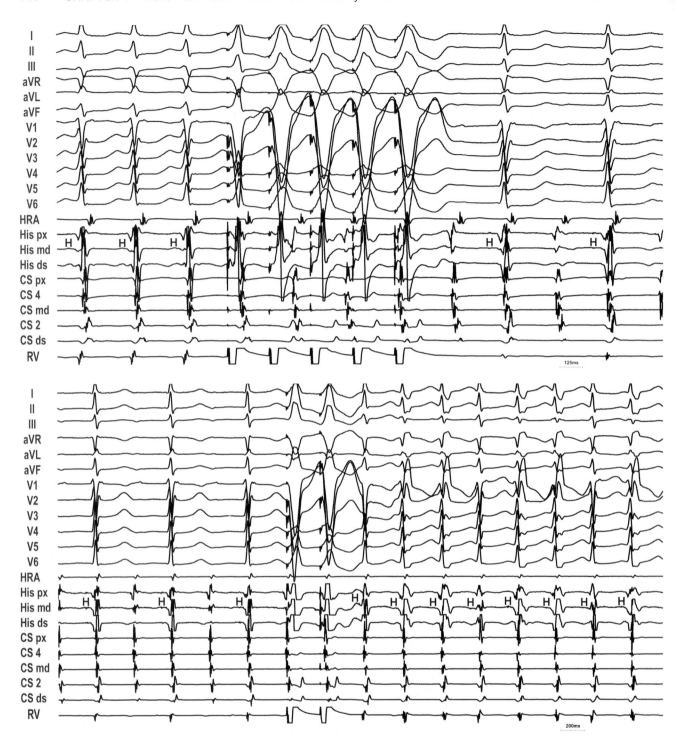

FIGURE 7-16 Typical AVNRT with 2:1 block above the His bundle. *Top*: Overdrive ventricular pacing fails to accelerate the atrium to the pacing cycle length but retrogradely penetrates the LCFP, rendering it functionally refractory upon pacing cessation and inducing LCFP block. Exposure of the LCFP to a "long–short" sequence initiates and perpetuates 2:1 LCFP block until interrupted by two ventricular paced complexes with resumption of 1:1 conduction (albeit with 3:2 RBBB).

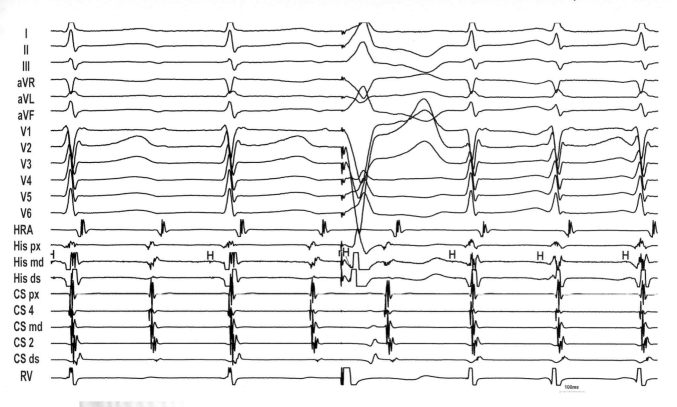

FIGURE 7-17 Typical AVNRT with 2:1 block above the His bundle. A single PVC retrogradely penetrates the His bundle and advances the atrium. This interrupts the "long–short" H–H cycle perpetuating 2:1 LCFP block and causes a momentary "frameshift" in the pattern of conduction. After the PVC, exposure of the LCFP to a shorter "long" cycle (rH–H interval) reduces LCFP refractoriness and allows resumption of 1:1 conduction.

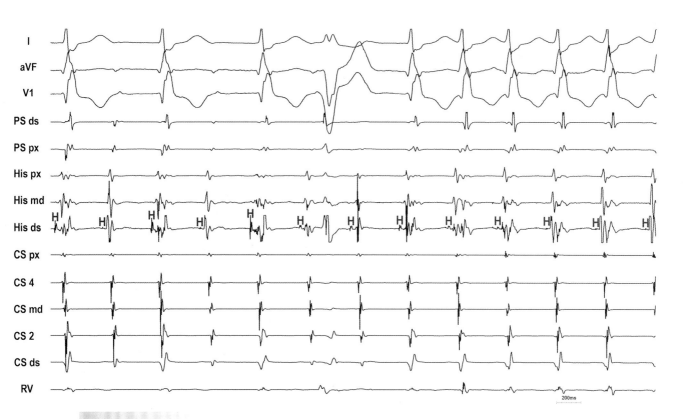

FIGURE 7-18 Typical AVNRT with 2:1 block below the His bundle. A single PVC retrogradely penetrates the LCFP below the His bundle, interrupting the "long–short" sequence perpetuating 2:1 LCFP block Nodal allowing 1:1 conduction.

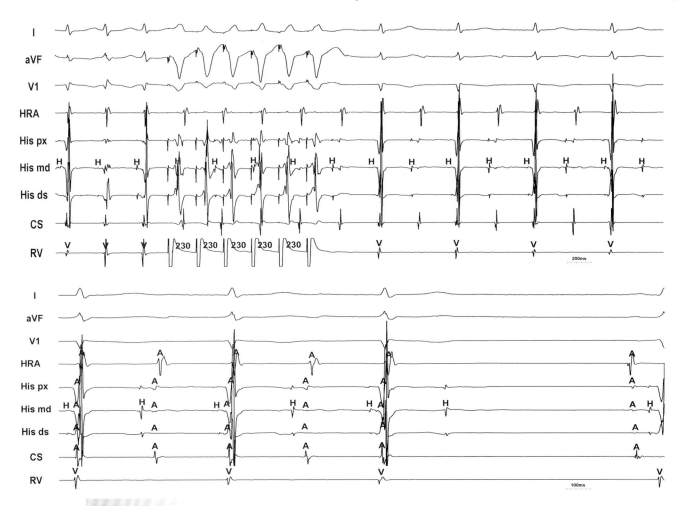

FIGURE 7-19 Typical AVNRT with 2:1 block below the His bundle. Overdrive ventricular pacing fails to accelerate the atrium to the pacing cycle length but retrogradely penetrates the LCFP below the His bundle, rendering it functionally refractory upon pacing cessation. Exposure of the LCFP to "long–short" sequences initiates and perpetuates 2:1 LCFP block. Tachycardia terminates with retrograde block in the FP coincident with LCFP block. Spontaneous termination with HA block excludes JT.

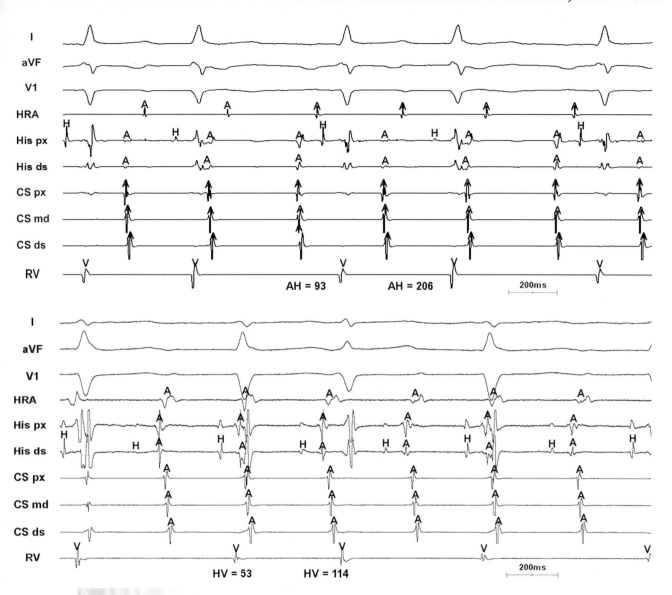

FIGURE 7-20 AVNRT with 3:2 suprahisian (*top*) and infrahisian (*bottom*) Wenckebach block. During suprahisian block, the AH interval increases from 93 to 206 ms before block, while the HV interval remains constant. During infrahisian block, the HV interval increases from 53 to 114 ms before block, while the AH interval remains constant. The QRS complex is narrow despite HV prolongation, indicating that the site of delay is either in the distal His bundle (beyond its recording site) or simultaneously in both bundle branches.

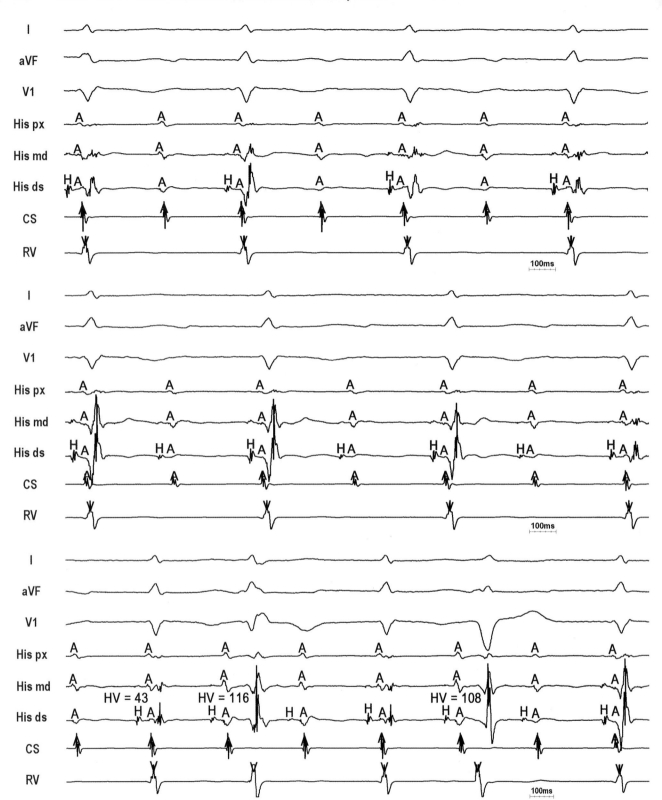

FIGURE 7-21 Typical AVNRT with 2:1 suprahisian (*top*), 2:1 infrahisian (*middle*), and 3:2 infrahisian Wenckebach (*bottom*) block. Infrahisian Wenckebach is associated with RBBB and LBBB.

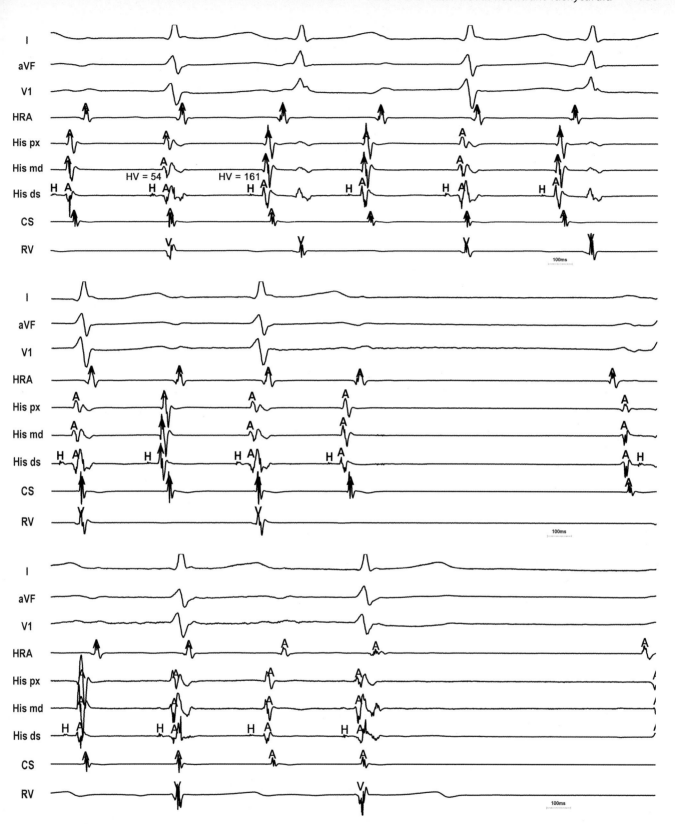

FIGURE 7-22 Typical AVNRT with 3:2 Wenckebach and 2:1 infrahisian block. During 3:2 Wenckebach, the HV interval increases from 54 to 161 ms accompanied by incomplete RBBB before block. Block in the SP terminates tachycardia with and without simultaneous infrahisian block.

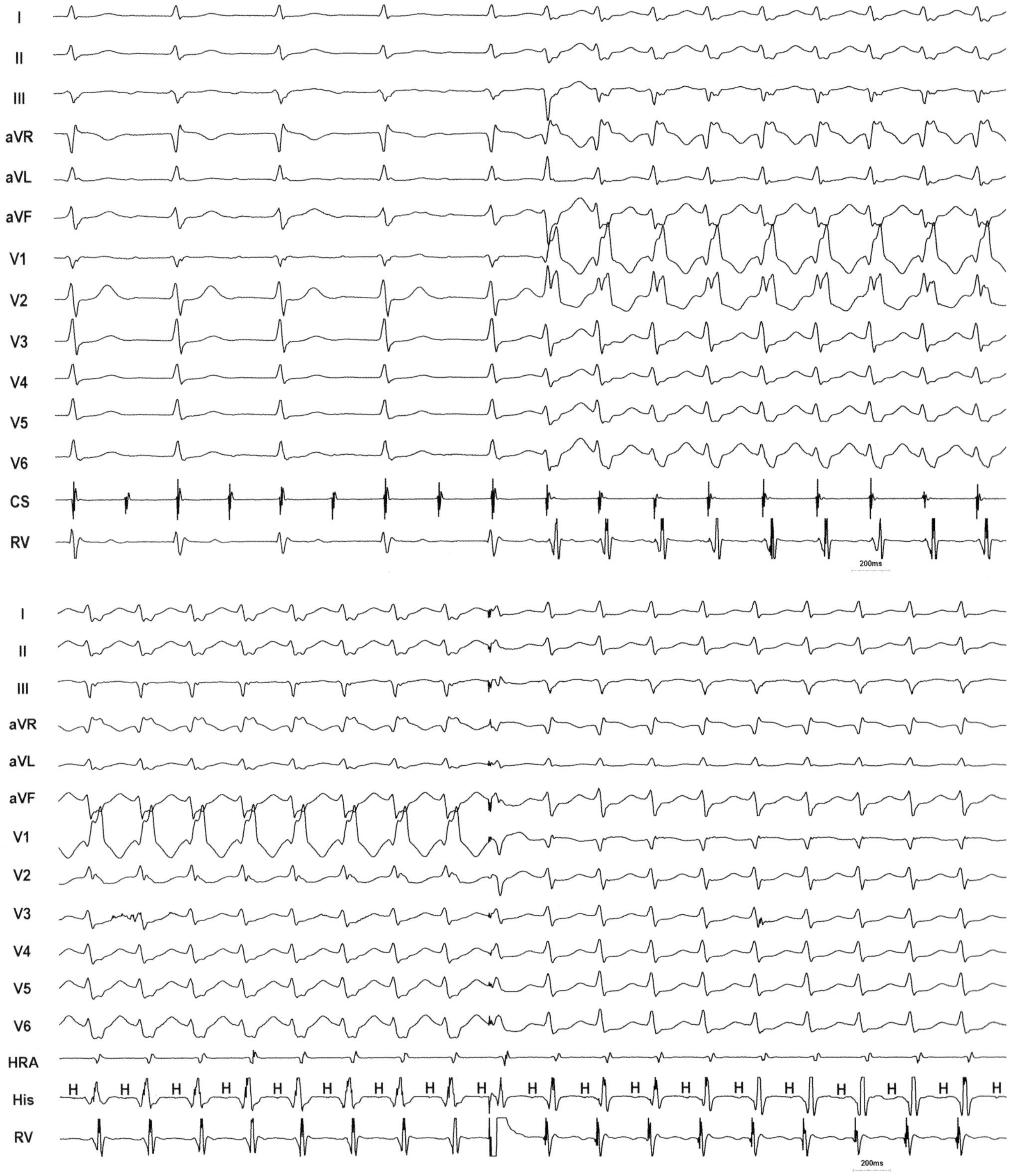

FIGURE 7-23 Typical AVNRT with 2:1 LCFP block transitioning to 1:1 conduction. The long–short sequence accompanying 1:1 conduction induces RBBB, which is perpetuated by transeptal linking. A single RV PVC prematurely penetrates the right bundle shifting its refractoriness leftward ("peeling back of refractoriness"), breaks the transeptal link, and causes loss of RBBB.

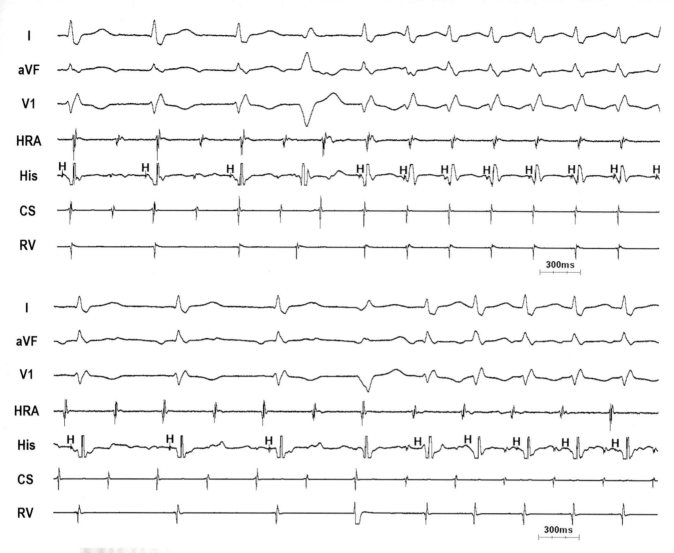

FIGURE 7-24 Typical (*top*) and atypical (*bottom*) AVNRT with 2:1 block above the His bundle. Atrial activation is earliest at the antero- and posteroseptum, respectively. A single VPD retrogradely penetrates the LCFP, "peeling back" its refractoriness and shifting the timing and pattern of block. This interrupts the long–short sequence perpetuating 2:1 block, allowing 1:1 conduction.

Typical AVNRT with 2:1 LCFP Block

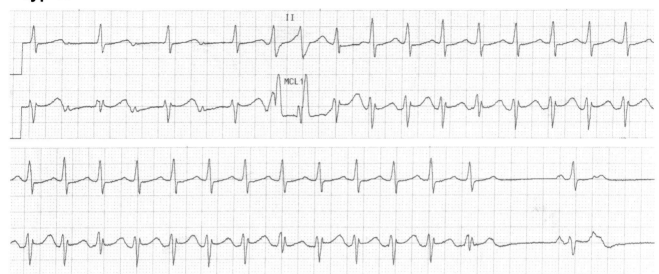

Atypical AVNRT with 2:1 LCFP Block

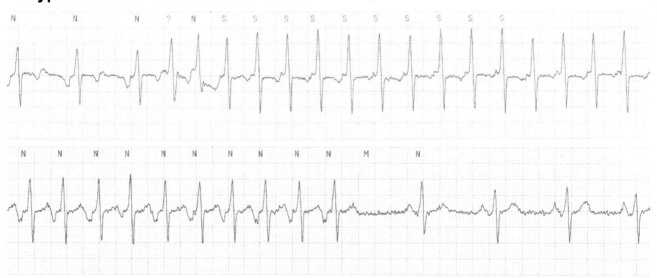

FIGURE 7-25 Typical and atypical AVNRT with 2:1 LCFP block. During typical AVNRT, narrow, retrograde P waves are buried exactly in mid-diastole. Transient aberration accompanies onset of 1:1 conduction.

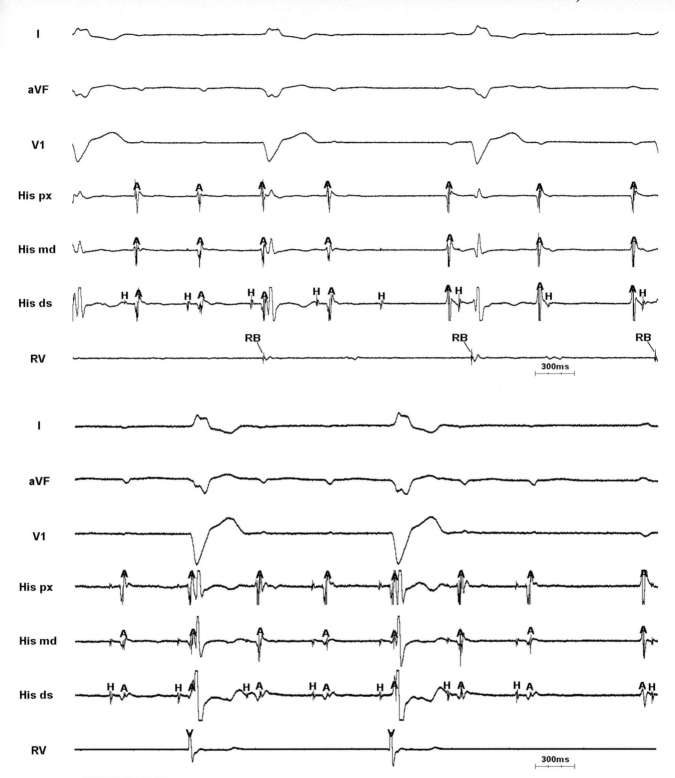

FIGURE 7-26 Typical AVNRT with pathologic high-grade infrahisian block and LBBB. HV intervals preceding LBBB measure 83 ms. During tachycardia and sinus rhythm, block occurs below the His bundle. Tachycardia terminates with block in the FP (*top*) and SP (*bottom*) excluding JT and AT, respectively.

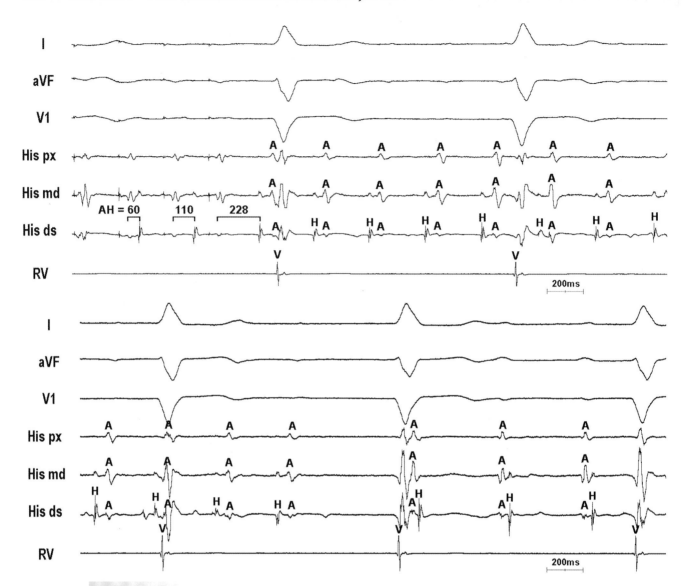

FIGURE 7-27 Typical AVNRT with pathologic third-degree infrahisian block and an RV escape rhythm. Rapid atrial pacing (cycle length = 250 ms) causes decrement in the FP and a switch to the SP (AH = 228 ms) initiating tachycardia. Tachycardia terminates with antegrade block in the SP excluding AT.

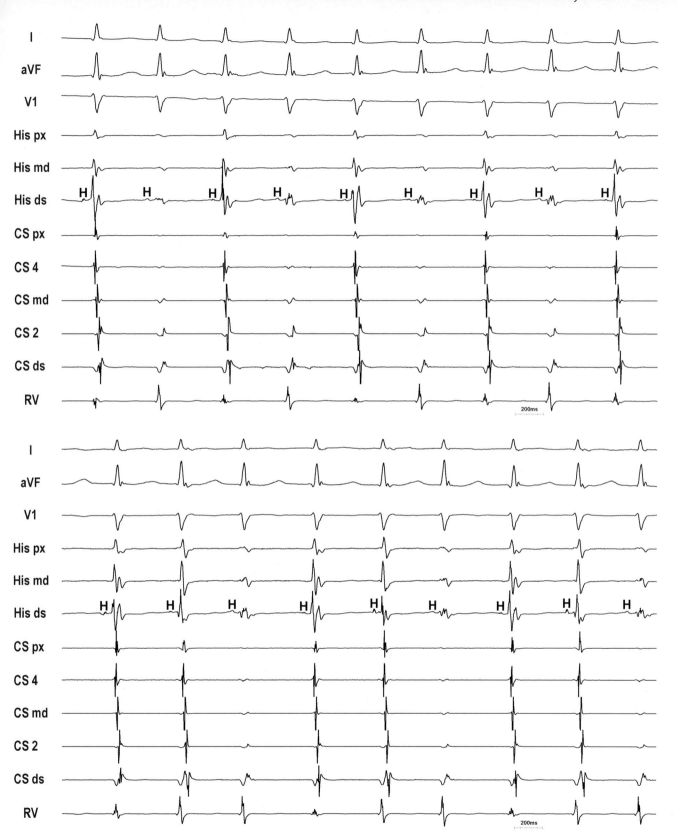

FIGURE 7-28 Typical AVNRT with 2:1 (*top*) and 3:1 (*bottom*) UCFP block.

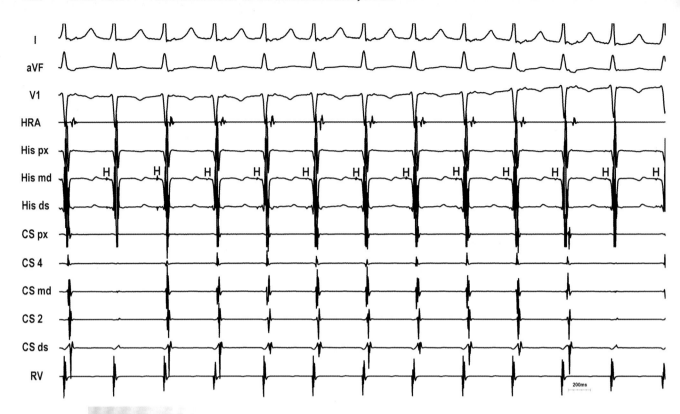

FIGURE 7-29 Typical AVNRT with long cycle UCFP Wenckebach block. VA (HA) intervals progressively increase until UCFP block without change in TCL.

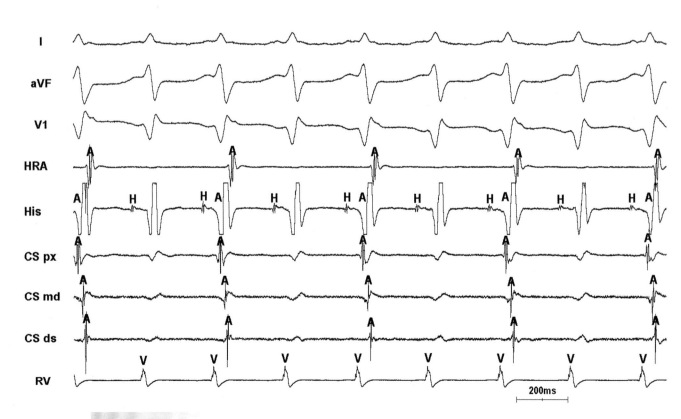

FIGURE 7-30 Typical AVNRT with 2:1 UCFP block.

Bundle Branch Block

The His-Purkinje system is not an integral part of the tachycardia mechanism so that development of bundle branch block (BBB) does not affect AVNRT (**Fig. 7-31**).[28]

ZONES OF TRANSITION

INITIATION

Induction of typical AVNRT is easier with atrial rather than ventricular stimulation (**Figs. 7-32 and 7-33**). A critically-timed atrial impulse falls into the tachycardia window (defined by the difference in antegrade refractory periods of the FP and SP). The impulse 1) fails to conduct over the FP (unidirectional block) and 2) conducts exclusively over the SP (slow conduction). A critical AH delay is required to allow sufficient time for the FP to recover excitability, conduct retrogradely, and initiate tachycardia.[29] Less commonly, typical AVNRT can be initiated by ventricular stimulation or after a dual antegrade response (**Figs. 7-11 and 7-34**). In contrast, atypical AVNRT is easier to induce with ventricular rather than atrial stimulation (**Figs. 7-32 and 7-33**).

TERMINATION

The FP and SP of the AV node are critical components of the tachycardia mechanism, and block in either pathway terminates tachycardia. Spontaneous termination with AV block demonstrates dependence on the AV node and excludes an AT (**Fig. 7-35**). Spontaneous termination with JA block argues against JT (**Figs. 7-19 and 7-26**).

PACING MANEUVERS FROM THE VENTRICLE

The diagnosis of a narrow complex tachycardia is facilitated by pacing maneuvers delivered from the ventricle (inverse rule).

DIASTOLIC VPDs

Single extrastimuli delivered during the diastolic period of AVNRT (diastolic scanning) can penetrate its circuit and reset or terminate tachycardia (**see Fig. 5-8**). However, in contrast to ORT, early VPDs (non–His refractory) are required because of the large distance between the right ventricular (RV) pacing site and AV node.

AVNRT with 2:1 RBBB

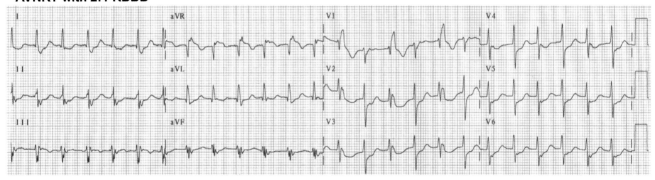

AVNRT with 2:1 LBBB

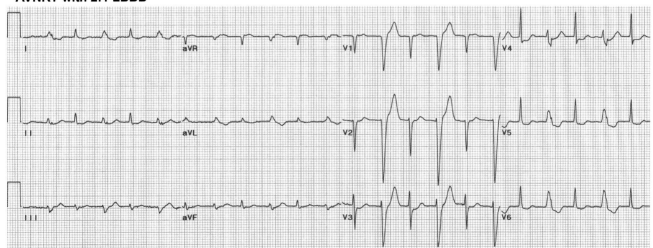

FIGURE 7-31 Typical AVNRT with 2:1 RBBB (*top*) and LBBB (*bottom*). TCL is unaffected by BBB.

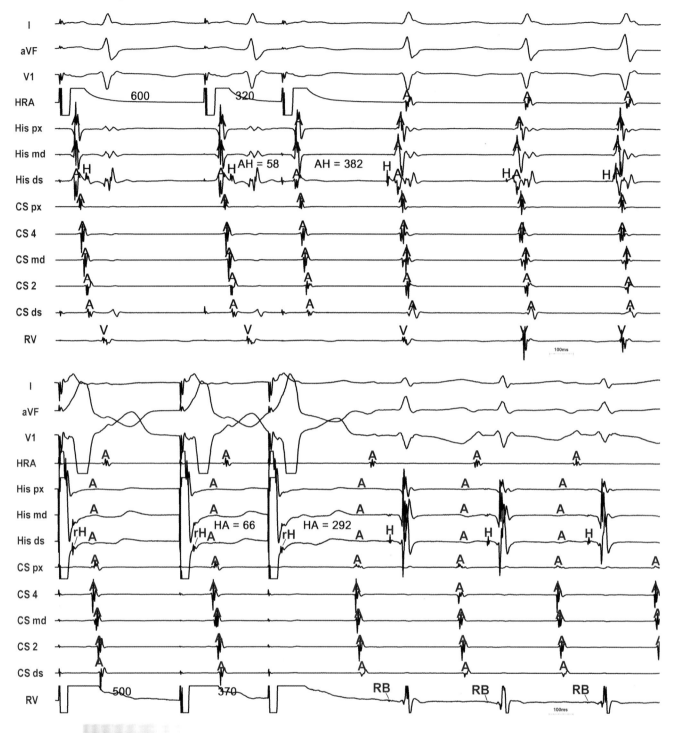

FIGURE 7-32 Induction of typical (*top*) and atypical (*bottom*) AVNRT by programmed extrastimulation after an antegrade (AH) and retrograde (HA) jump, respectively. Note that in the bottom tracing, switch from retrograde FP to SP is accompanied by 1) prolongation of the HA interval and 2) change in earliest atrial activation from anteroseptum (His bundle region) to posteroseptum (CS os region).

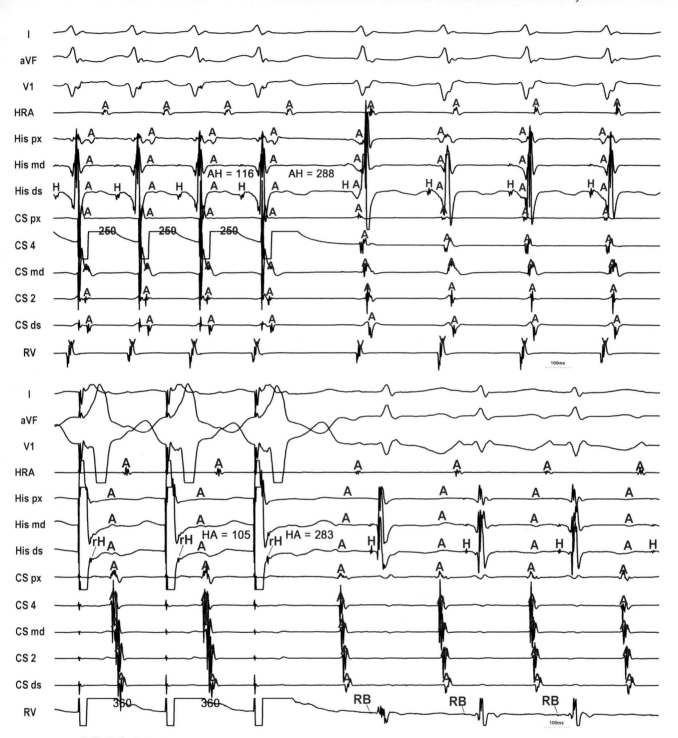

FIGURE 7-33 Induction of typical (*top*) and atypical (*bottom*) AVNRT by rapid pacing after an antegrade (AH) and retrograde (HA) jump, respectively. Note that in the bottom tracing, switch from retrograde FP to SP is accompanied by 1) prolongation of the HA interval and 2) change in earliest atrial activation from anteroseptum (His bundle region) to posteroseptum (CS os region).

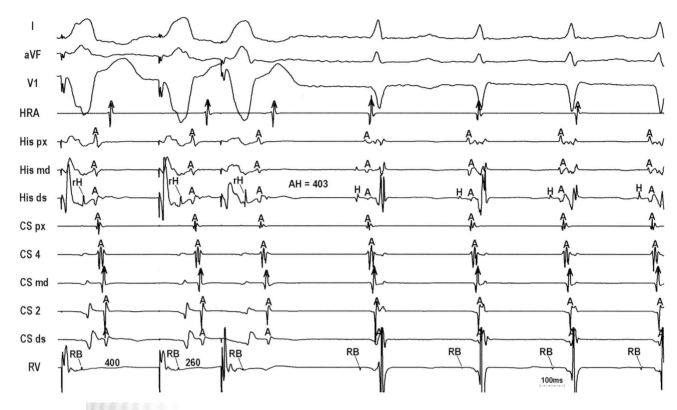

FIGURE 7-34 Induction of typical AVNRT by programmed ventricular extrastimulation. The extrastimulus conducts retrogradely over the FP (earliest atrial activation at the His bundle region) and conceals into the SP. Subsequent conduction from FP into the relative refractory SP results in prolonged AH interval (403 ms) and initiation of slow–fast AVNRT.

Preexcitation Index

During diastolic scanning, the longest coupling interval that preexcites the atrium establishes the preexcitation index (PI). The PI is equal to TCL minus the longest coupling interval advancing the atrium. Because of the large distance between the RV apex and AVNRT circuit, the PI for AVNRT is ≥100 ms.[30]

HIS Refractory VPD ("V on H" Maneuver)

His refractory VPDs fail to affect AVNRT unless a nodo-fascicular/nodo-ventricular AP is present (**Figs. 6-12, 6-13, and 11-16 to 11-19**).[31–35]

ENTRAINMENT FROM THE VENTRICLE

Ventricular overdrive pacing can penetrate the reentrant circuit in the AV node and accelerate the atrium to the pacing cycle length without terminating tachycardia. Because entrainment requires retrograde activation of the His bundle to reach the AV node, all QRS complexes are fully paced ("concealed entrainment").

"AV" Response

The response of AVNRT to entrainment from the ventricle is "AV" (**Figs. 7-36 and 7-37**).[36] However, AVNRT can generate "AAV" responses in the following settings: 1) typical AVNRT when HV is greater than HA interval, 2) atypical AVNRT when

retrograde VA (SP) is greater than VV (pacing cycle length) (classic pseudo AAV), 3) atypical AVNRT with retrograde dual (FP and SP) response (true AAV), 4) atypical AVNRT with LCFP block, and 5) atypical AVNRT when AH is greater than TCL (see Table 5-2) (see Fig. 6-16).[32,37–41] During typical AVNRT with HV greater than HA, the position of the His bundle within the response establishes the diagnosis (AHA and AAH responses for AVNRT and AT, respectively). During the classic pseudo AAV response with atypical AVNRT, identifying the last atrial activation sequence that is accelerated to the pacing cycle length (last entrained atrium) shows a true AV response. True AAV responses after entrainment of atypical AVNRT are either due to pacing-induced termination followed by a dual retrograde response (FP and SP) and re-initiation of tachycardia or entrainment of an atypical AVNRT with a large excitable gap so that collision between orthodromic and antidromic wavefronts occurs in the SP (not FP). Upon pacing cessation, the last antidromic wavefront conducts over the FP, while its orthodromic counterpart conducts over the SP, generating a dual response.

Post-pacing Interval (PPI)

The PPI following entrainment of AVNRT from the RV apex is long relative to the TCL (PPI − TCL >115 ms) because of the large distance between the pacing site and AVNRT circuit (**Figs. 7-36 and 7-37**).[42]

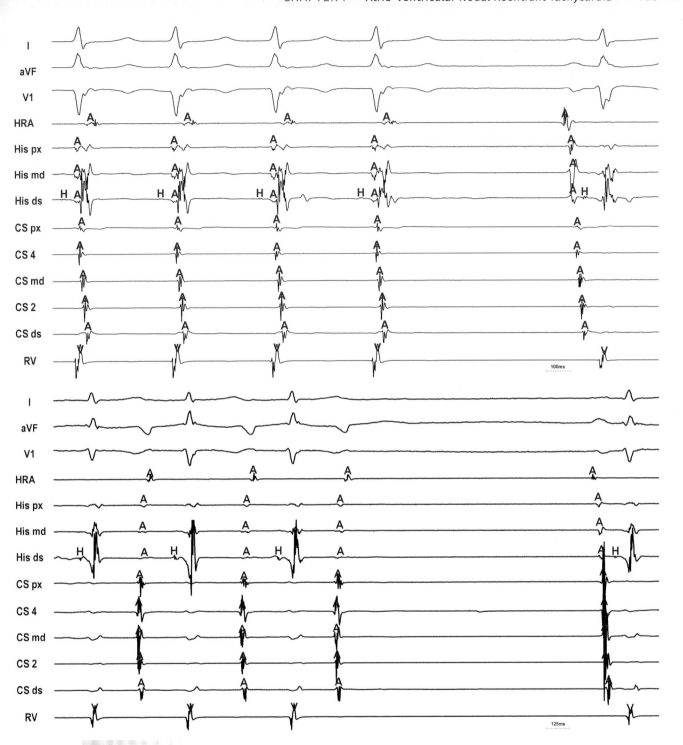

FIGURE 7-35 Termination of typical (*top*) and atypical (*bottom*) AVNRT with AV block (SP and FP, respectively).

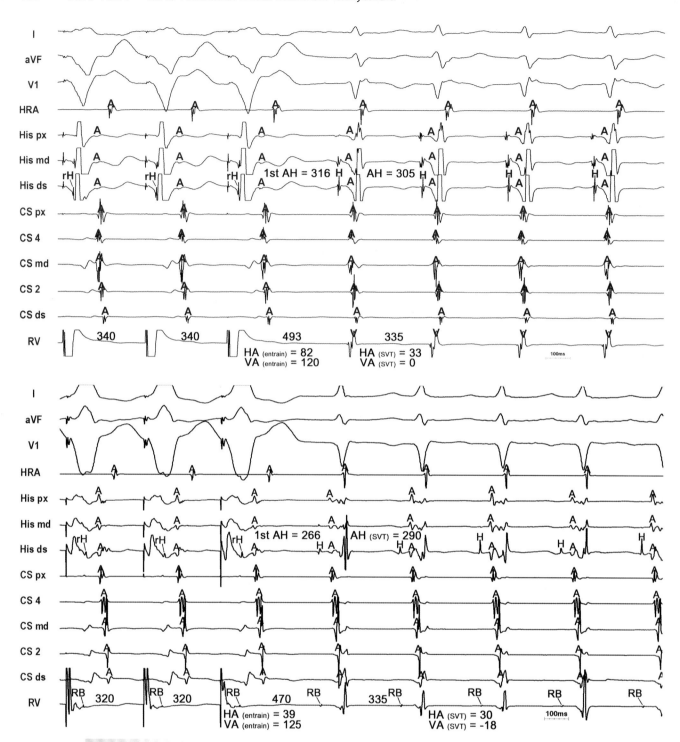

FIGURE 7-36 Entrainment of typical AVNRT from the RV apex (*top*) and base (*bottom*), respectively. The response upon pacing cessation is "AV" (or AH). *Top*: The PPI − TCL = 158 ms, cPPI = 147 ms, ΔHA = 49 ms, ΔVA = 120 ms. *Bottom*: The PPI − TCL = 135 ms, cPPI = 159 ms, ΔHA = 9 ms, ΔVA = 143 ms (VA[SVT] is negative excluding ORT). The first AH is paradoxically 24 ms shorter because tachycardia accelerated for one cycle following entrainment. Note that retrograde His bundle potentials precede and follow the local ventricular electrogram during RV apical and basal pacing, respectively.

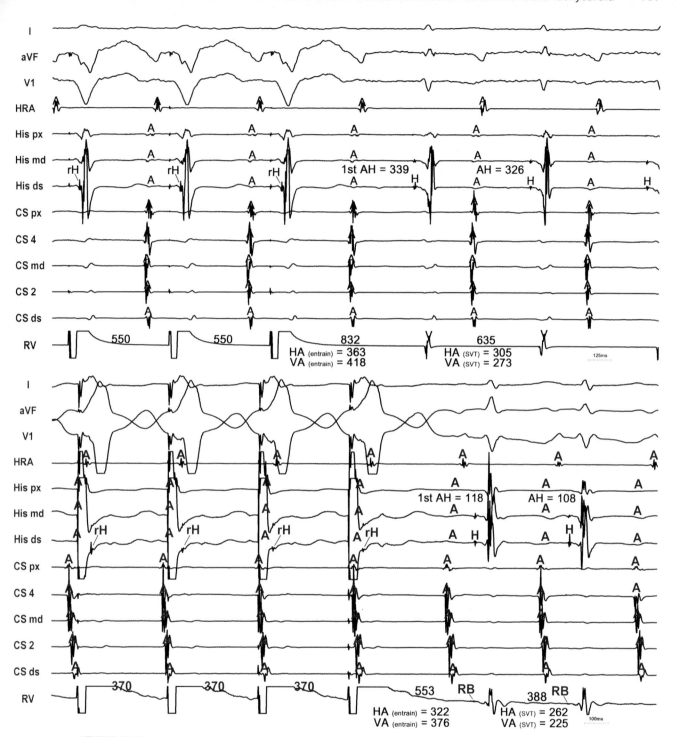

FIGURE 7-37 Entrainment of atypical AVNRT from the RV apex (*top*) and base (*bottom*), respectively. The response upon pacing cessation is "AV" (or AH). *Top:* The PPI − TCL = 197 ms, cPPI = 184 ms, ΔHA = 58 ms, ΔVA = 145 ms. *Bottom:* Only the last two paced complexes accelerate the atrium to the pacing cycle length after a long VA interval. The ability of the first two paced complexes to retrogradely capture the His bundle and yet not accelerate the atrium to the pacing cycle length, itself, argues against permanent form of junctional reciprocating tachycardia. The PPI − TCL = 165 ms, cPPI = 155 ms, ΔHA = 60 ms, ΔVA = 151 ms. Note that retrograde His bundle potentials precede and follow the local ventricular electrogram during RV apical and basal pacing, respectively.

ΔHA Value

The His bundle and atria are activated sequentially over the AV node during entrainment of AVNRT from the ventricle (true HA interval) but simultaneously during tachycardia (pseudo HA interval). Therefore, the $HA_{(entrainment)} > HA_{(AVNRT)}$ or $\Delta HA = HA_{(entrainment)} - HA_{(AVNRT)} > 0$ (**Figs. 7-36 and 7-37**).[43,44]

ΔVA Value

Similarly, the difference between the stimulus-A interval (SA) during entrainment of AVNRT (true interval) and the VA interval during tachycardia (pseudo-interval) ($\Delta VA = SA - VA$) > 85ms (**Figs. 7-36 and 7-37**).[42]

ONSET OF VENTRICULAR OVERDRIVE PACING

Narrow complex tachycardia cannot always be entrained because of repeated pacing-induced termination, but identifying when tachycardia is perturbed or terminates can differentiate AVNRT from ORT. Resetting or termination of AVNRT requires a fully paced ventricular complex to retrogradely penetrate the His bundle and AV node. Therefore, advancement/delay of the atrium or VA block with tachycardia termination cannot occur during the transition zone or within one fully paced QRS complex.[45,46]

PACING MANEUVERS FROM THE ATRIUM

While pacing maneuvers in the ventricle differentiate AVNRT versus ORT/AT, pacing maneuvers in the atrium can further separate AVNRT versus AT as well as AVNRT versus JT.

AVNRT VERSUS AT (VA LINKING)

VA intervals one beat after atrial overdrive pacing are linked to tachycardia (conventional method) or following decremental or differential atrial pacing: $\Delta VA < 10$ ms for AVNRT and >10 ms for AT. For AT, the VA is not a true conduction interval but a value dependent on the AT return interval at the pacing site (which itself depends on the proximity of the pacing site to the AT site of origin) and AV conduction time.[24,47–49]

AVNRT VERSUS JT

Atrial Overdrive Pacing

The response to atrial overdrive pacing is "AHA" for AVNRT and "AHH" for JT (**Figs. 7-38 to 7-40**).[50] However, while an "AHA" response is specific for AVNRT, "AHH" responses are less specific for JT and can be seen with AVNRT: 1) pseudo AHH response when AH (SP conduction) is greater than AA (atrial pacing cycle length) and 2) true AHH due to dual antegrade response (FP and SP) (atrial overdrive pacing stopped AVNRT, which then restarted after a dual antegrade response or AVNRT has a large excitable gap so that the collision point between orthodromic and antidromic wavefronts occurs in the SP resulting in a dual antegrade response upon pacing cessation).

Diastolic APDs

Late-coupled (His refractory) APDs that reset (advance/delay) or terminate tachycardia with AV block excludes JT (**Figs. 7-41 and 7-42**).[51–55] An early-coupled APD that resets tachycardia

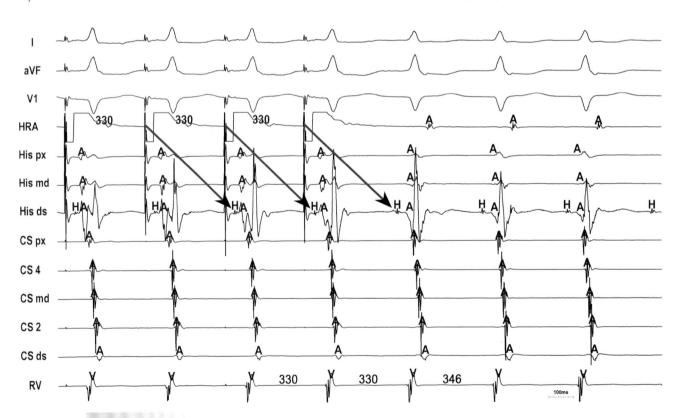

FIGURE 7-38 "AHA" response during atrial overdrive pacing (entrainment) of typical AVNRT.

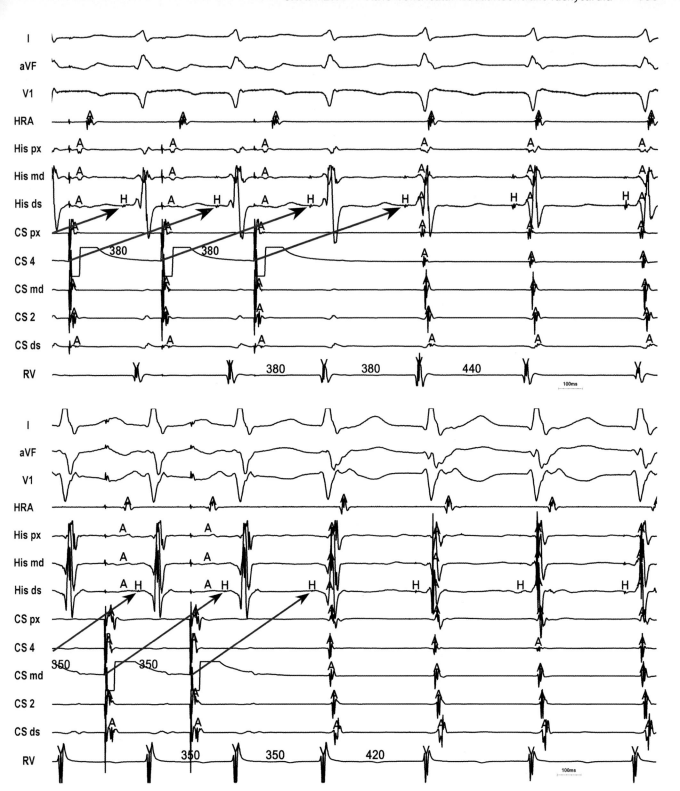

FIGURE 7-39 Pseudo "AHH" responses during atrial overdrive pacing (entrainment) of typical AVNRT. This is a true AHA response with an "AHH" pattern resulting from markedly prolonged SP conduction.

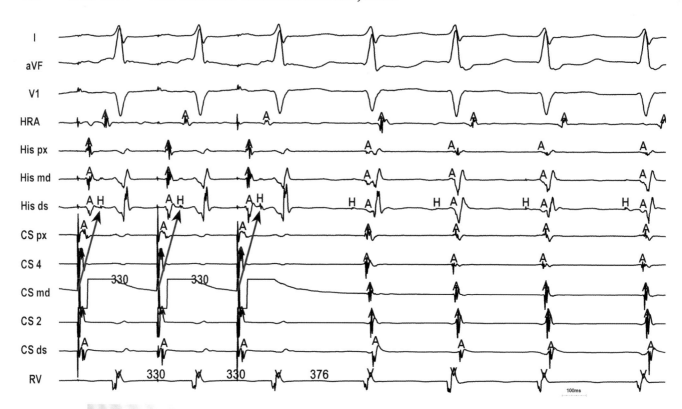

FIGURE 7-40 True "AHH" response during atrial overdrive pacing of JT. An alternative possibility is a dual AV nodal response (FP and SP) with typical AVNRT.

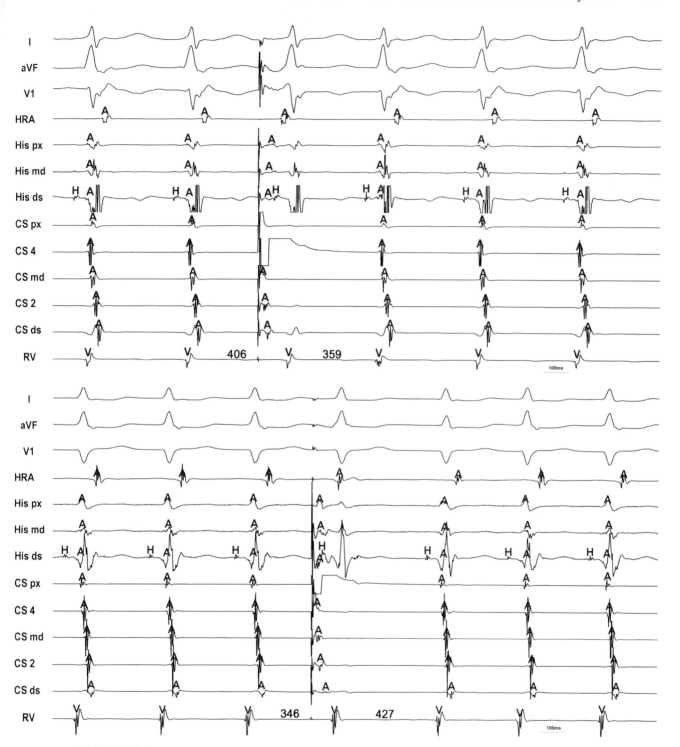

FIGURE 7-41 His refractory APDs advance (*top*) and delay (*bottom*) the His bundle during typical AVNRT. Such findings exclude JT.

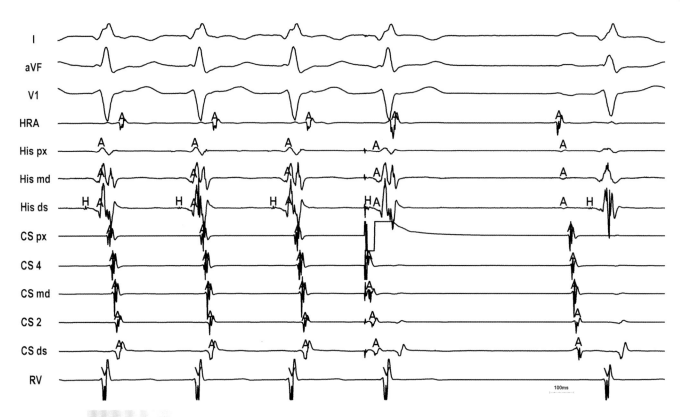

FIGURE 7-42 A His refractory APD terminates typical AVNRT with block in the SP. Such a finding excludes JT.

by conducting over the FP without terminating tachycardia favors JT because during typical AVNRT, the diastolic interval is occupied by the SP (**Figs. 7-43 and 7-44**) (another possibility, however, is that an early-coupled APD resets AVNRT with a dual antegrade response).[52–54]

A third maneuver to differentiate AVNRT from JT is to evaluate ΔHA values during ventricular overdrive pacing/entrainment, but this is less well established.[56,57]

UNUSUAL ELECTROPHYSIOLOGIC PHENOMENA

CYCLE LENGTH ALTERNANS

AVNRT with multiple separate or longitudinally dissociated AV nodal pathways or simply interplay between SP and FP conduc-

tion (PR/RP reciprocity or "sanctity of the PR/RP relationship") can cause variability in TCL including cycle length alternans (**Figs. 7-45 and 7-46**).[58]

DUAL TACHYCARDIAS

AVNRT can coexist with other tachycardias including idiopathic VT, AT, and, rarely, atrial fibrillation (**Fig. 7-47**).[59–62] Atrial fibrillation with AVNRT supports the concept that AVNRT is a "subatrial" circuit with an UCFP.

CTI/SVC BLOCK

Conduction block in bystander sites (SVC, cavo-tricuspid isthmus [CTI]) can occur during AVNRT but does not affect tachycardia (**Figs. 7-48 and 7-49**).

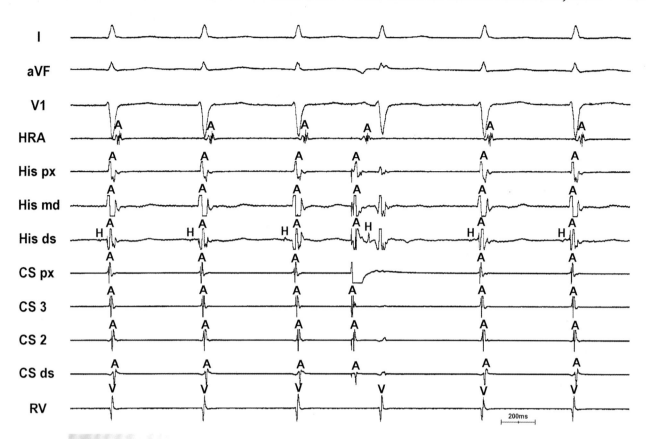

FIGURE 7-43 An early APD conducts over the FP and resets JT. An alternative possibility is an early APD conducts with a dual AV nodal response (FP and SP) resetting typical AVNRT.

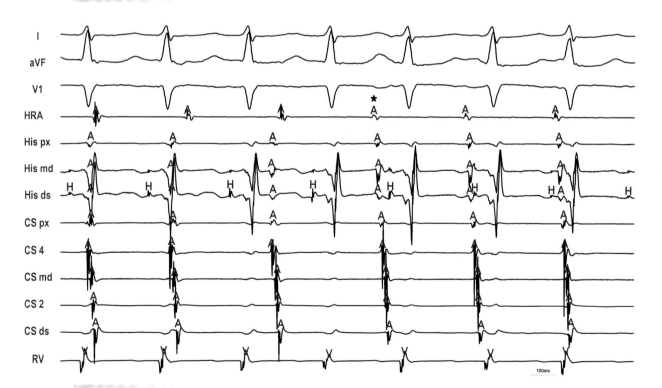

FIGURE 7-44 JT with JA Wenckebach. HA intervals prolong until block occurs, allowing appearance of sinus rhythm—the first beat (*asterisk*) of which conducts over the FP and resets JT. Absence of subsequent JA conduction results from atrial or FP refractoriness during superimposed sinus rhythm. An alternative possibility is typical AVNRT with UCFP Wenckebach block. The first sinus complex conducts with a dual AV nodal response (FP and SP) during AVNRT.

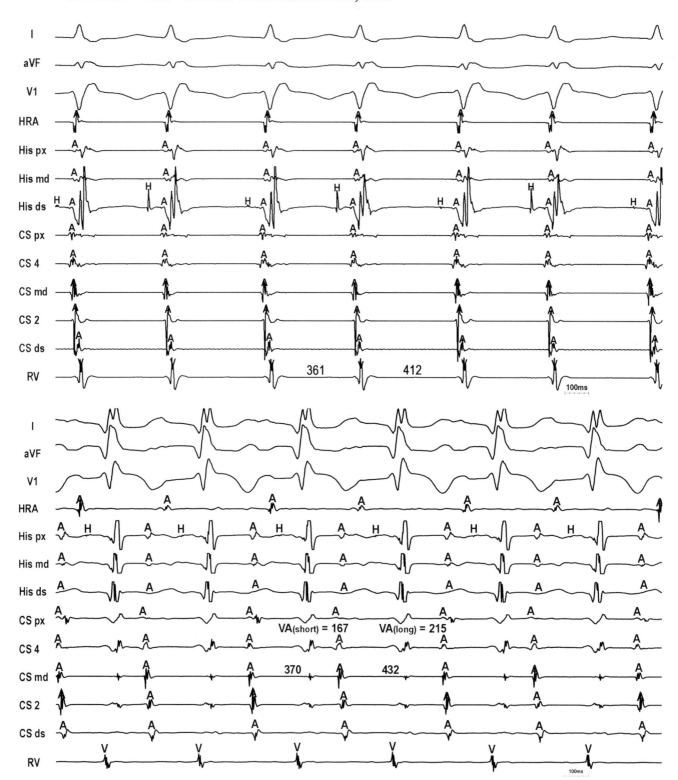

FIGURE 7-45 Typical (*top*) and atypical (*bottom*) AVNRT with cycle length alternans. *Top*: typical AVNRT with alternating antegrade conduction over two SPs (slow and slower) or a longitudinally dissociated SP. *Bottom*: atypical AVNRT with alternating retrograde conduction over two SPs or a longitudinally dissociated SP. VA intervals alternate between long (215 ms) and short (167 ms) producing atrial alternans. Longer and shorter VA intervals are followed by shorter (119 ms) and longer (151 ms) AH intervals, respectively (AH/HA reciprocity), so that ventricular alternans is less prominent (VV short/long = 392 ms/408 ms).

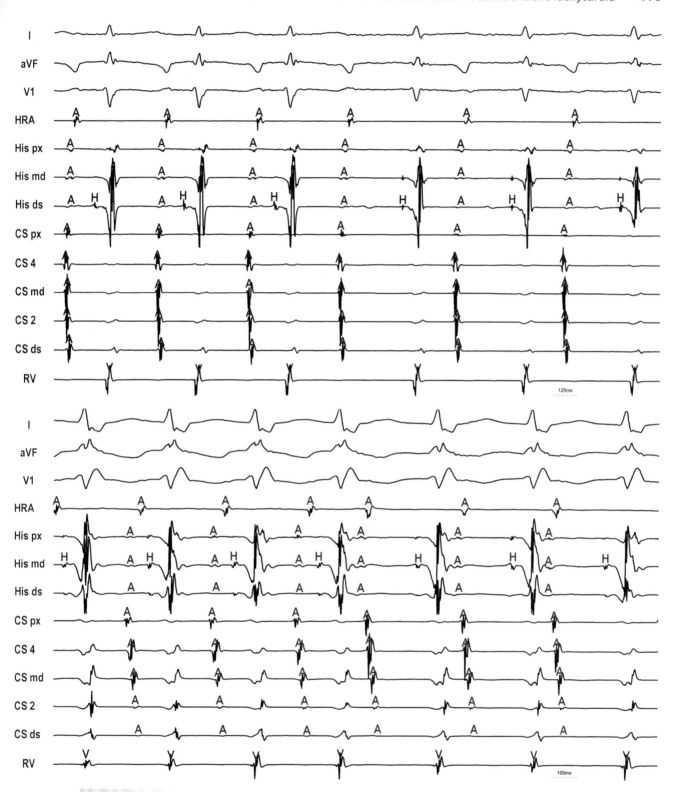

FIGURE 7-46 Triple AV node physiology. *Top*: Atypical (fast–slow) AVNRT abruptly transitions to a slower (slow–slow) AVNRT without change in retrograde (SP) atrial activation pattern: one retrograde (SP) and two antegrade (FP and different SP). Note PR/RP reciprocity. *Bottom*: Atypical (fast–slow) AVNRT abruptly transitions to a slower (slow–"superior" slow) AVNRT. Retrograde atrial activation changes from earliest at the posteroseptum (SP at CS os) to anteroseptum ("superior" SP at His bundle). It is possible that the retrograde SP for fast–slow AVNRT is the antegrade SP for slow–"superior" slow AVNRT.

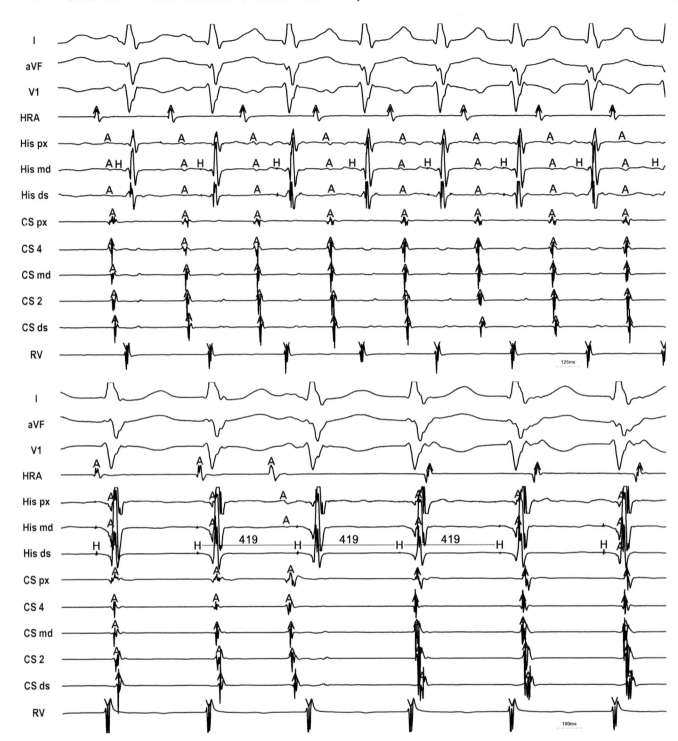

FIGURE 7-47 Double tachycardia (right AT and typical AVNRT). *Top:* transition from a long RP to short RP tachycardia because the atrium (controlled by AT) is beating faster than the ventricle (controlled by AVNRT). *Bottom:* A spontaneous His refractory APD fails to affect AVNRT but terminates AT, allowing retrograde atrial activation from the FP to become manifest. This indicates that JA block in the top tracing was due to physiologic refractoriness of the atrium or UCFP because of superimposed AT (pseudo JA block rather than true JA block).

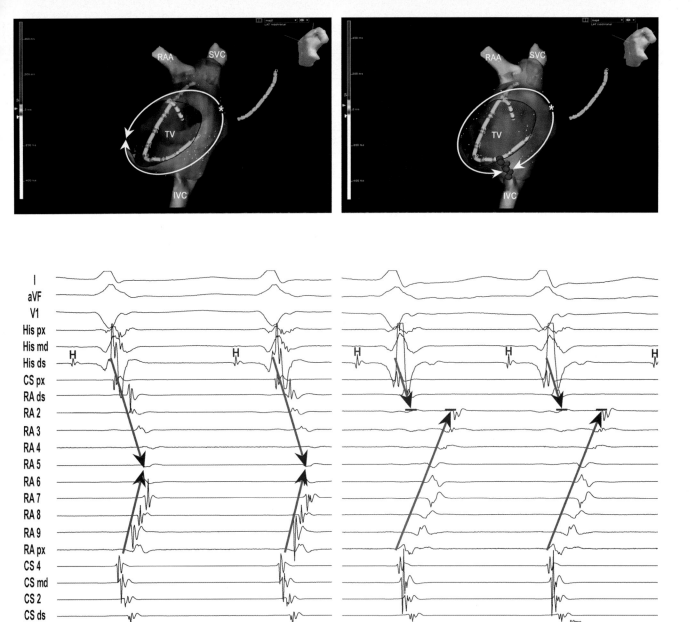

FIGURE 7-48 Typical AVNRT without (*left*) and with (*right*) CTI block. During tachycardia, the earliest site of atrial activation is at the anteroseptum (*asterisk*).

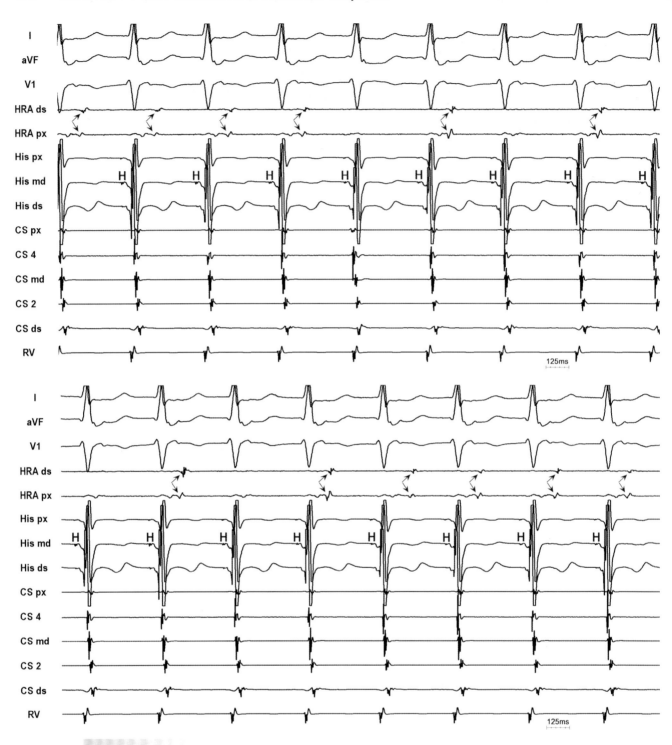

FIGURE 7-49 Typical AVNRT with transient 2:1 block to the SVC. *Arrows* denote SVC potentials.

REFERENCES

1. Moe GK, Preston JB, Burlington H. Physiologic evidence for a dual A-V transmission system. Circ Res 1956;4:357–375.
2. Anselme F, Papageorgiou P, Monahan K, et al. Presence and significance of the left atrionodal connection during atrioventricular nodal reentrant tachycardia. Am J Cardiol 1999;83:1530–1536.
3. Fisch C, Knoebel S. Dual atrioventricular conduction. In: Fisch C, Knoebel S, eds. Electrocardiography of Clinical Arrhythmias. Armonk, NY: Futura Publishing Company, 2000:345–356.
4. Itagaki T, Ohnishi Y, Inoue T, Yokoyama M. Linking phenomenon in dual atrioventricular nodal pathways. Jpn Circ J 2001;65:937–940.
5. Fisch C, Steinmetz EF. Supernormal phase of atrioventricular (A-V) conduction due to potassium. A-V alternans with first-degree A-V block. Am Heart J 1961;62:211–220.
6. Csapo G. Paroxysmal nonreentrant tachycardia due to simultaneous conduction in dual atrioventricular nodal pathways. Am J Cardiol 1979;43:1033–1045.
7. Massumi RA. Interpolated His bundle extrasystoles. An unusual cause of tachycardia. Am J Med 1970;49:265–270.
8. Gaba D, Pavri BB, Greenspon AJ, Ho RT. Dual antegrade response tachycardia induced cardiomyopathy. Pacing Clin Electrophysiol 2004;27:533–536.

9. Lin FC, Yeh SJ, Wu D. Determinants of simultaneous fast and slow pathway conduction in patients with dual atrioventricular nodal pathways. Am Heart J 1985;109:963–970.

10. Wang NC. Dual atrioventricular nodal nonreentrant tachycardia: a systematic review. Pacing Clin Electrophysiol 2011;34:1671–1681.

11. Morris KE, Steinberg LA, Prystowsky EN, Padanilam BJ. Premature beats and unexpected heart block: an unusual mechanism confirmed by ablation. Circ Arrhythm Electrophysiol 2012;5:e44–e45.

12. Otomo K, Wang Z, Lazzara R, Jackman W. Atrioventricular nodal reentrant tachycardia: electrophysiological characteristics of four forms and implications for the reentrant circuit. In: Zipes D, Jalife J, eds. Cardiac Electrophysiology: From Cell to Bedside. 3rd ed. Philadelphia, PA: WB Saunders Company, 2000:504–521.

13. Baker JH II, Plumb VJ, Epstein AE, Kay GN. PR/RR interval ratio during rapid atrial pacing: a simple method for confirming the presence of slow AV nodal pathway conduction. J Cardiovasc Electrophysiol 1996;7:287–294.

14. Katritsis DG, Camm AJ. Atrioventricular nodal reentrant tachycardia. Circulation 2010;122:831–840.

15. Hwang C, Martin DJ, Goodman JS, et al. Atypical atrioventricular node reciprocating tachycardia masquerading as tachycardia using a left-sided accessory pathway. J Am Coll Cardiol 1997;30:218–225.

16. Kaneko Y, Naito S, Okishige K, et al. Atypical fast-slow atrioventricular nodal reentrant tachycardia incorporating a "superior" slow pathway: a distinct supraventricular tachyarrhythmia. Circulation 2016;133:114–123.

17. Josephson M, Kastor J. Paroxysmal supraventricular tachycardia: is the atrium a necessary link? Circulation 1976;54:430–435.

18. Miller J, Rosenthal M, Vassallo J, Josephson M. Atrioventricular nodal reentrant tachycardia: studies on upper and lower 'common pathways.' Circulation 1987;75:930–940.

19. DiMarco J, Sellers T, Belardinelli L. Paroxysmal supraventricular tachycardia with Wenckebach block: evidence for reentry within the upper portion of the atrioventricular node. J Am Coll Cardiol 1984;3:1551–1555.

20. Hariman R, Chen C, Caracta A, Damato A. Evidence that AV nodal re-entrant tachycardia does not require participation of the entire AV node. Pacing Clin Electrophysiol 1983;6:1252–1257.

21. Wellens H, Wesdorp J, Düren D, Lie K. Second degree block during reciprocal atrioventricular nodal tachycardia. Circulation 1976;4:595–599.

22. Willems S, Shenasa M, Borggrefe M, et al. Atrioventricular nodal reentry tachycardia: electrophysiologic comparisons in patients with and without 2:1 infra-His block. Clin Cardiol 1993;16:883–888.

23. Benditt D, Pritchett E, Smith W, Gallagher J. Ventriculoatrial intervals: diagnostic use in paroxysmal supraventricular tachycardia. Ann Intern Med 1979;91:161–166.

24. Knight BP, Ebinger M, Oral H, et al. Diagnostic value of tachycardia features and pacing maneuvers during paroxysmal supraventricular tachycardia. J Am Coll Cardiol 2000;36:574–582.

25. Amat-y-Leon F, Dhingra R, Wu D, Denes P, Wyndham C, Rosen K. Catheter mapping of retrograde atrial activation. Observations during ventricular pacing and AV nodal re-entrant paroxysmal tachycardia. Br Heart J 1976;38:355–362.

26. Ravindran BK, Pavri BB, Greenspon AJ, Ho RT. Tachycardia during bradycardia: what is the mechanism? J Cardiovasc Electrophysiol 2003;14(8):894–896.

27. Das M, Gizurarson S, Roshan J, Nair K. Spontaneous ECG observations during an incessant long RP tachycardia—what is the tachycardia mechanism? Heart Rhythm 2014;11:325–327.

28. Barold HS, Newman M, Flanagan M, Barold SS. Two-to-one bundle branch block during atrioventricular nodal reentrant tachycardia: what is the mechanism? Heart Rhythm 2007;4:371–373.

29. Goldreyer B, Damato A. The essential role of atrioventricular conduction delay in the initiation of paroxysmal supraventricular tachycardia. Circulation 1971;43:679–687.

30. Miles W, Yee R, Klein G, Zipes D, Prystowsky E. The preexcitation index: an aid in determining the mechanism of supraventricular tachycardia and localizing accessory pathways. Circulation 1986;74:493–500.

31. Ho RT, Frisch DR, Pavri BB, Levi SA, Greenspon AJ. Electrophysiological features differentiating the atypical atrioventricular node-dependent long RP supraventricular tachycardias. Circ Arrhythm Electrophysiol 2013;6:597–605.

32. Ho RT, Fischman DL. Entrainment versus resetting of a long RP tachycardia: what is the diagnosis? Heart Rhythm 2012;9:312–314.

33. Ho RT, Levi SA. An atypical long RP tachycardia—what is the mechanism? Heart Rhythm 2013;10:1089–1090.

34. Ho RT, Kenia AS, Chhabra SK. Resetting and termination of a short RP tachycardia: what is the mechanism? Heart Rhythm 2013;10:1927–1929.

35. Ho RT. Unusual termination of a short RP tachycardia: what is the mechanism? Heart Rhythm 2017;14:935–937.

36. Knight B, Zivin A, Souza J, et al. A technique for the rapid diagnosis of atrial tachycardia in the electrophysiology laboratory. J Am Coll Cardiol 1999;33:775–781.

37. Kaneko Y, Nakajima T, Irie T, Iizuka T, Tamura S, Kurabayashi M. Atrial and ventricular activation sequence after ventricular induction/entrainment pacing during fast-slow atrioventricular nodal reentrant tachycardia: new insight into the use of V-A-A-V for the differential diagnosis of supraventricular tachycardia. Heart Rhythm 2017;14:1615–1622.

38. Kaneko Y, Nakajima T, Irie T, Kato T, Iljima T, Kurabayashi M. Long RP' tachycardia with an initial A-A-V activation sequence: what is the mechanism? J Cardiovasc Electrophysiol 2011;22:945–947.

39. Vijayaraman P, Lee BP, Kalahasty G, Wood MA, Ellenbogen KA. Reanalysis of the "pseudo A-A-V" response to ventricular entrainment of supraventricular tachycardia: importance of His-bundle timing. J Cardiovasc Electrophysiol 2006;17:25–28.

40. Vijayaraman P, Kok LC, Rhee B, Ellenbogen KA. Wide complex tachycardia: what is the mechanism? Heart Rhythm 2005;2:107–109.

41. Crawford TC, Morady F, Pelosi F Jr. A long R-P paroxysmal supraventricular tachycardia: what is the mechanism? Heart Rhythm 2007;4:1364–1365.

42. Michaud GF, Tada H, Chough S, et al. Differentiation of atypical atrioventricular node re-entrant tachycardia from orthodromic reciprocating tachycardia using a septal accessory pathway by the response to ventricular pacing. J Am Coll Cardiol 2001;38:1163–1167.

43. Ho RT, Mark GE, Rhim ES, Pavri BB, Greenspon AJ. Differentiating atrioventricular nodal reentrant tachycardia from atrioventricular reentrant tachycardia by ΔHA values during entrainment from the ventricle. Heart Rhythm 2008;5:83–88.

44. Mark GE, Rhim ES, Pavri BB, Greenspon AJ, Ho RT. Differentiation of atrio-ventricular nodal reentrant tachycardia from orthodromic atrioventricular reentrant tachycardia by ΔHA intervals during entrainment from the ventricle [abstract]. Heart Rhythm 2006;3:S321.

45. AlMahameed ST, Buxton AE, Michaud GF. New criteria during right ventricular pacing to determine the mechanism of supraventricular tachycardia. Circ Arrhythm Electrophysiol 2010;3:578–584.

46. Dandamudi G, Mokabberi R, Assal C, et al. A novel approach to differentiating orthodromic reciprocating tachycardia from atrioventricular nodal reentrant tachycardia. Heart Rhythm 2010;7:1326–1329.

47. Kadish AH, Morady F. The response of paroxysmal supraventricular tachycardia to overdrive atrial and ventricular pacing: can it help determine the tachycardia mechanism? J Cardiovasc Electrophysiol 1993;4:239–252.

48. Maruyama M, Kobayashi Y, Miyauchi Y, et al. The VA relationship after differential atrial overdrive pacing: a novel tool for the diagnosis of atrial tachycardia in the electrophysiologic laboratory. J Cardiovasc Electrophysiol 2007;18:1127–1133.

49. Sarkozy A, Richter S, Chierchia G, et al. A novel pacing manoeuvre to diagnose atrial tachycardia. Europace 2008;10:459–466.

50. Fan R, Tardos JG, Almasry I, Barbera S, Rashba EJ, Iwai S. Novel use of atrial overdrive pacing to rapidly differentiate junctional tachycardia from atrioventricular nodal reentrant tachycardia. Heart Rhythm 2011;8:840–844.

51. Padanilam BJ, Manfredi JA, Steinberg LA, Olson JA, Fogel RI, Prystowsky EN. Differentiating junctional tachycardia and atrioventricular node re-entry tachycardia based on response to atrial extrastimulus pacing. J Am Coll Cardiol 2008;52:1711–1717.

52. Ho RT, Pietrasik G, Greenspon AJ. A narrow complex tachycardia with intermittent atrioventricular dissociation: what is the mechanism? Heart Rhythm 2014;11(11):2116–2119.

53. Chen H, Shehata M, Cingolani E, Chugh SS, Chen M, Wang X. Differentiating atrioventricular nodal re-entrant tachycardia from junctional tachycardia: conflicting responses? Circ Arrhythm Electrophysiol 2015;8:232–235.

54. Roberts-Thomson KC, Seiler J, Steven D, et al. Short AV response to atrial extrastimuli during narrow complex tachycardia: what is the mechanism? J Cardiovasc Electrophysiol 2009;20:946–948.

55. Boonyapisit W, Chalfoun N, Morady F, Jongnarangsin K. Supraventricular tachycardia with simultaneous atrial and ventricular activation: what is the mechanism? Heart Rhythm 2008;5:622–623.

56. Srivathsan K, Gami AS, Barrett R, Monahan K, Packer DL, Asirvatham SJ. Differentiating atrioventricular nodal reentrant tachycardia from junctional tachycardia: novel application of the delta H-A interval. J Cardiovasc Electrophysiol 2008;19:1–6.

57. Luebbert J, Greenspon AJ, Pavri BB, Frisch DR, Ho RT. Do ΔHA values differentiate slow-fast atrio-ventricular nodal reentrant tachycardia from automatic junctional tachycardia arising from the slow pathway of the AV node. Heart Rhythm 2011;8:S302.

58. Buch E, Tung R, Shehata M, Shivkumar K. Alternating cycle length during supraventricular tachycardia: what is the mechanism? J Cardiovasc Electrophysiol 2009;20:1071–1073.

59. Ho RT, Idris S, Joshi N, Mehrotra P. A narrow complex tachycardia with varying RP intervals: what is the mechanism? Heart Rhythm 2015;12:1878–1881.

60. Saluja D, Beauregard L, Patel A, Coromilas J. The simultaneous presence of sustained atrial fibrillation and atrioventricular nodal reentrant tachycardia. Heart Rhythm 2015;12:229–233.

61. Richter S, Brugada P. Atrioventricular nodal reentry: the atrium is not a necessary link. J Cardiovasc Electrophysiol 2009;20:697–698.

62. Chen J, Josephson ME. Atrioventricular nodal tachycardia occurring during atrial fibrillation. J Cardiovasc Electrophysiol 2000;11:812–815.

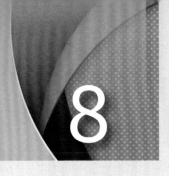

8 Ablation of Atrio-ventricular Nodal Reentrant Tachycardia

Introduction

Catheter ablation is a highly effective treatment for atrio-ventricular nodal reentrant tachycardia (AVNRT). While ablation of the fast pathway (FP) was initially performed, slow pathway (SP) ablation is preferred because it 1) carries a lower risk of causing atrio-ventricular (AV) block, 2) does not prolong the PR interval, and 3) treats atypical forms of AVNRT (e.g., slow–slow) that do not use the FP.[1–8]

The purpose of this chapter is to:

1. Describe the anatomy of the AV node and its atrial approaches (SP and FP).
2. Discuss the technique of SP ablation.
3. Define endpoints for ablation of AVNRT.

ANATOMY OF THE AV NODE

The compact AV node and its perinodal structures are contained within the triangle of Koch, which is defined by the 1) tendon of Todaro, 2) septal leaflet of the tricuspid valve, and 3) coronary sinus ostium (CS os) (base of the triangle).[9,10] The central fibrous body and penetrating His bundle lie at the apex of the triangle. The compact AV node is located along the right interatrial septum posterior and inferior to the His bundle and superior to the CS os. The SP (right inferior extension) is located at the level of the CS os, while the FP (superior extensions) lies superior to the His bundle above the tendon of Todaro and outside of the triangle of Koch.[11] Left atrio-nodal inputs (left inferior extensions, inferolateral inputs) course along the CS.

ABLATION OF THE SLOW PATHWAY (RIGHT INFERIOR EXTENSION)

Properly positioned His bundle and CS catheters are useful landmarks to identify the triangle of Koch and the His bundle during ablation. The His bundle catheter, however, does not define the entire location of the His bundle, and electro-anatomic mapping of the His bundle (His bundle cloud) identifies additional sites that should be avoided during ablation. Additionally, the CS catheter positioned from the femoral versus internal jugular vein outlines the CS differently (roof versus floor of the CS, respectively).

The baseline PR interval should be analyzed prior to ablation. While SP ablation can be successful in patients with first-degree AV block, PR prolongation (especially >300 ms)

suggests impaired or absent FP conduction where ablation of the SP in the latter can cause acute or delayed AV block.[12–14]

SINUS RHYTHM MAPPING OF THE SLOW PATHWAY

Anatomic SP ablation targeting the right inferior extension treats the majority of AVNRT (slow–fast, fast–slow, slow–slow, and even AVNRT using left atrio-nodal inputs).[15,16] The ablation catheter is advanced across the tricuspid valve into the right ventricle. With clockwise torque, it is slowly pulled back along the posteroseptum until a small atrial and large ventricular electrogram is recorded inferior to the His bundle and slightly anterior to the CS os. Target site criteria for the SP are 1) a low-amplitude (far-field) atrial electrogram; 2) a late, sharp, high-frequency (near-field) SP potential; 3) a moderate to large ventricular electrogram (AV ratio ≤0.5); and 4) an absent His bundle potential (**Figs. 8-1 to 8-6**).[1,2] Sharp "SP-type" potentials, however, can be found at multiple different sites within the triangle of Koch.[17] In the absence of a discrete SP potential, the atrial signal is often a low-amplitude, multicomponent electrogram. Because the compact AV node is posterior and inferior to the His bundle, the roof of the CS and sites with large atrial electrograms should be avoided for ablation.

RETROGRADE MAPPING OF THE SLOW PATHWAY

The SP can also be mapped when it conducts retrogradely during ventricular pacing or atypical AVNRT (fast–slow, slow–slow) by identifying the earliest site of atrial activation (**Figs. 8-7 to 8-10**). Because retrograde SP conduction precedes

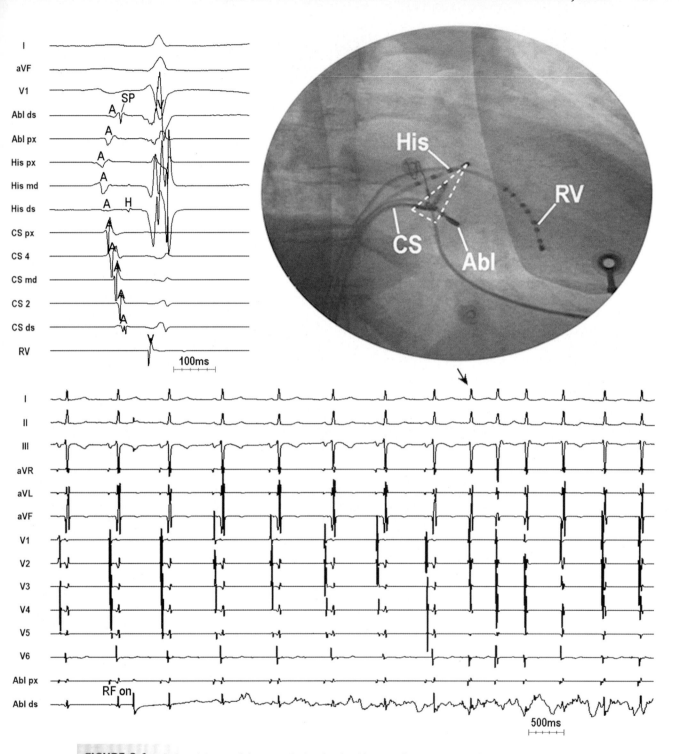

FIGURE 8-1 Ablation of the SP of the AV node (NSR). The ablation catheter is positioned along the posteroseptum where it records a low-amplitude (far-field) atrial electrogram followed by a high-frequency (near-field) SP potential. The ventricular electrogram is large, and a His bundle signal is absent. Application of RF energy causes junctional tachycardia (*arrow*) with preserved JA conduction. Dashed lines denote the triangle of Koch.

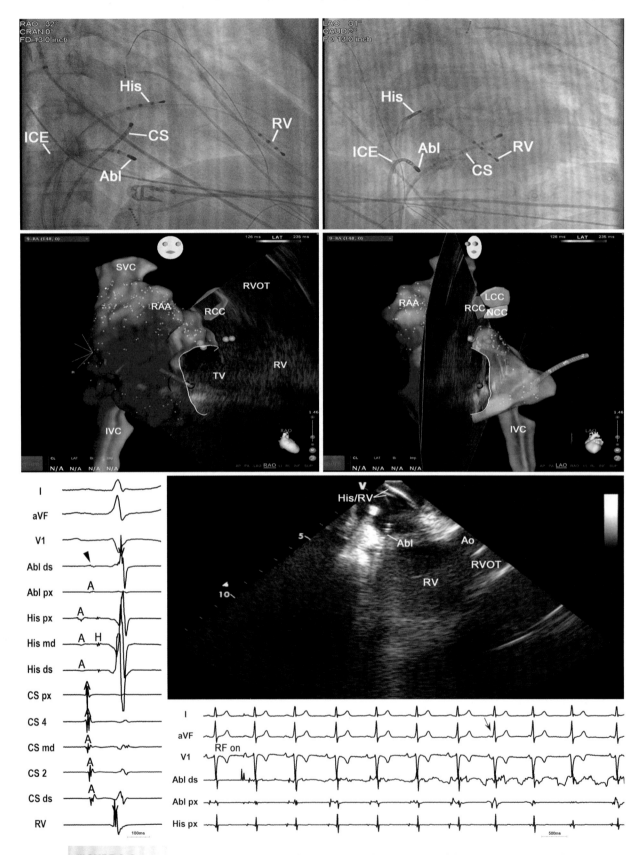

FIGURE 8-2 Ablation of the SP of the AV node (NSR). The ablation catheter is positioned along the posteroseptum where it records a low-amplitude atrial electrogram (*arrowhead*) and a large ventricular electrogram. A His bundle signal is absent. The earliest site of atrial activation during typical AVNRT (*red*) is along the anteroseptum (His bundle region). Application of RF energy to the posteroseptum (CS os region) causes a slow junctional rhythm (*arrow*). *Yellow tags* denote His bundle sites.

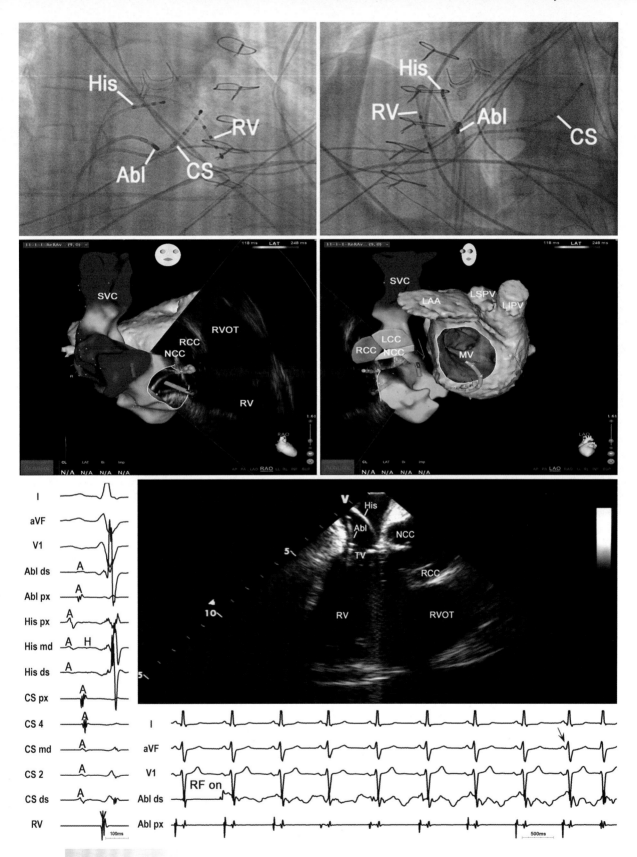

FIGURE 8-3 Ablation of the SP of the AV node (NSR). The ablation catheter is positioned along the posteroseptum where it records a low-amplitude atrial electrogram and a large ventricular electrogram. A His bundle signal is absent. The earliest site of atrial activation during typical AVNRT (*red*) is along the anteroseptum (His bundle region). Application of RF energy to the posteroseptum (CS os region) causes junctional rhythm (*arrow*) with JA conduction. Yellow tags denote His bundle sites.

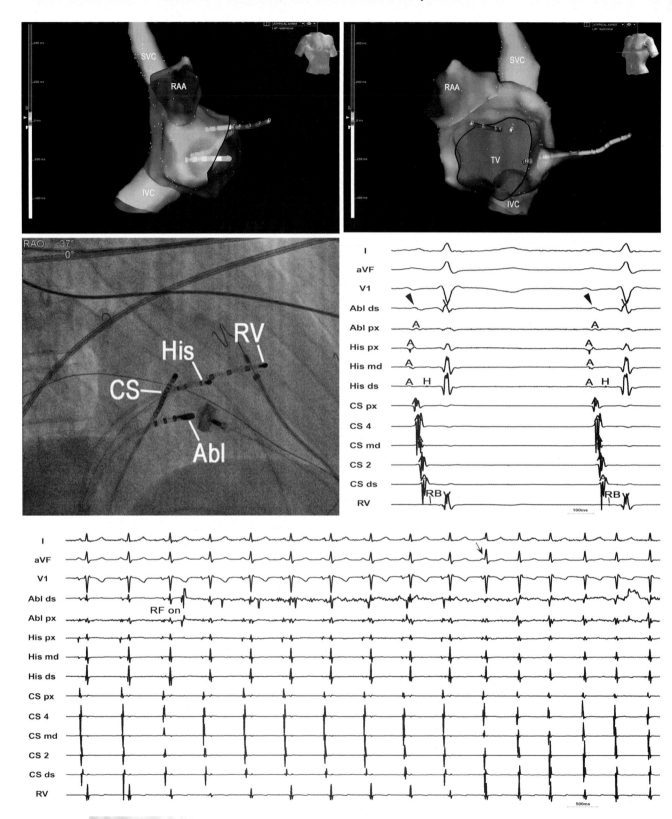

FIGURE 8-4 Ablation of the SP of the AV node (NSR). The ablation catheter is positioned along the posteroseptum where it records a low-amplitude atrial electrogram (*arrowheads*) and a moderate-sized ventricular electrogram. A His bundle signal is absent. The earliest site of atrial activation during atypical AVNRT (*white*) is along the posteroseptum (CS os region) where application of RF energy during NSR causes a junctional rhythm (*arrow*) with intact JA conduction.

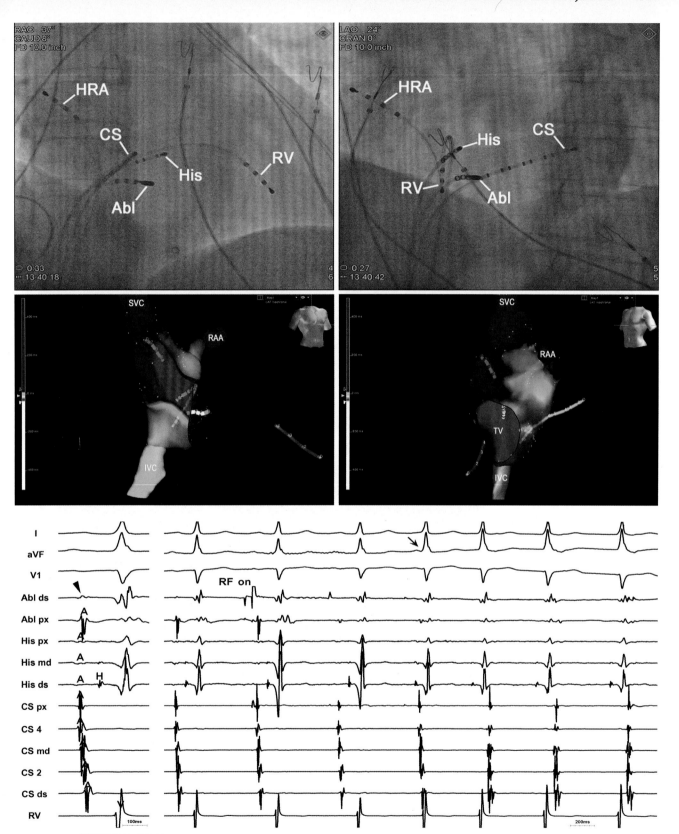

FIGURE 8-5 Ablation of the SP of the AV node (NSR). The ablation catheter is positioned along the posteroseptum where it records a low-amplitude, multicomponent atrial electrogram (*arrowhead*) and a moderate-sized ventricular electrogram. A His bundle signal is absent. The earliest site of atrial activation during atypical AVNRT (*white*) is along the posteroseptum (CS os region) where application of RF energy during NSR causes a slow junctional rhythm (*arrow*) with intact JA conduction.

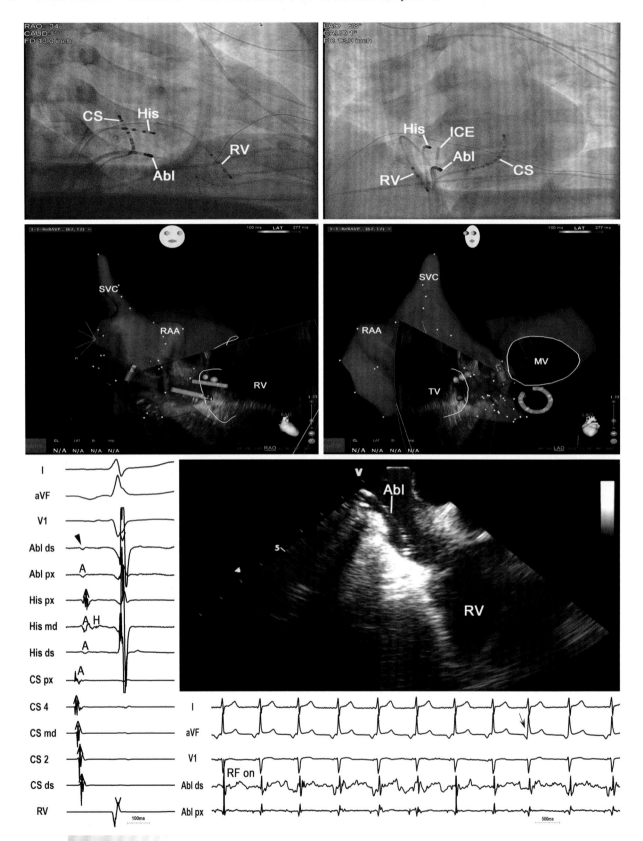

FIGURE 8-6 Ablation of the SP of the AV node. The ablation catheter is positioned along the posteroseptum where it records a low-amplitude atrial electrogram (*arrowhead*) during a persistent ectopic atrial rhythm and large ventricular electrogram. The atrial electrogram at the SP site is later than at CS px (site closest to atrial tachycardia [AT] origin). A His bundle signal is absent. The earliest site of atrial activation during typical AVNRT (*red*) is along the anteroseptum (His bundle region). Application of RF energy to the posteroseptum (CS os region) causes a slow junctional rhythm (*arrow*). Yellow tags denote His bundle sites.

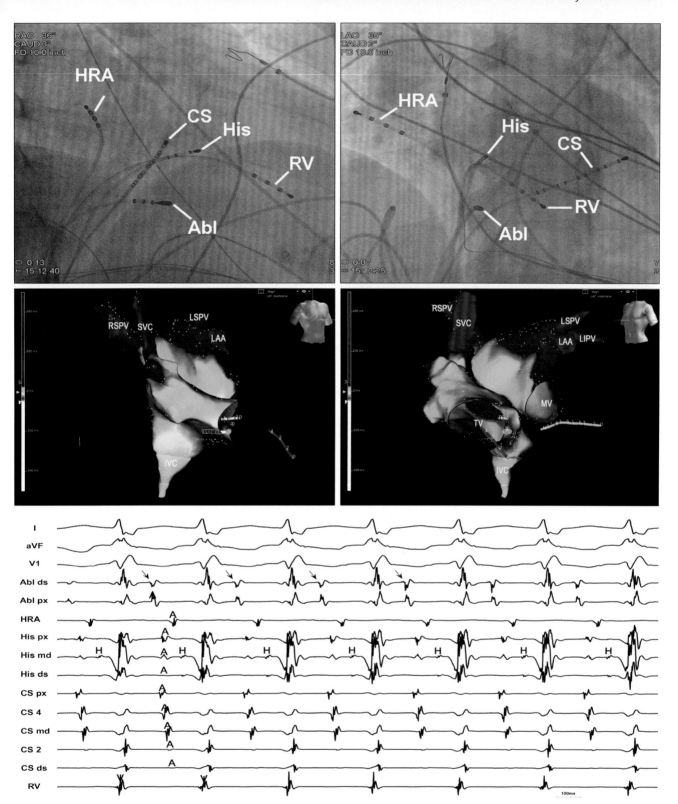

FIGURE 8-7 Ablation of the SP of the AV node (atypical AVNRT). The ablation catheter is positioned near the CS os along the posteroseptum where it records a low-amplitude atrial electrogram (*arrows*) and a moderate to large ventricular electrogram at the earliest site of atrial activation (*white*) during atypical AVNRT. A His bundle signal is absent. Application of RF energy to this site successfully ablated AVNRT.

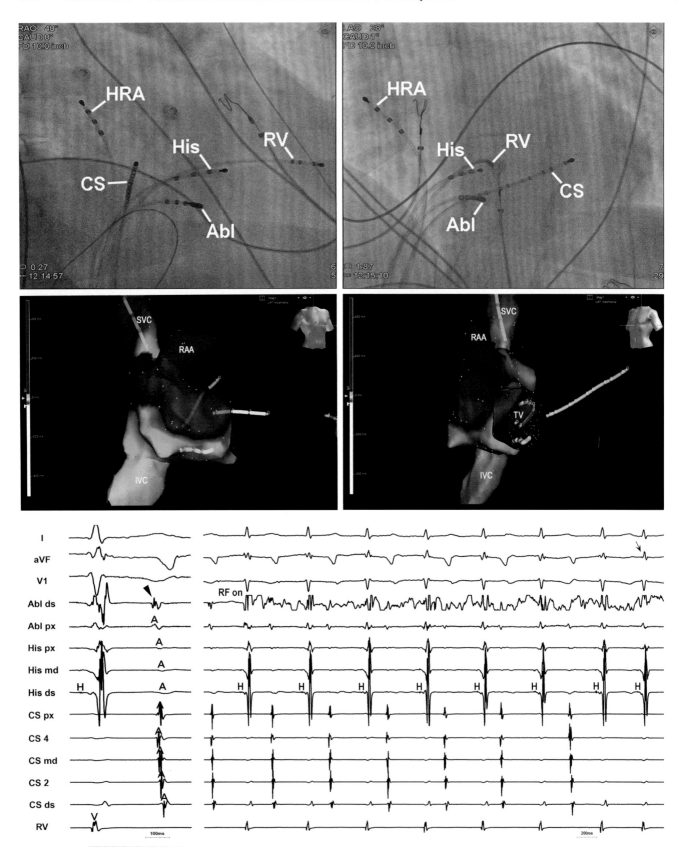

FIGURE 8-8 Ablation of the SP of the AV node (atypical AVNRT). The ablation catheter is positioned along the right posteroseptum where it records a low-amplitude atrial electrogram (*arrowhead*) and a large ventricular electrogram at the earliest site of atrial activation (*white*, pre–P wave × 32 ms) during atypical AVNRT. A His bundle signal is absent. Application of RF energy caused retrograde delay and block in the SP terminating AVNRT followed by a premature junctional complex (*arrow*). Note that the junctional complex is nod associated with JA conduction because retrograde FP conduction was absent at baseline, making monitoring of JA conduction during RF delivery difficult.

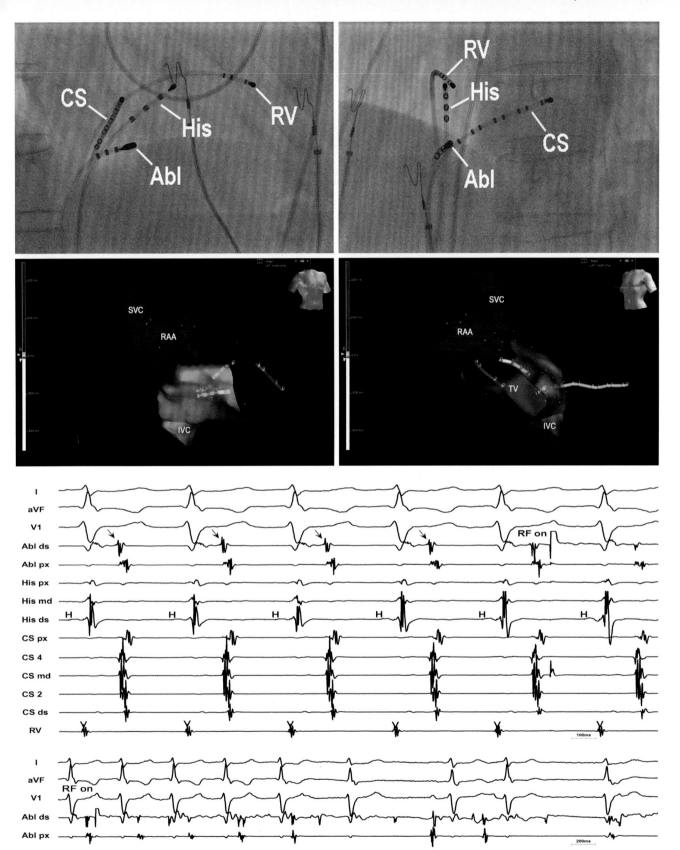

FIGURE 8-9 Ablation of the SP of the AV node (atypical AVNRT). The ablation catheter is positioned at the CS os along the posteroseptum where it records the earliest site of atrial activation (*white, arrows*) during atypical AVNRT. A His bundle signal is absent. Application of RF energy terminates tachycardia. A junctional escape complex with JA conduction occurs at the end of the tracing.

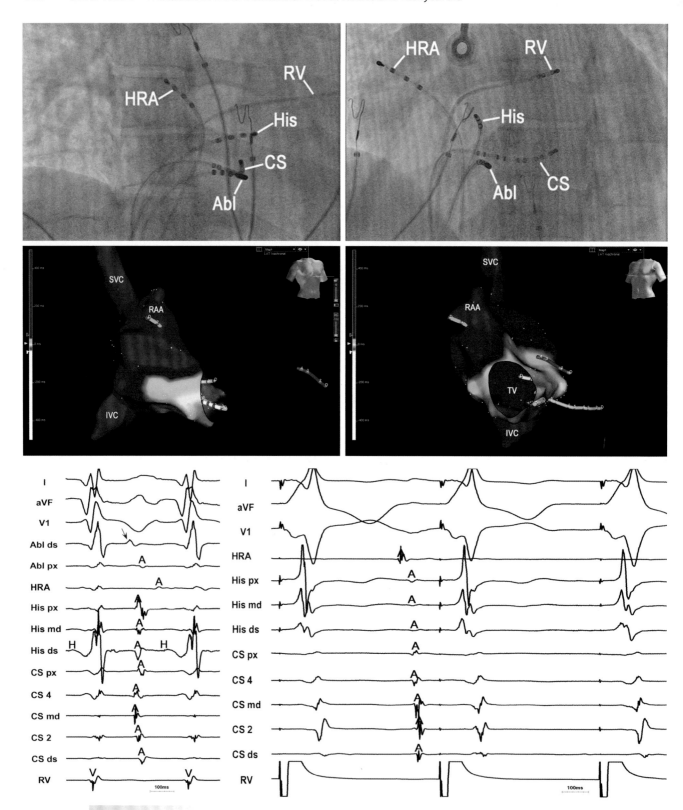

FIGURE 8-10 Ablation of the SP of the AV node (atypical AVNRT). The ablation catheter is positioned near the CS os along the posteroseptum where it records a small atrial (*arrow*) and large ventricular electrogram at the earliest site of atrial activation (*white*) during atypical AVNRT. A His bundle signal is absent. Application of RF terminated tachycardia and abolished retrograde SP conduction (VA dissociation).

atrial activation, the order of the high frequency (near-field) SP potential relative to the low-amplitude (far-field) atrial electrogram is reversed compared to sinus rhythm.[1]

LEFT-SIDED ABLATION

Rarely, AVNRT is refractory to right-sided ablation and requires ablation within the CS or endocardially along the left posteroseptum (left inferior extension) or lateral mitral annulus (inferolateral inputs).[18–21] Sinus rhythm target site criteria (small, multicomponent atrial electrogram, large ventricular electrogram) are similar along the left posteroseptum resulting in junctional rhythm. Because the exact location of an antegradely conducting inferolateral input integral to tachycardia is unknown, it can be mapped along the mitral annulus by identifying the atrial site with the longest coupling interval that resets tachycardia.

MONITORING DURING RF DELIVERY

Ablation of the SP characteristically induces junctional ectopy (a sensitive but nonspecific marker of success).[22] Safe junctional ectopy is 1) slow and 2) associated with JA conduction. Rarely, successful ablation can be achieved without junctional ectopy.[23] Because of the risk of AV block, catheter movement (fluoroscopy, electro-anatomic mapping) and the junctional rhythm should be monitored continuously during RF delivery. Signs predicting AV block and necessitating immediate termination of RF energy include 1) rapid (<350 ms) junctional tachycardia, 2) JA block, 3) PR prolongation (suggesting injury to the compact AV node), and 4) widening of QRS morphology (due to accelerated ventricular rhythm from a more distal ablation location) (**Fig. 8-11**).[22,24–26] One useful technique for SP ablation is a piecemeal approach with initial immediate discontinuation of RF energy upon onset of junctional ectopy followed by repeated ablation of progressively longer durations.[27]

When baseline retrograde VA conduction is poor, monitoring JA conduction during RF delivery can be difficult as both safe and malignant junctional ectopy show no JA conduction. Either low-dose isoproterenol (to improve retrograde AV nodal conduction) or atrial overdrive pacing with onset of junctional rhythm (pacing rate faster than junctional rhythm to monitor antegrade AV conduction) can be employed to help ensure that AV node function remains intact during continued RF delivery (**Fig. 8-12**).[28] Isoproterenol, in particular, can facilitate SP ablation during dual antegrade response tachycardia by 1) abolishing antegrade SP conduction (which itself mimics junctional ectopy with JA block) and 2) facilitating retrograde FP conduction (which is characteristically absent during DART).[29–31]

PROCEDURAL ENDPOINTS

Ablation of the SP is effective therapy for patients who have AVNRT or dual AV nodal physiology with a documented but noninducible supraventricular tachycardia that is consistent with AVNRT.[32] The endpoint for successful SP ablation is either 1) total abolition (complete elimination of SP conduction) or 2) modification (residual SP conduction with at most single AV nodal echoes but not repetitive AV nodal reentry).[33]

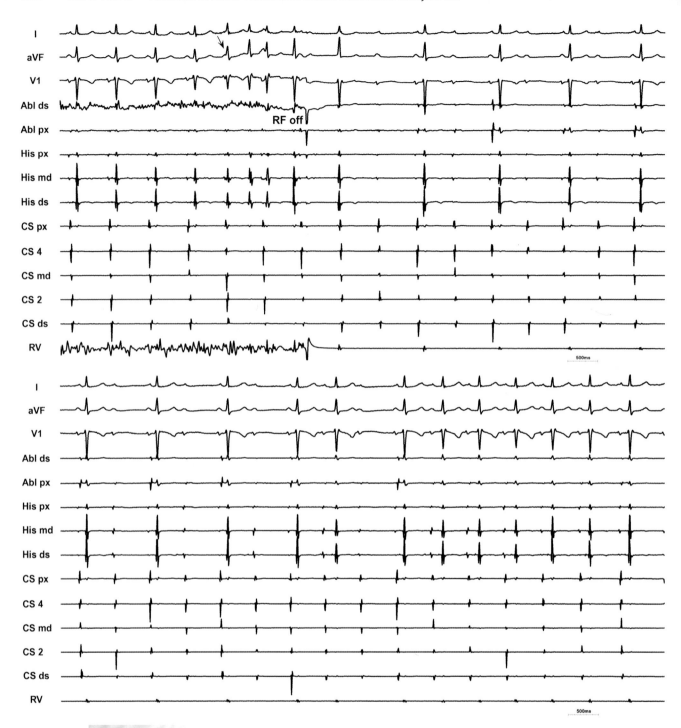

FIGURE 8-11 Inadvertent AV block during ablation of AVNRT. Application of RF energy results in rapid junctional tachycardia (*arrow*) with JA block. Despite discontinuation of RF energy within 0.94 sec, transient AV block occurred.

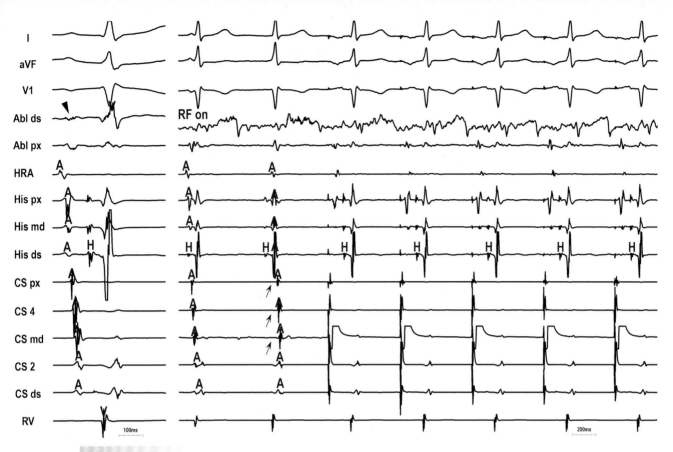

FIGURE 8-12 Atrial overdrive pacing during SP ablation. The ablation catheter is positioned along the posteroseptum where it records a low-amplitude, fractionated atrial (*arrowhead*) and large ventricular electrogram. A His bundle signal is absent. Application of RF energy causes junctional rhythm, but rapid JA conduction is absent (*arrows*). Atrial overdrive pacing (faster than the junctional rhythm) with intact 1:1 AV conduction ensures antegrade integrity of the AV node during continued RF delivery.

REFERENCES

1. Jackman WM, Beckman KJ, McClelland JH, et al. Treatment of supraventricular tachycardia due to atrioventricular nodal reentry by radiofrequency catheter ablation of slow-pathway conduction. N Engl J Med 1992;327:313–318.
2. Haissaguerre M, Gaita F, Fischer B, et al. Elimination of atrioventricular nodal reentrant tachycardia using discrete slow potentials to guide application of radiofrequency energy. Circulation 1992;85:2162–2175.
3. Kay GN, Epstein AE, Dailey SM, Plumb VJ. Selective radiofrequency ablation of the slow pathway for the treatment of atrioventricular nodal reentrant tachycardia. Evidence for involvement of perinodal myocardium within the reentrant circuit. Circulation 1992;85:1675–1688.
4. Roman CA, Wang X, Friday KJ, et al. Catheter technique for selective ablation of slow pathway in AV nodal reentrant tachycardia [abstract]. Pacing Clin Electrophysiol 1990;13:498.
5. Haissaguerre M, Warin JF, Lemetayer P, Saoudi N, Guillem JP, Blanchot P. Closed-chest ablation of retrograde conduction in patients with atrioventricular nodal reentrant tachycardia. N Engl J Med 1989;320:426–433.
6. Goy JJ, Fromer M, Schlaepfer J, Kappenberger L. Clinical efficacy of radiofrequency current in the treatment of patients with atrioventricular node reentrant tachycardia. J Am Coll Cardiol 1990;16:418–423.
7. Lee MA, Morady F, Kadish A, et al. Catheter modification of the atrioventricular junction with radiofrequency energy for control of atrioventricular nodal reentry tachycardia. Circulation 1991;83:827–835.
8. Jazayeri MR, Hempe SL, Sra JS, et al. Selective transcatheter ablation of the fast and slow pathways using radiofrequency energy in patients with atrioventricular nodal reentrant tachycardia. Circulation 1992;85:1318–1328.
9. Cox JL, Holman WL, Cain ME. Cryosurgical treatment of atrioventricular node reentrant tachycardia. Circulation 1987;76:1329–1336.
10. Ross DL, Johnson DC, Denniss AR, Cooper MJ, Richards DA, Uther JB. Curative surgery for atrioventricular junctional ("AV nodal") reentrant tachycardia. J Am Coll Cardiol 1985;6:1383–1392.
11. Katritsis DG, Becker A. The atrioventricular nodal reentrant tachycardia circuit: a proposal. Heart Rhythm 2007;4:1354–1360.
12. Sra JS, Jazayeri MR, Blanck Z, Deshpande S, Dhala AA, Akhtar M. Slow pathway ablation in patients with atrioventricular node reentrant tachycardia and a prolonged PR interval. J Am Coll Cardiol 1994;24:1064–1068.
13. Reithmann C, Remp T, Oversohl N, Steinbeck G. Ablation for atrioventricular nodal reentrant tachycardia with a prolonged PR interval during sinus rhythm: the risk of delayed higher-degree atrioventricular block. J Cardiovasc Electrophysiol 2006;17:973–979.
14. Rigden LB, Klein LS, Mitrani RD, Zipes DP, Miles WM. Increased risk of heart block following slow pathway ablation for AV nodal reentrant tachycardia in patients with marked PR interval prolongation during sinus rhythm [abstract]. Pacing Clin Electrophysiol 1995;18:II-918.
15. Katritsis DG, Marine JE, Contreras FM, et al. Catheter ablation of atypical atrioventricular nodal reentrant tachycardia. Circulation 2016;134:1655–1663.
16. Hwang C, Martin DJ, Goodman JS, et al. Atypical atrioventricular node reciprocating tachycardia masquerading as tachycardia using a left-sided accessory pathway. J Am Coll Cardiol 1997;30:218–225.
17. Asirvatham SJ, Stevenson WG. Atrioventricular nodal block with atrioventricular nodal reentrant tachycardia ablation. Circ Arrhythm Electrophysiol 2015;8:745–747.
18. Jais P, Haissaguerre M, Shah DC, et al. Successful radiofrequency ablation of a slow atrioventricular nodal pathway on the left posterior atrial septum. Pacing Clin Electrophysiol 1999;22:525–527.
19. Katritsis DG, Giazitzoglou E, Zografos T, Ellenbogen KA, Camm AJ. An approach to left septal slow pathway ablation. J Interv Card Electrophysiol 2011;30:73–79.

20. Green J, Aziz Z, Nayak HM, Upadhyay GA, Moss JD, Tung R. "Left ventricular" AV nodal reentrant tachycardia: case report and review of the literature. HeartRhythm Case Rep 2016;2:367–371.

21. Otomo K, Nagata Y, Uno K, Fujiwara H, Iesaka Y. Atypical atrioventricular nodal reentrant tachycardia with eccentric coronary sinus activation: electrophysiological characteristics and essential effects of left-sided ablation inside the coronary sinus. Heart Rhythm 2007;4:421–432.

22. Jentzer JH, Goyal R, Williamson BD, et al. Analysis of junctional ectopy during radiofrequency ablation of the slow pathway in patients with atrioventricular nodal reentrant tachycardia. Circulation 1994;90:2820–2826.

23. Hsieh M, Chen S, Tai C, Yu W, Chen Y, Chang M. Absence of junctional rhythm during successful slow-pathway ablation in patients with atrioventricular nodal reentrant tachycardia. Circulation 1998;98:2296–2300.

24. Lipscomb KJ, Zaidi AM, Fitzpatrick AP, Lefroy D. Slow pathway modification for atrioventricular node re-entrant tachycardia: fast junctional tachycardia predicts adverse prognosis. Heart 2001;85:44–47.

25. Thakur RK, Klein GJ, Yee R, Stites HW. Junctional tachycardia: a useful marker during radiofrequency ablation for atrioventricular node reentrant tachycardia. J Am Coll Cardiol 1993;22:1706–1710.

26. Chen H, Shehata M, Ma W, et al. Atrioventricular block during slow pathway ablation: entirely preventable? Circ Arrhythm Electrophysiol 2015;8:739–744.

27. Meininger GR, Calkins H. One method to reduce heart block risk during catheter ablation of atrioventricular nodal reentrant tachycardia. J Cardiovasc Electrophysiol 2004;15:727–728.

28. Liberman L, Hordof AJ, Pass RH. Rapid atrial pacing: a useful technique during slow pathway ablation. Pacing Clin Electrophysiol 2007;30:221–224.

29. Wang NC, Razak EA, Jain SK, Saba S. Isoproterenol facilitation of slow pathway ablation in incessant dual atrioventricular nodal nonreentrant tachycardia. Pacing Clin Electrophysiol 2012;35:e31–e34.

30. Gaba D, Pavri BB, Greenspon AJ, Ho RT. Dual antegrade response tachycardia induced cardiomyopathy. Pacing Clin Electrophysiol 2004;27:533–536.

31. Lin F-C, Yeh S-J, Wu D. Determinants of simultaneous fast and slow pathway conduction in patients with dual atrioventricular nodal pathways. Am Heart J 1985;109:963–970.

32. Bogun F, Knight B, Weiss R, et al. Slow pathway ablation in patients with documented but noninducible paroxysmal supraventricular tachycardia. J Am Coll Cardiol 1996;28:1000–1004.

33. Lindsay BD, Chung MK, Gamache C, et al. Therapeutic end points for the treatment of atrioventricular node reentrant tachycardia by catheter-guided radiofrequency current. J Am Coll Cardiol 1993;22:733–740.

Basic Evaluation of Accessory Pathways

Introduction

The typical accessory pathway (AP) (bundle of Kent) is a muscle fiber bridging the atrio-ventricular (AV) groove and providing electrical continuity between the atrium and ventricle in parallel to the AV node–His-Purkinje axis.[1] It can conduct antegradely, retrogradely, or bidirectionally. Antegradely conducting APs show ventricular preexcitation on the 12-lead ECG and are therefore "manifest." If they conduct exclusively in the antegrade direction, they are "manifest only." If they conduct only in the retrograde direction, they do not cause preexcitation and are therefore called "concealed." Factors limiting antegrade conduction of concealed APs almost always occur at its ventricular insertion site (AP–ventricle [V] interface) and include 1) "impedance mismatch" (small AP fiber incapable of generating sufficient current to activate the large mass of ventricular muscle) and 2) retrograde concealment from sinus-driven AV node–His-Purkinje conduction into the AP with a prolonged anterograde refractory period (which can be unmasked if AV block occurs).[2–4] The Wolff-Parkinson-White (WPW) pattern refers to ventricular preexcitation on the ECG, while the WPW syndrome is the association of symptoms with the WPW pattern.

The purpose of this chapter is to:
1. Describe the 12-lead ECG and electrophysiologic hallmarks of manifest preexcitation.
2. Localize APs by the 12-lead ECG and intracardiac recordings.
3. Define the electrophysiologic properties of APs.
4. Discuss sudden death risk stratification of APs.

HALLMARKS OF MANIFEST PREEXCITATION

12-LEAD ECG

During sinus rhythm, the ECG signs of ventricular preexcitation are 1) short PR interval ($\leq$120 ms), 2) delta wave (slurring of the initial forces of the QRS complex), and 3) secondary ST–T wave abnormalities.[5,6] The PR interval is short because the AP "bypasses" the AV node–His-Purkinje system to prematurely activate the ventricle ("preexcite"). The PJ interval, however, is normal because the time required to complete ventricular activation is unchanged.[6] The QRS complex is a fusion between His-Purkinje and AP conduction, and the delta wave reflects the initial activation of the ventricle by the AP. During sinus rhythm, the degree of preexcitation is therefore primarily determined by 1) AP location relative to the sinus node and 2) status of AV nodal conduction. Preexcitation is greatest with right-sided APs near the sinus node because of the short conduction time to the AP relative to the AV node–His-Purkinje axis. Inapparent or minimal preexcitation can occur with left free wall APs because the large distance between the sinus node and AP causes

minimal activation of the ventricle by the AP. Inapparent preexcitation can be unmasked by adenosine/coronary sinus (CS) pacing or excluded by the presence of a septal q wave in lead V6 (unobscured normal left to right septal activation by the His-Purkinje system) (**Figs. 9-1 and 9-2**).[7–10] Latent preexcitation refers to preexcitation that is absent during sinus rhythm but becomes manifest only with atrial pacing and occurs with slow, decrementally conducting APs (e.g., atrio-fascicular AP). Intermittent preexcitation refers to abrupt loss of preexcitation during sinus rhythm that identifies a poorly conducting AP with a long antegrade refractory period and generally a low risk for sudden death (especially if present during catecholamine provocation (e.g., isoproterenol) (**Fig. 9-3**). Fixed preexcitation refers to constant preexcitation during sinus rhythm. Enhancing AV nodal conduction (exercise, isoproterenol) reduces the degree of preexcitation.

ELECTROPHYSIOLOGIC STUDY

The intracardiac hallmark of preexcitation is a short (<35 ms) or negative HV interval (**Fig. 9-3**).[11] It corresponds inversely

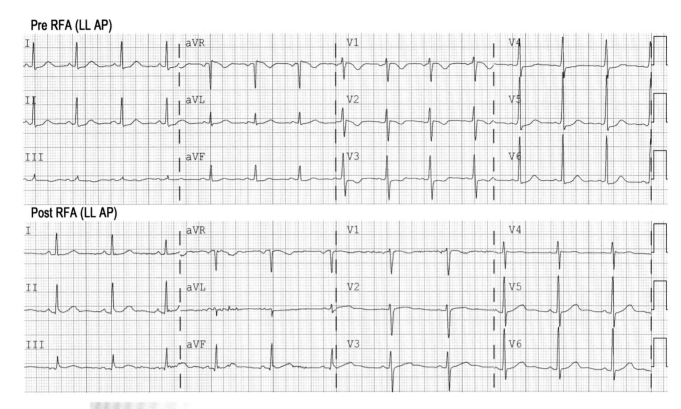

FIGURE 9-1 Inapparent preexcitation. *Top*: Preexcitation is subtle, and hint of a delta wave is seen only in leads V3 and V4. *Bottom*: After ablation of a left free wall AP, the delta wave is gone. Although a q wave in V6 is not seen, inferior q waves are now evident.

to the size of the delta wave on the surface ECG. Because AV APs originate above the His bundle, His extrasystoles conduct to the ventricle without preexcitation. A preexcited His bundle extrasystole identifies a fasciculo-ventricular AP that originates below the His bundle.

AP LOCALIZATION

APs can be found anywhere along the tricuspid or mitral annuli except classically at the fibrous aorto-mitral continuity (left anteroseptal region), although rare cases have been reported.[12] In decreasing order of frequency, AP sites include left free wall, posteroseptal, right free wall, and anteroseptal.[11] Rarely, APs are located in the atrial appendages, CS diverticulum, ligament of Marshall, and noncoronary cusp of the aortic valve.[13–17]

12-LEAD ECG

The ECG clues to identify the approximate location of an AP are its 1) delta-wave axis during manifest preexcitation and 2) P-wave axis during orthodromic reciprocating tachycardia (ORT).[11,18–23]

Delta-Wave Axis

The horizontal delta-wave transition in the anterior precordium (V1–V3) differentiates left-sided, septal, and right-sided APs,

while the vertical delta-wave axis determines its anterior or posterior location along the annulus **(Fig. 9-4)**.[11,18–22] Early delta-wave transition (at or before V1) indicates a left-sided AP because initial ventricular forces are directed anteriorly toward the right ventricle. Negative delta waves in the lateral (I, aVL) or inferior leads identify a left free wall or left posterior AP, respectively. Transition at V2 (overlying the interventricular septum) indicates a right postero- or midseptal AP. Posteroseptal APs show a sum of delta-wave polarities in the inferior leads (II, III, aVF) ≤ −2, while midseptal APs show a sum of −1, 0, or +1. In the absence of incomplete right bundle branch block (RBBB) or infundibular pattern, a terminal r wave in V1 raises the possibility of a left-sided septal AP (possibly due to early activation of the proximal left bundle by the left-sided AP with late activation of the right ventricle) **(Fig. 9-5)**.[24,25] A negative delta wave in II, steep (≥45 degrees) positive delta wave in aVR, and deep S wave (R ≤ S) in V6 suggest an epicardial posteroseptal AP within the CS or its branches.[26] Late transition (at or beyond V3) indicates a right-sided AP. Anteroseptal APs show a "left bundle branch block" ("LBBB") type pattern with a small narrow positive delta wave transitioning at V3, sum of delta-wave polarities in the inferior leads (II, III, aVF) ≥+2, and a frontal axis +30 to +120 degrees. Classic true parahisian APs, however, show negative delta waves in V1 and V2 or sum of initial r wave (V1 + V2) <0.5 mV (because initial forces are directed away from V1 and V2—both of which are

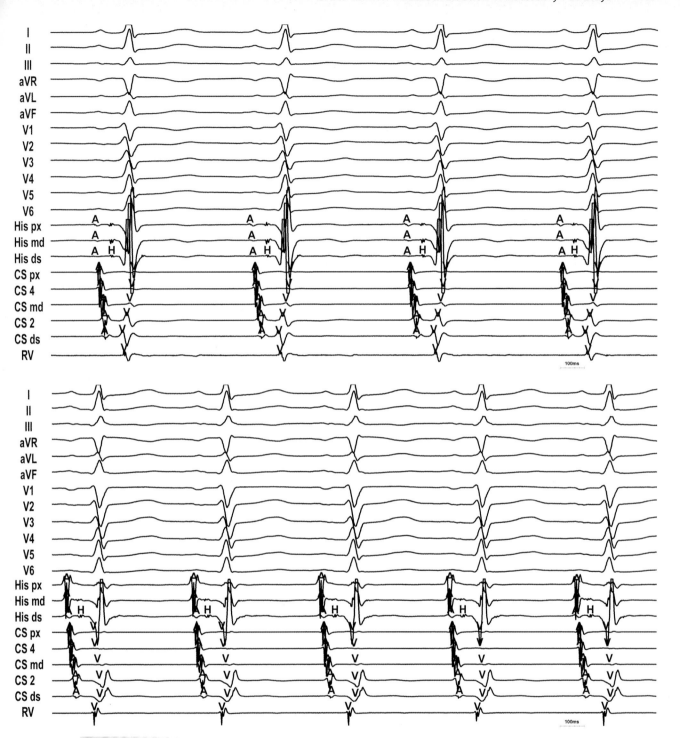

FIGURE 9-2 Inapparent preexcitation. *Top:* The HV is short (31 ms). Clue to the presence of a left free wall AP is the early ventricular electrogram on CS ds with distal to proximal ventricular activation along the CS. *Bottom:* After ablation of the left free wall AP, the HV normalizes (44 ms) and the ventricular electrogram on CS ds is now late.

equidistant from the midline sternum that overlies the membranous septum).[21] Right free wall APs generally transition later beyond V3 indicating that initial ventricular forces are directed posteriorly toward the left ventricle and demonstrate a frontal axis +30 to −60 degrees.

P-Wave Axis

P-wave polarities during ORT also differentiate left-sided, septal, and right-sided APs. A rightward axis (aVR [+], aVL [−]) indicates eccentric atrial activation arising from a left-sided AP, while a leftward axis (aVR [−], aVL [+]) identifies eccentric activation

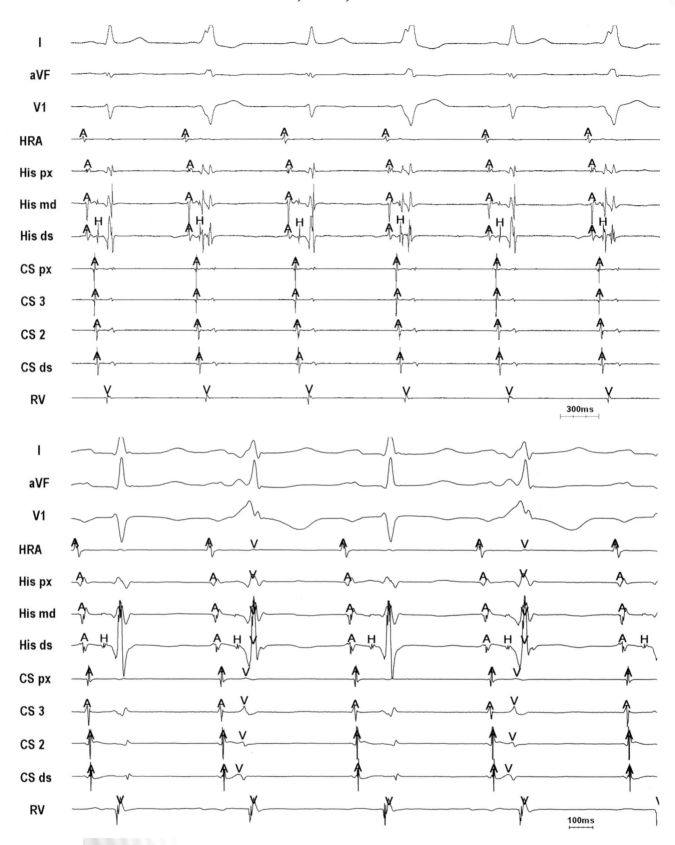

FIGURE 9-3 Intermittent (2:1) preexcitation over a right (*top*) and left (*bottom*) free wall AP. During preexcitation, the HV is short (negative).

Right free wall

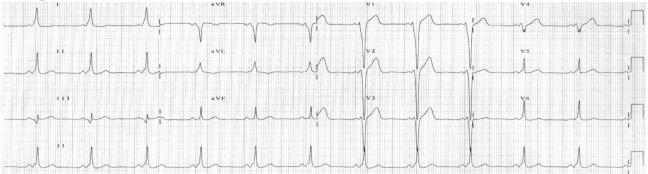

Posteroseptal

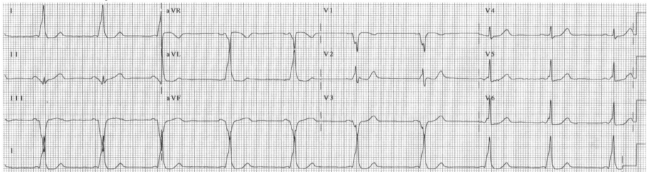

Anteroseptal

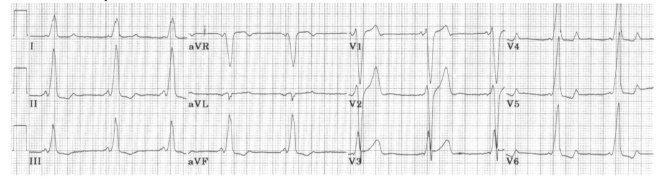

Left free wall

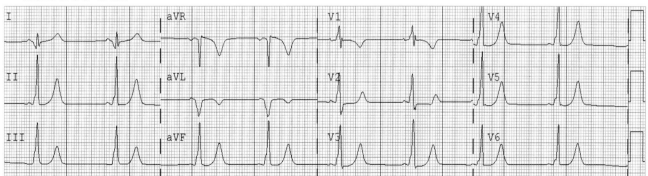

FIGURE 9-4 A 12-lead ECG of manifest preexcitation over a right free wall, posteroseptal, anteroseptal, and left free wall AP. The right free wall AP shows "LBBB" morphology with late precordial transition (V4–V5). The right posteroseptal AP shows transition at V2 (overlying the septum) and negative delta waves inferiorly. The anteroseptal AP shows "LBBB" morphology with positive delta waves inferiorly. The left free wall AP shows "RBBB" morphology and negative delta wave in lead I.

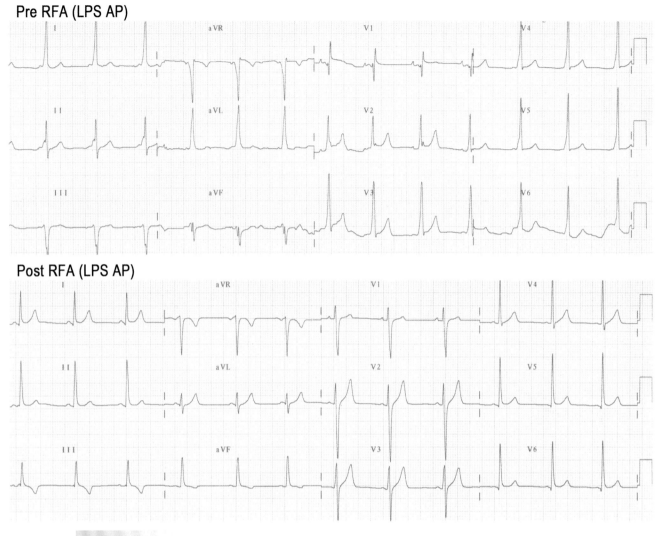

FIGURE 9-5 V1 terminal r wave (left septal AP). A 12-lead ECG before (*top*) and after (*bottom*) ablation of a left posteroseptal AP. Note the delta-wave transition (V1–V2) and QR complex (terminal R wave) in V1, which disappears after ablation. (The top ECG also has a limb lead reversal.)

from a right-sided AP. Postero- and midseptal APs generate a narrow P wave with a midline superior axis (aVR and aVL [+]), while anteroseptal APs can produce positive P waves inferiorly.[12,23]

ELECTROPHYSIOLOGIC STUDY

Location of the AP is determined by the 1) earliest site of ventricular activation during manifest preexcitation; 2) earliest site of atrial activation during retrograde AP conduction; and, if present, 3) AP potentials.[11,20] A less commonly used method for AP localization is differential atrial pacing, which identifies the AP atrial insertion site by identifying the atrial pacing site yielding the shortest stimulus–delta interval.[27] During the electrophysiologic study, multiple annular sites are mapped using catheters positioned at the His bundle region (anteroseptum) and within the CS (posteroseptum and left AV sulcus). While a venous equivalent to the CS is absent for the tricuspid annulus, its endocardium can be mapped using a multipolar "Halo" catheter.

Earliest Site of Ventricular Activation
Because the AP preexcites the ventricle, its ventricular insertion site is identified by locating the earliest ventricular electrogram relative to delta-wave onset ("pre-delta").

Earliest Site of Atrial Activation
Two patterns of retrograde AP conduction are 1) concentric (midline) or 2) eccentric. Septal APs generate concentric patterns earliest near the CS os (posteroseptal AP) or His bundle region (anteroseptal AP). Right and left free wall APs create eccentric patterns with earliest atrial sites away from the septum. During retrograde AP conduction (ventricular pacing, ORT), the earliest site of atrial activation identifies its atrial insertion site.

Accessory Pathway Potentials
Direct recordings of the AP can generate high-frequency deflections (AP or Kent potentials) between the atrial and ventricular electrograms during preexcited sinus rhythm and/or ORT (**see Figs. 10-20 and 12-10**).

ELECTROPHYSIOLOGIC PROPERTIES OF THE AP

ANTEGRADE AP ERP

During programmed atrial extrastimulation, the longest A_1A_2 interval that fails to conduct over the AP defines its antegrade effective refractory period (ERP) (**Figs. 9-6 to 9-10**).[28] At long A_1A_2 coupling intervals exceeding both AV node and AP ERP, A_2 conducts to the ventricle with fusion over the AP and His-Purkinje system. As the coupling interval shortens and encroaches on the AV node relative refractory period, the HV interval decreases, while the degree of preexcitation increases because the contribution by the AP to ventricular activation increases. At a critical coupling interval (AP ERP), conduction over the AP fails and occurs only over the AV node provided that the AV node ERP has not been reached.

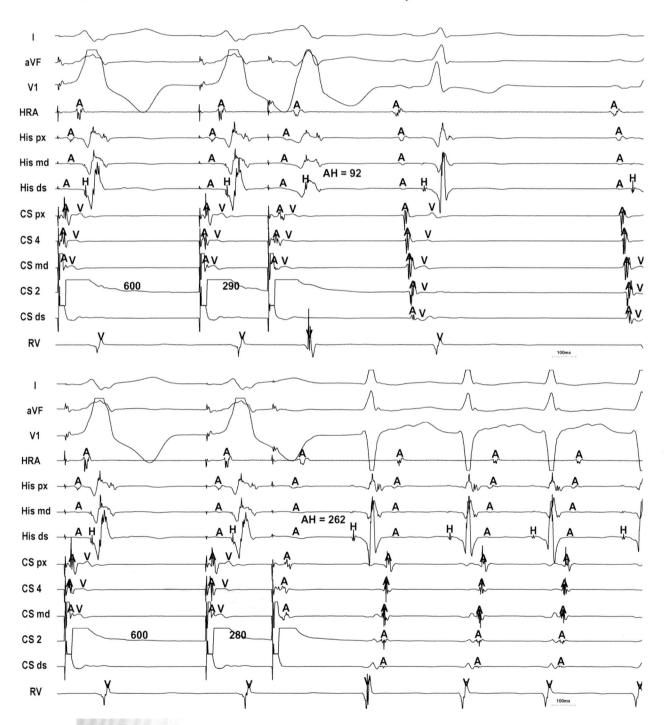

FIGURE 9-6 Antegrade AP ERP (left free wall AP). At a coupling interval of 290 ms, antegrade conduction occurs over the fast pathway (FP) (AH = 92 ms) and AP. At 280 ms, antegrade conduction blocks over the FP and AP (ERP), conducts only over the slow pathway (SP) (AH = 262 ms) causing sufficient AV delay to initiate ORT.

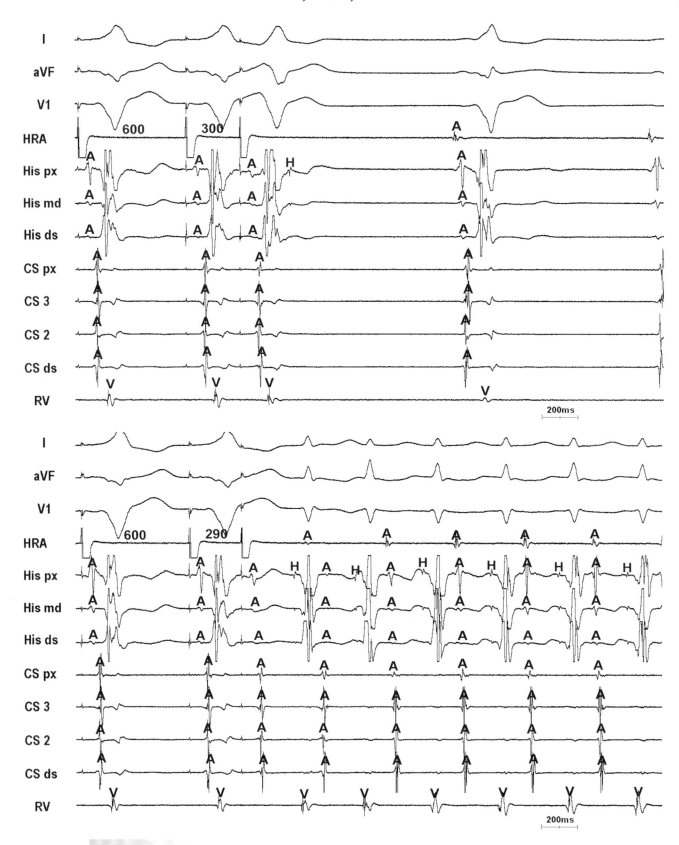

FIGURE 9-7 Antegrade AP ERP (right free wall AP). At a coupling interval of 300 ms, antegrade conduction occurs over the AV node and AP. At 290 ms, antegrade conduction blocks over the AP (ERP) and conducts only over the AV node. A subsequent atrial premature depolarization (APD) initiates ORT.

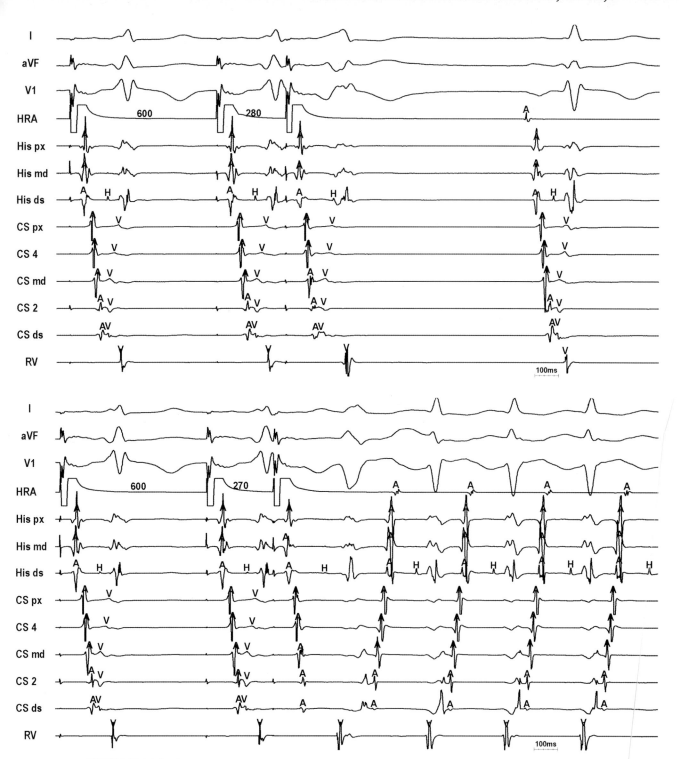

FIGURE 9-8 Antegrade AP ERP (left free wall AP). At a coupling interval of 280 ms, antegrade conduction occurs over the AV node and AP. At 270 ms, antegrade conduction blocks over the AP (ERP) and conducts only over the AV node–His-Purkinje axis. Exposure of the bundle branches to a long–short sequence inherent in programmed extrastimulation induces LBBB aberration, which facilitates induction of left-sided ORT.

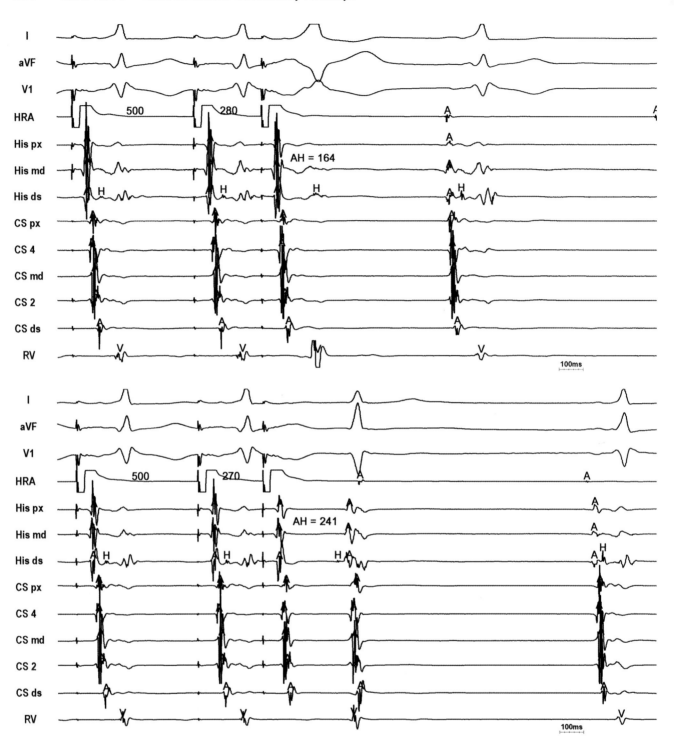

FIGURE 9-9 Antegrade AP ERP (left posterior AP). At a coupling interval of 280 ms, antegrade conduction occurs over the fast pathway (FP) (AH = 164 ms) and AP. At 270 ms, antegrade conduction blocks over the FP and AP (ERP), conducts only over the slow pathway (SP), and induces a single typical AV nodal echo (retrograde FP preempts AP).

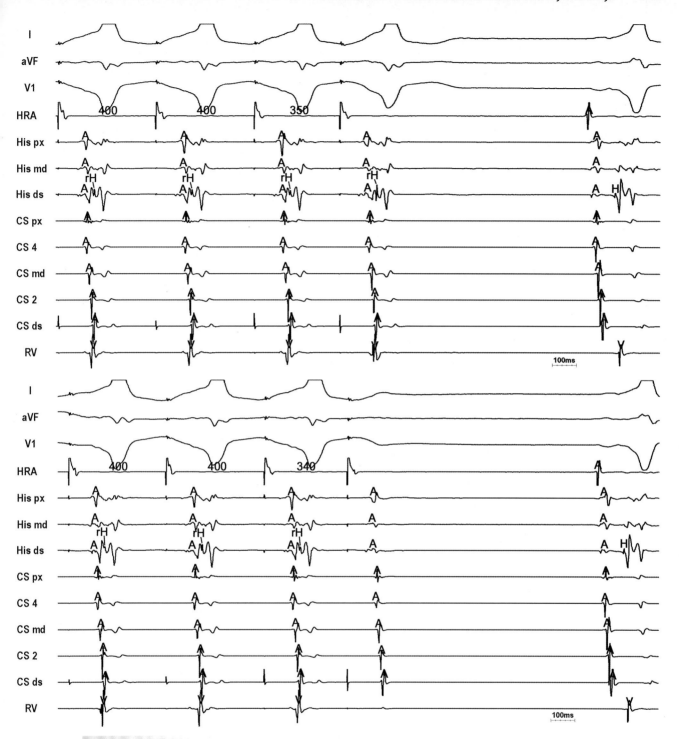

FIGURE 9-10 Antegrade AP ERP (right free wall AP). At a coupling interval of 350 ms, antegrade conduction occurs only over the AP followed by retrograde activation of the His bundle (rH). Note the short "AH" interval. At 340 ms, antegrade conduction blocks over the AP (ERP) resulting in no conduction to the ventricle and loss of the retrograde His bundle.

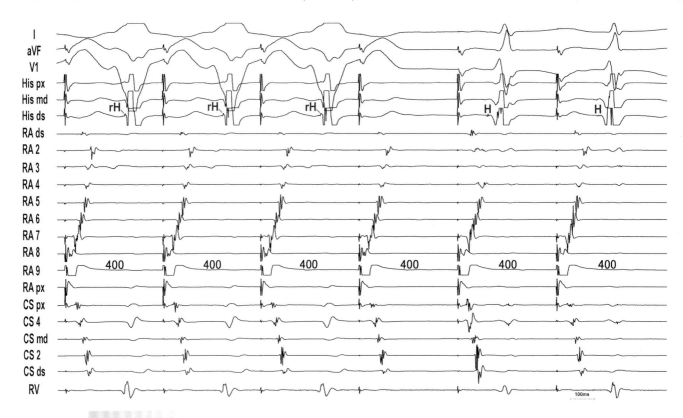

FIGURE 9-11 Antegrade AP block cycle length (right posterior). During atrial pacing at 400 ms, antegrade conduction occurs only over the slowly-conducting AP with a long stimulus–delta interval followed by retrograde activation of the His bundle (rH). The fourth paced complexes fail to conduct over the AP (with loss of retrograde activation of the His bundle), while subsequent paced complexes decrement over the AV node.

ANTEGRADE 1:1 CYCLE LENGTH

Decremental atrial pacing determines the shortest pacing cycle length maintaining 1:1 antegrade conduction over the AP (Fig. 9-11).

RETROGRADE AP ERP

During programmed ventricular extrastimulation with retrograde AP conduction, the longest V1–V2 interval that fails to conduct over the AP defines the retrograde AP ERP (Figs. 9-12 to 9-15).

RETROGRADE 1:1 CYCLE LENGTH

Decremental ventricular pacing determines the shortest pacing cycle length maintaining 1:1 retrograde AP conduction (Fig. 9-16).

RISK OF SUDDEN DEATH

Sudden death associated with WPW has been attributed to rapid preexcited atrial fibrillation degenerating into ventricular fibrillation.[28–31] Unlike the AV node, which serves as a filter manifesting rate-dependent, decremental conduction that slows with faster atrial rates, APs demonstrate fixed, nondecremental conduction that can generate rapid ventricular rates during atrial fibrillation especially with catecholamine surges (e.g., exercise). The risk of sudden death therefore is dependent on antegrade AP refractoriness. The following features identify a low-risk AP: 1) intermittent preexcitation; 2) abrupt, exercise-induced AP block; 3) shortest preexcited RR interval during atrial fibrillation >250 ms; and 4) loss of preexcitation with procainamide, ajmaline, or disopyramide.[32–38] Intermittent preexcitation (particularly on isoproterenol) demonstrates that the AP is incapable of sustaining 1:1 conduction during sinus rhythm and therefore unlikely to conduct rapidly during atrial fibrillation with exercise.[32] Similarly, abrupt loss of preexcitation with exercise demonstrates that the AP is incapable of sustaining 1:1 conduction during sinus tachycardia.[33] During exercise, abrupt loss of preexcitation (rate-dependent AP block) should be differentiated from gradual loss of preexcitation (pseudonormalization) due to enhanced AV nodal conduction. During pseudonormalization, the AP continues to conduct antegradely, but the delta wave slowly disappears as the relative contribution to ventricular activation by the AV node–His-Purkinje system increases. Because the antegrade refractory period correlates with the shortest preexcited RR interval during atrial fibrillation (equivalent to the antegrade AP functional refractory period), an antegrade AP ERP or a shortest atrial pacing cycle length maintaining 1:1 AP conduction >250 ms is a reasonable but not ideal surrogate to the shortest preexcited RR interval when atrial fibrillation is absent.[34,35] Lastly, the ability to alter AP conduction with sodium channel–blocking drugs suggests a low-risk AP, although this is controversial.[36–38]

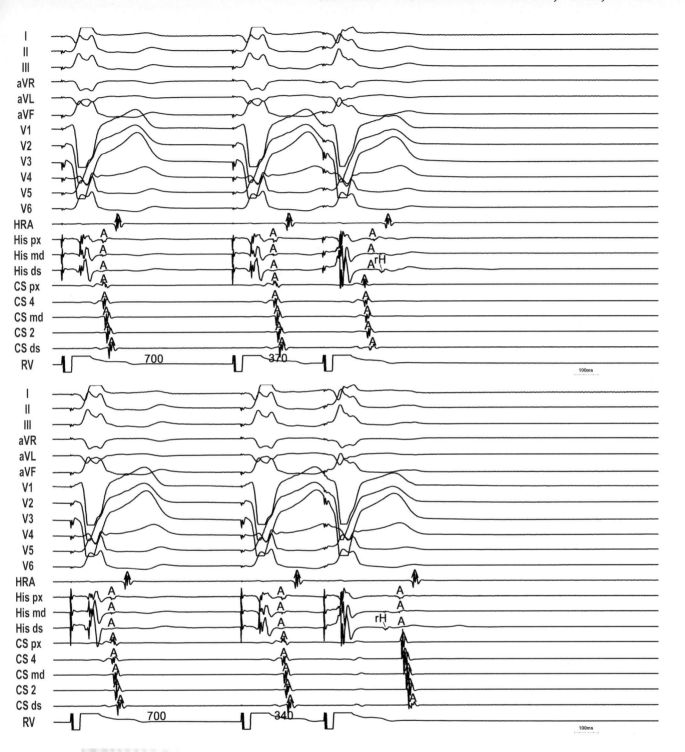

FIGURE 9-12 Retrograde AP ERP (right posteroseptal). During the drive train, retrograde conduction occurs over the fast pathway (FP) (earliest atrial activation at the His bundle region). At a coupling interval of 370 ms, retrograde right bundle (RB) refractoriness causes a "VH jump" exposing a posteroseptal AP (earliest atrial activation at CS px). At 340 ms, retrograde conduction blocks over the AP (ERP) and conducts exclusively over the His bundle and FP.

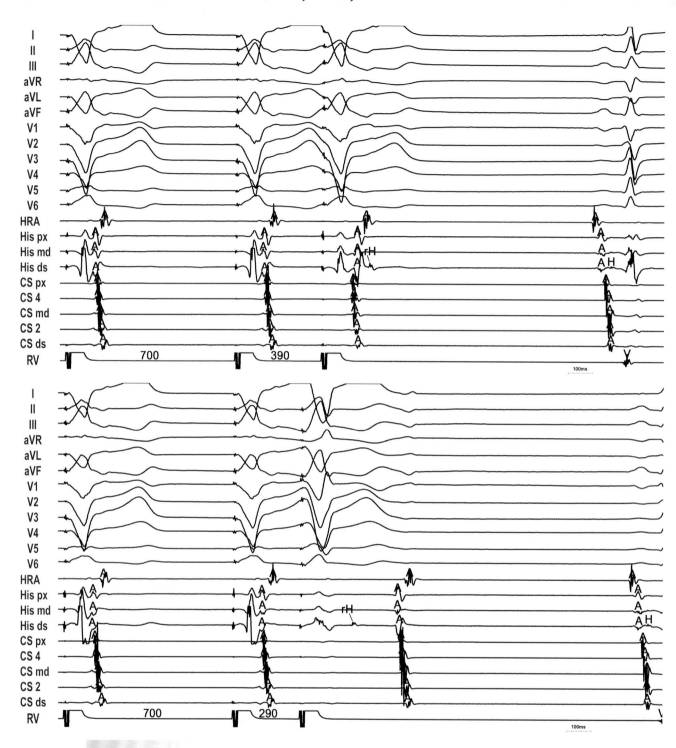

FIGURE 9-13 Retrograde AP ERP (left posteroseptal). During the drive train, retrograde conduction occurs over the fast pathway (FP) (earliest atrial activation at the His bundle region). At a coupling interval of 390 ms, retrograde right bundle (RB) refractoriness causes a "VH jump" exposing a left posteroseptal AP (earliest atrial activation at CS px). At 290 ms, retrograde conduction blocks over the AP (ERP) and conducts exclusively over the His bundle and a relative refractory FP resulting in a prolonged HA time.

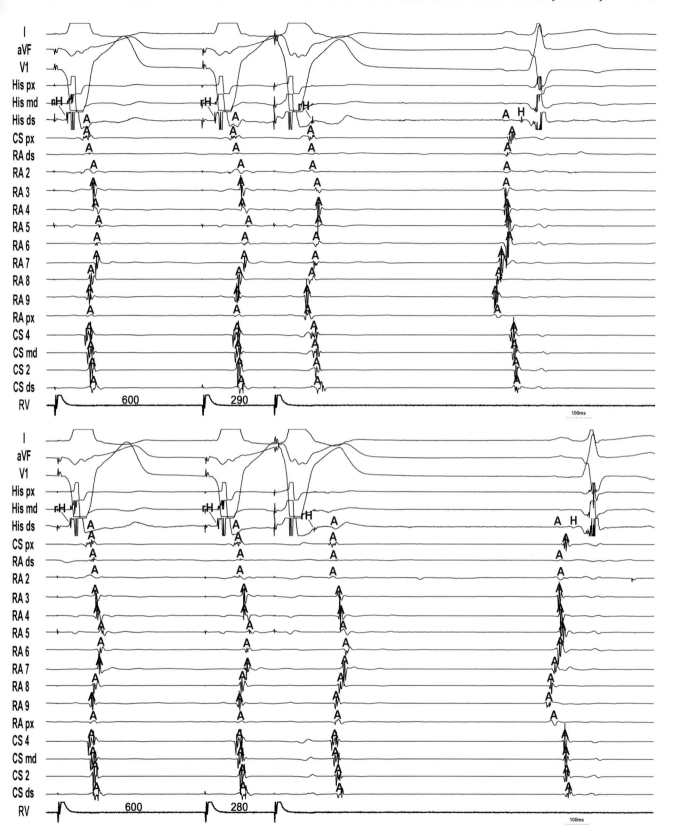

FIGURE 9-14 Retrograde AP ERP (anteroseptal). During the drive train, retrograde conduction occurs over the fast pathway (FP) (earliest atrial activation at the His bundle region). At a coupling interval of 290 ms, retrograde right bundle (RB) refractoriness causes a "VH jump" exposing an anteroseptal AP (earliest atrial activation also at the His bundle region but with a longer stimulus-A [St-A] interval and slightly different atrial activation pattern). At 280 ms, retrograde conduction blocks over the AP (ERP) and conducts exclusively over the His bundle and FP.

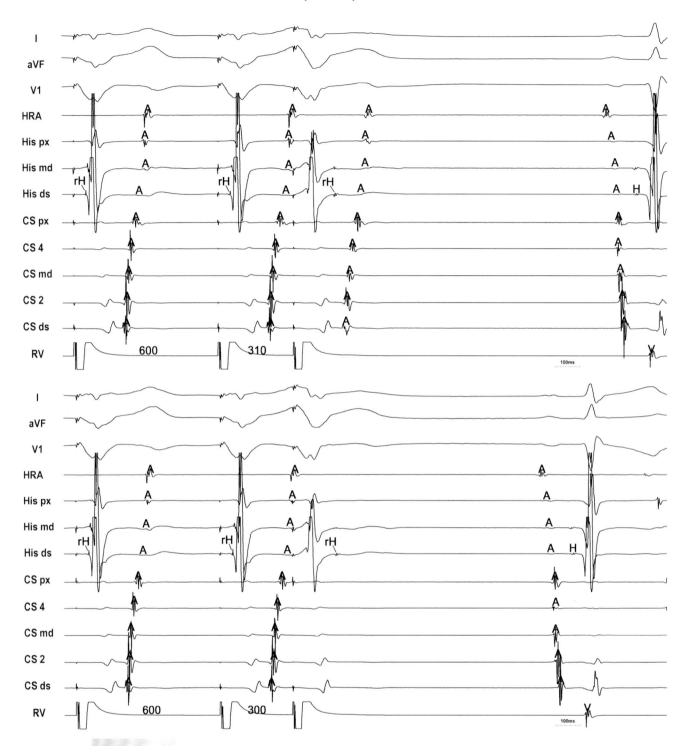

FIGURE 9-15 Retrograde AP ERP (left free wall). During the drive train, retrograde conduction occurs over a left free wall AP (earliest atrial activation at CS ds). At a coupling interval of 310 ms, retrograde right bundle (RB) refractoriness causes a "VH jump" without change in VA interval indicating that retrograde atrial activation is not linked to the His bundle and therefore confirms the presence of an AP. At 300 ms, retrograde conduction blocks over the AP (ERP).

UNUSUAL ELECTROPHYSIOLOGIC PHENOMENA

PHASE 4 BLOCK

Phase 3 AP block occurs when fast sinus or pacing rates encroach on AP refractoriness, while phase 4 AP block occurs at slower sinus rates when spontaneous diastolic depolarizations elevate AP membrane potentials above resting potential (Figs. 9-17 and 9-18).[39,40] The presence of both phase 3 and 4 AP block results in QRS normalization at faster and slower rates, respectively, so that ventricular preexcitation only occurs within a narrow window of heart rates (flanked by two zones of

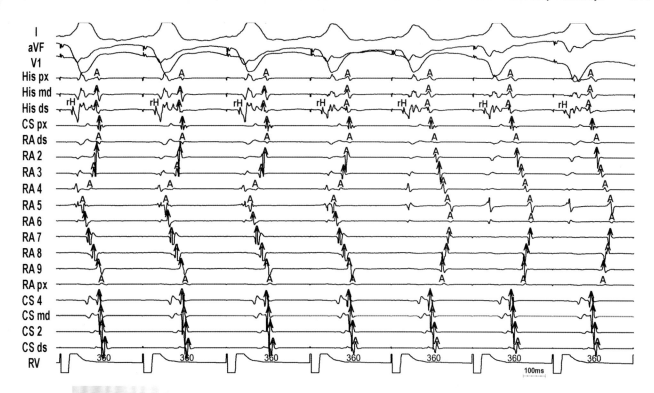

FIGURE 9-16 Retrograde AP block cycle length (right free wall). During ventricular pacing at 360 ms, retrograde conduction abruptly switches from a right free wall AP (earliest atrial activation at RA 5) to the fast pathway (FP) (earliest atrial activation at the His bundle region).

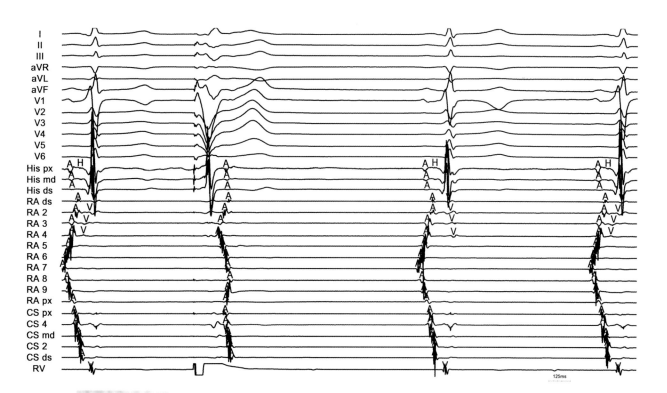

FIGURE 9-17 Phase 4 AP block. The first and last sinus beats conduct with a short HV interval and subtle preexcitation over a slowly conducting right posterolateral AP. A single ventricular extrastimulus conduct over the AP (earliest atrial activation at RA 4), resetting the sinus node and inducing a noncompensatory pause. The pause causes phase 4 block in the AP with normalization of the HV interval and loss of preexcitation (loss of early ventricular activation at RA 4). Note that AH intervals remain unchanged, further indicating that the loss of preexcitation was not pseudonormalization due to enhanced AV nodal conduction after the pause.

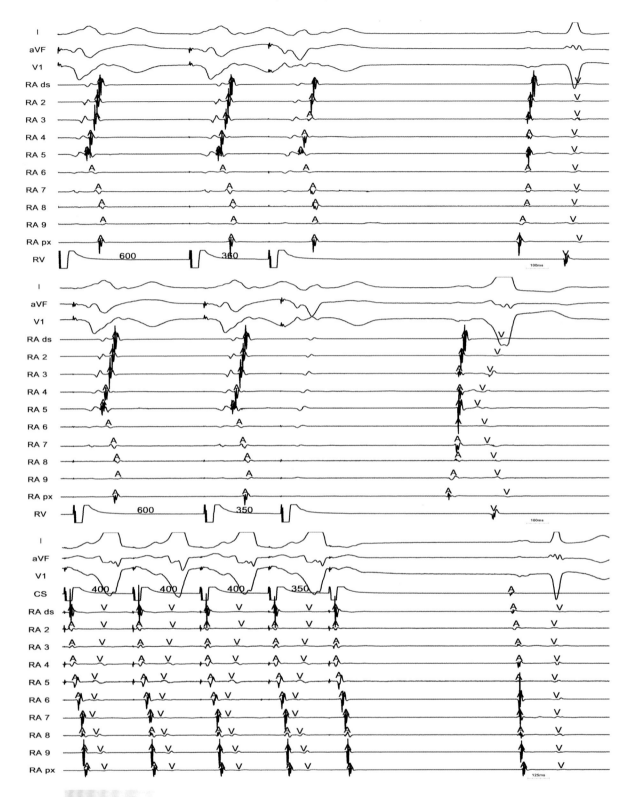

FIGURE 9-18 Phase 4 AP block. *Top panel*: At a ventricular coupling interval of 360 ms, retrograde conduction occurs over the AP followed by a sinus pause and phase 4 block in the AP. *Middle panel*: At 350 ms, retrograde block occurs in the AP (retrograde AP ERP) causing earlier return of the sinus beat and ventricular preexcitation. Although the sinus beat returns earlier, the AA interval between the two tracings are similar indicating that the ventricular extrastimulus at 350 ms concealed into (but failed to conduct over) the AP. *Bottom panel*: Preexcitation occurs during rapid atrial pacing but disappears after the extrastimulus (phase 3 block) and paradoxically after the sinus pause (phase 4 block). Loss of early ventricular activation along the lateral tricuspid annulus accompanying QRS normalization indicates that absence of preexcitation is not due to enhanced AV nodal conduction (pseudonormalization) following the pause. Overdrive suppression and fatigue in the AP is an alternative possibility.

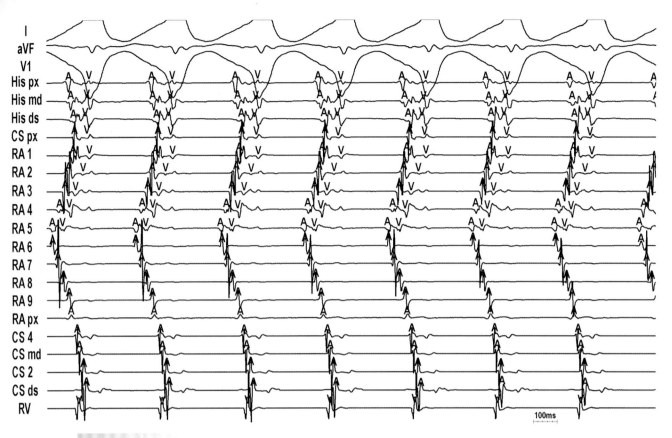

FIGURE 9-19 AP automaticity. Isoproterenol-induced automaticity of a right free wall AP results in a preexcited tachycardia where the earliest site of atrial and ventricular activation is the same. (An atrial tachycardia arising from the atrial insertion site of the AP cannot be definitively excluded.)

block or "accordion effect"). (In contrast, phase 3 and 4 bundle branch block (BBB) cause the opposite with BBB at fast and slow rates, respectively, and QRS normalization within a narrow window of heart rates.) Phase 4 AP block suggests a diseased AP, and its presence is supported by the presence of AP automaticity (spontaneous diastolic depolarizations reaching firing threshold).[41]

FATIGUE

In addition to phase 4 block, the fatigue phenomenon is an alternative explanation for loss of preexcitation after pacing.[42–44] Rapid atrial or ventricular pacing repetitively conceals into an AP and suppresses subsequent conduction (overdrive suppression).

AUTOMATICITY

Rarely, manifest APs show spontaneous automaticity (spontaneous preexcited QRS complex with or without simultaneous atrial activation arising from the AP) (Fig. 9-19).[41,45–47]

SUPERNORMALITY

The supernormal period of an AP is a brief window at the end of its recovery period during which, otherwise, subthreshold

sinus impulses unexpectedly show preexcitation and occur in APs with prolonged refractoriness. While supernormality in an AP has been described in the electrophysiology laboratory, spontaneous episodes are rare because they require a unique combination of both AV block and an AP with poor conduction (Fig. 9-20).[42,48–51] Preexcitation only occurs when sinus complexes fall into the supernormal window of the AP following escape complexes.

LONGITUDINAL DISSOCIATION

A longitudinally dissociated AP refers to an AP demonstrating both short and long conduction times without a change in preexcited QRS morphology (antegrade dissociation) or retrograde atrial activation (retrograde dissociation). It has been described for both AV and atrio-fascicular AP and is a cause for cycle length alternans during antidromic and orthodromic reciprocating tachycardia.[52–54]

AV BLOCK

Preexcitation during AV block is uncommon (**Figs. 9-21 and 9-22**). It has been described most commonly with left-sided APs with AV block being unmasked or caused by catheter ablation.[55,56]

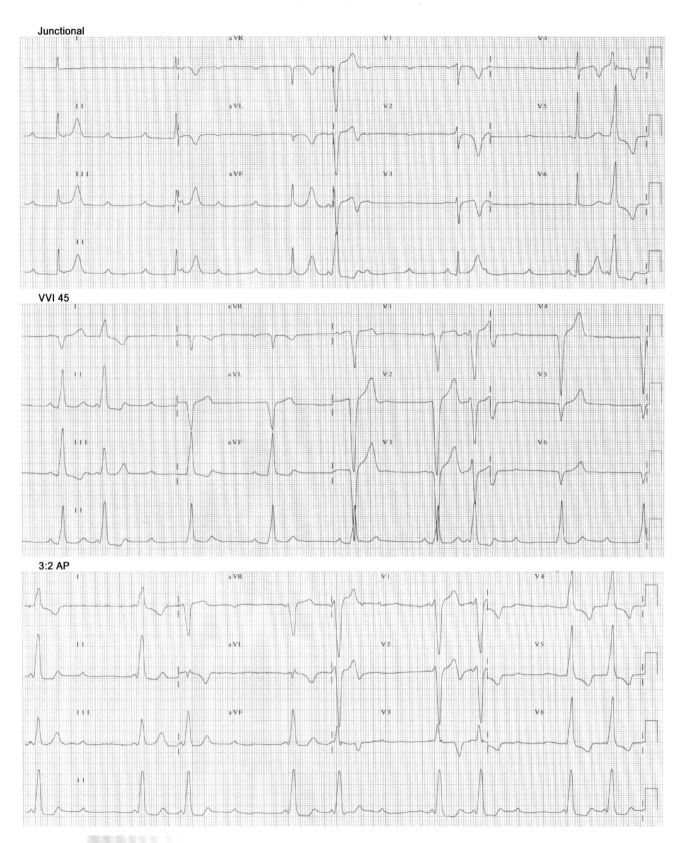

FIGURE 9-20 Supernormality in an AP during AV block. Preexcitation only occurs during critically-timed sinus impulses that fall into the supernormal window of AP excitability during junctional escape (*top*) and ventricular paced rhythm (*middle*). The supernormal window occurs late after the T wave because it widens and shifts rightward by the slow underlying ventricular rate. During 3:2 AP conduction, preexcitation occurs after a long pause (due to recovery of excitability) and immediately afterward (due to supernormal excitability). The third P wave of each cycle falls outside of the supernormal window because of ventriculophasic sinus arrhythmia and a narrowing and leftward shift of the supernormal window following successive activation of the AP.

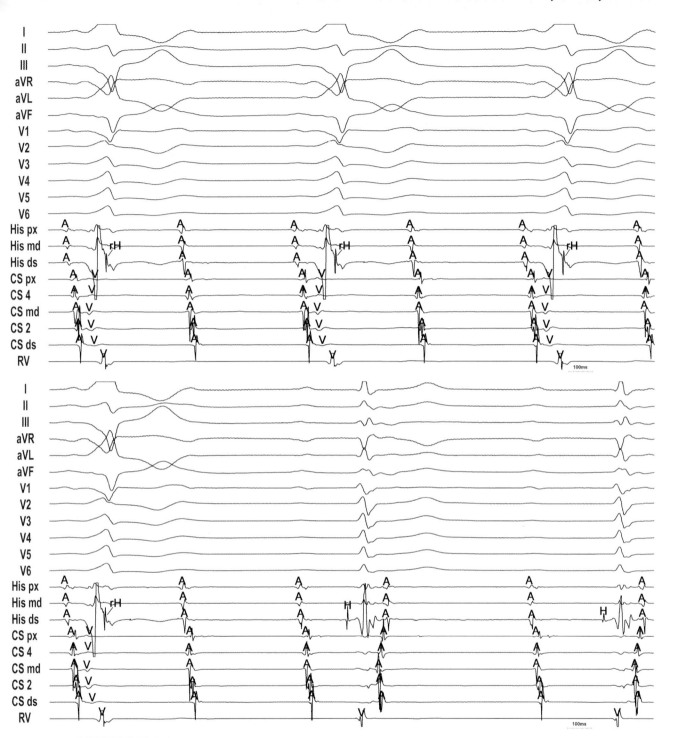

FIGURE 9-21 Preexcitation during AV block. *Top:* The 2:1 preexcitation in the setting of intranodal AV block. Note that after preexcited complexes, retrograde activation of the His bundle occurs, but antidromic reciprocating tachycardia fails to develop because of retrograde block in the AV node. *Bottom:* Preexcitation disappears, and a junctional escape rhythm emerges. Note that junctional escape complexes are followed by retrograde activation over the AP, but orthodromic reciprocating tachycardia fails to develop because of antegrade block in the AV node.

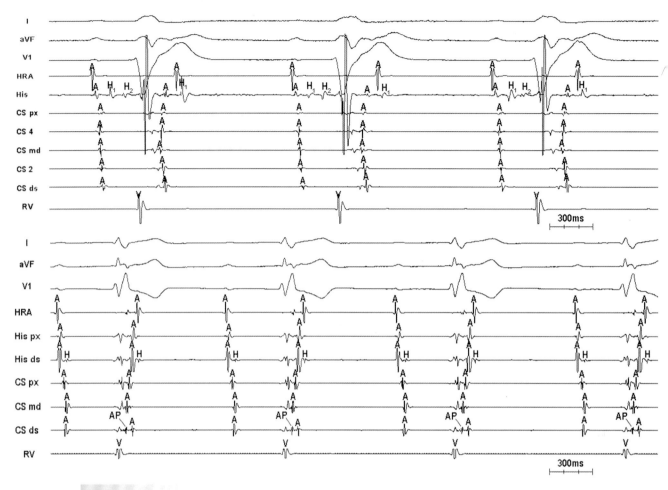

FIGURE 9-22 Concealed AP during AV block. *Top:* Sinus impulses conduct with intrahisian delay ($H_1H_2 = 110$ ms) and LBBB. This AV delay allows development of single orthodromic reciprocating echoes over a concealed left posterior AP, but ORT fails to develop because of intrahisian block. *Bottom:* Sinus rhythm with complete infrahisian AV block and a left ventricular escape rhythm. Each escape complex is followed by retrograde atrial activation over a concealed left free wall AP. Fixed coupling between ventricular escape complexes and subsequent P waves supports retrograde AP activation rather than atrial premature depolarizations. Despite retrograde AP conduction, ORT fails to develop because of infrahisian AV block. Note the AP potential between the ventricular and atrial electrograms at CS ds.

REFERENCES

1. Wood FC, Wolferth CC, Geckeler GD. Histologic demonstration of accessory muscular connections between auricle and ventricle in a case of short P-R interval and prolonged QRS complex. Am Heart J 1943;25:454–462.
2. Kuck K, Friday KJ, Kunze K, Schlüter M, Lazzara R, Jackman WM. Sites of conduction block in accessory atrioventricular pathways. Basis for concealed accessory pathways. Circulation 1990;82:407–417.
3. De la Fuente D, Sasyniuk B, Moe GK. Conduction through a narrow isthmus in isolated canine atrial tissue. A model of the W-P-W syndrome. Circulation 1971;44:803–809.
4. Prystowsky EN, Pritchett EL, Gallagher JJ. Concealed conduction preventing anterograde preexcitation in Wolff-Parkinson-White syndrome. Am J Cardiol 1984;53:960–961.
5. Wolff L, Parkinson J, White PD. Bundle-branch block with short P-R interval in healthy young people prone to paroxysmal tachycardia. Am Heart J 1930;5:685–704.
6. Wolferth CC, Wood FC. The mechanism of production of short P-R intervals and prolonged QRS complexes in patients with presumably undamaged hearts: hypothesis of an accessory pathway of auriculoventricular conduction (bundle of Kent). Am Heart J 1933;8:297–311.
7. Teo WS, Klein GJ, Yee R, Leitch JW, Murdock CJ. Significance of minimal preexcitation in Wolff-Parkinson-White syndrome. Am J Cardiol 1991;67:205–207.
8. Bogun F, Kalusche D, Li Y, Auth-Eisernitz S, Grönefeld G, Hohnloser SH. Septal Q waves in surface electrocardiographic lead V6 exclude minimal ventricular preexcitation. Am J Cardiol 1999;84:101–104, A9.

9. Liberman L, Pass RH, Starc TJ, Hordof AJ, Silver ES. Uncovering the septal Q wave and other electrocardiographic changes in pediatric patients with pre-excitation before and after ablation. Am J Cardiol 2010;105:214–216.
10. Garratt CJ, Antoniou A, Griffith MJ, Ward DE, Camm AJ. Use of intravenous adenosine in sinus rhythm as a diagnostic test for latent preexcitation. Am J Cardiol 1990;65:868–873.
11. Cain ME, Luke RA, Lindsay BD. Diagnosis and localization of accessory pathways. Pacing Clin Electrophysiol 1992;15:801–824.
12. Tada H, Naito S, Taniguchi K, Nogami A. Concealed left anterior accessory pathways: two approaches for successful ablation. J Cardiovasc Electrophysiol 2003;14:204–208.
13. Guo X, Sun Q, Ma J, et al. Electrophysiological characteristics and radiofrequency catheter ablation of accessory pathway connecting the right atrial appendage and the right ventricle. J Cardiovasc Electrophysiol 2015;26: 845–852.
14. Mah D, Miyake C, Clegg R, et al. Epicardial left atrial appendage and biatrial appendage accessory pathways. Heart Rhythm 2010;7:1740–1745.
15. Sun Y, Arruda M, Otomo K, et al. Coronary sinus-ventricular accessory connections producing posteroseptal and left posterior accessory pathways: incidence and electrophysiological identification. Circulation 2002;106: 1362–1367.
16. Hwang C, Peter CT, Chen PS. Radiofrequency ablation of accessory pathways guided by the location of the ligament of Marshall. J Cardiovasc Electrophysiol 2003;14:616–620.
17. Suleiman M, Brady PA, Asirvatham SJ, Friedman PA, Munger TA. The noncoronary cusp as a site for successful ablation of accessory pathways: electrogram characteristics in three cases. J Cardiovasc Electrophysiol 2011;22:203–209.

18. Fitzpatrick AP, Gonzales RP, Lesh MD, Modin GW, Lee RJ, Scheinman MM. New algorithm for the localization of accessory atrioventricular connections using a baseline electrocardiogram. J Am Coll Cardiol 1994;23:107–116.

19. Milstein S, Sharma AD, Guiraudon GM, Klein GJ. An algorithm for the electrocardiographic localization of accessory pathways in the Wolff-Parkinson-White syndrome. Pacing Clin Electrophysiol 1987;10:555–563.

20. Szabo TS, Klein GJ, Guiraudon GM, Yee R, Sharma AD. Localization of accessory pathways in the Wolff-Parkinson-White syndrome. Pacing Clin Electrophysiol 1989;12:1691–1705.

21. González-Torrecilla E, Peinado R, Almendral J, et al. Reappraisal of classical electrocardiographic criteria in detecting accessory pathways with a strict para-Hisian location. Heart Rhythm 2013;10:16–21.

22. Liu Q, Shehata M, Lan DZ, et al. Accurate localization and catheter ablation of superoparaseptal accessory pathways. Heart Rhythm 2018;15:688–695.

23. Tai C, Chen S, Chiang C, Lee S, Chang M. Electrocardiographic and electrophysiologic characteristics of anteroseptal, midseptal, and para-Hisian accessory pathways. Implications for radiofrequency catheter ablation. Chest 1996;109:730–740.

24. Young C, Lauer MR, Liem LB, Sung RJ. A characteristic electrocardiographic pattern indicative of manifest left-sided posterior septal/paraseptal accessory atrioventricular connections. Am J Cardiol 1993;72:471–475.

25. Liu E, Shehata M, Swerdlow C, et al. Approach to the difficult septal atrioventricular accessory pathway: the importance of regional anatomy. Circ Arrhythm Electrophysiol 2012;5:e63–e66.

26. Takahashi A, Shah DC, Jaïs P, et al. Specific electrocardiographic features of manifest coronary vein posteroseptal accessory pathways. J Cardiovasc Electrophysiol 1998;9:1015–1025.

27. Denes P, Wyndham CR, Amat-y-leon F, et al. Atrial pacing at multiple sites in the Wolff-Parkinson-White syndrome. Br Heart J 1977;39:506–514.

28. Klein GJ, Bashore TM, Sellers TD, Pritchett EL, Smith WM, Gallagher JJ. Ventricular fibrillation in the Wolff-Parkinson-White syndrome. N Engl J Med 1979;301:1080–1085.

29. Dreifus LS, Haiat R, Watanabe Y, Arriaga J, Reitman N. Ventricular fibrillation. A possible mechanism of sudden death in patients and Wolff-Parkinson-White syndrome. Circulation 1971;43:520–527.

30. Olen MM, Baysa SJ, Rossi A, Kanter RJ, Fishberger SB. Wolff-Parkinson-White syndrome: a stepwise deterioration to sudden death. Circulation 2016;133:105–106.

31. Sarrias A, Villuendas R, Bisbal F, et al. From atrial fibrillation to ventricular fibrillation and back. Circulation 2015;132:2035–2036.

32. Klein GJ, Gulamhusein SS. Intermittent preexcitation in the Wolff-Parkinson-White syndrome. Am J Cardiol 1983;52:292–296.

33. Strasberg B, Ashley WW, Wyndham C, et al. Treadmill exercise testing in the Wolff-Parkinson-White syndrome. Am J Cardiol 1980;45:742–748.

34. Wellens HJ, Durrer D. Wolff-Parkinson-White syndrome and atrial fibrillation. Relation between refractory period of accessory pathway and ventricular rate during atrial fibrillation. Am J Cardiol 1974;34:777–782.

35. Yee R, Klein GJ, Prystowsky E. The Wolff-Parkinson-White syndrome and related variants. In: Zipes DP, Jalife J, eds. Cardiac Electrophysiology: From Cell to Bedside. 3rd ed. Philadelphia, PA: WB Saunders, 2000:845–861.

36. Wellens HJ, Braat S, Brugada P, Gorgels AP, Bär FW. Use of procainamide in patients with the Wolff-Parkinson-White syndrome to disclose a short refractory period of the accessory pathway. Am J Cardiol 1982;50:1087–1089.

37. Sharma AD, Yee R, Guiraudon G, Klein GJ. Sensitivity and specificity of invasive and noninvasive testing for risk of sudden death in Wolff-Parkinson-White syndrome. J Am Coll Cardiol 1987;10:373–381.

38. Fananapazir L, Packer DL, German LD, et al. Procainamide infusion test: inability to identify patients with Wolff-Parkinson-White syndrome who are potentially at risk of sudden death. Circulation 1988;77:1291–1296.

39. Przybylski J, Chiale PA, Quinteiro RA, Elizari MV, Rosenbaum MB. The occurrence of phase-4 block in the anomalous bundle of patients with Wolff-Parkinson-White syndrome. Eur J Cardiol 1975;3:267–280.

40. Fujiki A, Tani M, Mizumaki K, Yoshida S, Sasayama S. Rate-dependent accessory pathway conduction due to phase 3 and phase 4 block. Antegrade and retrograde conduction properties. J Electrocardiol 1992;25:25–31.

41. Lerman BB, Josephson ME. Automaticity of the Kent bundle: confirmation by phase 3 and phase 4 block. J Am Coll Cardiol 1985;5:996–998.

42. Lum JJ, Ho RT. Dynamic effects of exercise and different escape rhythms on the supernormal period of an accessory pathway. J Cardiovasc Electrophysiol 2007;18:672–675.

43. Ohe T, Shimonura K, Shiroeda O. Fatigue phenomenon of the accessory pathway. Int J Cardiol 1985;8:211–214.

44. Fujimura O, Smith BA, Kuo CS. Effect of verapamil on an accessory pathway manifesting as "fatigue phenomenon" in Wolff-Parkinson-White syndrome. Chest 1993;104:305–307.

45. Tseng ZH, Yadav AV, Scheinman MM. Catecholamine dependent accessory pathway automaticity. Pacing Clin Electrophysiol 2004;27:1005–1007.

46. Przybylski J, Chiale PA, Halpern MS, Lázzari JO, Elizari MV, Rosenbaum MB. Existence of automaticity in anomalous bundle of Wolff-Parkinson-White syndrome. Br Heart J 1978;40:672–680.

47. Deam AG, Burton ME, Walter PF, Langberg JJ. Wide complex tachycardia due to automaticity in an accessory pathway. Pacing Clin Electrophysiol 1995;18:2106–2108.

48. McHenry PL, Knoebel SB, Fisch C. The Wolff-Parkinson-White (WPW) syndrome with supernormal conduction through the anomalous bypass. Circulation 1966;34:734–739.

49. Calabrò MP, Saporito F, Carerj S, Oreto G. "Early" capture beats in advanced A-V block: by which mechanism? J Cardiovasc Electrophysiol 2005;16:1108–1109.

50. Chang M, Miles WM, Prystowsky EN. Supernormal conduction in accessory atrioventricular connections. Am J Cardiol 1987;59:852–856.

51. Przybylski J, Chiale PA, Sánchez RA, et al. Supernormal conduction in the accessory pathway of patients with overt or concealed ventricular preexcitation. J Am Coll Cardiol 1987;9:1269–1278.

52. Belhassen B, Misrahi D, Shapira I, Laniado S. Longitudinal dissociation in an anomalous accessory atrioventricular pathway. Am Heart J 1983;106:1441–1443.

53. Atié J, Brugada P, Brugada J, et al. Longitudinal dissociation of atrioventricular accessory pathways. J Am Coll Cardiol 1991;17:161–166.

54. Sternick EB, Sosa E, Scanavacca M, Wellens HJ. Dual conduction in a Mahaim fiber. J Cardiovasc Electrophysiol 2004;15:1212–1215.

55. Barbhaiya C, Rosman J, Hanon S. Preexcitation and AV block. J Cardiovasc Electrophysiol 2012;23:106–107.

56. Seidl K, Hauer B, Zahn R, Senges J. Unexpected complete AV block following transcatheter ablation of a left posteroseptal accessory pathway. Pacing Clin Electrophysiol 1998;21:2139–2142.

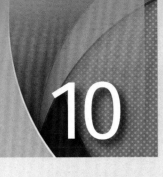

10 Orthodromic Reciprocating Tachycardia

Introduction

Orthodromic reciprocating tachycardia (ORT) is the second most common paroxysmal supraventricular tachycardia (SVT) and the prototypical accessory pathway (AP)-mediated tachycardia.

The purpose of this chapter is to:
1. Discuss the mechanism of ORT and its electrophysiologic features.
2. Diagnose ORT by analysis of transition zones (TZs).
3. Understand specific pacing maneuvers to diagnose ORT.

MECHANISM

ORT is a macroreentrant AP-mediated tachycardia utilizing the atrio-ventricular (AV) node–His-Purkinje axis as the antegrade limb (true or "ortho") and an AP as the retrograde limb of the circuit. The ventricles are activated by the His-Purkinje system, and therefore, QRS complexes are normal. After activation of the ventricle, the AP and atrium are activated sequentially ("in series"). P waves result from retrograde activation of the AP, and their axis reflects AP location.

ELECTROPHYSIOLOGIC FEATURES

12-LEAD ECG

The 12-lead ECG of ORT is a 1) regular narrow complex tachycardia (NCT), 2) short RP interval ≥70 ms, and 3) P-wave axis (generally superior) that reflects the AP location.[1,2] Retrograde AP conduction is typically rapid, but because the ventricles and atria are sequentially activated, the RP interval ≥70 ms with P wave buried within the ST segment. An NCT with an RP interval <70 ms therefore excludes ORT. Rightward (aVR [+], aVL [−]) and leftward (aVR [−], aVL [+]) P-wave axes identify left- and right-sided APs, respectively. A midline, superior P-wave axis (aVR [+], aVL [+]) suggests a septal AP. Anteroseptal APs can produce inferior P-wave axes.[3]

ELECTROPHYSIOLOGIC STUDY

The electrophysiologic features of ORT are 1) antegrade His bundle electrograms preceding QRS complexes, 2) VA interval ≥70 ms, and 3) earliest atrial activation at the site of the AP (**Figs. 10-1 and 10-2**).[1,2] The VA interval is the intracardiac equivalent of the

surface RP interval and is ≥70 ms. Atrial activation is either concentric or eccentric depending on AP location.[4] Septal APs generate concentric (antero- or posteroseptal) activation patterns, while right and left free wall APs produce right and left eccentric patterns, respectively. Because APs span the tricuspid or mitral annuli, earliest atrial activation occurs at the annulus. In general, a NCT with earliest atrial activation far from an annular site argues against ORT and suggests diagnosis of atrial tachycardia (AT), although nonannular APs (e.g., atrial appendage AP) have been described.

AV Relationship

Except for ORT using a nodo-fascicular/nodo-ventricular AP (nodo-fascicular reentrant tachycardia [NFRT]), all ORT requires participation of both the atrium and ventricle (obligatory 1:1 AV relationship).[5] ORT, therefore, cannot occur with AV block (**see Figs. 9-21 and 9-22**).[6,7] ORT, however, can occur with AV dissociation (NFRT) (**see Figs. 11-11 and 11-12**).[8] Because ORT is dependent on the AV node and retrograde AP conduction is generally rapid and fixed, oscillations in AH and HH intervals precede and predict VV and subsequent AA intervals.

Bundle Branch Block

Aberration-induced cycle length changes during NCT reflect His-Purkinje participation in tachycardia and are unique to ORT. ORT uses the shortest functional circuit capable of sustained reentry and, therefore, incorporates the bundle branch ipsilateral to the AP as an integral part of its circuit. During tachycardia, development of bundle branch block (BBB) ipsilateral to the AP forces antegrade conduction over the contralateral bundle and enlarges the circuit with transseptal conduction (**Fig. 10-3**). The addition of transseptal conduction causes an 1) obligatory increase in VA interval and generally 2) nonobligatory increase in tachycardia cycle length (TCL) (Coumel's sign) (**Figs. 10-4 to 10-7**).[9–13] The degree of VA interval increase depends on the

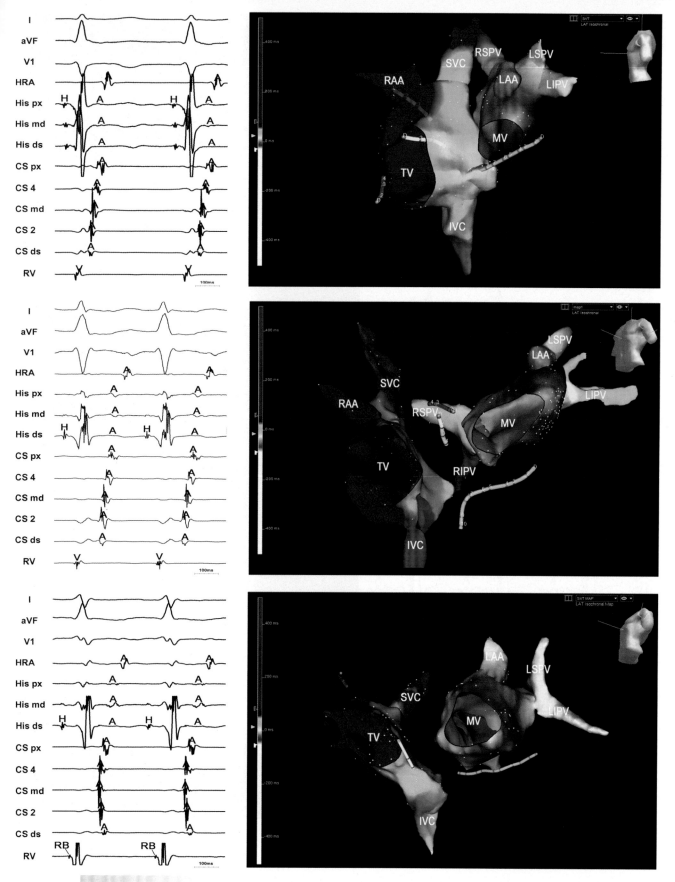

FIGURE 10-1 ORT using a left anterolateral (*top*), lateral (*middle*), and posterolateral (*bottom*) AP. Earliest site of atrial activation during retrograde AP conduction is depicted in white.

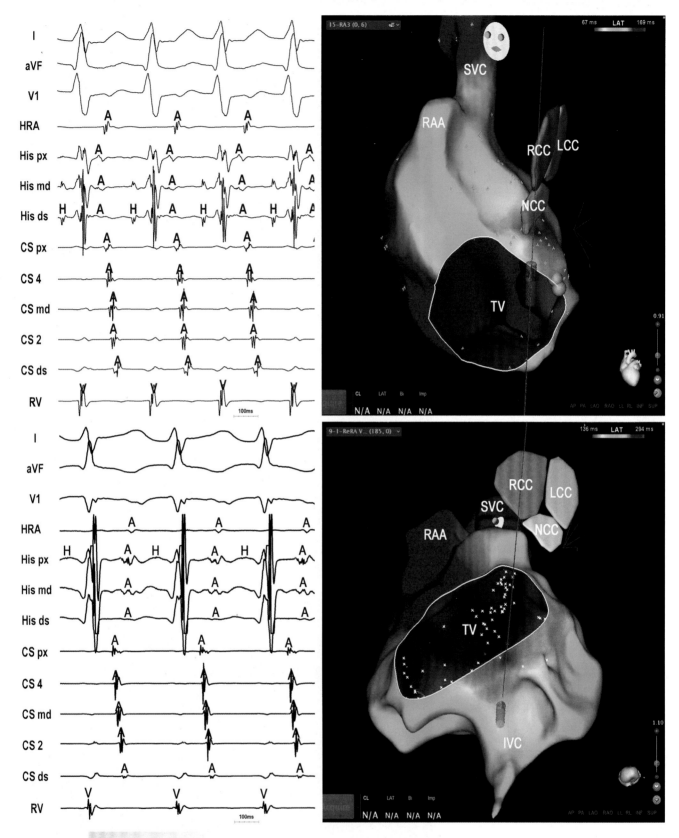

FIGURE 10-2 ORT using an anteroseptal (*top*) and posterior-posteroseptal (*bottom*) AP. Earliest site of atrial activation during retrograde AP conduction is depicted in red.

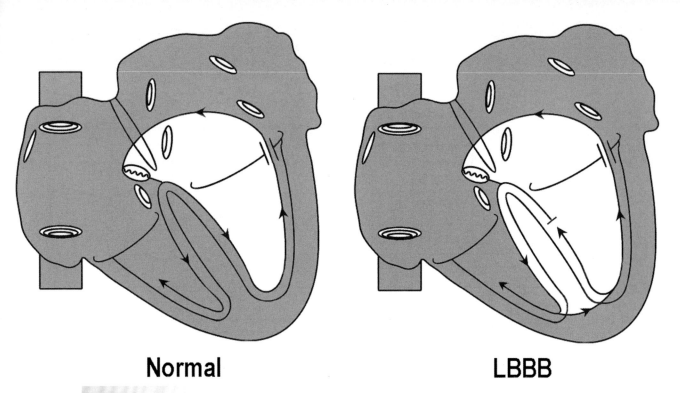

Normal   **LBBB**

FIGURE 10-3 Schematic diagram illustrating Coumel's sign. ORT using a left free wall AP. LBBB (ipsilateral to the AP) forces antegrade conduction over the RB and across the septum enlarging the circuit and obligating an increase in the VA interval. Concealed transeptal retrograde conduction ("transeptal linking") perpetuates BBB. Right bundle branch block (RBBB) (contralateral to the AP) does not affect the circuit.

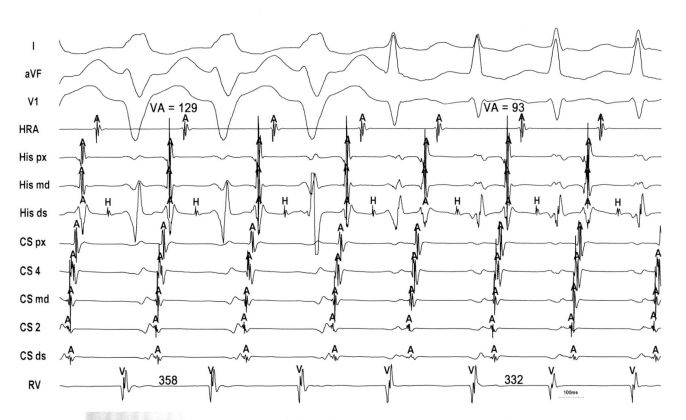

FIGURE 10-4 Coumel's sign (ORT using a left free wall AP). Atrial activation is left eccentric. Loss of LBBB causes a 36 ms shortening of the VA interval and acceleration of tachycardia.

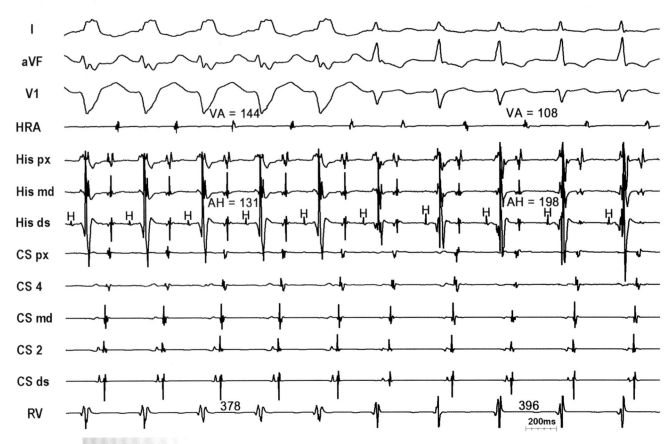

FIGURE 10-5 Coumel's sign (ORT using a left free wall AP). Atrial activation is left eccentric. Loss of LBBB results in 36 ms shortening of the VA interval but 67 ms lengthening of the AH interval (due to decremental conduction over the AV node), causing paradoxical slowing of tachycardia. The VA interval is more important than TCL to assess the effect of BBB on ORT.

AP location: Free wall APs increase the VA interval >35 ms, and septal APs increase the VA interval <25 ms.[10] TCL prolongs with ipsilateral BBB provided that the increase in VA interval is not counterbalanced by an equivalent decrease in the AV (generally, AH) interval. Conversely, loss of BBB ipsilateral to the AP causes tachycardia acceleration. Rarely, loss of BBB might cause paradoxical *slowing* of tachycardia if the decrease in VA interval is counterbalanced by a greater increase in the AV interval (decrement in the AV node or switch from fast pathway [FP] to slow pathway [SP]) (**Figs. 10-5 and 10-6**).[14] The VA interval (not TCL), therefore, is the important variable when assessing the effect of BBB on ORT. Once established, BBB is perpetuated by repetitive, concealed, transeptal conduction from unblocked to blocked bundle (transeptal linking).[15]

ZONES OF TRANSITION

INITIATION

Atrial Stimulation

Induction of ORT by atrial stimulation (programmed extrastimulation or burst pacing) requires that an impulse falls into the tachycardia window (defined as the difference in antegrade refractory periods between the AV node and AP). A critically timed impulse 1) fails to conduct over the AP (unidirectional block) and 2) conducts exclusively over the AV node–His-Purkinje system (slow conduction). For manifest APs, this atrial stimulus blocks in the AP, causing abrupt PR prolongation and normalization of the QRS complex at tachycardia onset. Critical AV delay over the AV node–His-Purkinje axis allows recovery of AP excitability and initiation of tachycardia.[16] This critical AV delay can occur in the 1) AV node, 2) His bundle, and/or 3) bundle branches (particularly, BBB ipsilateral to the AP) (**Figs. 10-8 to 10-10**). Sufficient AV node delay (AH prolongation) can occur by two mechanisms: physiologic decrement or switch from FP to SP. Delay in the His-Purkinje system facilitating ORT is manifested by HV prolongation and/or BBB ipsilateral to the AP. Ipsilateral BBB forces antegrade conduction over the contralateral bundle, and the addition of transeptal conduction to the circuit allows additional time for the AP to recover excitability. Restitution (cycle length dependency) and longitudinal dissociation of bundle branch refractory periods provide the conditions favorable to induce functional BBB using long–short sequences inherent in

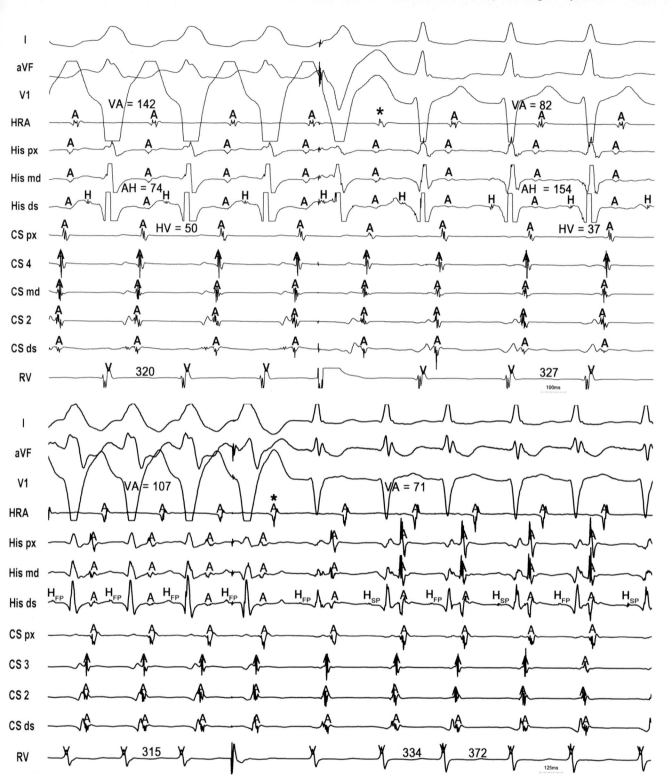

FIGURE 10-6 Coumel's sign (ORT using a left free wall AP). Atrial activation is left eccentric. *Top*: A His refractory right ventricular extrastimulus crosses the septum, advances the atrium (*asterisk*) over the AP, and breaks the transeptal link perpetuating LBBB. Loss of LBBB results in 60 ms shortening of the VA interval but 80 ms lengthening of the AH interval (due to decremental conduction over the AV node), causing paradoxical slowing of tachycardia. *Bottom*: A His refractory ventricular extrastimulus advances the atrium (*asterisk*) over the AP, breaks the transeptal link perpetuating LBBB, and induces dual AV node physiology (FP/SP alternans). Loss of LBBB results in 36 ms shortening of the VA interval, but FP/SP decrement causes paradoxical slowing of tachycardia and cycle length alternans.

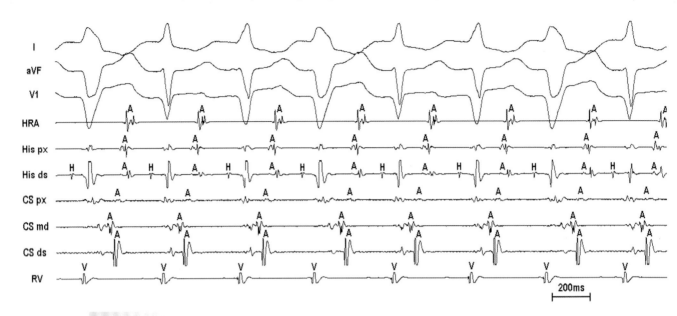

FIGURE 10-7 Coumel's sign with 3:2 LBBB Wenckebach (ORT using a left posterior AP). The earliest site of atrial activation is at CS md. VA intervals accompanying normal and incomplete LBBB are similar (VA = 93 ms) but longer with complete LBBB (VA = 147 ms). Note the repeating sequence of AA prolongation for three successive cycles accompanying LBBB Wenckebach as AA intervals bracketing normal and complete LBBB are the shortest and longest, respectively.

programmed atrial extrastimulation, particularly at long drive cycle lengths.[17]

Ventricular Stimulation

Induction of ORT by ventricular stimulation (programmed extrastimulation or burst pacing) require that an impulse fall into the tachycardia window (defined by the difference in retrograde refractory periods between the His-Purkinje–AV node axis and AP). A critically timed impulse 1) fails to conduct retrogradely over the His-Purkinje–AV node axis (unidirectional block) and 2) conducts exclusively over the AP.[18] A critical VA delay allows recovery of the AV node–His-Purkinje axis and initiation of tachycardia. The site of unidirectional block occurs either in the 1) His-Purkinje system or 2) AV node and can be determined by 1) retrograde His bundle potentials and 2) first $AH_{(ORT)}$ versus second $AH_{(ORT)}$ (**Figs. 10-11 to 10-15**). Absence of a retrograde His bundle potential following the last pacing stimulus (when retrograde His bundle potentials are otherwise present) and first $AH_{(ORT)}$ less than the second $AH_{(ORT)}$ indicates block in the His-Purkinje system and failure to retrogradely penetrate the AV node. Presence of a retrograde His bundle potential after the last pacing stimulus and first $AH_{(ORT)}$ greater than the second $AH_{(ORT)}$ indicates penetration of the AV node prior to block (unless the His bundle is orthodromically activated, [**Fig. 10-13**]).

Bundle Branch Reentrant Beats ("V3 Response")

A characteristic feature of ORT using a left-sided AP is its induction by bundle branch reentrant (BBR) beats during programmed ventricular extrastimulation (**Figs. 10-16 and 10-17**). Typical BBR beats 1) follow a "VH jump," 2) manifest left bundle branch block (LBBB) morphology, and 3) are preceded by His bundle electrograms ($HV_{[BBR]} ≥ HV_{[nonpreexcited NSR]}$). A single ventricular extrastimulus fails to conduct over the right bundle (retrograde right bundle effective refractory period) and crosses the interventricular septum to activate the left and His bundle ("VH jump"). Sufficient retrograde delay allows the RB to recover excitability, conduct antegradely, and induce a single BBR beat ("V3 response"). The single BBR beat crosses the septum, fails to conduct over the left bundle (unidirectional block), and conducts exclusively over the left-sided AP to initiate tachycardia (conditions similar to left-sided ORT induction by atrial stimulation with LBBB).

TERMINATION

The weak links for ORT are the AV node–His bundle axis and AP where block at either site terminates tachycardia.

Spontaneous

The obligatory 1:1 AV relationship during ORT implies that either AV or VA block precludes tachycardia induction or causes termination. Antegrade block occurs either in the 1) AV node or 2) His-Purkinje system. Spontaneous termination with block in the AV node demonstrates tachycardia dependence on the AV node and excludes AT (**Fig. 10-18**). The rare spontaneous termination with block below the AV node demonstrates tachycardia dependence on the His-Purkinje system and excludes both AV nodal reentrant tachycardia (AVNRT)

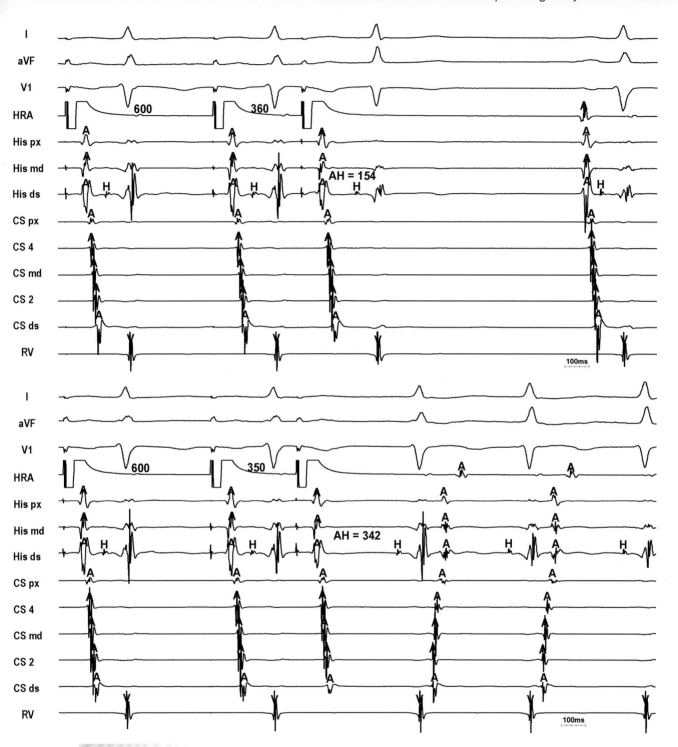

FIGURE 10-8 ORT induction facilitated by SP conduction. At a coupling interval of 360 ms, conduction occurs over the FP (AH = 154 ms). At 350 ms, the extrastimulus encounters FP refractoriness (antegrade FP ERP) and conducts over the SP (AH = 342 ms) with sufficient AV delay to initiate ORT using a left free wall AP.

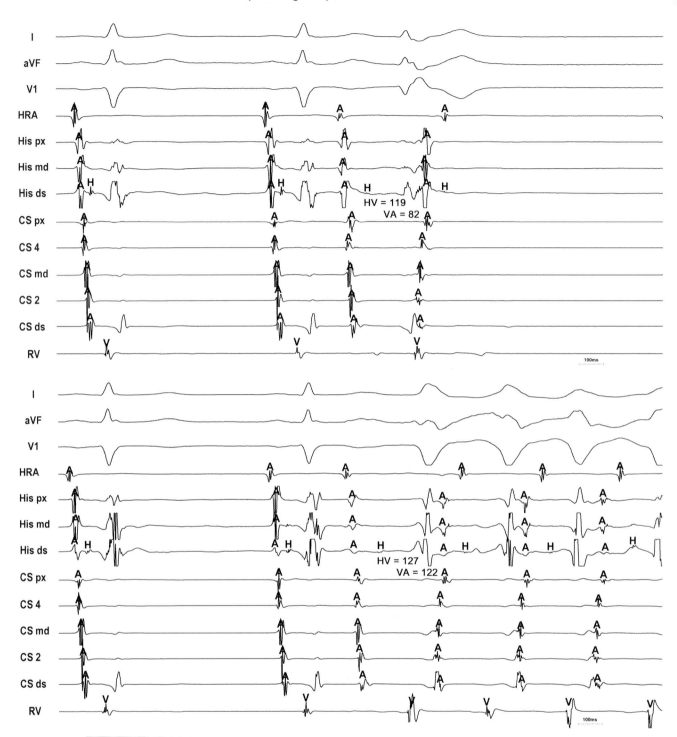

FIGURE 10-9 ORT induction facilitated by ipsilateral BBB. *Top:* During sinus rhythm, a spontaneous APC encroaches on His-Purkinje refractoriness, conducts with HV prolongation (119 ms)/right bundle branch block (RBBB), and induces a single orthodromic reciprocating echo over a left free wall AP that fails to initiate ORT because of infrahisian AV block. *Bottom:* A similarly coupled APC preceded by a slightly longer sinus cycle length conducts with HV prolongation (127 ms)/LBBB. LBBB increases the VA interval of the reciprocating echo, allowing sufficient time for the otherwise refractory His-Purkinje system to recover partial excitability initiating ORT with LBBB.

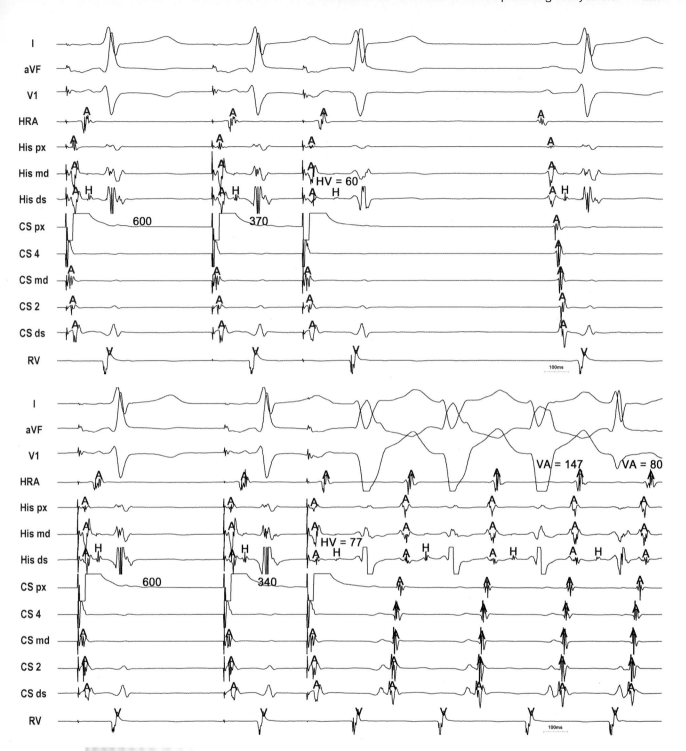

FIGURE 10-10 ORT induction facilitated by ipsilateral BBB. At a coupling interval of 370 ms, conduction occurs normally over the FP–His-Purkinje axis (HV = 60 ms). At 340 ms, conduction encroaches on His-Purkinje refractoriness, resulting in greater HV prolongation (77 ms)/LBBB, which allows sufficient AV delay to induce ORT using a left free wall AP. Note the shortening of the VA interval (67 ms) and TCL with loss of LBBB (Coumel's sign).

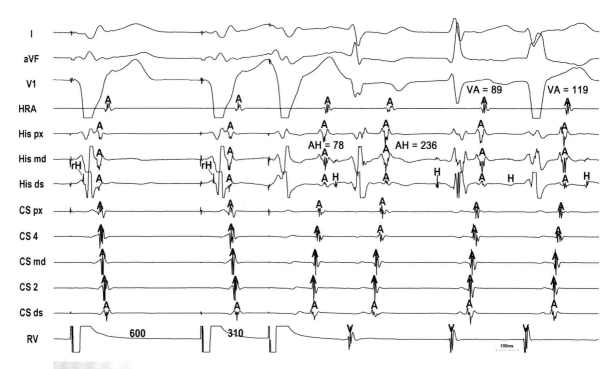

FIGURE 10-11 Induction of ORT by programmed ventricular extrastimulation with retrograde block in the His-Purkinje system. During the drive train, retrograde atrial activation is concentric (earliest at the His bundle region) due to conduction over the FP. The extrastimulus encounters retrograde His-Purkinje refractoriness exposing a left free wall AP (left eccentric atrial activation earliest at CS ds). Lack of retrograde concealment into the AV node allows subsequent antegrade FP conduction (AH = 78 ms) followed by SP conduction (AH = 236 ms) at tachycardia onset. Concealment from SP into FP ("linking") causes partial FP refractoriness and subsequent mild prolongation of the third AH interval. This long–short sequence causes LBBB aberration with prolongation of the VA interval (Coumel's sign). Note that the His bundle morphology after the extrastimulus is similar to tachycardia and different from the drive train indicating antegrade (not retrograde) activation.

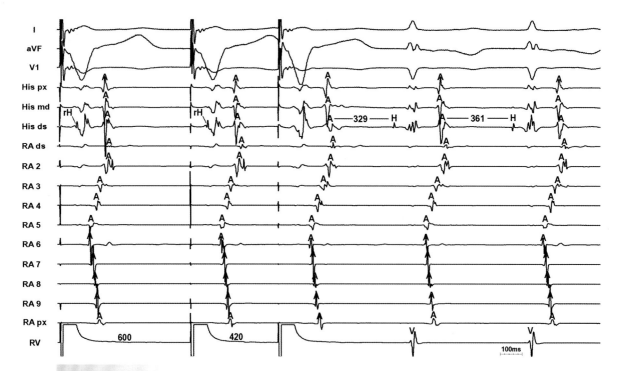

FIGURE 10-12 Induction of ORT by programmed ventricular extrastimulation with retrograde block in the His-Purkinje system. During the drive train, retrograde conduction occurs over a right free wall AP (right eccentric atrial activation earliest at RA 6). The extrastimulus encounters retrograde His-Purkinje refractoriness and initiates slow ORT. Lack of retrograde concealment into the AV node allows the first AH (329 ms) to be shorter than the subsequent AH interval (361 ms).

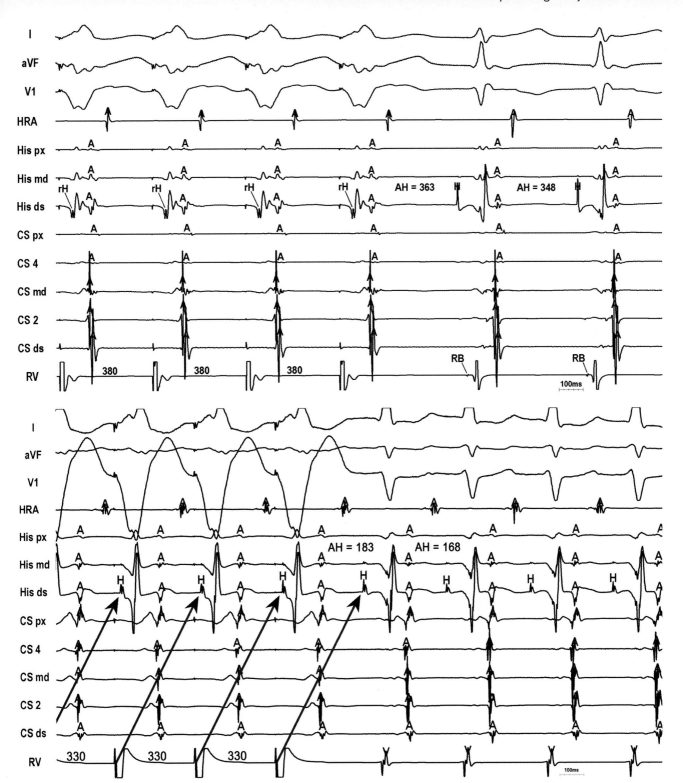

FIGURE 10-13 Induction of ORT by rapid ventricular pacing with retrograde block in the AV node (*top*) and His-Purkinje system (*bottom*). *Top:* During rapid ventricular pacing, retrograde conduction occurs over the His bundle and a posteroseptal AP with onset of ORT upon pacing cessation. Retrograde concealment into the AV node causes a longer AH interval at tachycardia onset (363 ms) than the subsequent AH interval (348 ms). *Bottom:* During rapid ventricular pacing, retrograde conduction occurs over a left posteroseptal AP but blocks in the distal His-Purkinje system causing orthodromic capture of the His bundle at tachycardia onset. The first AH (183 ms) is longer than subsequent AH intervals (168 ms) because acceleration of the atrial rate by ventricular pacing encroaches on relative refractoriness of the AV node. Ventricular pacing that orthodromically captures the His bundle indicates the presence of an AP.

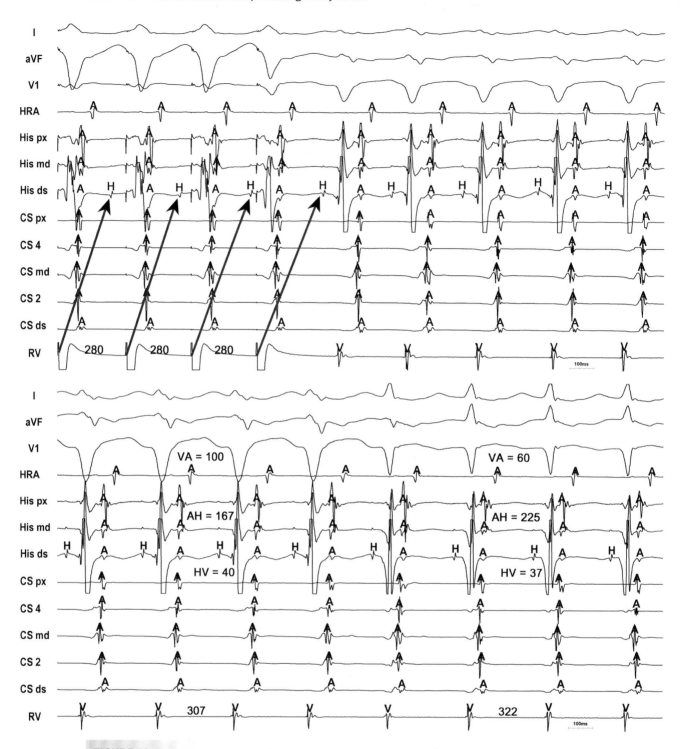

FIGURE 10-14 *Top*: Induction of ORT by rapid ventricular pacing with retrograde block in the His-Purkinje system. During rapid ventricular pacing, retrograde conduction occurs over a left posterior AP but blocks in the distal His-Purkinje system causing orthodromic capture of the His bundle. Encroachment of the accelerated atrium on AV nodal refractoriness causes progressive AH prolongation until pacing cessation. Sufficient AH delay initiates ORT with LBBB (late retrograde penetration of the LB by RV stimulation results in persistent LB refractoriness at tachycardia onset). *Bottom*: Loss of LBBB causes 40 ms shortening of the VA interval but 58 ms lengthening of the AH interval and, therefore, paradoxical slowing of tachycardia.

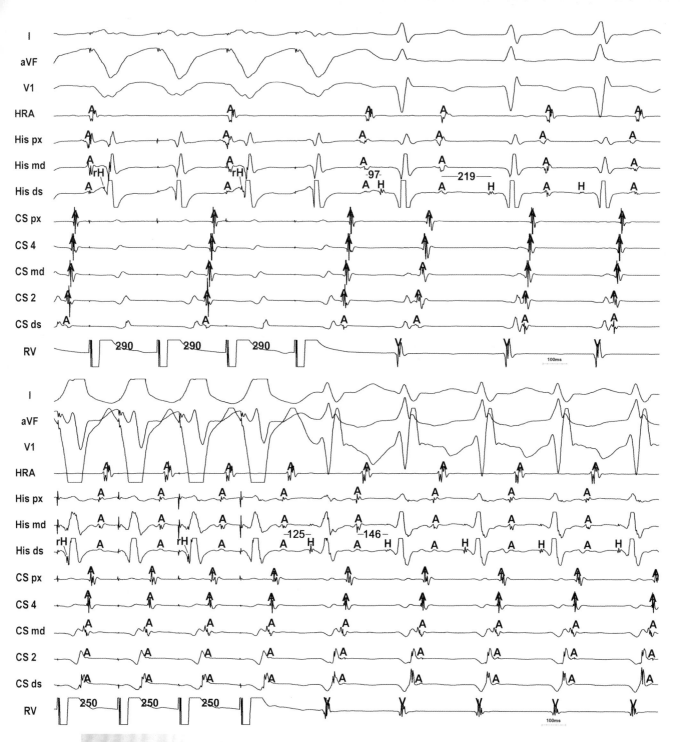

FIGURE 10-15 Induction of ORT by rapid ventricular pacing with retrograde block in the His-Purkinje system. *Top:* During rapid ventricular pacing, retrograde conduction alternates between a left free wall AP and the His bundle. The last paced complex blocks retrogradely over the His-Purkinje system (unidirectional block) and conducts over a left free wall AP after transeptal conduction (conduction delay) initiating ORT. Lack of retrograde concealment into the AV node allows subsequent antegrade FP conduction (AH = 97 ms) followed by SP conduction (AH = 219 ms) at tachycardia onset. Concealment from SP to FP ("linking") renders the FP relatively refractory causing mild prolongation of the third AH interval. *Bottom:* During rapid ventricular pacing, 1:1 retrograde conduction occurs over a left free wall AP but 2:1 over the His bundle. After the last paced complex, lack of retrograde concealment into the AV node allows a shorter first AH interval at tachycardia onset (125 ms) than subsequent AH intervals (146 ms).

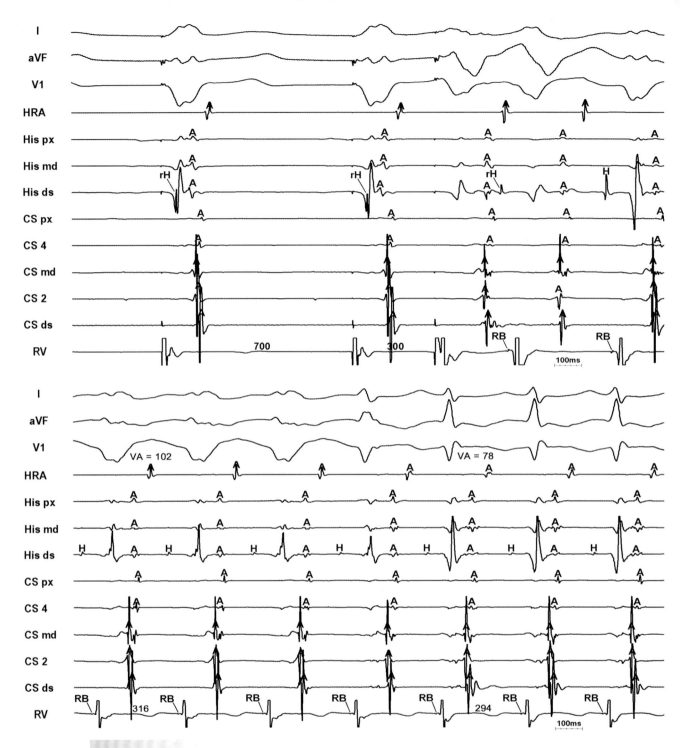

FIGURE 10-16 Induction of left-sided ORT by BBR beats. During the drive train, retrograde atrial activation is concentric (earliest at the His bundle region) due to conduction over the FP. The extrastimulus encounters retrograde RB refractoriness inducing a "VH jump" (226 ms) and exposing a left posterior AP (earliest atrial activation at CS md). Note that atrial activation preceded retrograde His bundle (rH) activation indicating an extranodal AP. The "VH jump" causes a single BBR beat that fails to conduct retrogradely over the LB to the His bundle (unidirectional block) and conducts exclusively over the AP with sufficient transseptal delay (slow conduction) to initiate ORT. Persistent refractoriness of the recently depolarized LB causes LBBB at tachycardia onset, which is perpetuated by transseptal linking. Subsequent accommodation and shortening of LB refractory periods normalize the QRS complex. Loss of LBBB aberration causes shortening of the VA interval (24 ms) and TCL (22 ms) (Coumel's sign).

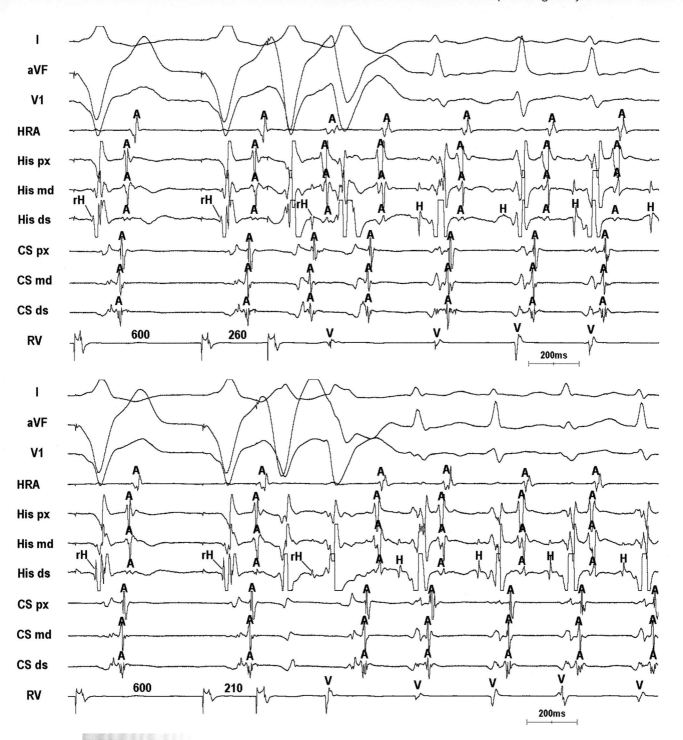

FIGURE 10-17 Induction of left-sided ORT by BBR beats. During the drive train, retrograde atrial activation occurs over a left free wall AP (earliest at CS ds). *Top*: The ventricular extrastimulus conducts over the AP but encounters RB refractoriness, inducing a "VH jump" (VH = 175 ms) and BBR beat. The BBR beat crosses the septum and fails to conduct retrogradely over the LB to activate the His bundle (unidirectional block) but conducts over the AP with sufficient transeptal delay to initiate ORT. *Bottom*: A shorter coupled ventricular extrastimulus encounters AP and RB refractoriness inducing a longer "VH jump" (VH = 220 ms) and BBR beat, which again initiates ORT. Note that the AH interval at tachycardia onset is shorter in the bottom compared to top tracing because the lack of retrograde AP conduction following the extrastimulus eliminates subsequent antegrade concealment into the AV node.

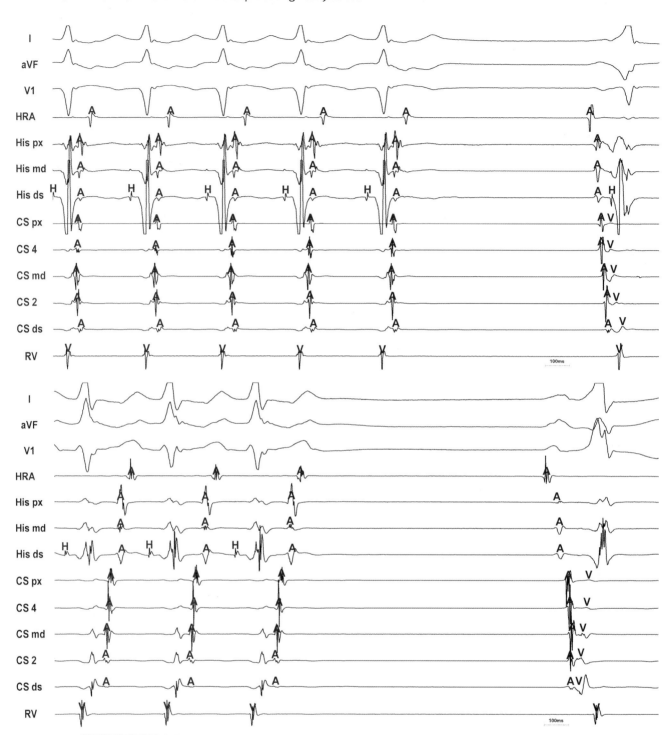

FIGURE 10-18 Termination of ORT with intranodal AV block. Tachycardia slows prior to termination because of AH prolongation preceding block (AV node Wenckebach) indicating dependence on the AV node. The earliest site of atrial and ventricular activation during ORT and preexcited sinus rhythm, respectively, are along the right posteroseptum (*top*) and left free wall (*bottom*).

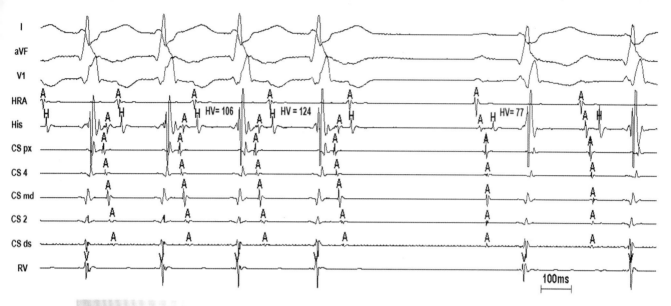

FIGURE 10-19 Termination of ORT with infrahisian AV block. During ORT using a right posteroseptal AP (earliest atrial activation at CS px), the HV interval is markedly prolonged with underlying right bundle branch block/left posterior fascicular block (RBBB/LPFB).Tachycardia slows prior to termination because of HV prolongation preceding block (LAFB Wenckebach), indicating dependence on the His-Purkinje system (excluding both AVNRT and AT).

and AT (**Fig. 10-19**).[7] Retrograde AP block can occur either at its atrial or ventricular insertion sites (**Fig. 10-20**).[6,19,20]

Induced

Single ventricular premature depolarizations (VPDs) delivered during the diastolic period of the tachycardia (diastolic scanning) can penetrate the reentrant circuit and extinguish reentry. Its antidromic wavefront collides with tachycardia, while its orthodromic wavefront encounters AP refractoriness, fails to reach the atrium (VA block), and terminates tachycardia. Termination of an NCT by an early VPD with VA block excludes AT.

His Refractory VPD

His refractory VPDs are late-coupled VPDs whose antidromic wavefront collides with the tachycardia wavefront below the His bundle (the His bundle itself having been "committed" by tachycardia). Such VPDs cannot conduct over the His bundle and, therefore, can only reach the atrium over an AP. Termination of a NCT by a His refractory VPD with VA block indicates the presence of an AP, excludes pure AT and AVNRT, and strongly favors a diagnosis of ORT (**Figs. 10-21 to 10-23**). However, a His refractory VPD can terminate AVNRT in the presence of a bystander nodo-fascicular/nodo-ventricular AP (see **Figs. 6-12 and 11-16**).[21]

PACING MANEUVERS FROM THE VENTRICLE

Diagnosis of ORT is facilitated by pacing maneuvers delivered from the ventricle (inverse rule).

DIASTOLIC VPDs

Single extrastimuli delivered from the right ventricle (RV) during diastole can penetrate the ORT circuit and perturb (reset or terminate) tachycardia.[22,23]

Preexcitation Index

During diastolic scanning, the longest coupling interval that preexcites the atrium over the AP establishes the preexcitation index (PI).[24] The PI (PI = TCL − longest coupling interval preexciting the atrium) is directly related to distance between the RV pacing site and AP. Septal and left free wall APs are associated with a small (<45 ms) and large (>75 ms) PI, respectively.

His Refractory VPD ("V on H" Maneuver)

In addition to termination of NCT with VA block, His refractory VPD that reset tachycardia also indicates the presence of an AP. Resetting can be either 1) advancement (preexcitation) of the atrium or 2) delay (postexcitation) of the atrium (**Figs. 10-22 to 10-26**). Resetting and termination are both proof of the presence of an AP but not necessarily that the AP participates in tachycardia (a His refractory VPD can reset or terminate AVNRT in the presence of a bystander nodo-fascicular/nodo-ventricular AP). Postexcitation delay is seen with slowly conducting decremental APs (long RP tachycardias) (see Chapter 6).

ENTRAINMENT FROM THE VENTRICLE

Ventricular overdrive pacing delivered at a cycle length shorter than TCL can penetrate the ORT circuit and accelerate the

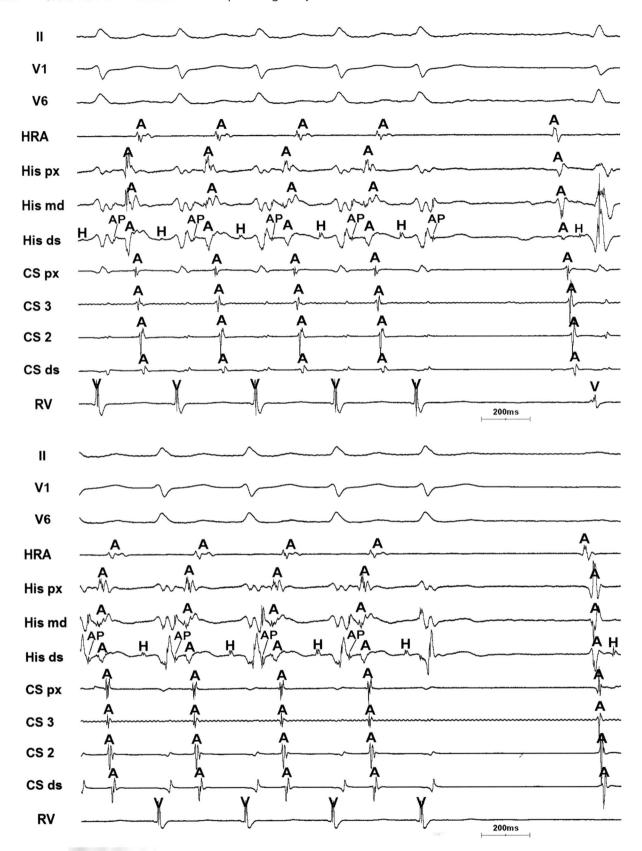

FIGURE 10-20 Termination of ORT with retrograde block at the atrial (*top*) and ventricular (*bottom*) insertion sites of a parahisian AP. A high-frequency AP potential is recorded between ventricular and atrial electrograms on the His bundle channel that records a His bundle potential. Persistence and disappearance of the potential accompanying VA block indicates that it is not a part of the atrial or ventricular electrogram, respectively, and therefore represents a true AP potential. In the bottom tracing, slower ORT results in longer AP refractoriness facilitating block at its ventricular insertion site.

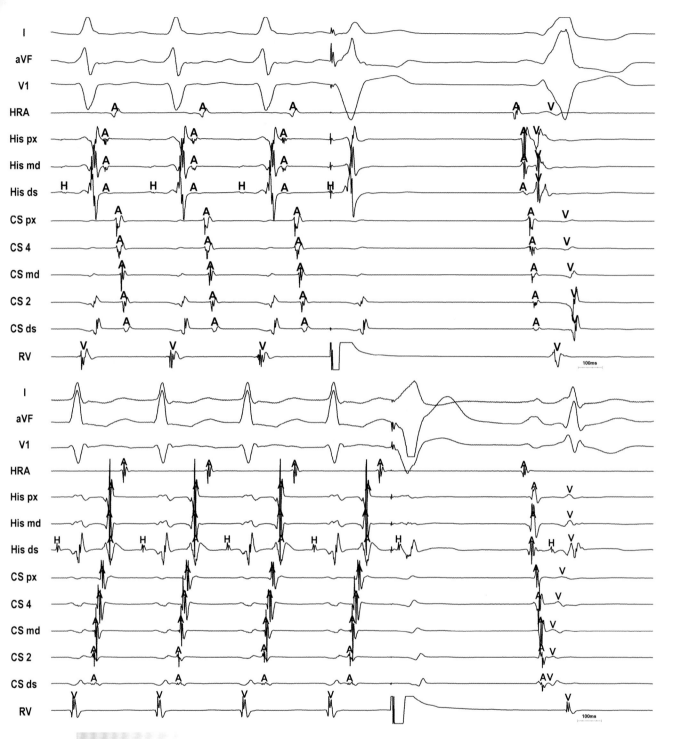

FIGURE 10-21 Termination of ORT by His refractory VPDs with VA block. The earliest site of atrial and ventricular activation during ORT and preexcited sinus rhythm are identical: anteroseptal (*top*) and left free wall (*bottom*) regions.

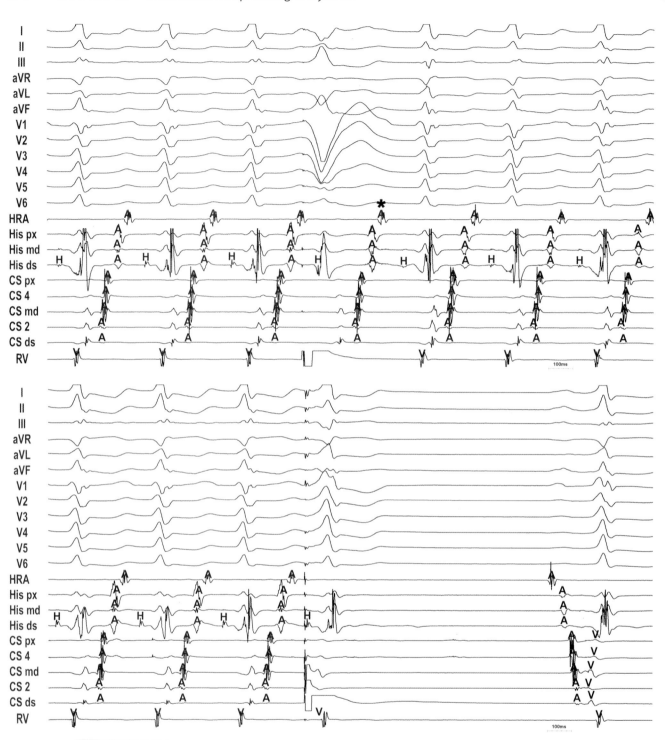

FIGURE 10-22 Resetting (*top*) and termination (*bottom*) of left-sided ORT by His refractory RV and LV VPDs, respectively. A His refractory RV apical VPD advances the atrium (*asterisk*). A His refractory LV basal VPD (delivered from a ventricular branch of the coronary sinus) terminates tachycardia with VA block. Closer proximity of the LV VPD to the AP allows it to terminate tachycardia despite its longer coupling interval. The earliest site of atrial and ventricular activation during ORT and preexcited sinus rhythm is at CS 2 indicating a left posterolateral AP.

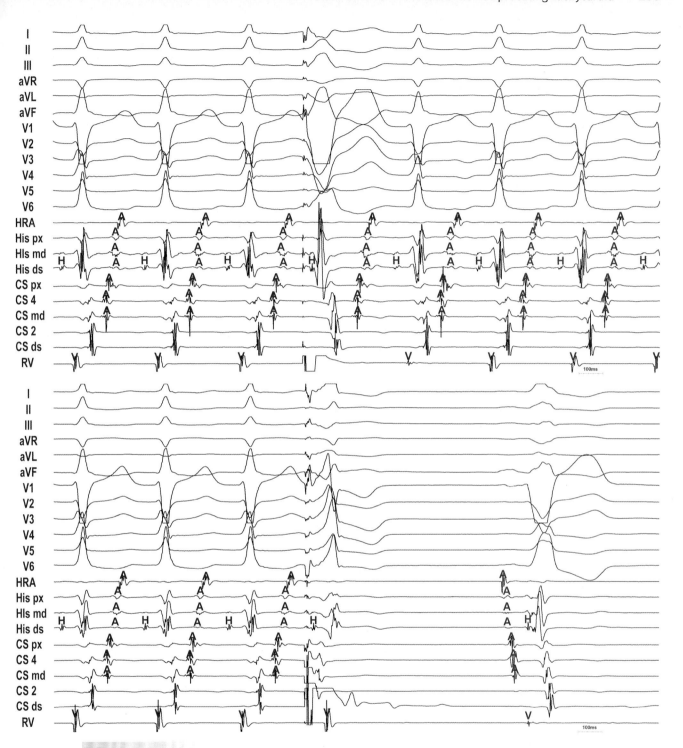

FIGURE 10-23 Negative (*top*) and positive (*bottom*) responses of left-sided ORT to His refractory RV and LV VPDs, respectively. During ORT using a left posterior AP (earliest atrial activation at CS md), a His refractory RV apical VPD fails to penetrate the circuit and affects tachycardia. However, a His refractory LV basal VPD (delivered from a ventricular branch of the coronary sinus) closer to the AP terminates tachycardia with VA block. A spontaneous RV VPD occurs during sinus rhythm.

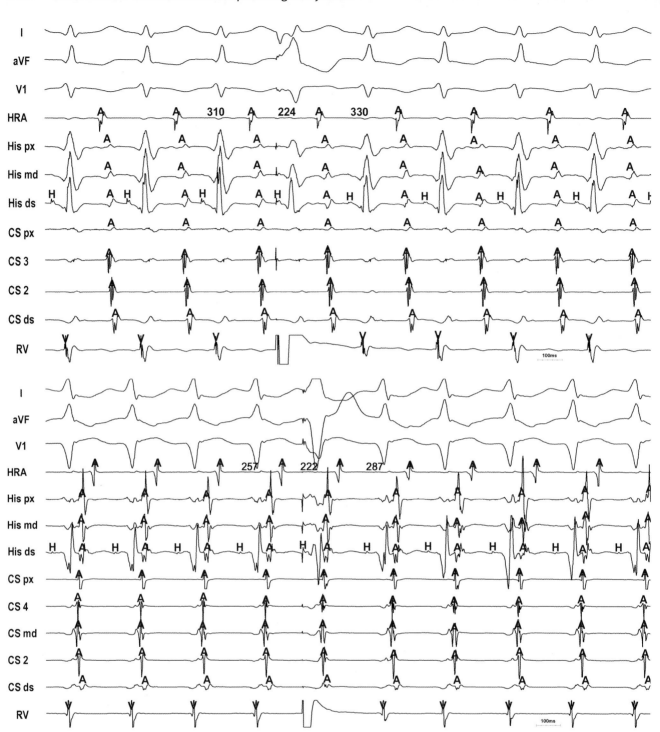

FIGURE 10-24 Resetting of ORT using right free wall (*top*) and left posterior (*bottom*) APs by His refractory RV VPDs. *Top*: A His refractory VPD advances the atrium (earliest at HRA) by 86 ms. *Bottom*: A His refractory VPD advances the atrium (earliest at CS md) by 35 ms. Note that for similarly timed RV VPDs (relative to the His bundle), the right-sided AP is advanced to a greater degree.

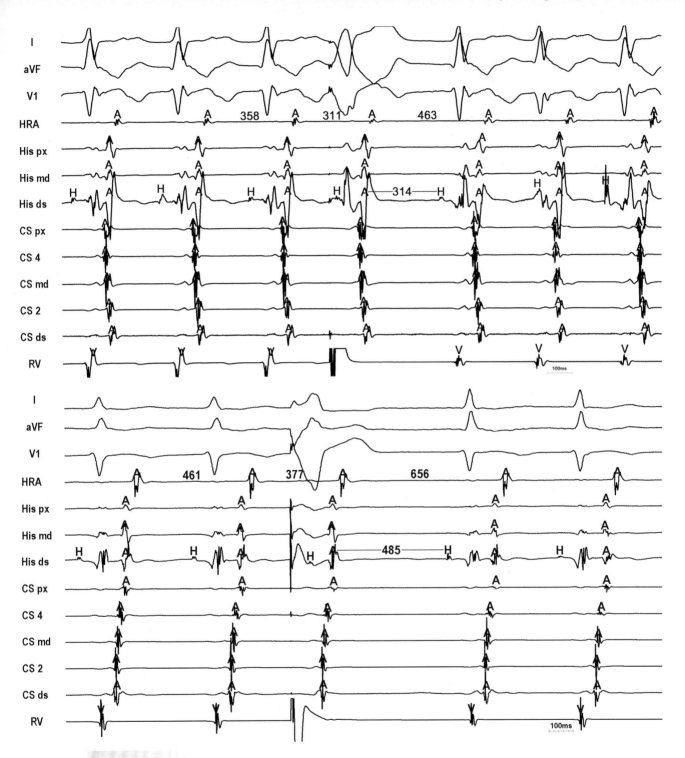

FIGURE 10-25 Resetting of ORT using left posteroseptal (*top*) and left free wall (*bottom*) APs by His refractory VPDs. In both cases, the advanced atrium encroaches on relative refractoriness of the AV node causing resetting with significant antegrade (AH) delay.

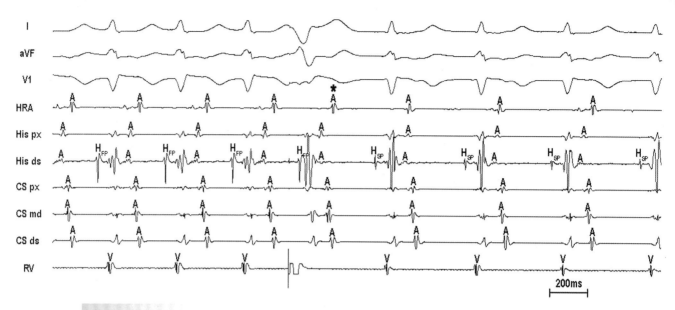

FIGURE 10-26 ORT with longitudinal dissociation of the AV node. During ORT using an anteroseptal AP (earliest atrial activation at the His bundle region), a His refractory VPD advances the atrium (*asterisk*), which then encounters FP refractoriness (longer ERP) and conducts over the SP (shorter ERP), causing abrupt deceleration of tachycardia. Concealment from SP into FP ("linking") maintains SP conduction and the slower tachycardia.

atrium to the pacing cycle length without terminating tachycardia. During entrainment, each *n* orthodromic wavefront collides with the *n* + 1 antidromic wavefront. Collision between orthodromic and antidromic wavefronts can occur either below (slower pacing rates) or above (faster pacing rates) the His bundle recording site (progressive fusion) (fourth criteria of transient entrainment) (see Fig. 2-6).[25–28]

Orthodromic Capture of the His Bundle

Orthodromic capture of the His bundle (equivalent to continuous resetting by repetitive His refractory VPDs) is indicative of an AP and a likely diagnosis of ORT (**Figs. 10-27 and 10-28; see also Fig. 5-21**). Important clues to orthodromic capture of the His bundle is the presence of paced QRS fusion (facilitated by basal sites pacing near the AP) and identifying the last His bundle electrogram accelerated to the pacing cycle length (which has the same morphology as tachycardia).[29]

"AV" Response

The response of ORT to entrainment from the ventricle is "AV" fulfilling its obligatory 1:1 AV relationship (**Figs. 10-27 and 10-28; see also Fig. 5-21**).[30]

Post-pacing Interval

The post-pacing interval (PPI) following entrainment of ORT from the right ventricular apex is short relative to the TCL (PPI − TCL ≤115 ms) because of the close proximity between the pacing site and tachycardia circuit (**Fig. 10-27; see also Fig. 5-21**).[31] However, rapid pacing rates particularly with

antidromic capture of the His bundle can cause PPI − TCL >115 ms because of both retrograde penetration and antegrade acceleration of the AV node (**Fig. 10-27**).[32,33] This error can be minimized by pacing at cycle lengths only 10–20 ms shorter than TCL or correcting the PPI for the delay in the AV node.[34,35]

ΔHA Value

The His bundle and atria are activated in parallel over the His bundle and AP during entrainment of ORT (antidromic capture of the His bundle) but sequentially during tachycardia. Therefore, the $HA_{(entrainment)} < HA_{(ORT)}$ or $\Delta HA = HA_{(entrainment)} - HA_{(ORT)} < 0$ (**Fig. 10-27; see also Fig. 5-21**).[25,32,36] (With orthodromic capture of the His bundle, the $HA_{[entrainment]}$ is still $< HA_{[ORT]}$ or $\Delta HA < 0$ because the atrium is accelerated by ventricular pacing relative to the preceding orthodromically captured His bundle electrogram.)

ΔVA Value

The difference between the stimulus-A (SA) interval during entrainment of ORT and the VA interval during tachycardia ($\Delta VA = SA - VA \leq 85$ ms) (**Fig. 10-27; see also Fig. 5-21**).[31]

ONSET OF VENTRICULAR OVERDRIVE PACING

When tachycardia cannot be entrained because of repeated pacing-induced termination, ORT can be diagnosed by resetting (advancement/delay of the atrium) or termination (VA block) within the TZ (progressive paced QRS fusion) or by one fully

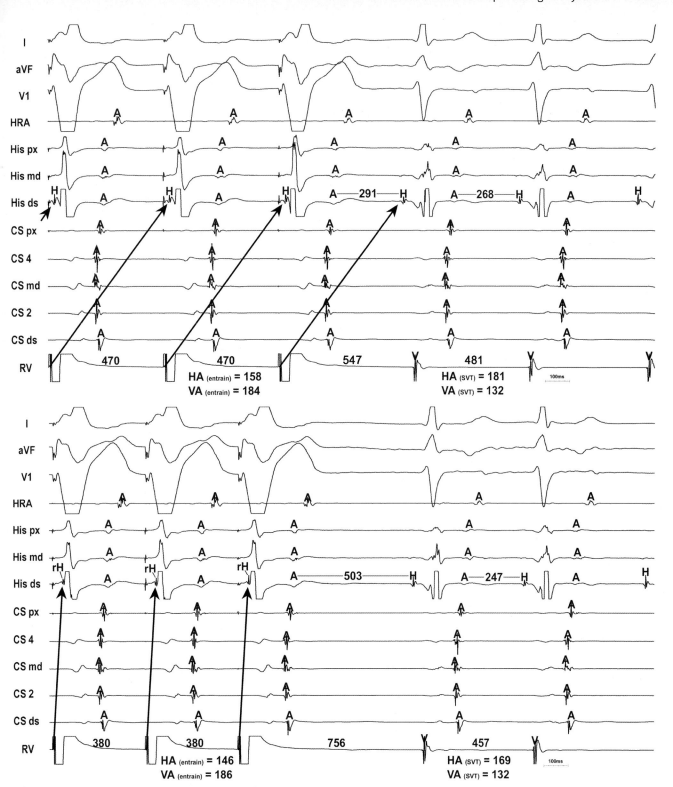

FIGURE 10-27 Entrainment of ORT using a left free wall AP with orthodromic (*top*) and antidromic (*bottom*) capture of the His bundle. *Top*: Entrainment with orthodromic capture of the His bundle alone indicates the presence of an AP. The PPI − TCL = 66 ms, corrected PPI [cPPI] = 43 ms, ΔHA = −23 ms, and ΔVA = 52 ms confirm ORT. *Bottom*: A faster pacing rate results in antidromic capture of the His bundle and very long PPI − TCL = 299 ms. The cPPI = 43 ms, ΔHA = −23 ms, and ΔVA = 54 ms indicate ORT. Note that the His bundle morphology during orthodromic capture and tachycardia are identical.

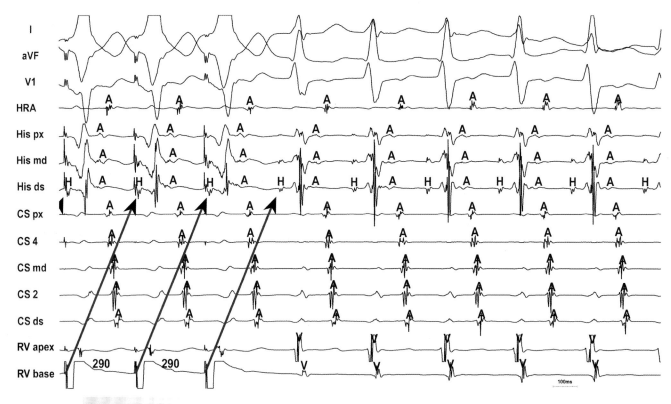

FIGURE 10-28 Entrainment of ORT using an anteroseptal AP with orthodromic capture of the His bundle. Paced ventricular complexes show constant QRS fusion (first criteria of transient entrainment). Entrainment with orthodromic capture of the His bundle alone indicates the presence of an AP and strong diagnosis of ORT without the need to measure PPI, corrected PPI, ΔVA, and ΔHA values. Note that the His bundle morphology during orthodromic capture and tachycardia are identical.

paced QRS complex (Fig. 10-29; see Figs. 5-24 and 5-25).[37,38] (Paced ventricular complexes within the TZ are fused and therefore "His-refractory.")

PACING MANEUVERS FROM THE ATRIUM

ORT VERSUS AT (VA LINKING)

VA intervals one beat after atrial overdrive pacing are linked to tachycardia (conventional method) or following decremental or differential atrial pacing: ΔVA <10 ms for ORT and >10 ms for AT (see Fig. 5-26). For AT, the VA is not a true conduction interval but a value dependent on the AT return interval at the pacing site (which itself depends on the proximity of the pacing site to the AT site of origin) and AV interval.[2,39–41]

UNUSUAL ELECTROPHYSIOLOGIC PHENOMENA

CYCLE LENGTH ALTERNANS

Cycle length alternans is beat-to-beat variability in ORT cycle length, which can result from a longitudinally-dissociated

AV node (antegradely [FP and SP]) or a longitudinally dissociated AP (retrogradely) (Figs. 10-30 and 10-31).[42–44]

QRS ALTERNANS

QRS alternans is beat-to-beat variability in the R wave amplitude (≥1 mm) during stable tachycardia. Although it has been suggested that the presence of QRS alternans indicates ORT, it is more likely a rate-related phenomenon (occurring at faster rates) and not specific for a particular tachycardia mechanism.[45–47]

CTI/MITRAL ISTHMUS/SVC BLOCK

Because the atrium is integral to the ORT circuit, cavo-tricuspid isthmus (CTI) or mitral isthmus block septal (medial) to a right- or left-sided AP, respectively, causes a change in atrial activation ("pseudo-concentric" pattern if there are no recording electrodes lateral to the AP) and enlarges the ORT circuit, causing an 1) obligatory increase in the AV interval and 2) nonobligatory increase in TCL, provided that the increase in AV interval is not counterbalanced by an equivalent decrease in the VA interval (e.g., decremental AP) ("Coumel's law in the atrium") (see Fig. 6-22).[48–51] Conduction block to bystander sites (e.g., SVC) does not affect ORT (Fig. 10-32).

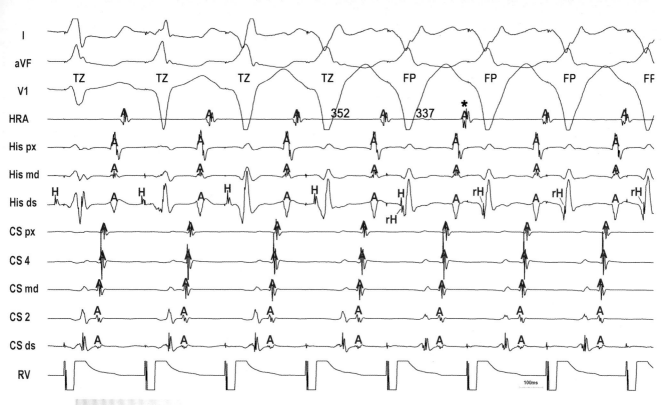

FIGURE 10-29 Onset of ventricular overdrive pacing during ORT using a left free wall AP. The first fully paced (FP) complex after the TZ remains His refractory and advances the atrium (*asterisk*) by 15 ms indicating the presence of an AP. Note that the index His bundle electrogram is a fusion potential with antegrade and retrograde components.

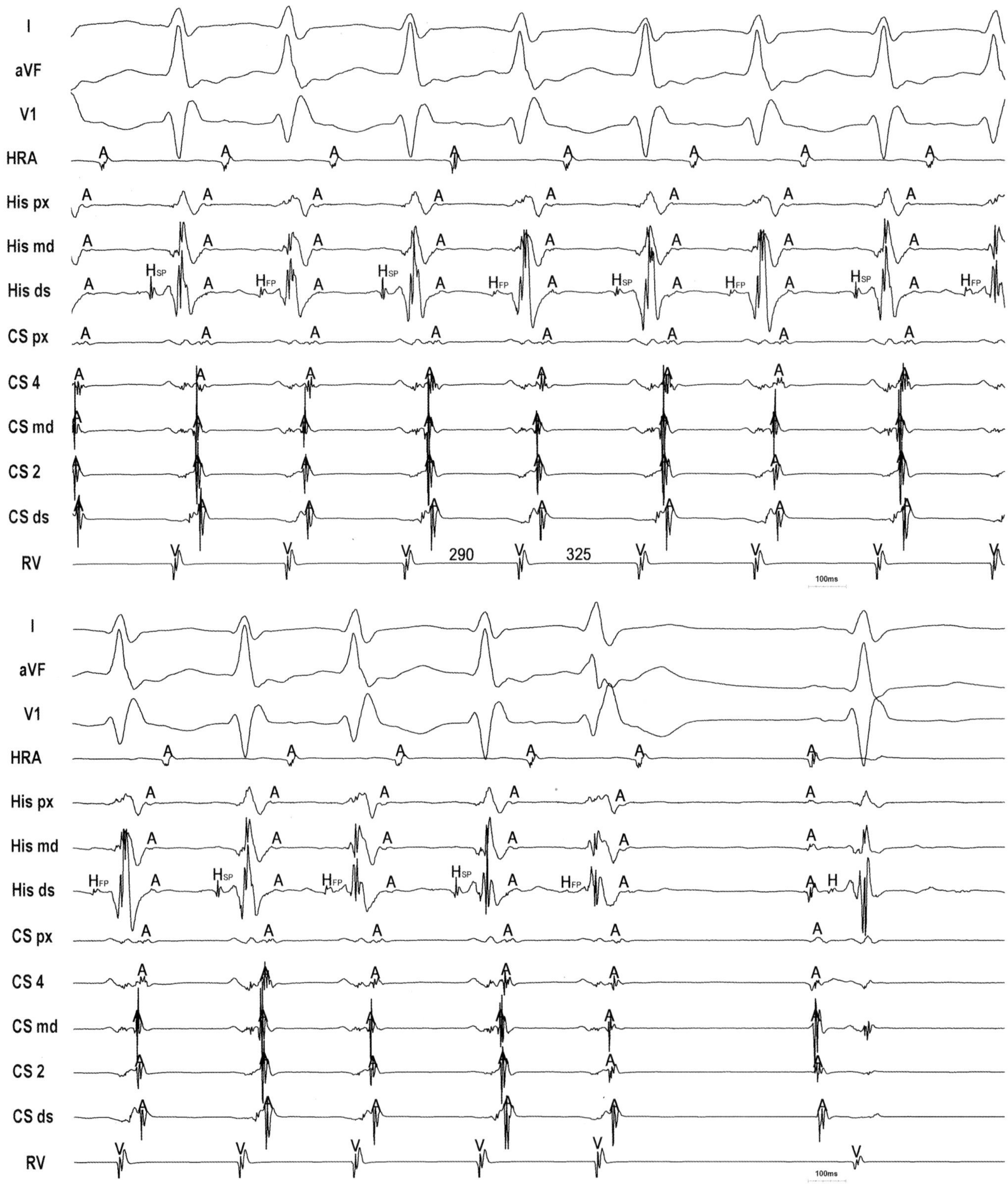

FIGURE 10-30 Termination of ORT with cycle length alternans and SP Wenckebach. *Top*: Longitudinal dissociation of the AV node (FP/SP alternans) causes cycle length alternans during ORT using a right posteroseptal AP (earliest atrial activation at CS px). Long–short sequence induces a greater degree of right bundle branch block (RBBB) aberration (but no change in VA interval). SP Wenckebach causes tachycardia slowing on alternate cycles prior to termination.

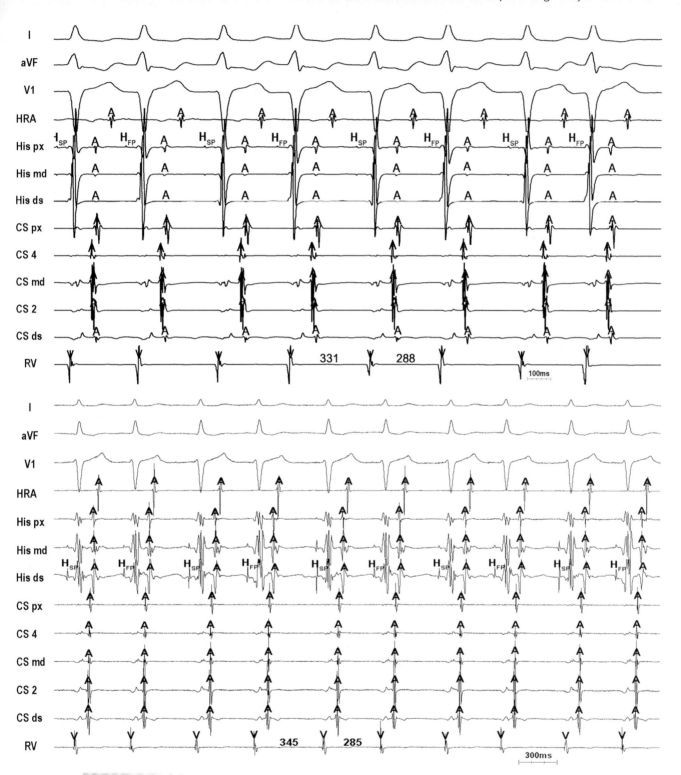

FIGURE 10-31 ORT with longitudinal dissociation of the AV node. Alternating conduction over the FP and SP (FP/SP alternans) during ORT using a left posterior (*top*) and left free wall (*bottom*) AP causes cycle length alternans.

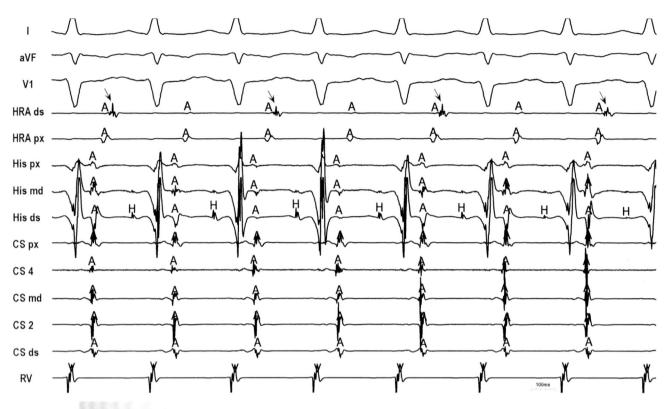

FIGURE 10-32 ORT with 2:1 block to the SVC. Arrows denote SVC potentials.

REFERENCES

1. Benditt D, Pritchett E, Smith W, Gallagher J. Ventriculoatrial intervals: diagnostic use in paroxysmal supraventricular tachycardia. Ann Intern Med 1979;91:161–166.
2. Knight BP, Ebinger M, Oral H, et al. Diagnostic value of tachycardia features and pacing maneuvers during paroxysmal supraventricular tachycardia. J Am Coll Cardiol 2000;36:574–582.
3. Tai C, Chen S, Chiang C, Lee S, Chang M. Electrocardiographic and electrophysiologic characteristics of anteroseptal, midseptal, and para-Hisian accessory pathways. Implication for radiofrequency catheter ablation. Chest 1996;109:730–740.
4. Josephson M, Scharf D, Kastor J, Kitchen J. Atrial endocardial activation in man. Electrode catheter technique of endocardial mapping. Am J Cardiol 1977;39:972–981.
5. Wellens H, Durrer D. The role of an accessory atrioventricular pathway in reciprocal tachycardia. Observations in patients with and without the Wolff-Parkinson-White syndrome. Circulation 1975;52:58–72.
6. Ho RT, DeCaro M. Narrow QRS complex tachycardia with a high-frequency potential recorded near the His bundle: what is the mechanism? Heart Rhythm 2005;2:664–666.
7. Chan KH, Obeyesekere M, Klein GJ, Sy RW. Wide complex tachycardia with telltale termination: what is the mechanism? Heart Rhythm 2013;10:1730–1731.
8. Ho RT. A narrow complex tachycardia with atrioventricular dissociation: what is the mechanism? Heart Rhythm 2017;14:1570–1573.
9. Coumel P, Attuel P. Reciprocating tachycardia in overt and latent preexcitation. Influence of functional bundle branch block on the rate of the tachycardia. Eur J Cardiol 1974;1:423–436.
10. Kerr C, Gallagher J, German L. Changes in ventriculoatrial intervals with bundle branch block aberration during reciprocating tachycardia in patients with accessory atrioventricular pathways. Circulation 1982;66:196–201.
11. Pritchett E, Tonkin A, Dugan F, Wallace A, Gallagher J. Ventriculo-atrial conduction time during reciprocating tachycardia with intermittent bundle-branch block in Wolff-Parkinson-White syndrome. Br Heart J 1976;38:1058–1064.
12. Jazayeri M, Caceres J, Tchou P, Mahmud R, Denker S, Akhtar M. Electrophysiologic characteristics of sudden QRS axis deviation during orthodromic tachycardia. Role of functional fascicular block in localization of accessory pathway. J Clin Invest 1989;83:952–959.
13. Ho RT, Rhim ES. Metamorphosis of a tachycardia: what is the mechanism? Heart Rhythm 2008;5:155–157.
14. Sauer WH, Jacobson JT. Paradoxical slowing of orthodromic reciprocating tachycardia with loss of bundle branch block ipsilateral to the accessory pathway. J Cardiovasc Electrophysiol 2009;20:347–348.
15. Spurrell R, Krikler D, Sowton E. Retrograde invasion of the bundle branches producing aberration of the QRS complex during supraventricular tachycardia studied by programmed electrical stimulation. Circulation 1974;50:487–495.
16. Goldreyer B, Damato A. The essential role of atrioventricular conduction delay in the initiation of paroxysmal supraventricular tachycardia. Circulation 1971;43:679–687.
17. Lehmann M, Denker S, Mahmud R, Tchou P, Dongas J, Akhtar M. Electrophysiologic mechanisms of functional bundle branch block at onset of induced orthodromic tachycardia in the Wolff-Parkinson-White syndrome. Role of stimulation method. J Clin Invest 1985;76:1566–1574.
18. Akhtar M, Shenasa M, Schmidt D. Role of retrograde His Purkinje block in the initiation of supraventricular tachycardia by ventricular premature stimulation in the Wolff-Parkinson-White syndrome. J Clin Invest 1981;67:1047–1055.
19. Jackman W, Friday K, Scherlag B, et al. Direct endocardial recording from an accessory atrioventricular pathway: localization of the site of block, effect of antiarrhythmic drugs, and attempt at nonsurgical ablation. Circulation 1983;68:906–916.
20. Kuck K, Friday K, Kunze K, Schlüter M, Lazzara R, Jackman W. Sites of conduction block in accessory atrioventricular pathways. Basis for concealed accessory pathways. Circulation 1990;82:407–417.
21. Ho RT, Levi SA. An atypical long RP tachycardia—what is the mechanism? Heart Rhythm 2013;10:1089–1090.
22. Zipes DP, DeJoseph RL, Rothbaum DA. Unusual properties of accessory pathways. Circulation 1974;49:1200–1211.
23. Benditt D, Benson DW Jr, Dunnigan A, et al. Role of extrastimulus site and tachycardia cycle length in inducibility of atrial preexcitation by premature ventricular stimulation during reciprocating tachycardia. Am J Cardiol 1987;60:811–819.
24. Miles W, Yee R, Klein G, Zipes D, Prystowsky E. The preexcitation index: an aid in determining the mechanism of supraventricular tachycardia and localizing accessory pathways. Circulation 1986;74:493–500.
25. Ho RT, Mark GE, Rhim ES, Pavri BB, Greenspon AJ. Differentiating atrioventricular nodal reentrant tachycardia from atrioventricular reentrant tachycardia by ΔHA values during entrainment from the ventricle. Heart Rhythm 2008;5:83–88.

26. Nagashima K, Kumar S, Stevenson WG, et al. Anterograde conduction to the His bundle during right ventricular overdrive pacing distinguishes septal pathway atrioventricular reentry from atypical atrioventricular nodal reentrant tachycardia. Heart Rhythm 2015;12:735–743.

27. Waldo AL, Maclean WA, Karp RB, Kouchoukos NT, James TN. Entrainment and interruption of atrial flutter with atrial pacing: studies in man following open heart surgery. Circulation 1977;56:737–745.

28. Waldo AL, Plumb VJ, Arciniegas JG, et al. Transient entrainment and interruption of the atrioventricular bypass pathway type of paroxysmal atrial tachycardia. A model for understanding and identifying reentrant arrhythmias. Circulation 1983;67:73–83.

29. Boyle PM, Veenhuyzen GD, Vigmond EJ. Fusion during entrainment of orthodromic reciprocating tachycardia is enhanced for basal pacing sites but diminished when pacing near Purkinje system end points. Heart Rhythm 2013;10:444–451.

30. Knight B, Zivin A, Souza J, et al. A technique for the rapid diagnosis of atrial tachycardia in the electrophysiology laboratory. J Am Coll Cardiol 1999;33: 775–781.

31. Michaud GF, Tada H, Chough S, et al. Differentiation of atypical atrioventricular node re-entrant tachycardia from orthodromic reciprocating tachycardia using a septal accessory pathway by the response to ventricular pacing. J Am Coll Cardiol 2001;38:1163–1167.

32. Rhim ES, Hillis MB, Mark GE, Ho RT. The ΔHA value during entrainment of a long RP tachycardia: another useful criterion for diagnosis of supraventricular tachycardia. J Cardiovasc Electrophysiol 2008;19:559–561.

33. Michaud GF. Entrainment of a narrow QRS complex tachycardia from the right ventricular apex: what is the mechanism? Heart Rhythm 2005;2:559–560.

34. Michaud GF, Morady F. Letters to the editor. Heart Rhythm 2006;7:1114–1115.

35. González-Torrecilla E, Arenal A, Atienza F, et al. First postpacing interval after tachycardia entrainment with correction for atrioventricular node delay: a simple maneuver for differential diagnosis of atrioventricular nodal reentrant tachycardias versus orthodromic reciprocating tachycardias. Heart Rhythm 2006;3:674–679.

36. Mark GE, Rhim ES, Pavri BB, Greenspon AJ, Ho RT. Differentiation of atrioventricular nodal reentrant tachycardia from orthodromic atrioventricular reentrant tachycardia by ΔHA intervals during entrainment from the ventricle [abstract]. Heart Rhythm 2006;3:S321.

37. AlMahameed ST, Buxton AE, Michaud GF. New criteria during right ventricular pacing to determine the mechanism of supraventricular tachycardia. Circ Arrhythm Electrophysiol 2010;3:578–584.

38. Dandamudi G, Mokabberi R, Assal C, et al. A novel approach to differentiating orthodromic reciprocating tachycardia from atrioventricular nodal reentrant tachycardia. Heart Rhythm 2010;7:1326–1329.

39. Kadish AH, Morady F. The response of paroxysmal supraventricular tachycardia to overdrive atrial and ventricular pacing: can it help determine the tachycardia mechanism? J Cardiovasc Electrophysiol 1993;4:239–252.

40. Maruyama M, Kobayashi Y, Miyauchi Y, et al. The VA relationship after differential atrial overdrive pacing: a novel tool for the diagnosis of atrial tachycardia in the electrophysiologic laboratory. J Cardiovasc Electrophysiol 2007;18:1127–1133.

41. Sarkozy A, Richter S, Chierchia G, et al. A novel pacing manoeuvre to diagnose atrial tachycardia. Europace 2008;10:459–466.

42. Csanadi Z, Klein GJ, Yee R, Thakur RK, Li H. Effect of dual atrioventricular node pathways on atrioventricular reentrant tachycardia. Circulation 1995; 91:2614–2618.

43. Sung R, Styperek J. Electrophysiologic identification of dual atrioventricular nodal pathway conduction in patients with reciprocating tachycardia using anomalous bypass tracts. Circulation 1979;60:1464–1476.

44. Atié J, Brugada P, Brugada J, et al. Longitudinal dissociation of atrioventricular accessory pathways. J Am Coll Cardiol 1991;17:161–166.

45. Green M, Heddle B, Dassen W, et al. Value of QRS alteration in determining the site of origin of narrow QRS supraventricular tachycardia. Circulation 1983;68:368–373.

46. Kay G, Pressley J, Packer D, Pritchett E, German L, Gilbert M. Value of the 12-lead electrocardiogram in discriminating atrioventricular nodal reciprocating tachycardia from circus movement atrioventricular tachycardia utilizing a retrograde accessory pathway. Am J Cardiol 1987;59:296–300.

47. Morady F. Significance of QRS alternans during narrow QRS tachycardias. Pacing Clin Electrophysiol 1991;14:2193–2198.

48. Ho RT, Yin A. Spontaneous conversion of a long RP to short RP tachycardia: what is the mechanism? Heart Rhythm 2014;11:522–525.

49. Ilkhanoff L, Couchonnal LF, Goldberger JJ. Implications of cavotricuspid isthmus block complicating ablation of a posteroseptal accessory pathway. J Interv Card Electrophysiol 2012;35:81–83.

50. Bulava A, Hanis J, Sitek D. Mitral isthmus conduction block: intriguing result of radiofrequency catheter ablation for a left concealed accessory pathway. Europace 2010;12:579–581.

51. Mahajan R, Rohit M, Talwar K. Activation sequence change during left free wall pathway ablation: what is the mechanism? J Cardiovasc Electrophysiol 2009;20:1174–1175.

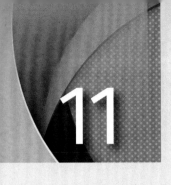

11 Unusual Types of Accessory Pathways

Introduction

Typical accessory pathways (APs) (bundle of Kent) are nondecremental muscle fibers spanning the tricuspid or mitral annulus. In contrast to single APs, multiple APs produce unusual patterns of ventricular preexcitation and/or retrograde atrial activation with both orthodromic and antidromic tachycardia circuits. Atypical APs include those exhibiting decremental conduction and/or originate/insert into the atrio-ventricular (AV) node–His-Purkinje axis (e.g., nodo-fascicular [NF] AP).

The purpose of this chapter is to:
1. Discuss the 12-lead ECG and electrophysiologic clues to the presence of multiple APs.
2. Describe the electrophysiologic features of the permanent form of junctional reciprocating tachycardia (PJRT).
3. Describe the electrophysiologic features of APs that originate/insert into the AV node–His-Purkinje axis.

MULTIPLE APs

Multiple APs can cause different orthodromic reciprocating tachycardia (ORT) and antidromic reciprocating tachycardia (ART) circuits. Antidromic reciprocating tachycardia itself should raise suspicion that more than one AP is present.[1,2] Right free wall and posteroseptal APs are a frequent combination, and Ebstein's anomaly is associated with multiple APs perhaps due to abnormal development of the tricuspid annulus.[2] Several 12-lead ECG and electrophysiologic clues indicate the presence of multiple APs.

12-LEAD ECG

Electrocardiographic clues to the presence of multiple APs include 1) an atypical or unusual pattern of preexcitation not explained by a single AP, 2) ≥2 preexcited QRS morphologies, 3) ≥2 P-wave morphologies during ORT, and 4) spontaneous change from ORT to preexcited tachycardia (ORT with bystander preexcitation).[3–5] Two or more preexcited QRS morphologies might be observed during atrial fibrillation and simulate polymorphic ventricular tachycardia, occur during different preexcited tachycardias, or follow administration of procainamide or ajmaline due to selective block in one AP.

ELECTROPHYSIOLOGIC STUDY

Electrophysiologic clues to the presence of multiple APs include 1) antegrade–retrograde mismatch (discrepancy between the earliest site of ventricular activation during manifest preexcitation and atrial activation during ORT), 2) ≥2 preexcited QRS morphologies, 3) ≥2 atrial exit sites or atrial activation patterns during ORT, and 4) antidromic tachycardia with retrograde conduction over another AP (duodromic tachycardia) **(Figs. 11-1 to 11-3)**.[3,4,6,7]

PERMANENT FORM OF JUNCTIONAL RECIPROCATING TACHYCARDIA

PJRT is a nearly incessant form of long RP ORT using a concealed, slowly conducting, decremental AV AP (see Chapter 6).[8–13] Its incessant behavior can cause a tachycardia-mediated cardiomyopathy. These APs are classically located in the posteroseptal region near the ostium (os) of the coronary sinus (CS), but other locations have been reported.[10] Absence of manifest preexcitation during sinus rhythm has been attributed to repetitive retrograde concealment from the AV node–His-Purkinje system into the AP with prolonged antegrade refractoriness rather than "impedance mismatch" at the AP ventricular insertion site because manifest preexcitation can develop with AV block.[11] A sinuous, tortuous course within the posterior pyramidal space causing changes in axial resistivity might explain its rate-dependent properties.[11]

ELECTROPHYSIOLOGIC FEATURES

12-lead ECG
The characteristic 12-lead ECG of PJRT is a regular, long RP narrow complex tachycardia with inverted P waves inferiorly

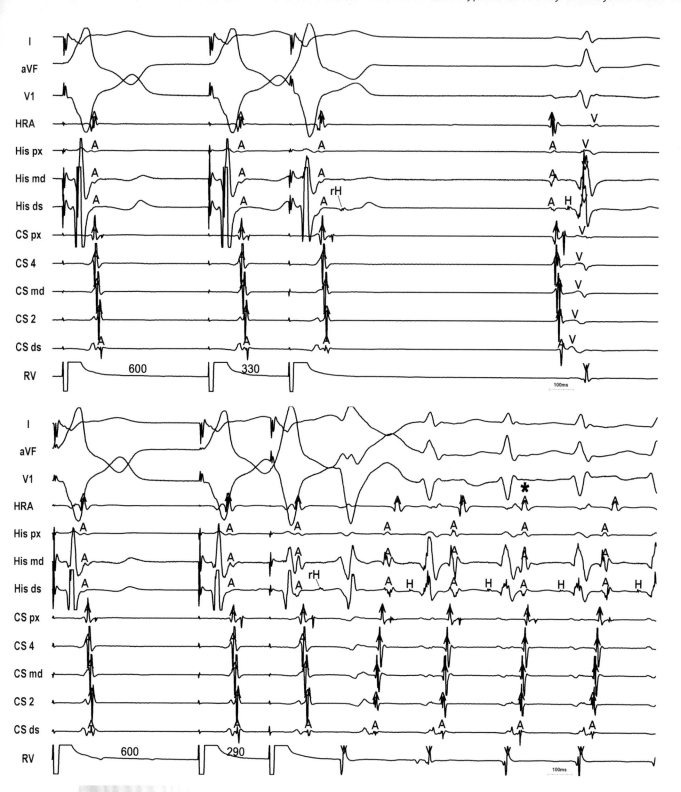

FIGURE 11-1 Multiple APs. *Top*: During programmed ventricular extrastimulation, retrograde atrial activation is right eccentric due to conduction over a right free wall AP. Further proof of an AP is established by the extrastimulus that induces a "VH jump" (rH), which allows retrograde atrial activation to precede His bundle activation. During sinus rhythm, the HV is short (32 ms) and ventricular activation is early along the lateral mitral annulus (CS ds) identifying a concomitant left free wall AP. *Bottom*: Despite retrograde conduction over the right free wall AP during the drive train, a single BBR beat induces ORT using the left free wall AP. The third atrial complex (*asterisk*) represents fusion over both APs.

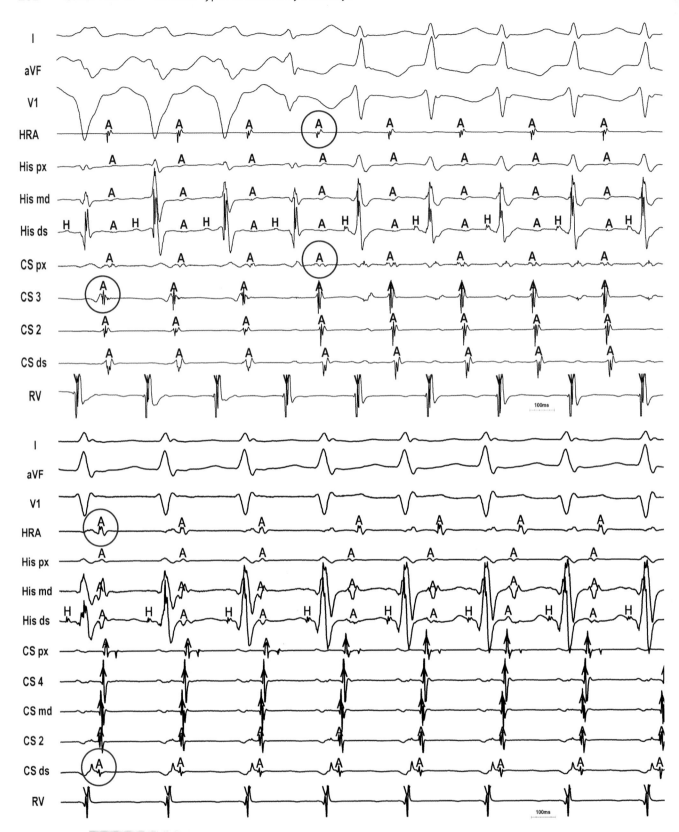

FIGURE 11-2 Multiple APs. *Top*: During ORT with LBBB, retrograde atrial activation is driven by a left posterior AP (earliest atrial activation at CS 3). Loss of LBBB and transeptal conduction shortens the ORT circuit, which encroaches on left posterior AP refractoriness and causes a shift to right posteroseptal and right free wall APs (early at CS px and HRA). (Note that the HRA during LBBB is also early indicating fusion with the right free wall AP.) *Bottom*: ORT with retrograde fusion over a right and left free wall AP for three beats. Subsequent loss of conduction over the right free wall AP without change in tachycardia indicates that the left free wall Pathway is dominant and responsible for ORT.

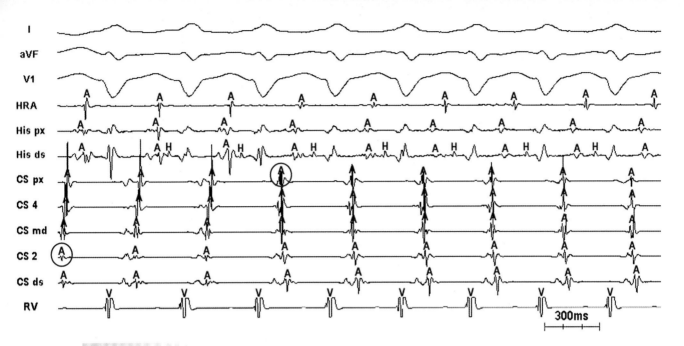

FIGURE 11-3 Multiple APs. Spontaneous shift of LBBB ORT using a left posterolateral AP (earliest atrial activation at CS 2) to a right posteroseptal AP (earliest at CS px). Note that LBBB ORT using the right-sided AP is faster due to loss of transeptal conduction.

and slightly positive P waves in V1 (due to AP location near the CS os) (see Fig. 6-3).[9]

Electrophysiologic Study

The ventriculo-atrial (VA) interval is long, and the earliest site of retrograde atrial activation is typically near the os of the CS (see Figs. 6-8 to 6-10).[9,11] A 1:1 AV relationship is mandatory.

ZONES OF TRANSITION

Initiation

Unlike classic ORT, induction of PJRT can occur spontaneously during sinus rhythm without the need for prematurity, which contributes to its incessant behavior (Fig. 11-4).[9] Initiation is dependent on achieving a critical sinus rate and not necessarily

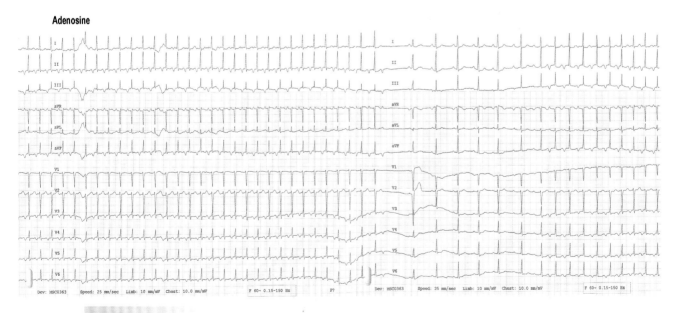

FIGURE 11-4 Adenosine-induced termination of PJRT. Adenosine causes PR prolongation and AV block resulting in slowing and termination of tachycardia, respectively, which demonstrates tachycardia dependence on the AV node. Spontaneous re-initiation without the need for prematurity contributes to its incessant behavior.

on a critical AV delay. Because the slow and decremental retrograde properties of the AP allow it to continually accept sinus impulses conducting over the AV node–His-Purkinje system, tachycardia is triggered when block occurs antegradely in the AP (e.g. AP-V interface) at a critical sinus rate.

Termination

The obligatory 1:1 AV relationship implies that PJRT terminates with either AV or VA block. Spontaneous termination with AV block excludes atrial tachycardia (AT). Termination by early-coupled ventricular premature depolarizations (VPDs) with VA block also excludes AT. Termination by His refractory VPDs with VA block excludes both pure atypical AV nodal reentrant tachycardia (AVNRT) and AT (but not NF reentrant tachycardia [NFRT] or atypical AVNRT with a bystander NF AP inserting into the slow pathway [SP]) (**Fig. 11-5; see also Figs. 6-11 and 6-12**).

PACING MANEUVERS FROM THE VENTRICLE

His Refractory VPD

His refractory VPDs can advance or paradoxically delay the atrium—the latter due to significant decremental properties of the AP (**Fig. 11-6; see also Fig. 6-14**).[14,15]

Entrainment from the Ventricle

Ventricular overdrive pacing accelerates PJRT to the pacing cycle length and the response to entrainment is "AV."[16] Slow retrograde AP conduction, however, can produce pseudo "AAV" responses yielding a false diagnosis of AT (**Fig. 11-7; see also Fig. 6-14**). Entrainment with orthodromic capture of the His bundle indicates the presence of an AP (**see Fig. 2-6**). While PJRT can cause post-pacing interval (PPI) − tachycardia cycle length (TCL) ≤115 ms, corrected PPI <110 ms, ΔHA ($HA_{[entrainment]}$ − $HA_{[SVT]}$) <0, and ΔVA (SA − VA) ≤85 ms, significant decrement in the AP can also generate large values for all these criteria yielding a false diagnosis of atypical AVNRT (**Figs. 11-7 to 11-9**).[17–21]

Onset of Ventricular Overdrive Pacing

Similar to classic ORT, PJRT can be reset (advanced or delayed) or terminated by paced ventricular complexes within the transition zone (the equivalent of a His refractory VPD) (**Fig. 11-10**).

ACCESSORY PATHWAYS ORIGINATING/INSERTING INTO THE AV NODE–HIS-PURKINJE SYSTEM

Atrio-nodal (James fibers) and atrio-His AP are rare. ORT, using a concealed atrio-nodal AP, shares features common to 1) AT (eccentric atrial activation [particularly, right-sided] and peristence despite AV block [block distal to the nodal input]), 2) AVNRT (long PPI following entrainment from the ventricle, no effect by His refractory VPDs), and 3) ORT (eccentric VA conduction during ventricular pacing).[22,23] Clues to an atrio-His AP include 1) short AH (PR) interval, 2) lack of AH prolongation

(decremental conduction) with premature atrial stimulation, and 3) rapid ventricular rates during supraventricular tachycardia (SVT)/atrial tachyarrhythmias.[24] Mahaim fibers refer collectively to variant APs that share several common electrophysiologic features: 1) classic origin (e.g., AV node) and/or insertion in (nodo-fascicular [NF]) or near (nodo-ventricular [NV]) the right bundle (RB) causing typical LBBB QRS complexes (although left-sided fibers have also been reported), 2) rate-dependent (decremental), antegrade-only conduction (although concealed retrogradely, conducting NF/NF APs have been described), and 3) minimal (fasciculo-ventricular) or even absent (NF/NV or atrio-fascicular [AF]) preexcitation during sinus rhythm (because of slow antegrade AP conduction) exposed only by atrial pacing or during antidromic tachycardia (latent AP). These include nodo-fascicular/nodo-ventricular, atrio-fascicular (or a long AV fiber inserting near the RB), and fasciculo-ventricular APs. Nodo-fascicular/nodo-ventricular APs originate in the AV node (often SP) and insert into the antero-apical region of the right ventricle in or near the RB. Atrio-fascicular (or long AV) APs originate along the lateral tricuspid annulus (posterolateral to anterolateral region) and insert in or near the RB. Fasciculo-ventricular APs originate in the RB and insert into the right ventricle.

NODO-FASCICULAR/NODO-VENTRICULAR AP

These APs are associated with dual AV nodal physiology and other AV connections.[25,26]

Electrophysiologic Features

The HV interval can be normal, and baseline preexcitation is often absent.[25,26] Decremental atrial pacing or atrial extrastimulation reveals typical LBBB preexcitation with prolonging St-delta intervals because of decremental conduction over the AP. During maximal preexcitation, block in the AV node distal to origin of the AP causes exclusive conduction over the AP with subsequent retrograde activation of the His bundle ("VH" interval). Further shortening of the atrial pacing cycle length or coupling interval causes increase in the St-delta interval, but the VH interval and degree of preexcitation remain the same. Because the AP bypasses the His bundle, His bundle extrasystoles normalize the QRS complex if preexcitation is present (unless the extrasystoles arise from the AV node proximal to the nodal origin of the AP).[26] Parahisian pacing can differentiate a nodo-fascicular ("AV nodal response") from a nodo-ventricular AP ("AP response").[27,28]

AV Block

Spontaneous episode of AV block is unique to NF/NV APs.[29,30] A sinus impulse conducts over the AV node–His-Purkinje axis and then reciprocates retrogradely over the nodal AP to render the AV node physiologically refractory for the next sinus beat (pseudo AV block). Single reciprocation can cause isolated episodes of AV block, but repetitive reciprocation leads to NFRT.

Orthodromic NFRT

ORT using a NF/NV AP is the only ORT that can be associated with AV dissociation. It is diagnosed by His refractory VPDs that

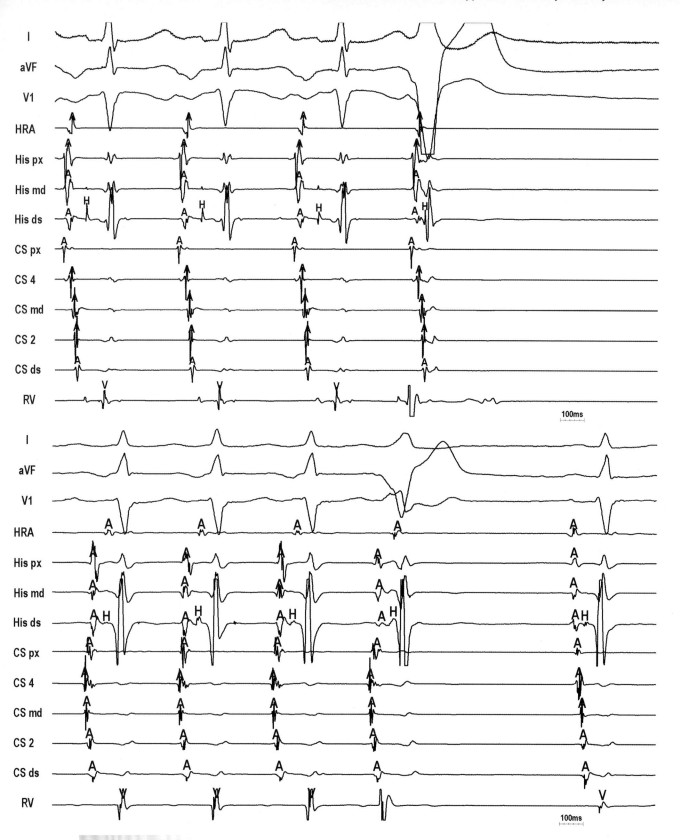

FIGURE 11-5 Termination of PJRT by His refractory VPDs with VA block. The RP interval is long, and earliest atrial activation is near the CS os (CS px [*top*], and CS 4 [*bottom*]). VPDs delivered during His bundle refractoriness terminate tachycardia with retrograde block in the AP.

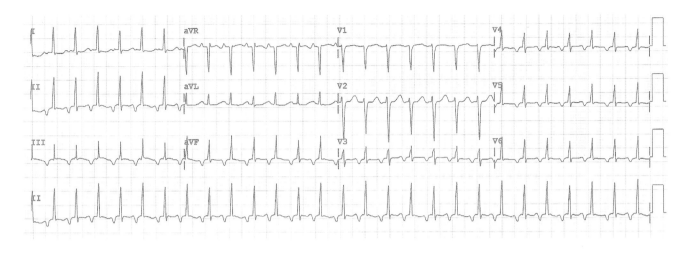

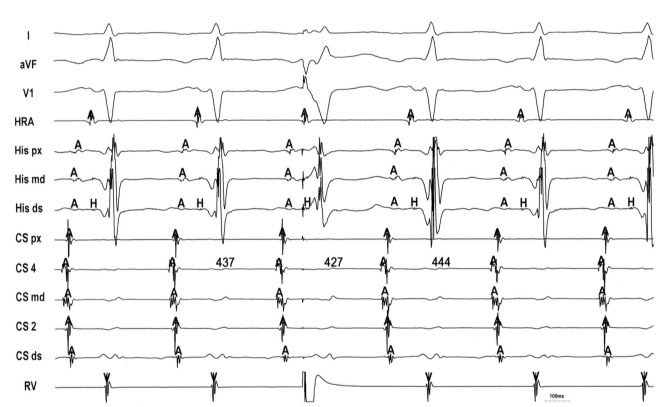

FIGURE 11-6 Resetting of PJRT by His refractory VPDs. P waves are inverted inferiorly and isoelectric/slightly positive in V1. The earliest site of atrial activation is near the CS os. A His refractory VPD advances the atrium by 10 ms.

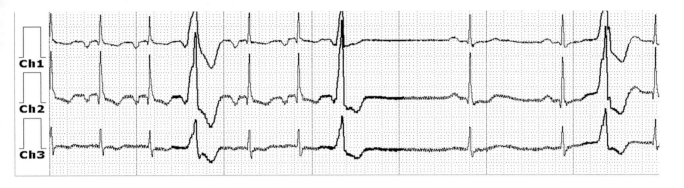

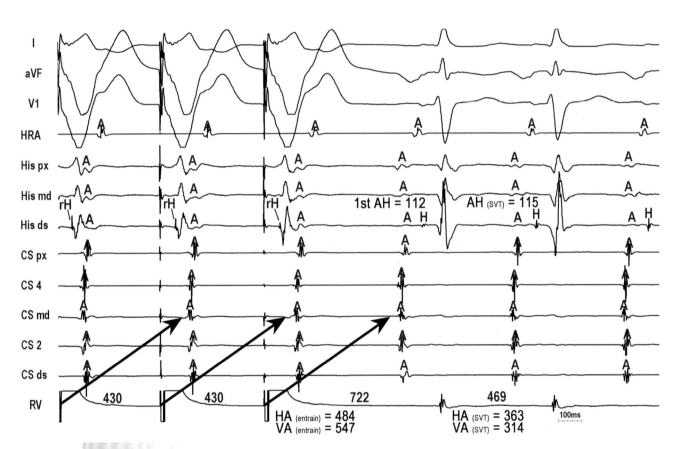

FIGURE 11-7 "Pseudo AAV" response during PJRT. *Top*: A spontaneous His refractory VPD (fused QRS) terminates PJRT with VA block, indicating the presence of an AP. The response to entrainment from the ventricle with antidromic capture of the His bundle is a "pseudo AAV" (true AV) response. Note that decremental conduction over the AP produces a long PPI − TCL = 253 ms, cPPI = 256 ms, ΔHA = 121 ms, and ΔVA = 233 ms yielding a false diagnosis of atypical AVNRT.

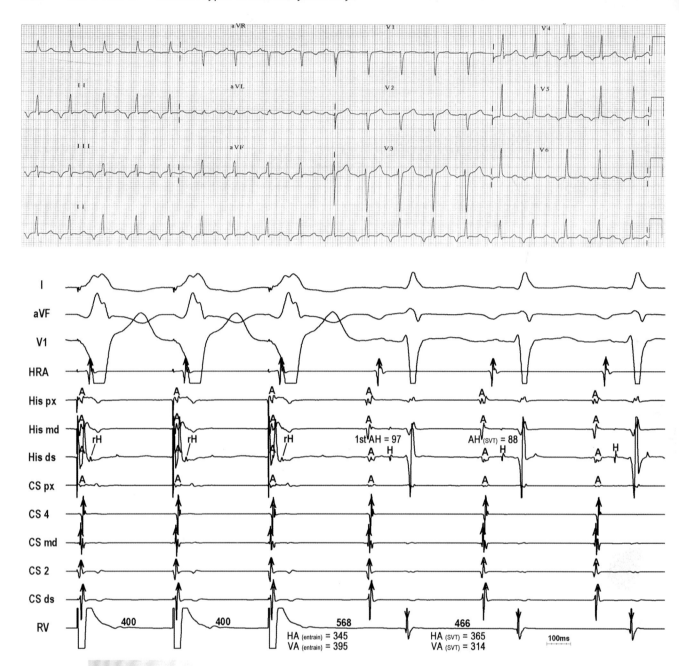

FIGURE 11-8 Entrainment of PJRT from the ventricle with antidromic capture of the His bundle. P waves are inverted inferiorly and isoelectric/slightly positive in V1. The response to entrainment from the ventricle is "AV." The PPI − TCL = 102 ms, cPPI = 93 ms, ΔHA = −20 ms, and ΔVA = 81 ms.

reset (advance or delay) the subsequent His bundle or terminate tachycardia (**Figs. 11-11 to 11-13**).[31–35] In the absence of AV dissociation, orthodromic NFRT is differentiated from PJRT (AV AP) by ΔAH (AH$_{[entrainment/\ pace\ @\ TCL]}$ − AH$_{[SVT]}$) >40 ms or paradoxically, AH$_{(SVT)}$ < AH$_{(NSR)}$ (**Figs. 11-14 and 11-15**) (see also **Table 6-1**).[27,36,37]

It has been suggested that orthodromic NVRT can be differentiated from orthodromic NFRT by the presence of manifest fusion during RV entrainment.[38] Because the circuit

for orthodromic NFRT is contained within the specialized conduction system, penetration of its excitable gap and entrainment of tachycardia requires penetration of the His-Purkinje system and fully paced ventricular complexes (analogous to concealed entrainment of AVNRT) so that ventricular fusion should not occur. This is true when the collision point between orthodromic and antidromic wavefronts is proximal to the His bundle bifurcation (AV node or His bundle) but not when collision occurs distal to the

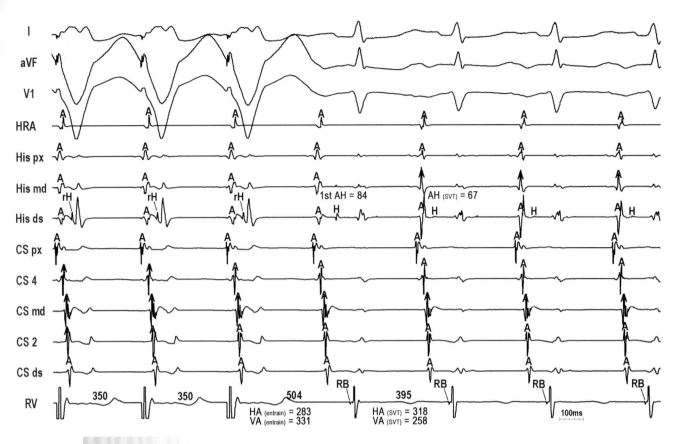

FIGURE 11-9 Entrainment of PJRT from the ventricle with antidromic capture of the His bundle. The earliest site of atrial activation is at the CS os (CS px). The response to entrainment is "AV." The PPI − TCL = 109 ms, cPPI = 92 ms, ΔHA = −35 ms, ΔVA = 73 ms.

His bundle bifurcation (RB close to insertion of the NF AP). In the latter case, the His bundle–left bundle–left ventricular axis can be orthodromically activated and fuse with paced right ventricular complexes.

Antidromic NFRT

Electrophysiologic features of antidromic tachycardia using a NF AP are 1) fixed, maximally preexcited typical LBBB QRS complexes; 2) short, negative HV interval (<30 ms); 3) retrograde His-RB activation sequence (proximal RB-His ds-His px); and 4) concentric atrial activation (retrograde conduction over the AV node) with a long A-delta interval (due to decremental AP conduction) or VA dissociation (nodal–atrial block).[25,26,39,40] Because the AP inserts in/near the RB, preexcited QRS complexes show typical LBBB morphology. Close proximity between the distal RB insertion site and His bundle coupled with simultaneous activation of the His bundle retrogradely and ventricle antegradely over the RB (pseudo HV interval) results in His bundle potentials occurring just after QRS onset (VH <30 ms) (which is in contrast to the longer true VH interval of classic antidromic tachycardia using an AV AP). Proximal retrograde RBBB, however, can cause switch from short to long VH tachycardia

and prolongation of the TCL as the left bundle becomes incorporated into the circuit ("reverse Coumel's sign"). Antidromic NFRT is the only antidromic tachycardia that can be associated with AV dissociation because the atrium is not an integral part of the circuit.[26,41]

AVNRT with Manifest/Concealed Bystander NF AP

Electrophysiologic clues supporting AVNRT with manifest bystander nodo-fascicular preexcitation over antidromic NFRT are 1) variable preexcitation or loss of preexcitation without affecting tachycardia; 2) short, positive HV interval (≥0); and 3) antegrade His-RB activation sequence (His px-His ds-proximal RB).[25,26,39,40] (RB potentials might coincide with His bundle potentials [His − RB = 0] if the former is activated retrogradely by the NF AP and the latter is activated antegradely by the AV node.)

The best method to diagnose the presence of concealed bystander NF APs is the delivery of His refractory VPDs, which reset or terminate AVNRT (or terminate ORT with antegrade block in the AV node).[27,42,43] Insertion of the NF AP into the SP is most common and identified by His refractory VPDs that 1) reset or terminate atypical (fast–slow) AVNRT with VA block (retrograde limb) or 2) reset or terminate typical

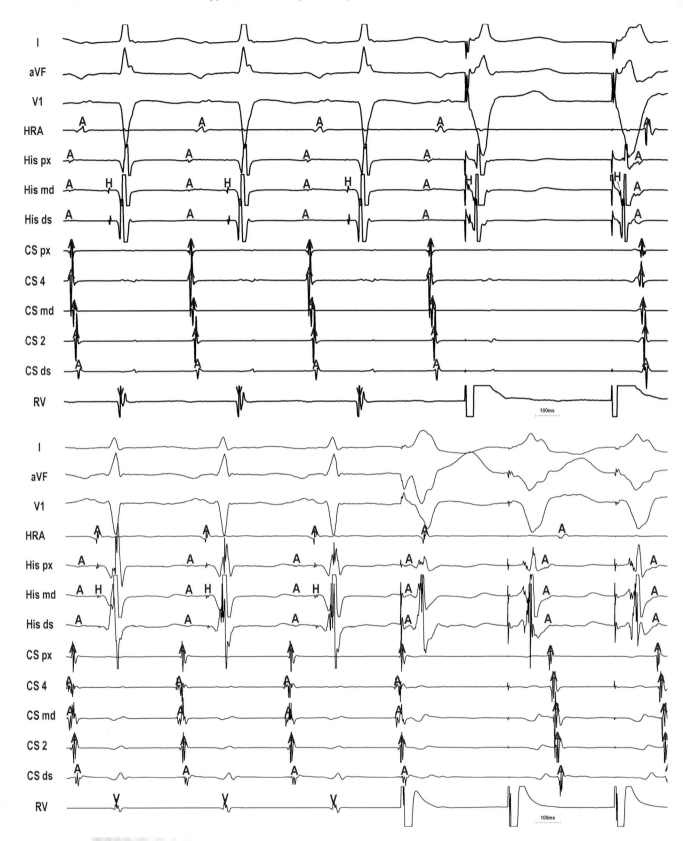

FIGURE 11-10 Termination of PJRT at onset of ventricular overdrive pacing. In both cases, the first paced complex is fused (His refractory), terminating tachycardia with VA block. After tachycardia terminates, retrograde conduction occurs over the FP.

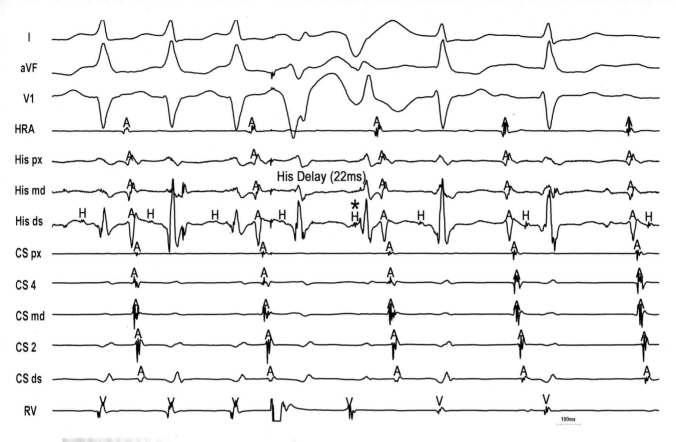

FIGURE 11-11 Resetting of NFRT by a His refractory VPD. AV dissociation is present. A His refractory VPD delays the His bundle (*asterisk*) by 22 ms. Tachycardia terminates following a second spontaneous VPD (also His bundle refractory). The subsequent sinus beat conducts over a partial refractory AV node with mild AH prolongation.

(slow–fast) AVNRT with AV block (antegrade limb) (**Figs. 11-16 to 11-18**).[44–47] Insertion of the NF AP into the fast pathway (FP) is less common and identified by His refractory VPDs that 1) affect atypical (fast–slow) AVNRT in the antegrade limb (FP) or 2) typical (slow–fast) AVNRT in the retrograde limb (FP) one cycle later (the His refractory VPD does not affect typical AVNRT immediately because retrograde FP preempts NF AP–FP conduction) (**Fig. 11-19**).[48]

ATRIO-FASCICULAR AP (OR LONG ATRIO-VENTRICULAR AP)

Electrophysiologic Features

Similar to NF APs, the HV can be normal and baseline preexcitation is often absent (an rS pattern in lead III suggests minimal preexcitation).[49] Atrial pacing exposes typical LBBB preexcitation with long St-delta intervals (latent preexcitation), but in contrast to NF/NV APs, preexcitation of an atrio-fascicular AP is preferentially greater with right atrial versus CS pacing because these APs typically originate from the lateral tricuspid annulus.[50,51] The distal insertion can be either in the RB (atrio-fascicular) or ventricular myocardium near the RB ("long AV").[52] Clues favoring a fascicular insertion

include 1) rapid intrinsicoid with typical LBBB QRS complexes, 2) shorter QRS duration (<140 ms), and 3) very short VH interval (<30 ms) during antidromic tachycardia.[53,54] His bundle extrasystoles normalize the QRS complex if preexcitation is present. Automaticity (perhaps because of AV node–like properties) and longitudinal dissociation in these pathways have been described.[55,56]

Antidromic AFRT

The classic tachycardia associated with atrio-fascicular APs is antidromic atrio-fascicular reentrant tachycardia (AFRT), which shares features similar to antidromic NFRT including 1) fixed, maximally preexcited typical LBBB QRS complexes; 2) short, negative HV interval (<30 ms); 3) retrograde His-RB activation sequence (proximal RB-His ds-His px); and 4) concentric atrial activation (retrograde conduction over the AV node) with a long A-delta interval (≥150 ms or AV/TCL ≥55% due to decremental AP conduction) (**Fig. 11-20**).[57] Proximal retrograde RBBB causes conversion from short to long VH tachycardia and prolongation of the TCL as the left bundle becomes incorporated into the circuit ("reverse Coumel's sign"). This is associated with widening of the QRS complex and leftward shift in axis (due to loss of ventricular fusion over

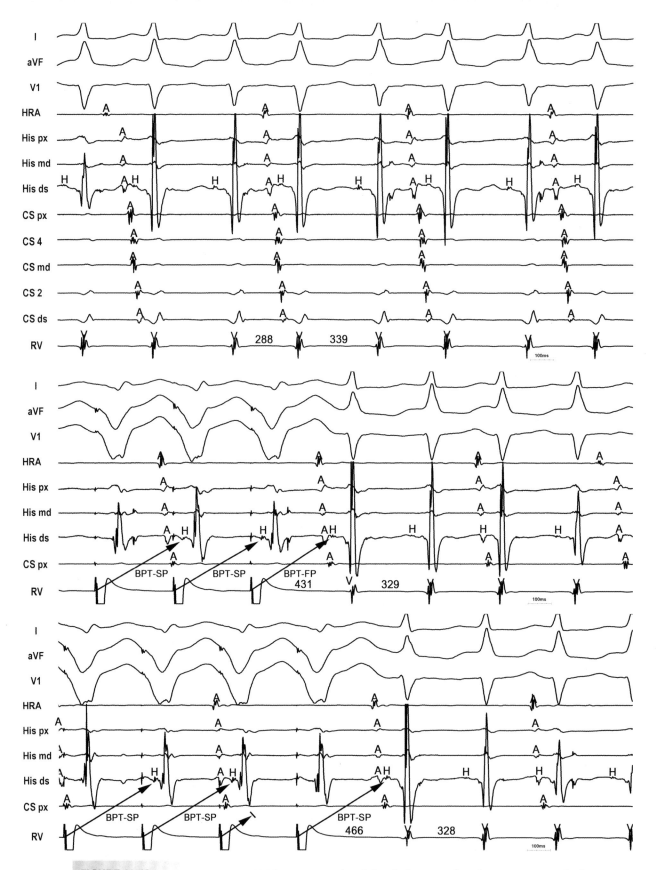

FIGURE 11-12 Same patient as **Figure 11-11**. *Top*: NFRT with cycle length alternans and AV dissociation. Longitudinal dissociation in the NF AP (retrogradely) or AV node (antegradely) explains cycle length alternans. *Middle* and *bottom*: Induction of NFRT by rapid ventricular pacing with orthodromic capture of the His bundle and short/long PPI (PPI − TCL = 102 ms/138 ms) due to antegrade FP/SP conduction, respectively (or retrogradely over a longitudinally dissociated NF AP).

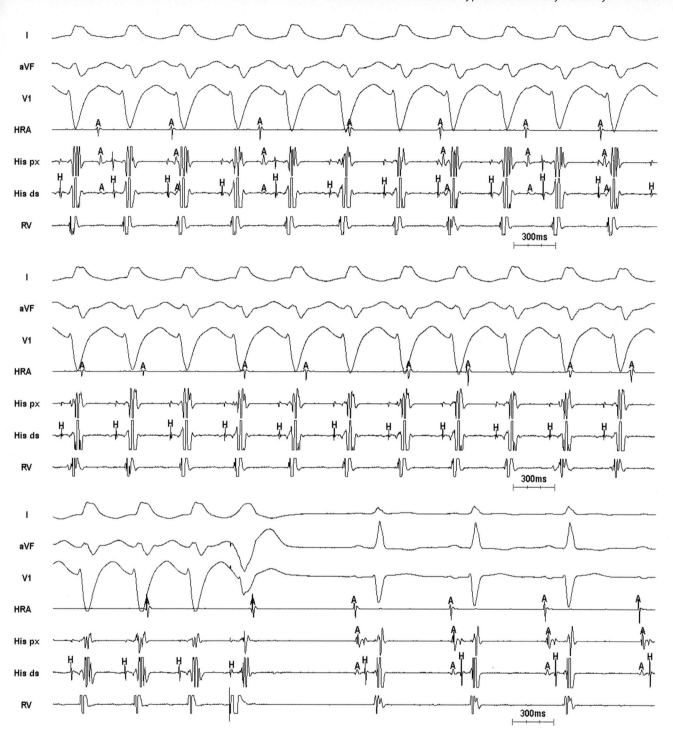

FIGURE 11-13 Orthodromic NFRT with AV dissociation (*top*) and 3:2 nodo-atrial Wenckebach (*middle*). His bundle potentials preceding typical LBBB QRS complexes with normal HV intervals identifying LBBB aberration and excluding a preexcited NF tachycardia. A His refractory VPD terminates tachycardia (*bottom*) proving presence of an AP, which in the presence of AV dissociation indicates a NF AP.

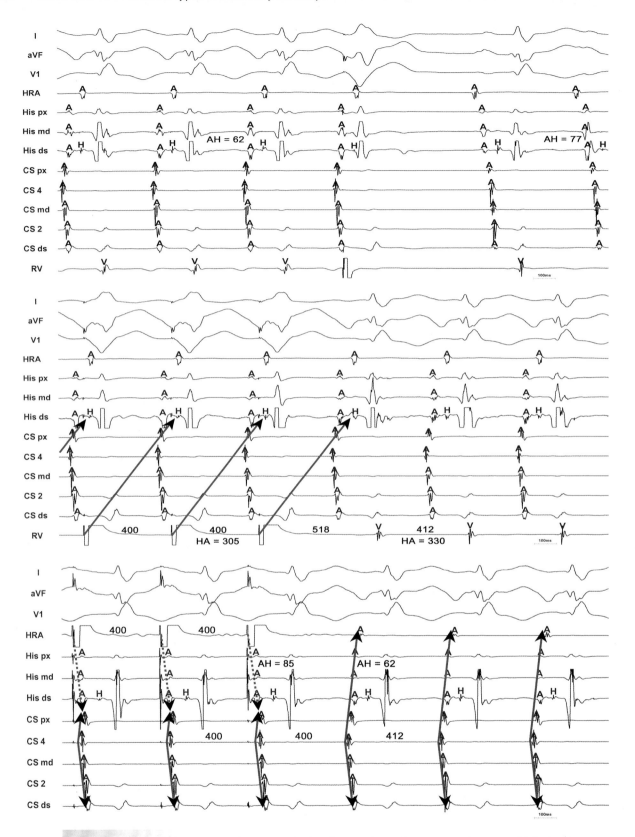

FIGURE 11-14 Orthodromic NFRT. The RP interval is long because the NF AP inserts into the atrio-nodal SP. *Top*: A His refractory VPD terminates tachycardia with VA block proving presence of an AP. Paradoxically, $AH_{(SVT)} < AH_{(NSR)}$ excluding PJRT. *Middle*: Entrainment from the ventricle with orthodromic capture of the His bundle again proves presence of an AP. The PPI − TCL = 106 ms and $\Delta HA = -25$ ms. *Bottom*: Entrainment from the atrium with constant manifest atrial fusion and the last orthodromically entrained electrograms occurring at the pacing cycle length (first criteria of transient entrainment). These findings indicate macroreentry and exclude atypical AVNRT with a bystander NF AP.

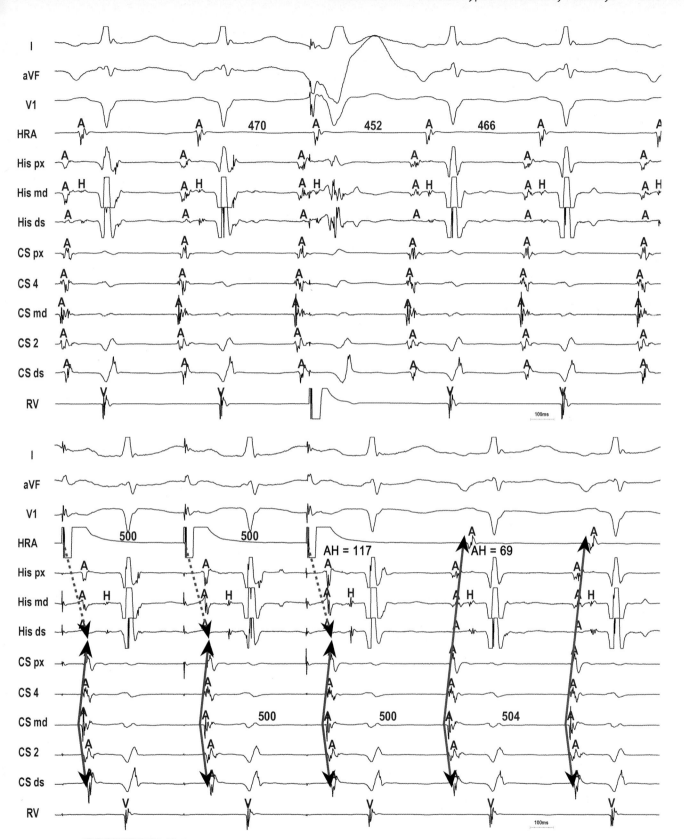

FIGURE 11-15 Orthodromic NFRT. The RP interval is long because the NF AP inserts into the atrio-nodal SP. *Top*: A His refractory VPD advances the atrium by 18 ms proving the presence of an AP. *Bottom*: Entrainment from the atrium with constant manifest atrial fusion and the last orthodromically entrained electrograms occurring at the pacing cycle length proving macroreentry (first criteria of transient entrainment) and excluding atypical AVNRT with a bystander NF AP. The ΔAH = to 48 ms excludes PJRT.

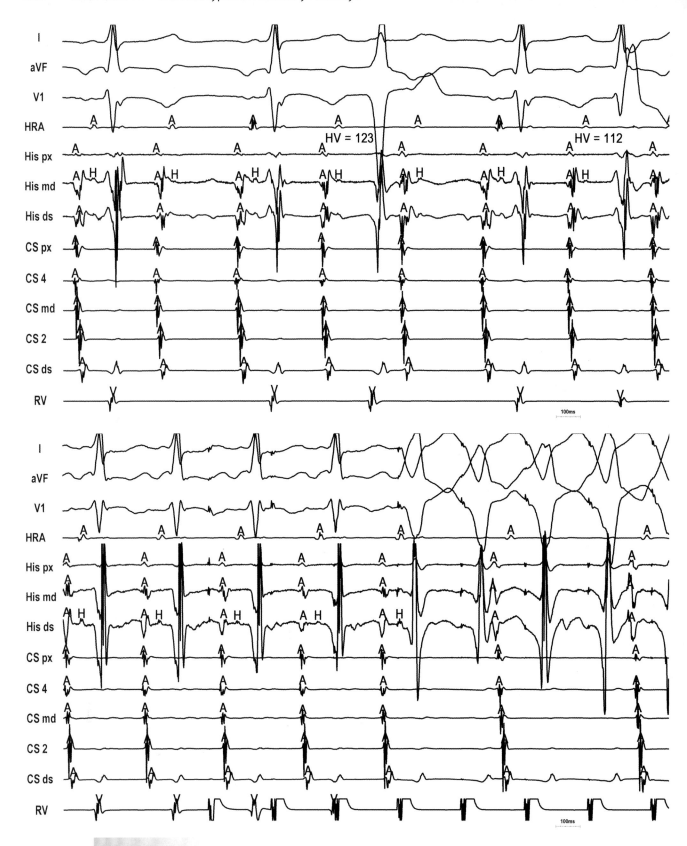

FIGURE 11-16 Atypical AVNRT with a bystander NF AP–SP. *Top:* During tachycardia, the presence of 2:1 and 3:2 infrahisian Wenckebach AV block with alternating LBBB/RBBB excludes ORT (PJRT/NFRT). *Bottom:* During onset of ventricular overdrive pacing, the first paced complex is His refractory and terminates tachycardia with VA block excluding AT. This finding indicates the existence of an AP—in this case, specifically a NF AP inserting into the SP (retrograde limb of atypical AVNRT).

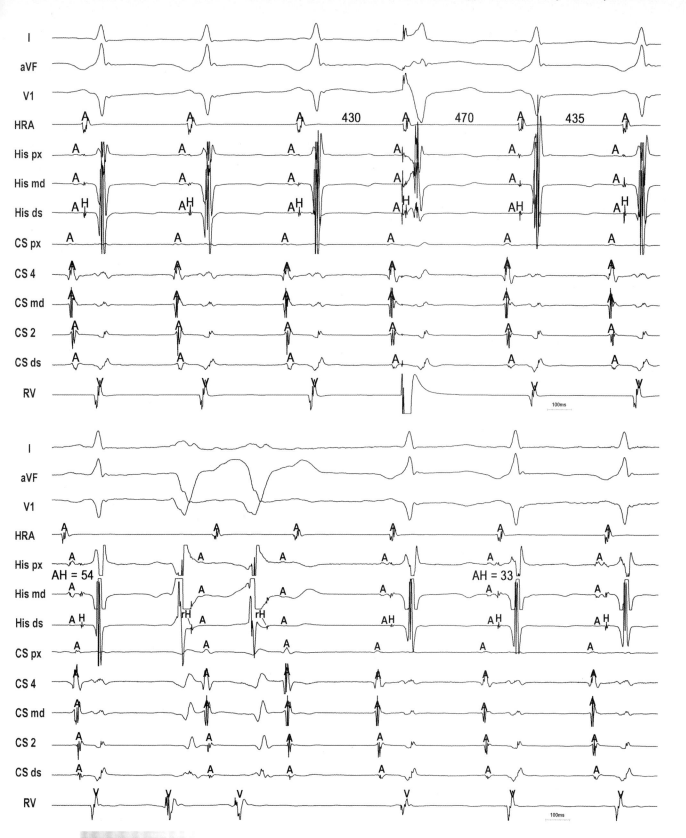

FIGURE 11-17 Atypical AVNRT with a bystander NF AP–SP. *Top*: A His refractory VPD delays the atrium by 40 ms proving presence of an AP. *Bottom*: Initiation by a ventricular couplet generates a "true AAV" response (double fire over the FP and NF AP–SP) and very long PPI—the latter favoring atypical AVNRT. Additionally, the $AH_{(SVT)}$ is very short (33 ms) and paradoxically, $AH_{(SVT)} < AH_{(NSR)}$. The bystander NF AP inserts into the SP (retrograde limb of atypical AVNRT).

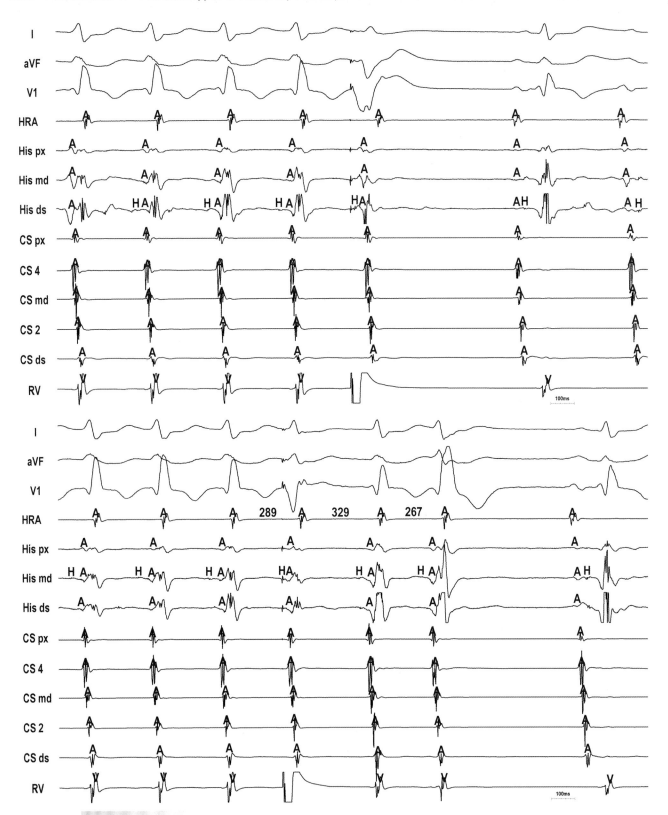

FIGURE 11-18 Typical AVNRT with a bystander NF AP–SP. *Top*: A His refractory VPD terminates typical (slow–fast) AVNRT with AV block indicating NF AP insertion into the SP of the AV node (antegrade limb of typical AVNRT). The fascicular insertion in the RB is beyond the site of proximal RBBB. *Bottom*: A His refractory VPD resets typical AVNRT with antegrade delay in the SP followed by termination with AV block two cycles later.

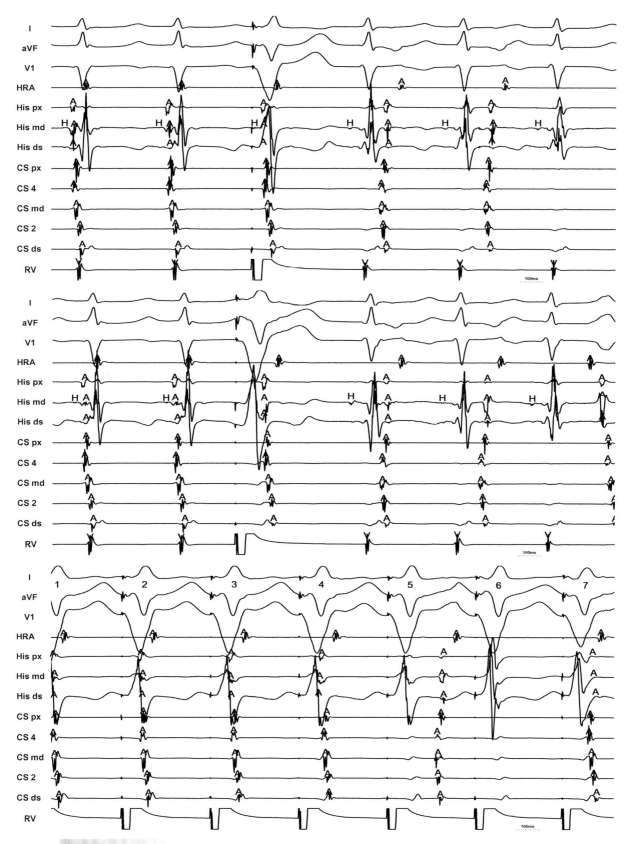

FIGURE 11-19 Typical AVNRT with a bystander NF AP–FP. Both a His refractory (*top*) and early-coupled (*middle*) VPD convert typical (slow–fast) AVNRT to an atypical (slow–slow) AVNRT by causing retrograde FP block—not immediately but one cycle later. Attempt to entrain typical AVNRT from the ventricle (*bottom*) failed to accelerate the atrium to the pacing cycle length. The fourth paced complex, however, conducted over the NF AP and concealed into the FP causing block one cycle later so that the fifth paced complex conducted over the SP before tachycardia termination.

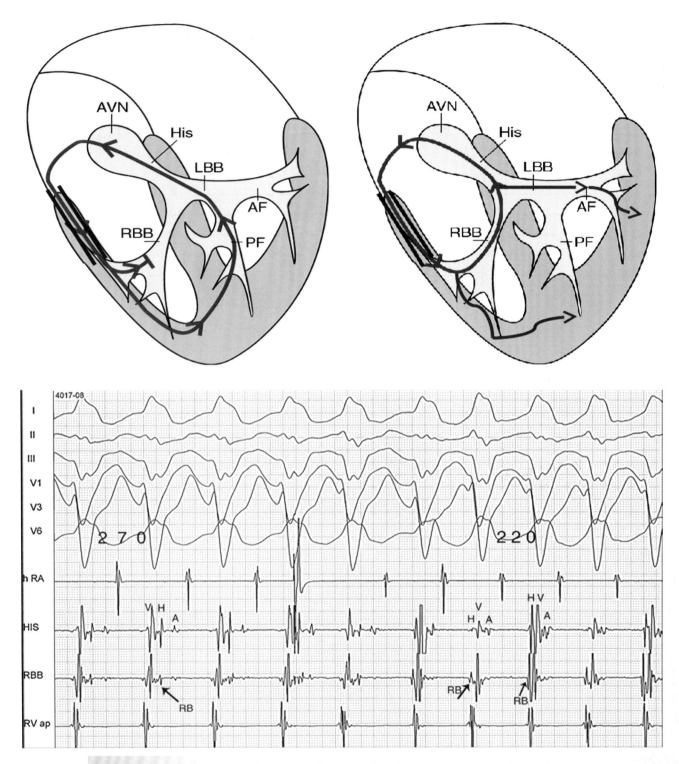

FIGURE 11-20 Antidromic AFRT (reverse Coumel's sign). Tachycardia shows long AV intervals, typical LBBB QRS complexes and a retrograde RB–His bundle activation sequence. Retrograde RB conduction causes a short VH tachycardia (220 ms) with His bundles potentials preceding local ventricular electrograms and RB potentials at/near QRS onset (fascicular insertion of the AP). Retrograde RBBB creates a long VH tachycardia (270 ms) by forcing conduction across the interventricular septum so that His bundle potentials now follow local ventricular electrograms and tachycardia slows by 50 ms. The increase in VH interval and TCL with retrograde bundle branch block (BBB) ipsilateral to the AP shows tachycardia dependence on the His-Purkinje system and is unique to antidromic tachycardia (reverse Coumel's sign). (Reprinted from Gandhavadi M, et al. Characterization of the distal insertion of atriofascicular accessory pathways and mechanisms of QRS patterns in atriofascicular antidromic tachycardia. Heart Rhythm 2013;10:1385–1392, with permission from Elsevier.)

the left anterior fascicle that occurs when retrograde RB conduction is present).[53,58] Antidromic AFRT and NFRT, however, can be differentiated by 1) VA dissociation and 2) AVJ-refractory APDs. While VA dissociation is possible with antidromic NFRT, antidromic AFRT requires a 1:1 AV relationship. An APD delivered from the lateral tricuspid annulus after inscription of the septal atrial electrogram (AVJ-refractory) can reset (advance or delay) or terminate antidromic tachycardia using an atriofascicular but not NF AP.[50,54,59,60]

FASCICULO-VENTRICULAR AP

Electrophysiologic Features

The hallmark of a fasciculo-ventricular AP is a short, fixed HV interval and constant degree of preexcitation (Fig. 11-21).[40,61,62] Because fasciculo-ventricular APs do not bypass the AV node, the degree of preexcitation can be minimal with narrow (~120 ms) preexcited QRS complexes compared to anteroseptal APs.[63] Decremental atrial pacing or atrial extrastimulation causes parallel prolongation of AH and St-delta intervals so that the HV intervals and the degree of preexcitation remain fixed until block occurs in the AP (unless the AP shows decremental

conduction in which case HV intervals prolong and the degree of preexcitation paradoxically decreases).[64] Unlike AV APs, antegrade conduction is linked to the AV node, and therefore, His bundle extrasystoles fail to normalize the QRS complex. Adenosine is useful to differentiate fasciculo-ventricular from AV APs by demonstrating 1) fixed preexcitation during PR prolongation or adenosine-induced atrial fibrillation, 2) loss of preexcitation with AV block, and 3) persistent preexcitation accompanying junctional escape complexes.[61] Fasciculo-ventricular APs have not been implicated as a mechanism for tachycardia but can serve as a bystander to other tachycardias.

UNUSUAL ELECTROPHYSIOLOGIC PHENOMENA

DOUBLE TACHYCARDIA (ORT AND AVNRT)

An unusual manifestation of AP-mediated tachycardias is the combination of dual AV node physiology and AP, which can cause cycle length alternans during ORT or uncommonly coexistence of ORT with AVNRT (Figs. 11-22 and 11-23).[65,66]

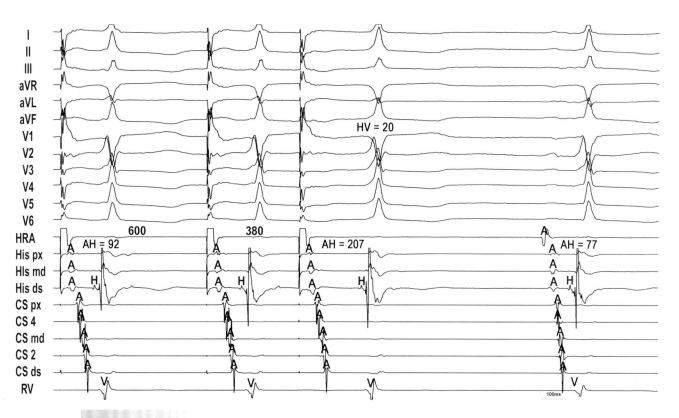

FIGURE 11-21 Fasciculo-ventricular AP. During programmed atrial extrastimulation, HV intervals are short (20 ms) and QRS complexes are minimally preexcited. Despite three different AH intervals (drive train, extrastimulus, and sinus rhythm), the short HV and degree of preexcitation remained fixed excluding an extranodal AP and indicating AP origin distal to the His bundle.

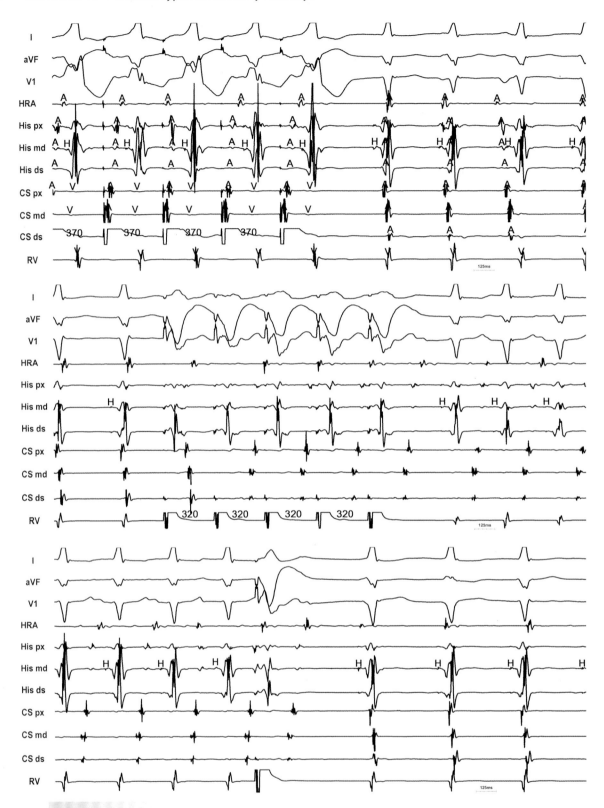

FIGURE 11-22 Conversion of typical AVNRT to ORT (and vice versa). *Top:* Rapid atrial pacing conducts with preexcitation over a left posterolateral AP initiating typical AVNRT after a triple antegrade response (FP, SP, and AP). Retrograde concealment from the His-Purkinje system into AP prevents bystander preexcitation during AVNRT. *Middle:* Ventricular overdrive pacing converts typical AVNRT to ORT. The second paced complex terminates AVNRT by causing retrograde block in the FP exposing conduction over the AP. Cessation of pacing results in an "AV" response, long PPI (due to antegrade AV node delay), and ORT. *Bottom:* An early-coupled VPD converts ORT to typical AVNRT. The VPD advances the atrium over the AP with significant prematurity to encroach on absolute FP refractoriness (longer ERP). Conduction, therefore, occurs exclusively over the SP (shorter ERP) re-initiating typical AVNRT (retrograde FP preempts AP).

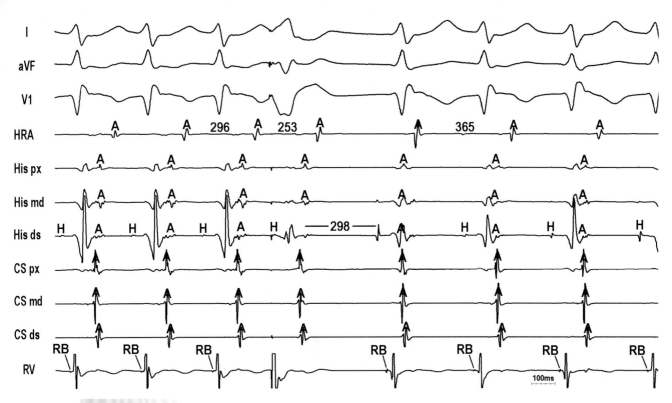

FIGURE 11-23 Conversion of ORT to typical AVNRT by a His refractory VPD. A His refractory VPD advances the atrium over a right posteroseptal AP with sufficient prematurity (43 ms) to encroach on absolute FP refractoriness (longer ERP). Conduction occurs exclusively over the SP (shorter ERP) (AH = 298 ms) to initiate a slower typical AVNRT (retrograde FP preempts AP).

REFERENCES

1. Bardy GH, Packer DL, German LD, Gallagher JJ. Preexcited reciprocating tachycardia in patients with Wolff-Parkinson-White syndrome: incidence and mechanisms. Circulation 1984;70:377–391.

2. Colavita PG, Packer DL, Pressley JC, et al. Frequency, diagnosis and clinical characteristics of patients with multiple accessory atrioventricular pathways. Am J Cardiol 1987;59:601–606.

3. Wellens HJ, Atié J, Smeets JL, Cruz FE, Gorgels AP, Brugada P. The electrocardiogram in patients with multiple accessory atrioventricular pathways. J Am Coll Cardiol 1990;16:745–751.

4. Akiyama T. Electrocardiographic clues for multiple accessory pathways in patients with pre-excitation syndromes. J Am Coll Cardiol 1990;16:1029–1031.

5. Fananapazir L, German LD, Gallagher JJ, Lowe JE, Prystowsky EN. Importance of preexcited QRS morphology during induced atrial fibrillation to the diagnosis and localization of multiple accessory pathways. Circulation 1990;81:578–585.

6. Heddle WF, Brugada P, Wellens HJ. Multiple circus movement tachycardias with multiple accessory pathways. J Am Coll Cardiol 1984;4:168–175.

7. Buch E, Nakahara S, Shivkumar K. Diagnostic maneuver during narrow-complex tachycardia: what is the arrhythmia mechanism? Heart Rhythm 2009;6:716–717.

8. Coumel P, Cabrol C, Fabiato A, Gourgon R, Slama R. Tachycardie permanente par rhythme reciproque. Arch Mal Coeur 1967;60:1830–1864.

9. Coumel P. Junctional reciprocating tachycardias. The permanent and paroxysmal forms of A-V nodal reciprocating tachycardias. J Electrocardiol 1975;8:79–90.

10. Ticho BS, Saul JP, Hulse E, De W, Lulu J, Walsh EP. Variable location of accessory pathways associated with the permanent form of junctional reciprocating tachycardia and confirmation with radiofrequency ablation. Am J Cardiol 1992;70:1559–1564.

11. Critelli G, Gallagher JJ, Monda V, Coltorti F, Scherillo M, Rossi L. Anatomic and electrophysiologic substrate of the permanent form of junctional reciprocating tachycardia. J Am Coll Cardiol 1984;4:601–610.

12. Gallagher JJ, Sealy WC. The permanent form of junctional reciprocating tachycardia: further elucidation of the underlying mechanism. Eur J Cardiol 1978;8:413–430.

13. Klein GJ, Kostuk WJ, Ko P, Gulamhusein S. Permanent junctional reciprocating tachycardia in an asymptomatic adult: further evidence for an accessory ventriculoatrial nodal structure. Am Heart J 1981;102:282–286.

14. Ho RT, Patel U, Weitz HH. Entrainment and resetting of a long RP tachycardia: which trumps which for diagnosis? Heart Rhythm 2010;7:714–715.

15. Bardy G, Packer D, German L, Coltorti F, Gallagher J. Paradoxical delay in accessory pathway conduction during long R-P' tachycardia after interpolated ventricular premature complexes. Am J Cardiol 1985;55:1223–1225.

16. Knight B, Zivin A, Souza J, et al. A technique for the rapid diagnosis of atrial tachycardia in the electrophysiology laboratory. J Am Coll Cardiol 1999;33:775–781.

17. Michaud GF, Tada H, Chough S, et al. Differentiation of atypical atrioventricular node re-entrant tachycardia from orthodromic reciprocating tachycardia using a septal accessory pathway by the response to ventricular pacing. J Am Coll Cardiol 2001;38:1163–1167.

18. Ho RT, Mark GE, Rhim ES, Pavri BB, Greenspon AJ. Differentiating atrioventricular nodal reentrant tachycardia from atrioventricular reentrant tachycardia by ΔHA values during entrainment from the ventricle. Heart Rhythm 2008;5:83–88.

19. Mark GE, Rhim ES, Pavri BB, Greenspon AJ, Ho RT. Differentiation of atrio-ventricular nodal reentrant tachycardia from orthodromic atrio-ventricular reentrant tachycardia by ΔHA intervals during entrainment from the ventricle [abstract]. Heart Rhythm 2006;3:S321.

20. Ho RT, Rhim ES. The ΔHA interval during entrainment of a long RP tachycardia—another useful criterion for the diagnosis of supraventricular tachycardia. J Cardiovasc Electrophysiol 2008;19:559–561.

21. Arias MA, Castellanos E, Puchol A, Rodríguez-Padial L. Ventricular entrainment of a long-RP supraventricular tachycardia. J Cardiovasc Electrophysiol 2010;21:466–468.

22. Zivin A, Morady F. Incessant tachycardia using a concealed atrionodal bypass tract. J Cardiovasc Electrophysiol 1998;9:191–195.

23. Okabe T, Tyler J, Daoud EG, Kalbfleisch SJ. An incessant repetitive tachycardia in a patient with prior AVNRT ablation: what is the mechanism? Heart Rhythm 2015;12:1395–1397.

24. Brechenmacher CJ. Atrio-hisian fibers anatomy and electrophysiology. Pacing Clin Electrophysiol 2013;36:137–141.

25. Ellenbogen KA, Ramirez NM, Packer DL, et al. Accessory nodoventricular (Mahaim) fibers: a clinical review. Pacing Clin Electrophysiol 1986;9:868–884.

26. Hoffmayer KS, Lee BK, Vedantham V, et al. Variable clinical features and ablation of manifest nodofascicular/ventricular pathways. Circ Arrhythm Electrophysiol 2015;8:117–127.

27. Ho RT, Frisch DF, Pavri BB, Levi SA, Greenspon AJ. Electrophysiological features differentiating the atypical atrioventricular node-dependent long RP supraventricular tachycardia. Circ Arrhythm Electrophysiol 2013;6:597–605.

28. Ho RT, Pavri BB. A long RP-interval tachycardia: what is the mechanism? Heart Rhythm 2013;10:456–458.

29. Tuohy S, Saliba W, Pai M, Tchou P. Catheter ablation as a treatment of atrioventricular block. Heart Rhythm 2018;15:90–96.

30. Roberts-Thomson KC, Seiler J, Raymond JM, Stevenson WG. Exercise induced tachycardia with atrioventricular dissociation: what is the mechanism? Heart Rhythm 2009;6:426–428.

31. Ho RT. A narrow complex tachycardia with atrioventricular dissociation: what is the mechanism? Heart Rhythm 2017;14:1570–1573.

32. Shimizu A, Ohe T, Takaki H, et al. Narrow QRS complex tachycardia with atrioventricular dissociation. Pacing Clin Electrophysiol 1988;11:384–393.

33. Mantovan R, Verlato R, Corrado D, Buia G, Haissaguerre M, Shah DC. Orthodromic tachycardia with atrioventricular dissociation: evidence for a nodoventricular (Mahaim) fiber. Pacing Clin Electrophysiol 2000;23:276–279.

34. Gula LJ, Posan E, Skanes AC, Krahn AD, Yee R, Klein GJ. Tachycardia with VA dissociation: an unusual tachycardia mechanism. J Cardiovasc Electrophysiol 2005;16:663–665.

35. Hamdan MH, Kalman JM, Lesh MD, et al. Narrow complex tachycardia with VA block: diagnostic and therapeutic implications. Pacing Clin Electrophysiol 1998;21:1196–1206.

36. Ho RT, Luebbert J. An unusual long RP tachycardia: what is the mechanism? Heart Rhythm 2012;9:1898–1901.

37. Okabe T, Hummel JD, Kalbfleisch SJ. A long RP supraventricular tachycardia: what is the mechanism? Heart Rhythm 2017;14:462–464.

38. Quinn FR, Mitchell LB, Mardell AP, Dal Disler RN, Veenhuyzen GD. Entrainment mapping of a concealed nodoventricular accessory pathway in a man with complete heart block and tachycardia-induced cardiomyopathy. J Cardiovasc Electrophysiol 2008;19:90–94.

39. Bardy GH, German LD, Packer DL, Coltorti F, Gallagher JJ. Mechanism of tachycardia using a nodofascicular Mahaim fiber. Am J Cardiol 1984;54:1140–1141.

40. Gallagher JJ, Smith WM, Kasell JH, Benson DW Jr, Sterba R, Grant AO. Role of Mahaim fibers in cardiac arrhythmias in man. Circulation 1981;64:176–189.

41. Mark AL, Basta LL. Paroxysmal tachycardia with atrioventricular dissociation in a patient with a variant of pre-excitation syndrome. J Electrocardiol 1974;7:355–364.

42. Chugh A, Elmouchi D, Han J. Termination of tachycardia with a ventricular extrastimulus: what is the mechanism? Heart Rhythm 2005;2:1148–1149.

43. Kalbfleisch SJ, Tyler J, Weiss R. A supraventricular tachycardia terminated with ventricular pacing: what is the tachycardia mechanism? Heart Rhythm 2012;9:1163–1164.

44. Ho RT, Fischman DL. Entrainment versus resetting of a long RP tachycardia: what is the diagnosis? Heart Rhythm 2012;9:312–314.

45. Ho RT, Levi SA. An atypical long RP tachycardia—what is the mechanism? Heart Rhythm 2013;10:1089–1090.

46. Bansal S, Berger RD, Spragg DD. An unusual long RP tachycardia: what is the mechanism? Heart Rhythm 2015;12:845–846.

47. Ho RT, Kenia AS, Chhabra SK. Resetting and termination of a short RP tachycardia: what is the mechanism? Heart Rhythm 2013;10:1927–1929.

48. Ho RT. Unusual termination of a short RP tachycardia: what is the mechanism? Heart Rhythm 2017;14:935–937.

49. Sternick EB, Timmermans C, Sosa E, et al. The electrocardiogram during sinus rhythm and tachycardia in patients with Mahaim fibers: the importance of an "rS" pattern in lead III. J Am Coll Cardiol 2004;44:1626–1635.

50. Tchou P, Lehmann MH, Jazayeri M, Akhtar M. Atriofascicular connection or a nodoventricular Mahaim fiber? Electrophysiologic elucidation of the pathway and associated reentrant circuit. Circulation 1988;77:837–848.

51. Klein GJ, Guiraudon GM, Kerr CR, et al. "Nodoventricular" accessory pathway: evidence for a distinct accessory atrioventricular pathway with atrioventricular node-like properties. J Am Coll Cardiol 1988;11:1035–1040.

52. Sternick EB, Timmermans C, Rodriguez LM, Wellens HJ. Mahaim fiber: an atriofascicular or a long atrioventricular pathway? Heart Rhythm 2004;1:724–727.

53. Gandhavadi M, Sternick EB, Jackman WM, Wellens HJ, Josephson ME. Characterization of the distal insertion of atriofascicular accessory pathways and mechanisms of QRS patterns in atriofascicular antidromic tachycardia. Heart Rhythm 2013;10:1385–1392.

54. Sternick EB, Lokhandwala Y, Timmermans C, et al. Atrial premature beats during decrementally conducting antidromic tachycardia. Circ Arrhythm Electrophysiol 2013;6:357–363.

55. Sternick EB, Sosa EA, Timmermans C, et al. Automaticity in Mahaim fibers. J Cardiovasc Electrophysiol 2004;15:738–744.

56. Sternick EB, Sosa E, Scanavacca M, Wellens HJ. Dual conduction in a Mahaim fiber. J Cardiovasc Electrophysiol 2004;15:1212–1215.

57. Sternick EB, Lokhandwala Y, Timmermans C, et al. The atrioventricular interval during pre-excited tachycardia: a simple way to distinguish between decrementally or rapidly conducting accessory pathways. Heart Rhythm 2009;6:1351–1358.

58. Sternick EB, Rodriguez LM, Timmermans C, et al. Effects of right bundle branch block on the antidromic circus movement tachycardia in patients with presumed atriofascicular pathways. J Cardiovasc Electrophysiol 2006;17:256–260.

59. Grogin HR, Lee RJ, Kwasman M, et al. Radiofrequency catheter ablation of atriofascicular and nodoventricular Mahaim tracts. Circulation 1994;90:272–281.

60. Sternick EB, Scarpelli RB, Gerken LM, Wellens HJ. Wide QRS tachycardia with sudden rate acceleration: what is the mechanism? Heart Rhythm 2009;6:1670–1673.

61. Sternick EB, Gerken LM, Vrandecic MO, Wellens HJ. Fasciculoventricular pathways: clinical and electrophysiologic characteristics of a variant of pre-excitation. J Cardiovasc Electrophysiol 2003;14:1057–1063.

62. Ali H, Sorgente A, Lupo P, et al. Nodo- and fasciculoventricular pathways: electrophysiological features and a proposed diagnostic algorithm for preexcitation. Heart Rhythm 2015;12:1677–1682.

63. Sternick EB, Rodriguez LM, Gerken LM, Wellens HJ. Electrocardiogram in patients with fasciculoventricular pathways: a comparative study with anteroseptal and midseptal accessory pathways. Heart Rhythm 2005;2:1–6.

64. Dey S, Tschopp D, Morady F, Jongnarangsin K. Fasciculoventricular bypass tract with decremental conduction properties. Heart Rhythm 2006;3:975–976.

65. Ho RT, Rhim ES. Metamorphosis of a tachycardia: what is the mechanism? Heart Rhythm 2008;5:155–157.

66. Balog JD, Frisch D, Whellan DJ, Ho RT. Alternating short and long RP tachycardias: what are the mechanisms? Heart Rhythm 2010;7:1907–1909.

Ablation of Accessory Pathways

Introduction
Catheter ablation is a highly effective treatment for accessory pathways (APs) that are high risk or cause symptoms.

The purpose of this chapter is to:
1. Discuss mapping techniques and target site criteria for AP ablation.
2. Discuss ablation of APs with unusual anatomic locations or electrophysiologic properties.

CLASSIC ATRIO-VENTRICULAR ACCESSORY PATHWAYS (BUNDLE OF KENT)

The classic atrio-ventricular (AV) AP (bundle of Kent) is a muscle fiber bridging the AV groove and inserting into the base of the ventricle near the tricuspid or mitral annulus. Access to the mitral annulus and a left-sided AP is achieved either by a transeptal (patent foramen ovale, transeptal puncture) or transaortic approach. With the transaortic approach, the tip of the ablation catheter is curved into a "pigtail" to avoid damaging the coronary arteries, prolapsed retrogradely across the aortic valve into the left ventricle, and positioned along the mitral annulus using posterior and counterclockwise torque. Mapping of a left-sided AP is facilitated by a recording catheter in the coronary sinus (CS) that provides a useful reference landmark and whose electrodes can bracket the AP in the left AV groove. While an equivalent venous structure is absent for the tricuspid annulus, a multipolar "Halo" catheter positioned along the endocardial aspect of the tricuspid annulus can guide ablation of a right-sided AP. The tricuspid annulus and a right-sided AP can be accessed either from the inferior vena cava (IVC) (inferior approach) or from the superior vena cava (SVC) (superior approach).

MAPPING

Antegrade
The earliest site of ventricular activation during manifest preexcitation (preexcited sinus rhythm, antidromic reciprocating tachycardia [ART]) identifies the ventricular insertion site of the AP. Target site criteria for AP ablation during antegrade mapping are 1) AP potentials (Kent potentials) and 2) earliest site of ventricular activation relative to delta wave onset (pre-delta) (**Figs. 12-1 to 12-9**).[1,2] AP potentials reflect rapid local AP activation and are sharp, high-frequency deflections sandwiched between atrial and ventricular electrograms preceding delta wave onset during preexcited sinus rhythm and atrial activation during orthodromic reciprocating tachycardia (ORT) (**Fig. 12-10**).[1–4] They can be recorded along the length of the AP and are differentiated from high-frequency components of the atrial or ventricular electrogram by demonstrating its dissociation from the atrium and ventricle, respectively (Kent validation) (**see Fig. 10-20**). The earlier the local ventricular electrogram precedes delta wave onset (pre-delta), the higher the probability of success, and a pre-delta value >10 ms has a 50% probability of successful ablation.[2] Annular (atrial and ventricular) electrograms are often fused and sometimes difficult to separate individually. Atrial or ventricular pacing maneuvers (rapid pacing/extrastimulation) to cause AV or VA block, respectively ("pacing to block"), or pacing from different sites to reverse the wavefront of activation, help to identify the atrial and ventricular components of the map electrogram.[3,3] AV fusion as a target site criteria can be misleading because of a slanting (oblique) AP. AV fusion occurs at sites downstream to the AP when the activation wavefront is in the direction of the slant (concurrent).[3] Conversely, fusion is absent at the AP (site recording an AP potential) when the activation wavefront is opposite the direction of the slant (countercurrent).

Retrograde
The earliest site of atrial activation during retrograde conduction over the AP (ventricular pacing, ORT) identifies the atrial insertion site of the AP. One limitation of mapping during ventricular pacing is rapid fast pathway (FP) conduction preempting AP conduction. This is particularly difficult for anteroseptal AP located near the His bundle. Potential solutions include 1) pacing at a fast rate (to cause delay/block in the FP), 2) pacing from a parahisian location with right ventricle (RV)-only capture (to delay conduction over the FP), 3) administration of negatively dromotropic

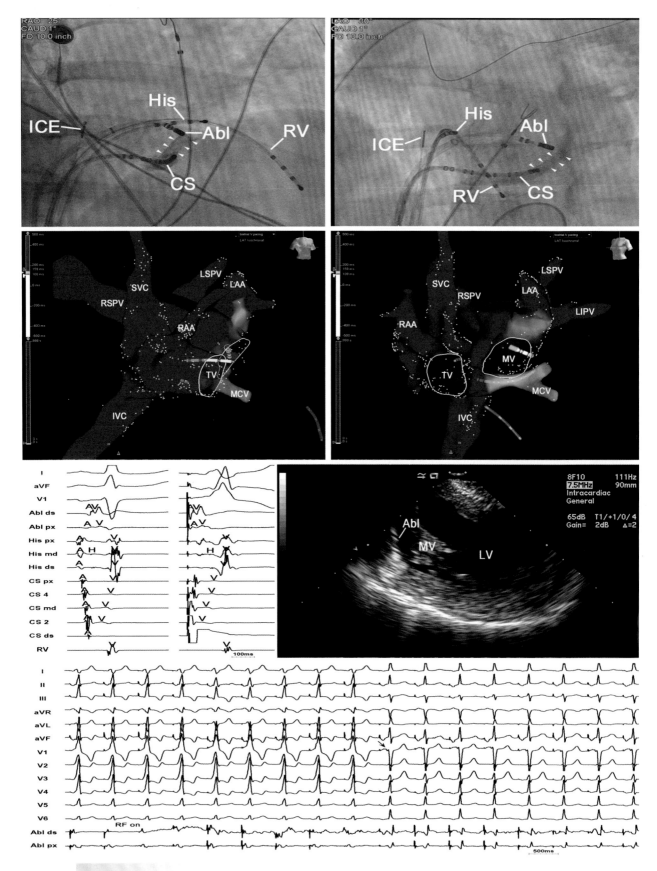

FIGURE 12-1 Ablation of a left free wall AP. The earliest site of atrial activation during retrograde AP conduction is at the lateral mitral annulus (*white*), which also records the earliest site of ventricular activation during preexcited sinus rhythm and CS pacing (pre-delta × 30 ms). Application of RF energy causes loss of preexcitation in 3.8 sec (*black arrow*). White arrowheads outline the CS during contrast angiography.

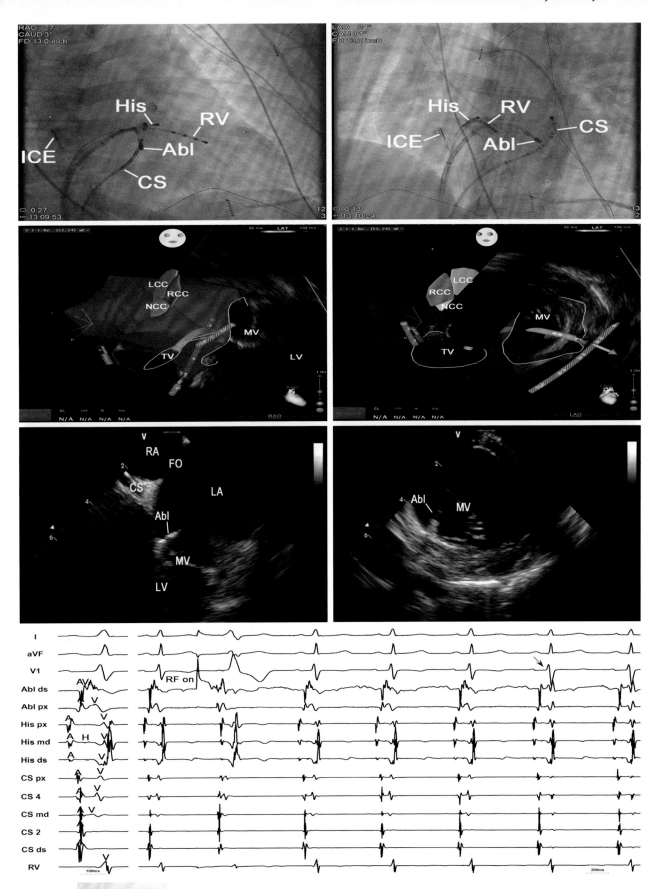

FIGURE 12-2 Ablation of a left posterolateral AP. The earliest site of atrial activation during retrograde AP conduction is at the posterolateral mitral annulus (*red*), which records the earliest site of ventricular activation during manifest preexcitation (pre-delta × 28 ms). Application of RF energy causes loss of preexcitation in 3.0 sec (*arrow*).

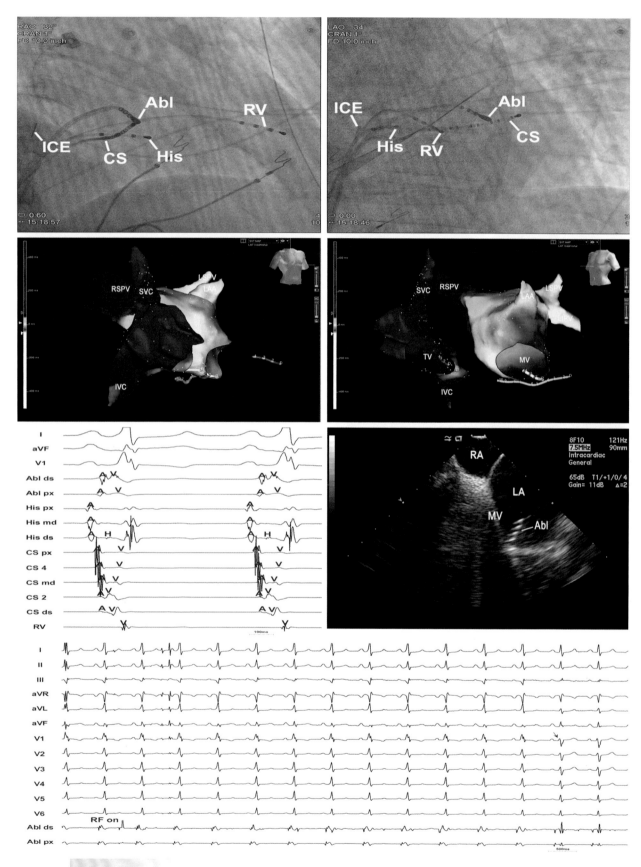

FIGURE 12-3 Ablation of a left posterolateral AP. The earliest site of atrial activation during retrograde AP conduction is at the posterolateral mitral annulus (*white*), which also records the earliest site of ventricular activation during manifest preexcitation (pre-delta × 21 ms). Application of RF energy causes loss of preexcitation in 7.7 sec (*arrow*).

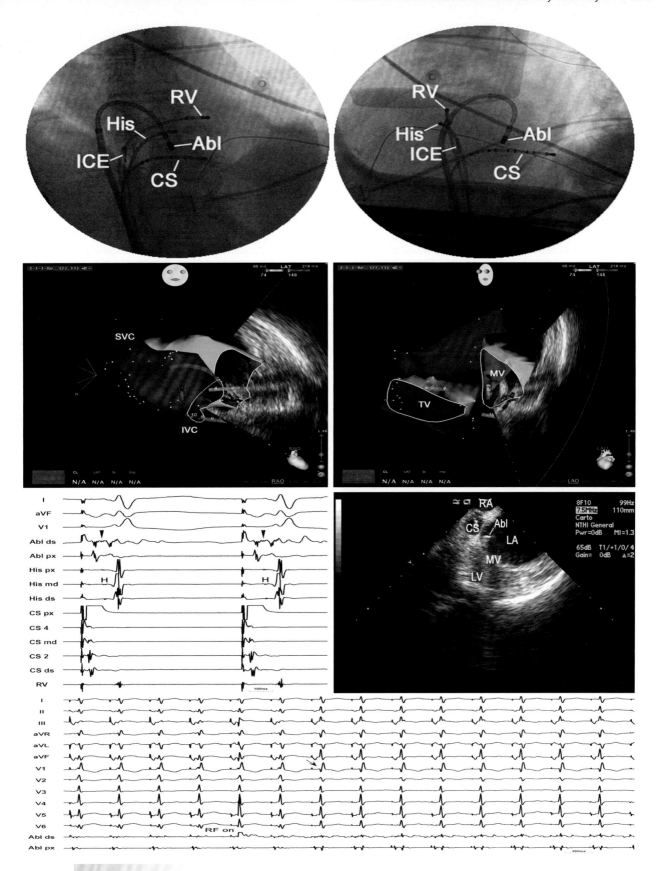

FIGURE 12-4 Ablation of a left posteroseptal AP. The earliest site of atrial activation during retrograde AP conduction is at the posteroseptal mitral annulus (*red*), which records a tiny AP potential (*vertical down arrowheads*) between atrial and ventricular electrograms during manifest preexcitation. Application of RF energy causes loss of preexcitation after 1 beat (*arrow*).

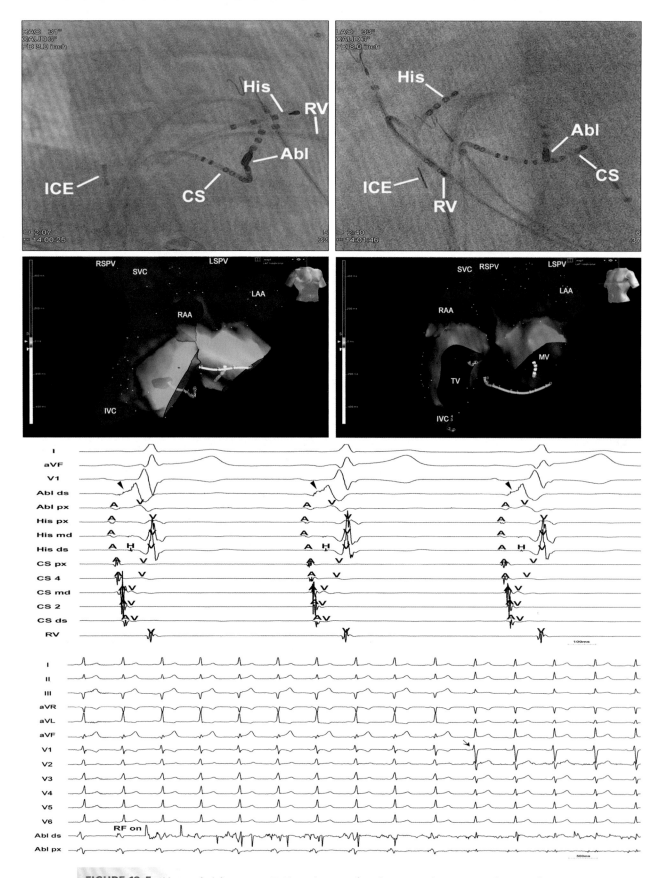

FIGURE 12-5 Ablation of a left posterior AP. The earliest site of atrial activation during retrograde AP conduction is at the posterior mitral annulus (*white*), which also records the earliest site of ventricular activation (*arrowheads*) during manifest preexcitation (pre-delta × 32 ms). Application of RF energy causes loss of preexcitation in 5.6 sec (*arrow*).

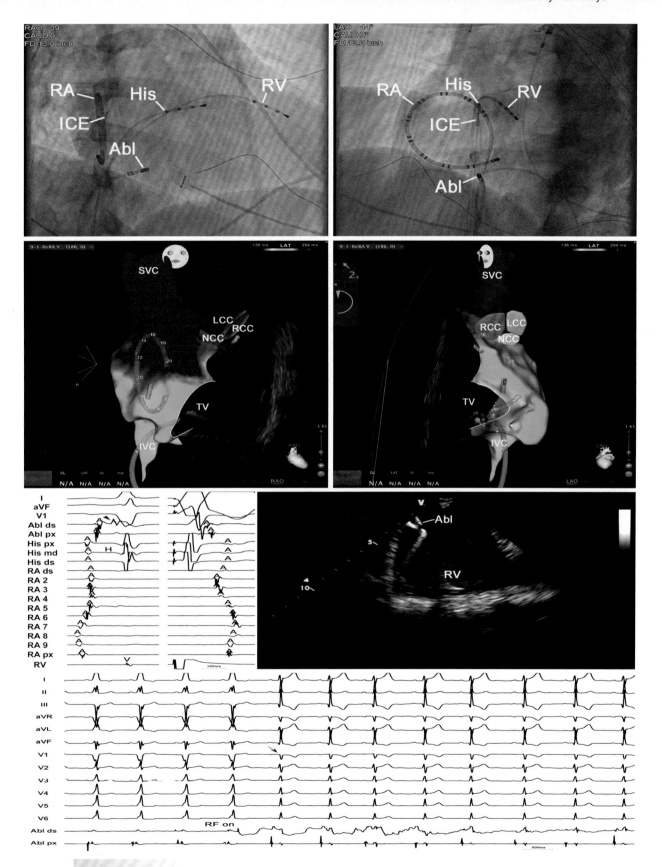

FIGURE 12-6 Ablation of a right posterior AP. The earliest site of atrial activation during retrograde AP conduction is at the inferior tricuspid annulus (*red*), which also records the earliest site of ventricular activation (*arrowhead*) during preexcited sinus rhythm (pre-delta × 20 ms). Application of RF energy causes immediate loss of preexcitation (*arrow*). Note that the ablation catheter is on the eustachian ridge.

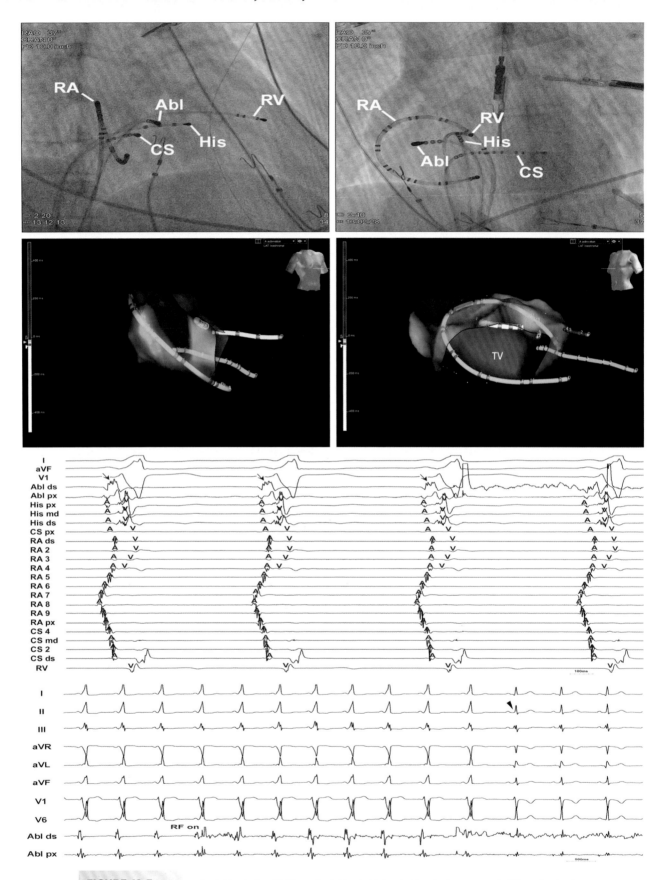

FIGURE 12-7 Ablation of a right anterior AP. The earliest site of atrial activation during retrograde AP conduction is at the anterior tricuspid annulus (*white*), which records continuous electric activity (*arrows*) between atrial and ventricular electrograms during manifest preexcitation. Application of RF energy causes loss of preexcitation in 5.3 sec (*arrowhead*).

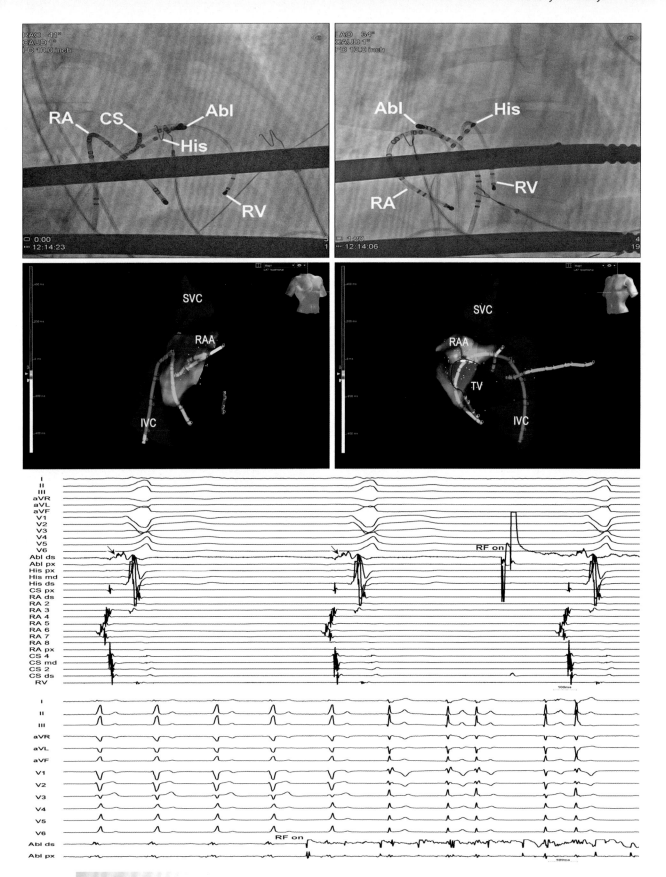

FIGURE 12-8 Ablation of a right anterolateral AP. The earliest site of atrial activation during retrograde AP conduction is at the anterolateral tricuspid annulus (*white*), which records continuous electric activity (*arrows*) between atrial and ventricular electrograms during manifest preexcitation. Application of RF energy causes loss of preexcitation after 1 beat.

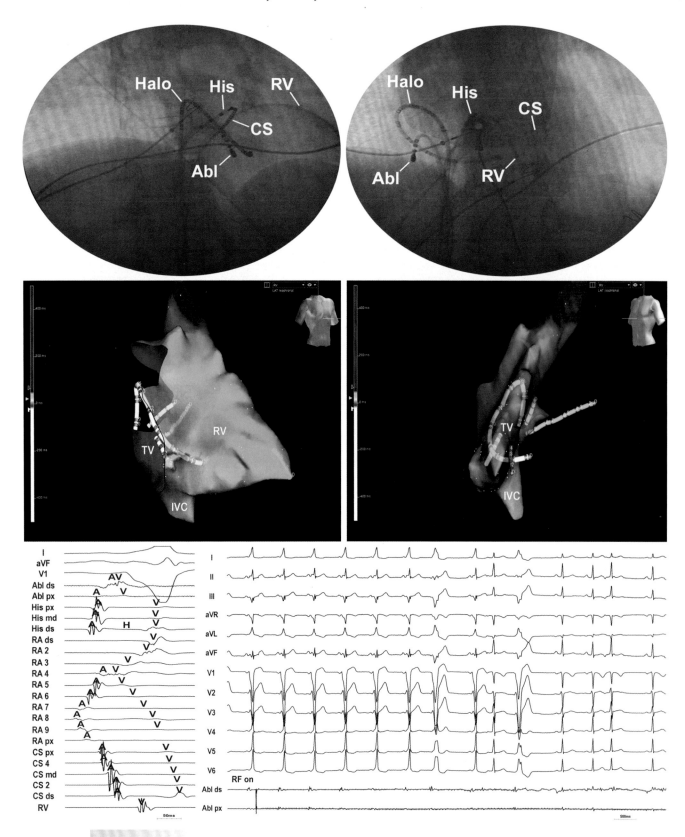

FIGURE 12-9 Ablation of a right posterolateral AP. The earliest site of ventricular activation during manifest preexcitation is at the posterolateral tricuspid annulus (*white*), where the local ventricular electrogram precedes delta wave onset by 26 ms. Application of RF energy causes loss of preexcitation in 6.9 sec.

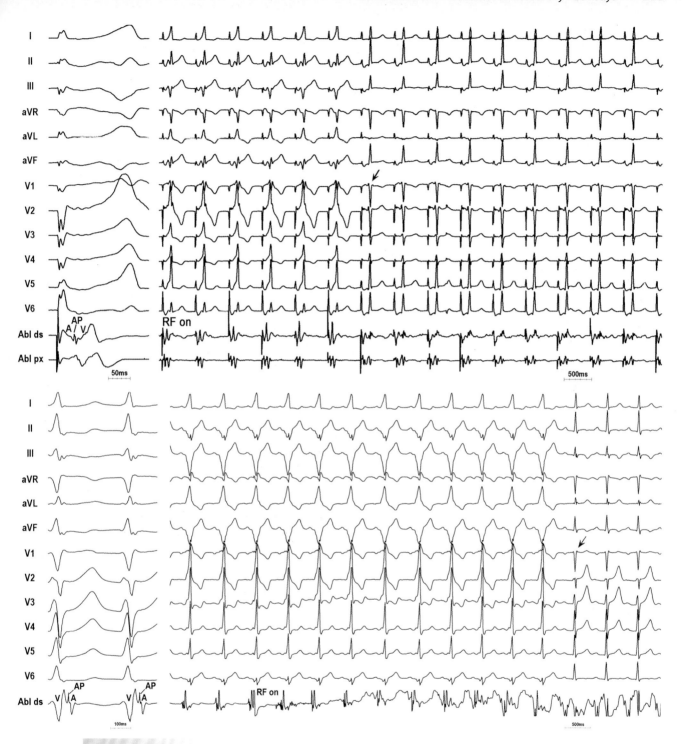

FIGURE 12-10 AP potentials during manifest preexcitation (*top*) and ORT (*bottom*). *Top:* The ablation catheter is positioned at the posterior mitral annulus where it records a sharp AP potential between atrial and ventricular electrograms during CS pacing. Application of RF causes loss of preexcitation (*arrow*). *Bottom:* The ablation catheter is positioned at the posterior mitral annulus where a sharp AP potential is recorded between ventricular and atrial electrograms during ORT. Application of RF energy causes loss of preexcitation in 5.9 sec (*arrow*).

medications (to slow FP conduction), and 4) mapping during ORT (where retrograde conduction occurs exclusively over the AP). Target site criteria for AP ablation during retrograde mapping are 1) AP potentials, 2) earliest site of atrial activation during AP conduction, and 3) site terminating ORT by an extrastimulus with nonglobal capture (**Figs. 12-6 and 12-10 to 12-20**).[1–7] When mapping retrogradely, analyzing electrograms during sinus rhythm or "pacing to block" helps define their atrial and ventricular components. VA fusion can be misleading for slanting APs and be absent for slow-conducting APs.

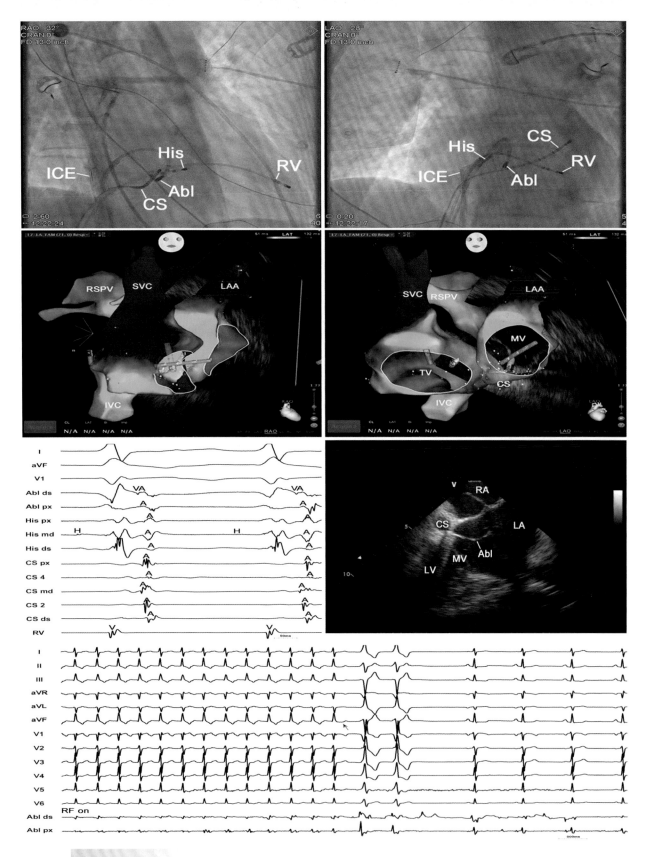

FIGURE 12-11 Ablation of a concealed left posteroseptal AP. The earliest site of atrial activation during ORT is at the posteroseptal mitral annulus (*red*). Application of RF energy causes termination of tachycardia with block in the AP (*arrow*). Note the proximity between the ablation catheter along the endocardial mitral annulus to the epicardial CS on intracardiac echocardiography (ICE).

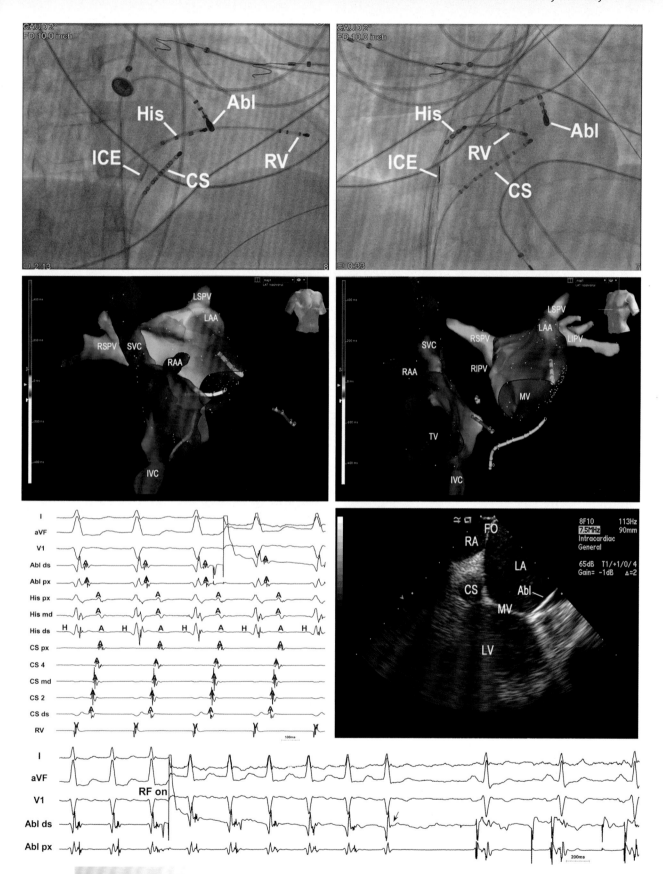

FIGURE 12-12 Ablation of a concealed left free wall AP. The earliest site of atrial activation during ORT is at the lateral mitral annulus (*white*). Application of RF energy terminates ORT with block in the AP (*arrow*). Note the increase in tissue echogenicity seen on intracardiac echocardiography (ICE) during RF delivery.

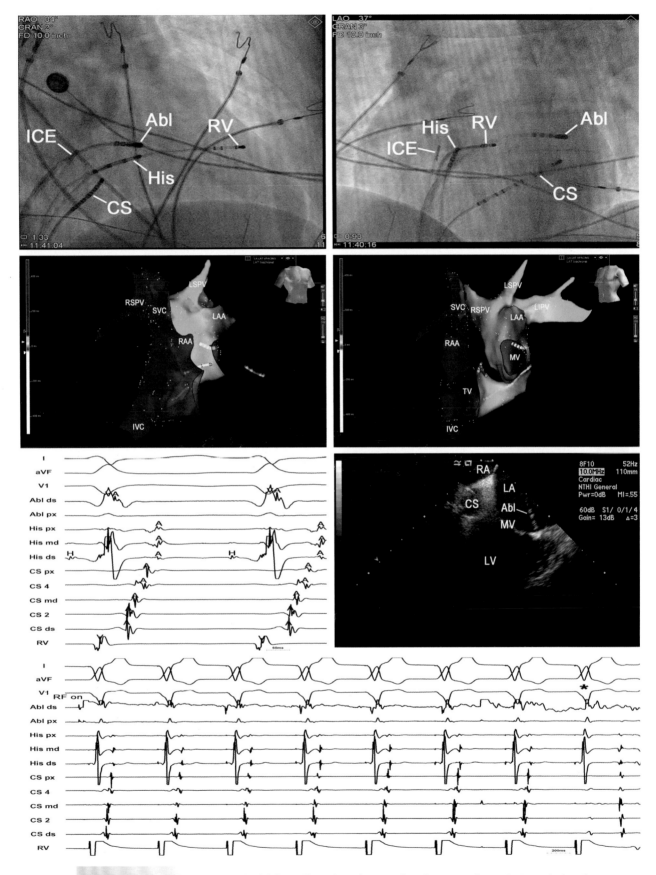

FIGURE 12-13 Ablation of a concealed left free wall AP. The earliest site of atrial activation during ORT is at the lateral mitral annulus (*white*). Application of RF energy during RV pacing causes retrograde block in the AP (*asterisk*) in 4.2 sec. Note the increase in tissue echogenicity seen on intracardiac echocardiography (ICE) during RF delivery.

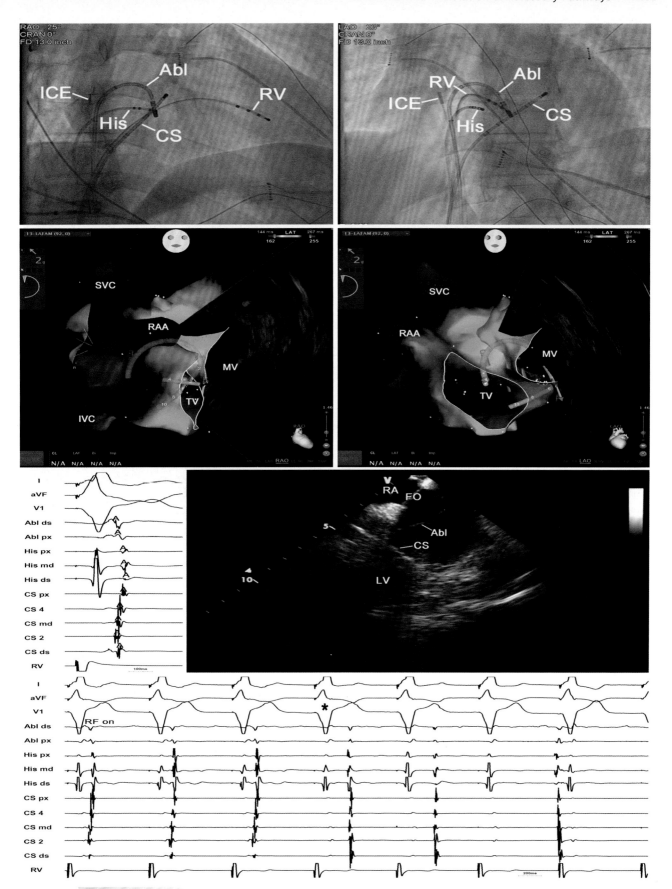

FIGURE 12-14 Ablation of a concealed left posterior AP. The earliest site of atrial activation during retrograde AP conduction is at the posterior mitral annulus (*red*). Application of RF energy causes loss of AP conduction in 6.7 sec (*asterisk*).

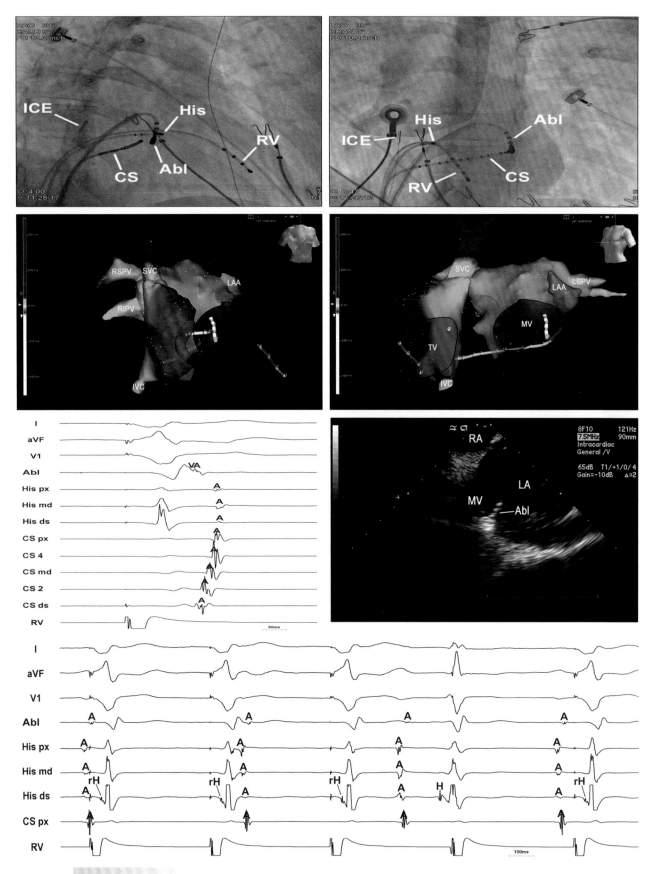

FIGURE 12-15 Ablation of a concealed left posterolateral AP. The earliest site of atrial activation during retrograde AP conduction is at the posterolateral mitral annulus (*white*). After RF ablation, VA dissociation is present. Note the increase in tissue echogenicity seen on intracardiac echocardiography (ICE) during RF delivery.

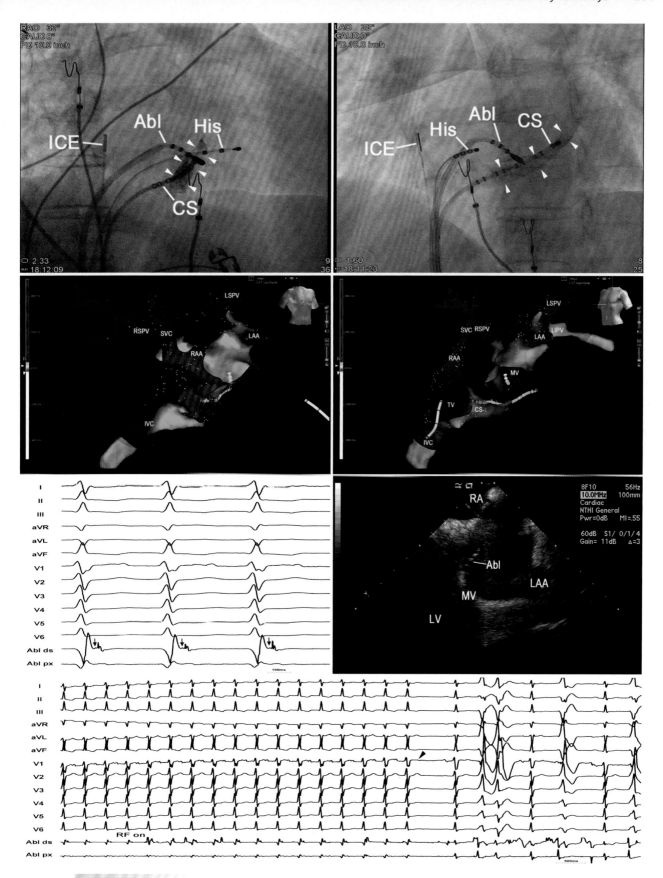

FIGURE 12-16 Ablation of a concealed left posterior AP. The earliest site of atrial activation during ORT is along the posterior mitral annulus (*white*), where tiny AP potentials (*vertical down arrows*) are recorded. RF delivery terminates ORT with retrograde block in the AP (*black arrowhead*). White arrowheads outline the CS during contrast angiography.

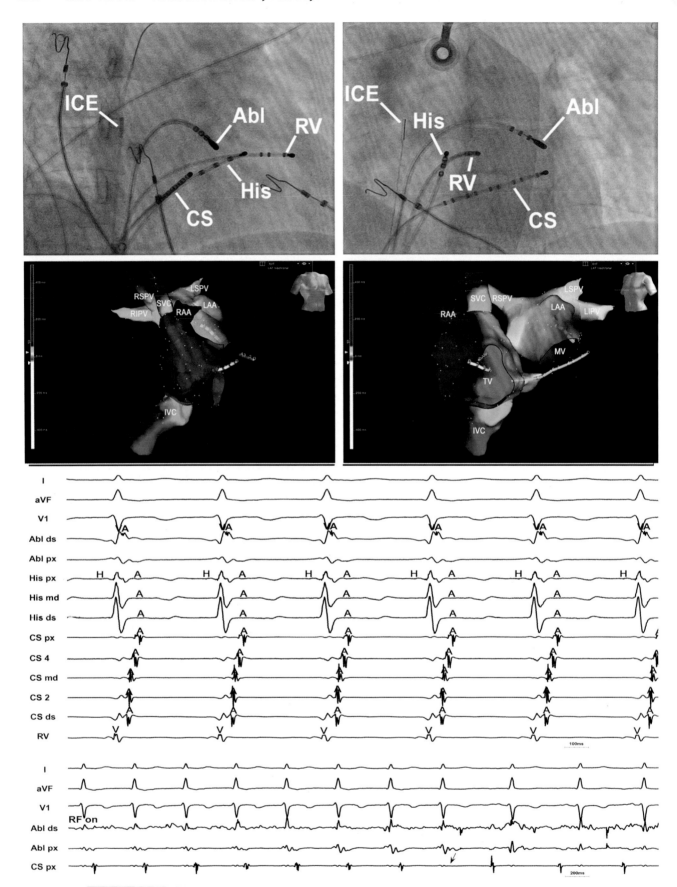

FIGURE 12-17 Ablation of a concealed left free wall AP. The earliest site of atrial activation during ORT is at the lateral mitral annulus (*white*). Application of RF energy terminates ORT with retrograde block in the AP (*arrow*).

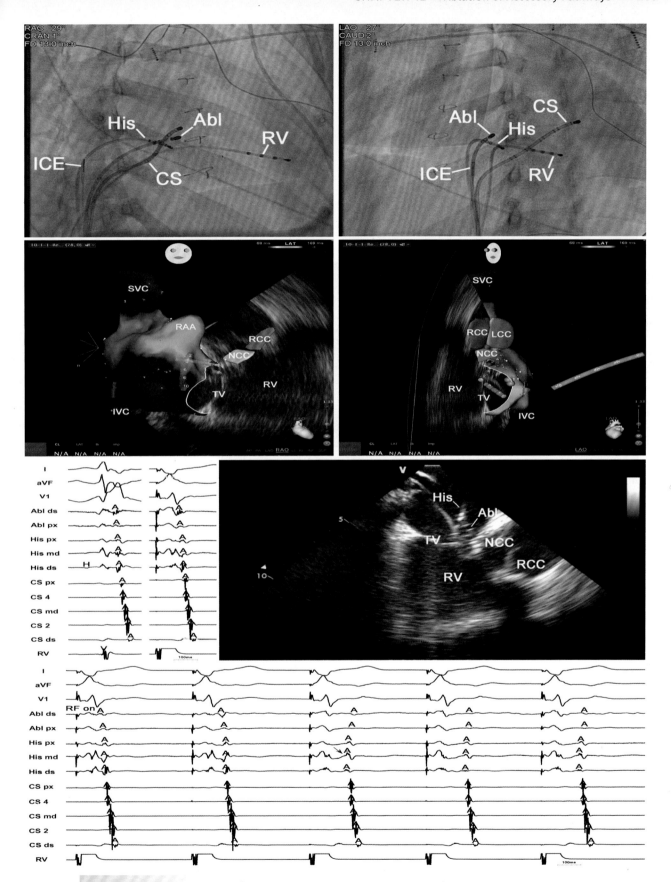

FIGURE 12-18 Ablation of an anteroseptal AP. The earliest site of atrial activation during retrograde AP conduction (*red*) is at the anteroseptal tricuspid annulus just beneath the NCC of the aortic valve where RF energy causes block in the AP and retrograde conduction over the FP (*arrow*). (Ablation from the NCC was unsuccessful.)

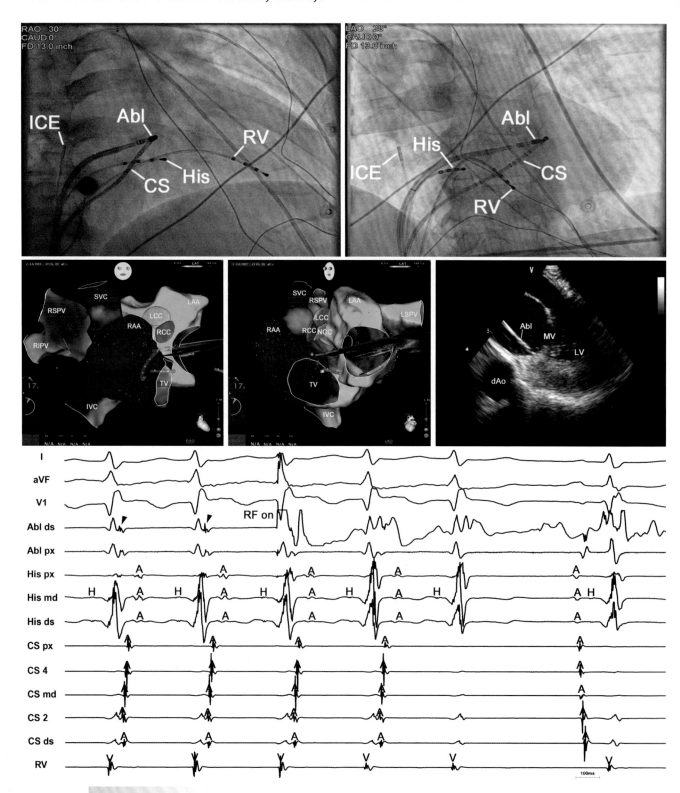

FIGURE 12-19 Ablation of a concealed left free wall AP. The earliest site of atrial activation during ORT is at the lateral mitral annulus (*red, arrowheads*, pre-CS 2 × 13 ms). Application of RF energy terminates ORT in 0.72 sec with retrograde block in the AP.

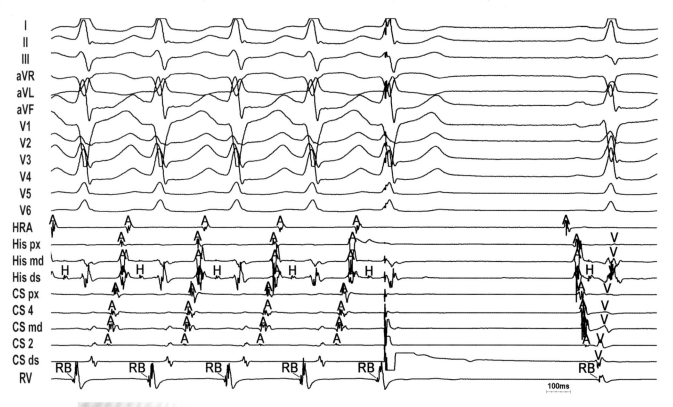

FIGURE 12-20 Termination of ORT by a nonpropagated extrastimulus. A His refractory extrastimulus delivered at the ventricular insertion site of a left free wall AP (CS ds) terminates tachycardia with nonglobal capture. During sinus rhythm, the local ventricular electrogram on CS ds precedes delta wave onset by 20 ms. The extrastimulus captures neither the atrium nor the ventricle but depolarizes the AP, rendering it refractory and terminating tachycardia.

ABLATION

Electrogram stability (<10% change in AV ratio/lack of appearance/disappearance of major deflections in the 3–5 beats preceding radiofrequency [RF] delivery) is an important determinant of durable success during RF ablation.[2] When ablation is performed during ORT, abrupt termination of tachycardia can result in catheter dislodgment from the successful ablation site. One strategy to maintain catheter stability throughout RF delivery is to entrain tachycardia from the ventricle during ablation.[8,9] If an AP is resistant to a particular ablation strategy, options include changing 1) mapping criteria (antegrade versus retrograde), 2) annular approach (transeptal versus transaortic), and 3) type of ablation catheter. Adenosine administration after ablation can help 1) confirm acute RF success (by inducing AV/VA block) and 2) predict AP recurrence (by causing AP membrane hyperpolarization and sodium channel reactivation, which directly restores AP excitability) **(Fig. 12-21)**.[10,11]

SPECIFIC LOCATIONS

Some resistant, seemingly free wall APs (right anterior, left anterolateral) can be difficult to ablate because they arise from the atrial appendages.[12,13] The atrial insertion of right atrial appendage (RAA) pathways can be targeted endocardially from the floor or inferior lobe of the RAA, but left atrial appendage (LAA) pathways

seem to require an epicardial approach. Septal pathways are also challenging because they can lie on either the right or the left side of the septum and near the AV node–His bundle axis.

Right versus Left versus CS Posteroseptal

Three anatomic compartments where posteroseptal APs are found include the 1) tricuspid annulus (right endocardial), 2) mitral annulus (left endocardial), and 3) CS/middle cardiac vein (epicardial).[14–18] APs can also be found within a CS diverticulum.[19–21] Clues to differentiate among these sites are 1) preexcited QRS morphology, 2) CS muscle atrial activation sequence, 3) ΔVA ($VA_{[His\ A]} - VA_{[earliest\ A]}$), and 4) atrial reset preceding advancement of the septal ventricular electrogram at the His bundle region during onset of ventricular overdrive pacing.[17,22–24]

The 12-lead ECG features suggesting a CS (epicardial) AP are 1) negative delta wave in lead II (which overlies the left-sided CS), 2) steep (≥45-degree angle) positive delta wave (initial 40 ms) in lead aVR, and 3) deep S wave (R ≤ S) in lead V6.[17] In addition to direct connections to the left atrium, the proximal CS is covered by a myocardial coat of striated muscle (continuous with right atrial myocardium proximally and extending to the middle cardiac vein distally) that is a potential source of epicardial APs. CS atrial electrograms, therefore, show a double component (blunt endocardial left atrial [LA] [far-field] and sharp epicardial CS [near-field]) during ORT/ventricular pacing.[22] A blunt/sharp activation sequence at the site of earliest atrial

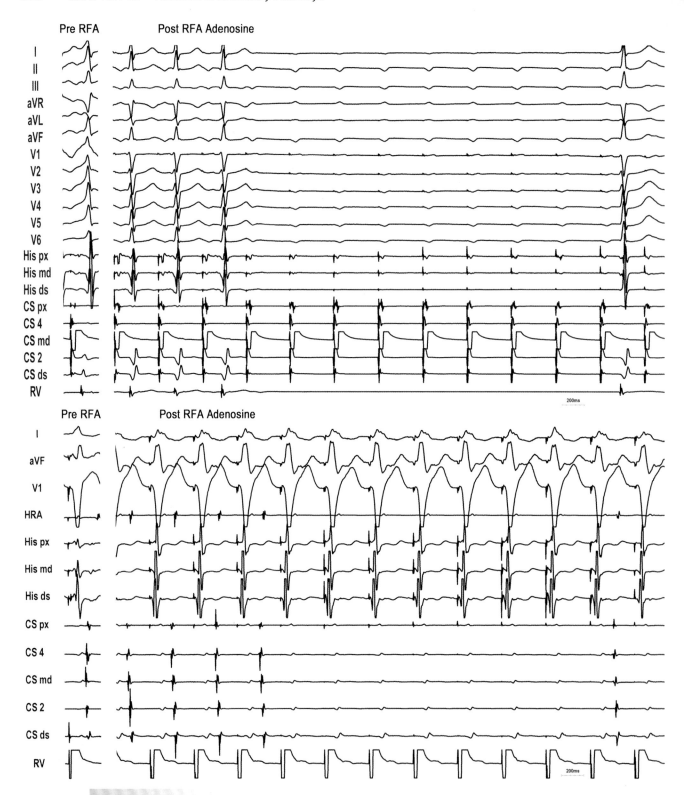

FIGURE 12-21 Adenosine after successful AP ablation. *Top*: Pre-RFA: Preexcitation occurs over a left free wall AP. Post-RFA: Preexcitation is absent. Adenosine induces transient AV block and fails to unmask preexcitation. *Bottom*: Pre-RFA: Retrograde conduction is eccentric over a left posterolateral AP. Post-RFA: Retrograde conduction is concentric over the AV node. Adenosine induces transient VA block and fails to unmask retrograde AP conduction.

activation (initial activation of endocardial LA relative to epicardial CS) indicates an endocardial mitral annular AP requiring a left-sided approach. A sharp/blunt activation sequence (initial activation of epicardial CS relative to endocardial LA) indicates either an endocardial tricuspid annular or epicardial CS AP that can be approached from the right side. Because the conduction time from the right posteroseptum to the right-sided His bundle region is shorter than from the left posteroseptum, the ΔVA (VA$_{[His\ A]}$ − VA$_{[earliest\ A]}$) <25 ms during ORT using right endocardial or CS ostium APs and ≥25 ms for left endocardial APs.[23] At the onset of entrainment from the ventricle, advancement of the atrium preceding advancement of the septal ventricular electrogram at the His bundle region (equivalent to atrial advancement by a late, fused His refractory ventricular premature depolarization [VPD]) is specific for a right posteroseptal AP.[24]

Distant proximity between the right ventricular pacing site and a left-sided AP makes resetting and entrainment of left-sided ORT more difficult than right-sided ORT (unless left bundle branch block [LBBB] is present). Although not specific for posteroseptal AP per se, the following favor a left-sided (compared to right-sided) AP: 1) preexcitation index >75 ms (because resetting of left-sided ORT requires earlier coupled VPDs), 2) corrected PPI − TCL >55 ms (because right ventricular stimulation is far from left-sided ORT), and 3) <2 paced complexes with fixed stimulus-A (St-A) intervals within the transition zone (because acceleration of left-sided ORT occurs later than right-sided ORT during ventricular overdrive pacing).[25–27]

Successful ablation sites within the middle cardiac vein can show relatively large AP potentials (AP/A and/or AP/V amplitude ratios ≥1).[16] Because of the proximity to the RCA or LCx and their branches, coronary angiography is recommended for ablation of APs in the middle cardiac vein. Coronary artery injury can occur if RF energy is delivered <5 mm (and in particular <2 mm) from the coronary artery; cryoablation might be safer alternative energy source.[28]

Parahisian versus NCC

Some APs are anteroseptal in location where RF delivery can damage the His bundle. Parahisian APs are defined as AP whose atrial or ventricular insertion sites are associated with a His bundle potential >0.1 mV. The 12-lead ECG features suggesting a parahisian AP are 1) positive delta waves in leads I, II, and aVF and 2) negative delta waves in V1 and V2 or sum of initial r wave (V1 + V2) <0.5 mV (because initial forces are directed away from V1 and V2, both of which are equidistant from the midline sternum that overlies the membranous septum).[29,30] Endocardial parahisian APs are prone to mechanical block during catheter manipulation, suggesting that they course superficially in the subendocardium in contrast to the deeper penetrating His bundle within the central fibrous body. Recording an AP potential and the smallest (far-field) His bundle potential possible are important target site criteria for successful ablation without causing AV block.[29,31] RF delivery with low, incremental energy ("slow and low") is important and should be terminated immediately with onset of a junctional rhythm or persistence of AP conduction after 10 sec.[29] However, before attempting ablation

of an AP near the right-sided His bundle, it would be important to map the noncoronary cusp (NCC) of the aortic valve as an alternative ablation site where the risk of AV block appears lower. The commissure of the NCC and right coronary cusp (RCC) sits directly above the His bundle as it penetrates the membranous septum. APs in the vicinity of the aortic cusps (trigone pathways) are most common from the NCC and rarely described for the left coronary cusp (LCC).[32–37]

ATYPICAL ACCESSORY PATHWAYS

PERMANENT FORM OF JUNCTIONAL RECIPROCATING TACHYCARDIA

The permanent form of junctional reciprocating tachycardia is a nearly incessant ORT utilizing a concealed, slowly conducting, decremental, AV AP. The AP is usually (but not always) located in the posteroseptal region and mapped by identifying the earliest site of atrial activation during ventricular pacing or tachycardia (see Figs. 6-18 to 6-20).[38,39]

MAHAIM FIBERS

Mahaim fibers refer collectively to variant APs that include 1) atrio-fascicular, 2) nodo-fascicular (or nodo-ventricular), and 3) fasciculo-ventricular APs. The classic description of a Mahaim fiber was a decremental, antegrade-only conducting pathway originating/inserting into (fascicular) or near (ventricular) the right bundle giving rise to typical LBBB preexcitation. Decrement can occur in the AP itself or its link (directly [nodo-fascicular/ nodo-ventricular] or indirectly [fasciculo-ventricular]) to the AV node. Concealed (retrograde-only) pathways responsible for ORT have been described. Rather than the older term Mahaim, these pathways are more precisely described by their anatomic sites of origin/insertion. The distal insertion site of these pathways can be mapped and targeted at/near the right bundle (at the risk of causing right bundle branch block [RBBB]) by identifying the ventricular site with 1) a perfect pacemap (concordance between paced and spontaneous LBBB QRS complexes); 2) earliest ventricular activation relative to the preexcited QRS complex; and 3) a steep QS electrogram pattern during unfiltered, unipolar recordings.[40] However, these pathways are more commonly mapped and targeted at their proximal origin. Most atrio-fascicular APs originate along the lateral tricuspid annulus (posterior to anterior), and its atrial insertion site is identified by 1) Mahaim potentials ("His bundle–like" potentials) between atrial and ventricular electrograms, 2) shortest stimulus-delta wave interval during constant atrial pacing, 3) longest coupled AVJ refractory atrial premature depolarization (APD) that preexcites the ventricle during antidromic tachycardia, and 4) site of mechanical block with catheter manipulation (Fig. 12-22).[41–44] Although rare, nodo-fascicular (or nodo-ventricular) APs seem to arise from the SP and therefore can be targeted by 1) identifying the site with earliest atrial activation or high-frequency AP potential during retrograde AP conduction or 2) selective ablation of the slow pathway of the AV node along the postero- or midseptum.[45,46]

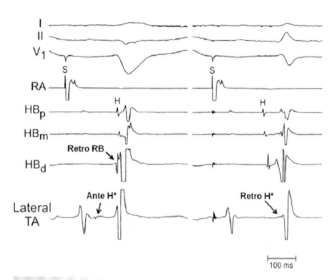

FIGURE 12-22 Ablation of an atrio-fascicular AP. Pre-RFA (*left*): Atrial pacing conducts over an atrio-fascicular AP with typical LBBB preexcitation. An antegrade Mahaim potential (H*) is recorded along the lateral tricuspid annulus with retrograde activation of the RB and His md. The proximal His bundle is activated antegradely by the AV node (His px precedes His md). Note that the RB is nearly simultaneous with QRS onset. Post-RFA (*right*): LBBB preexcitation is gone. The His and RB bundles are activated antegradely by the AV node followed by retrograde activation of the Mahaim. Note the polarity reversal of the His md and RB electrogram as activation shifts from retrograde to antegrade. (Reprinted from Gandhavadi M, et al. Characterization of the distal insertion of atrio-fascicular accessory pathways and mechanisms of QRS patterns in atrio-fascicular antidromic tachycardia. Heart Rhythm 2013;10:1385–1389, with permission from Elsevier.)

REFERENCES

1. Jackman WM, Wang X, Friday KJ, et al. Catheter ablation of accessory atrioventricular pathways (Wolff-Parkinson-White syndrome) by radiofrequency current. N Engl J Med 1991;324:1605–1611.
2. Calkins H, Kim Y, Schmaltz S, et al. Electrogram criteria for identification of appropriate target sites for radiofrequency catheter ablation of accessory atrioventricular connections. Circulation 1992;85:565–573.
3. Otomo K, Gonzalez MD, Beckman KJ, et al. Reversing the direction of paced ventricular and atrial wavefronts reveals an oblique course in accessory AV pathways and improves localization for catheter ablation. Circulation 2001;104:550–556.
4. Ho RT, DeCaro M. Narrow QRS complex tachycardia with a high-frequency potential recorded near the His bundle: what is the mechanism? Heart Rhythm 2005;2:664–666.
5. Jackman WM, Friday KJ, Yeung-Lai-Wah JA, et al. New catheter technique for recording left free-wall accessory atrioventricular pathway activation. Identification of pathway fiber orientation. Circulation 1988;78:598–611.
6. Logue JP, Greenspon AJ, Ho RT. Termination of a narrow complex tachycardia by a single extrastimulus: what is the mechanism? Heart Rhythm 2018;15:1889–1890.
7. Miller J, Suleman A, Hadian D. Termination of orthodromic supraventricular tachycardia with a nonpropagated stimulus. J Cardiovasc Electrophysiol 2003;14:439.
8. Okumura K, Yamabe H, Yasue H. Radiofrequency catheter ablation of accessory pathway during entrainment of the atrioventricular reciprocating tachycardia. Am J Cardiol 1993;72:188–193.
9. Li HG, Klein GJ, Zardini M, Thakur RK, Morillo CA, Yee R. Radiofrequency catheter ablation of accessory pathways during entrainment of AV reentrant tachycardia. Pacing Clin Electrophysiol 1994;17:590–594.
10. Keim S, Curtis AB, Belardinelli L, Epstein ML, Staples ED, Lerman BB. Adenosine-induced atrioventricular block: a rapid and reliable method to assess surgical and radiofrequency catheter ablation of accessory atrioventricular pathways. J Am Coll Cardiol 1992;19:1005–1012.
11. Spotnitz MD, Markowitz SM, Liu CF, et al. Mechanisms and clinical significance of adenosine-induced dormant accessory pathway conduction after catheter ablation. Circ Arrhythm Electrophysiol 2014;7:1136–1143.
12. Guo X, Sun Q, Ma J, et al. Electrophysiological characteristics and radiofrequency catheter ablation of accessory pathway connecting the right atrial appendage and the right ventricle. J Cardiovasc Electrophysiol 2015;26:845–852.
13. Mah D, Miyake C, Clegg R, et al. Epicardial left atrial appendage and biatrial appendage accessory pathways. Heart Rhythm 2010;7:1740–1745.
14. Wen MS, Yeh SJ, Wang CC, King A, Lin FC, Wu D. Radiofrequency ablation therapy of the posteroseptal accessory pathway. Am Heart J 1996;132:612–620.
15. Langberg JJ, Man KC, Vorperian VR, et al. Recognition and catheter ablation of subepicardial accessory pathways. J Am Coll Cardiol 1993;22:1100–1104.
16. Giorgberidze I, Saksena S, Krol RB, Mathew P. Efficacy and safety of radiofrequency catheter ablation of left-sided accessory pathways through the coronary sinus. Am J Cardiol 1995;76:359–365.
17. Takahashi A, Shah DC, Jaïs P, Hocini M, Clementy J, Haïssaguerre M. Specific electrocardiographic features of manifest coronary vein posteroseptal accessory pathways. J Cardiovasc Electrophysiol 1998;9:1015–1025.
18. Kobza R, Hindricks G, Tanner H, et al. Paraseptal accessory pathway in Wolff-Parkinson-White-Syndrom: ablation from the right, from the left or within the coronary sinus/middle cardiac vein? J Interv Card Electrophysiol 2005;12:55–60.
19. Lesh MD, Van Hare G, Kao AK, Scheinman MM. Radiofrequency catheter ablation for Wolff-Parkinson-White Syndrome associated with a coronary sinus diverticulum. Pacing Clin Electrophysiol 1991;14:1479–1484.
20. Lewalter T, Yang A, Schwab JO, Lüderitz B. Accessory pathway catheter ablation inside the neck of a coronary sinus diverticulum. J Cardiovasc Electrophysiol 2003;14:1386.
21. Morin DP, Parker H, Khatib S, Dinshaw H. Computed tomography of a coronary sinus diverticulum associated with Wolff-Parkinson-White syndrome. Heart Rhythm 2012;9:1338–1339.
22. Pap R, Traykov VB, Makai A, Bencsik G, Forster T, Sághy L. Ablation of posteroseptal and left posterior accessory pathways guided by left atrium-coronary sinus musculature activation sequence. J Cardiovasc Electrophysiol 2008;19:653–658.
23. Chiang CE, Chen SA, Tai CT, et al. Prediction of successful ablation site of concealed posteroseptal accessory pathways by a novel algorithm using baseline electrophysiological parameters: implication for an abbreviated ablation procedure. Circulation 1996;93:982–991.
24. Calvo D, Ávila P, García-Fernández FJ, et al. Differential responses of the septal ventricle and the atrial signals during ongoing entrainment: a method to differentiate orthodromic reciprocating tachycardia using septal accessory pathways from atypical atrioventricular nodal reentry. Circ Arrhythm Electrophysiol 2015;8:1201–1209.
25. Miles W, Yee R, Klein G, Zipes D, Prystowsky E. The preexcitation index: an aid in determining the mechanism of supraventricular tachycardia and localizing accessory pathways. Circulation 1986;74:493–500.
26. Akerström F, Pachón M, García-Fernández FJ, et al. Number of beats in the transition zone with fixed SA interval during right ventricular overdrive pacing determines accessory pathway location in orthodromic reentrant tachycardia. Pacing Clin Electrophysiol 2016;39:21–27.
27. Boonyapisit W, Methavigul K, Krittayaphong R, et al. Determining the site of accessory pathways in orthodromic reciprocating tachycardia by using the response to right ventricular pacing. Pacing Clin Electrophysiol 2016;39:115–121.
28. Stavrakis S, Jackman WM, Nakagawa H, et al. Risk of coronary artery injury with radiofrequency ablation and cryoablation of epicardial posteroseptal accessory pathways within the coronary venous system. Circ Arrhythm Electrophysiol 2014;7:113–119.
29. Haïssaguerre M, Marcus F, Poquet F, Gencel L, Le Métayer P, Clémenty J. Electrocardiographic characteristics and catheter ablation of parahissian accessory pathways. Circulation 1994;90:1124–1128.
30. Gonzalez-Torrecilla E, Peinado R, Almendral J, et al. Reappraisal of classical electrocardiographic criteria in detecting accessory pathways with a strict para-Hisian location. Heart Rhythm 2013;10:16–21.
31. Schlüter M, Kuck KH. Catheter ablation from right atrium of anteroseptal accessory pathways using radiofrequency current. J Am Coll Cardiol 1992;19:663–670.
32. Xu G, Liu T, Liu E, et al. Radiofrequency catheter ablation at the non-coronary cusp for the treatment of para-hisian accessory pathways. Europace 2015;17:962–968.
33. Tada H, Naito S, Nogami A, Taniguchi K. Successful catheter ablation of an anteroseptal accessory pathway from the noncoronary sinus of Valsalva. J Cardiovasc Electrophysiol 2003;14:544–546.
34. Suleiman M, Powell BD, Munger TM, Asirvatham SJ. Successful cryoablation in the noncoronary aortic cusp for a left anteroseptal accessory pathway. J Interv Card Electrophysiol 2008;23:205–211.
35. Suleiman M, Brady PA, Asirvatham SJ, Friedman PA, Munger TA. The noncoronary cusp as a site for successful ablation of accessory pathways: electrogram characteristics in three cases. J Cardiovasc Electrophysiol 2011;22:203–209.

36. Huang H, Wang X, Ouyang F, Antz M. Catheter ablation of anteroseptal accessory pathway in the non-coronary aortic sinus. Europace 2006;8: 1041–1044.

37. Shenthar J, Rai MK. Preexcited tachycardia mimicking outflow tract ventricular tachycardia ablated from the left coronary cusp. J Cardiovasc Electrophysiol 2014;25:653–656.

38. Ticho BS, Saul P, Hulse JE, De W, Lulu J, Walsh EP. Variable location of accessory pathways associated with the permanent form of junctional reciprocating tachycardia and confirmation with radiofrequency ablation. Am J Cardiol 1992;70:1559–1564.

39. Gaita F, Haissaguerre M, Guistetto C, et al. Catheter ablation of permanent junctional reciprocating tachycardia with radiofrequency current. J Am Coll Cardiol 1995;25:648–654.

40. Haissaguerre M, Warin JF, Le Metayer P, et al. Catheter ablation of Mahaim fibers with preservation of atrioventricular nodal conduction. Circulation 1990;82:418–427.

41. McClelland JH, Wang X, Beckman KJ, et al. Radiofrequency catheter ablation of right atriofascicular (Mahaim) accessory pathways guided by accessory pathway activation potentials. Circulation 1994;89:2655–2666.

42. Klein LS, Hackett FK, Zipes DP, Miles WM. Radiofrequency catheter ablation of Mahaim fibers at the tricuspid annulus. Circulation 1993;87:738–747.

43. Cappato R, Schlüter M, Weiss C, et al. Catheter-induced mechanical conduction block of right-sided accessory fibers with Mahaim-type preexcitation to guide radiofrequency ablation. Circulation 1994;90:282–290.

44. Mönnig G, Wasmer K, Milberg P, et al. Predictors of long-term success after catheter ablation of atriofascicular accessory pathways. Heart Rhythm 2012; 9:704–708.

45. Grogin HR, Lee RJ, Kwasman M, et al. Radiofrequency catheter ablation of atriofascicular and nodoventricular Mahaim tracts. Circulation 1994;90:272–281.

46. Hluchy J, Schlegelmilch P, Schickel S, et al. Radiofrequency ablation of a concealed nodoventricular Mahaim fiber guided by a discrete potential. J Cardiovasc Electrophysiol 1999;10:603–610.

13 Atrial Tachycardia

Introduction

Atrial tachycardia (AT) can be categorized into two general types: focal and macroreentrant. Focal ATs arise from a "point source" with centrifugal spread to the rest of the atria and due to enhanced automaticity, triggered activity, or microreentry. These tachycardias tend to cluster at specific anatomic sites that include the 1) crista terminalis ("crista tachycardia"), 2) tricuspid and mitral annuli, 3) atrial appendages, 4) interatrial septum, 5) coronary sinus ostium (CS os), and 6) pulmonary veins.[1] Macroreentrant ATs occur in the setting of atrial scar (e.g., surgery, prior ablation), which creates isthmuses of slow conduction that facilitate reentry.

The purpose of this chapter is to:
1. Localize focal AT by the 12-lead ECG.
2. Discuss the electrophysiologic features of AT.
3. Discuss mapping techniques for ablation of focal and macroreentrant AT.

12-LEAD ECG

The P-wave morphology during AT is determined by its anatomic site of origin and, therefore, valuable for localization.[2–5] It is best visualized during periods of atrio-ventricular (AV) block when not obscured by QRS complexes or T waves. (A burst of rapid ventricular pacing during tachycardia can dissociate P waves from QRS complexes/T waves.)

RIGHT VERSUS LEFT The most helpful leads to differentiate right from left ATs are V1 and aVL.[6] In general, because the right atrium is anterior relative to the left atrium (LA), right ATs generate posterior (V1: negative or biphasic [positive–negative]) and leftward (aVL: positive) P-wave axes.[2,6] In contrast, left ATs generate anterior (V1: positive or biphasic [negative–positive]) and rightward (aVL: negative or isoelectric) P-wave axes, (except for origin from the right superior pulmonary vein [RSPV] where P waves can be positive in aVL.)

SUPERIOR VERSUS INFERIOR Superior foci (e.g., high crista terminalis, superior pulmonary veins, atrial appendages) generate positive P wave in the inferior leads. As the tachycardia origin shifts downward (low crista terminalis, inferior pulmonary veins, CS os, inferior annuli), P-wave amplitudes decrease and even become negative in the inferior leads.

SEPTAL VERSUS FREE WALL Tachycardia P waves closer to the septum (e.g., right-sided pulmonary veins) tend to be narrower than those originating farther from the septum (e.g., left-sided pulmonary veins).

SPECIFIC P-WAVE MORPHOLOGIES

Sinus-Like Morphology

The crista terminalis is the most common site for right ATs. Because it is close to the sinus node, it generates sinus-like P waves (biphasic [positive–negative] in V1, inferior axis and negative in aVR) (Fig. 13-1).[7] Occasionally, a crista tachycardia shows a positive P wave in V1 in which case, the P wave is also positive in V1 during normal sinus rhythm (NSR) (due to the anatomic position of the heart relative to V1). This can be differentiated from the RSPV tachycardia, which shows the normal biphasic (positive–negative) P wave in V1 during NSR.[2] Right atrial appendage and superior tricuspid annular tachycardias demonstrate a negative P wave in V1 with variable precordial progression and an inferior axis, which can be difficult to differentiate from each other because of their close anatomic proximity.[8,9]

Atypical AVNRT-Like Morphology

Because the slow pathway (SP) of the AV node lies near the CS os, tachycardias originating from the CS os produce a similar characteristic morphology (isoelectric and then positive

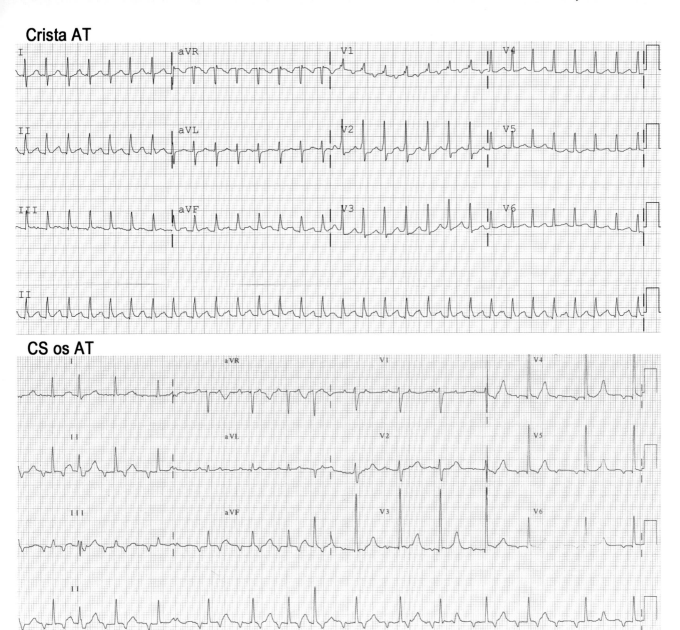

Crista AT

CS os AT

FIGURE 13-1 A 12-lead ECG of AT arising from the crista terminalis (*top*) and CS os (*bottom*). P waves of "crista tachycardias" resemble sinus tachycardia because of their close proximity to the SA node. P waves of CS tachycardias resemble atypical AVNRT because the SP lies near the ostium of the CS.

or biphasic [negative–positive] P waves in V1 and inverted P waves inferiorly) (**Fig. 13-1**).[10] CS tachycardias show precordial P-wave regression. Transition from positive to negative occurs earlier with tachycardia origin at CS os (V2) than in the body of the CS (V4).[11]

Biphasic (Negative–Positive) Morphology

The unusual narrow, biphasic (negative–positive) P-wave morphology in lead V1 and/or the inferior leads should raise suspicion of a septal origin: noncoronary cusp (NCC), aorto-mitral continuity (superior mitral annulus), perinodal, or interatrial septum (**Fig. 13-2**).[5,12–16]

Concordance

P waves inverted in the inferior leads and negatively concordant across the precordium are characteristic of origin from the inferior tricuspid annulus (the most anterior structure of the atrium) (**Fig. 13-3**).[9] Conversely, positive precordial P-wave concordance suggests origin from the pulmonary veins (the most posterior structure of the atrium and most common site for left ATs) (**Fig. 13-3**).[17] AT arising from the left-sided pulmonary veins are wider and more commonly notched than right-sided pulmonary veins. Because of their close anatomic proximity, differentiating the left superior

NCC AT

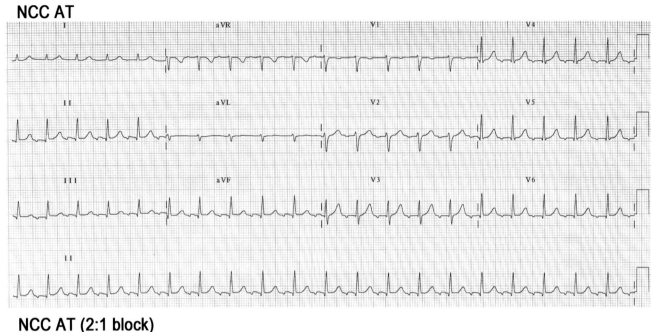

NCC AT (2:1 block)

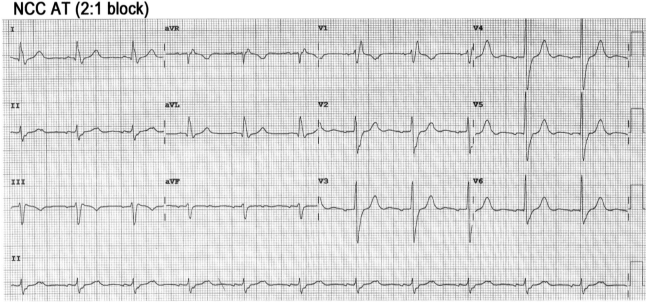

FIGURE 13-2 A 12-lead ECG of AT arising from the NCC of the aortic valve. 1:1 (*top*) and 2:1 (*bottom*) AV conduction. P waves show a characteristic biphasic (negative–positive) morphology in the inferior leads.

pulmonary vein (LSPV) from LA appendage tachycardias can be difficult. LA appendage tachycardias might show deeper negative P waves in aVL (because of its more leftward location) and less positive concordant (because of its more anterior location).

ELECTROPHYSIOLOGIC FEATURES

Intracardiac atrial activation patterns allow further localization of AT, particularly when P waves are difficult to identify on the 12-lead ECG. Certain features help differentiate AT from

atrio-ventricular nodal reentrant tachycardia (AVNRT) and orthodromic reciprocating tachycardia (ORT).

AV RELATIONSHIP

AV block is common during AT. In contrast, AV block is uncommon and usually transient during AVNRT and never occurs with ORT.

BUNDLE BRANCH BLOCK

In contrast to ORT, AT is not dependent on the His-Purkinje system and is therefore unaffected by development of bundle branch block.

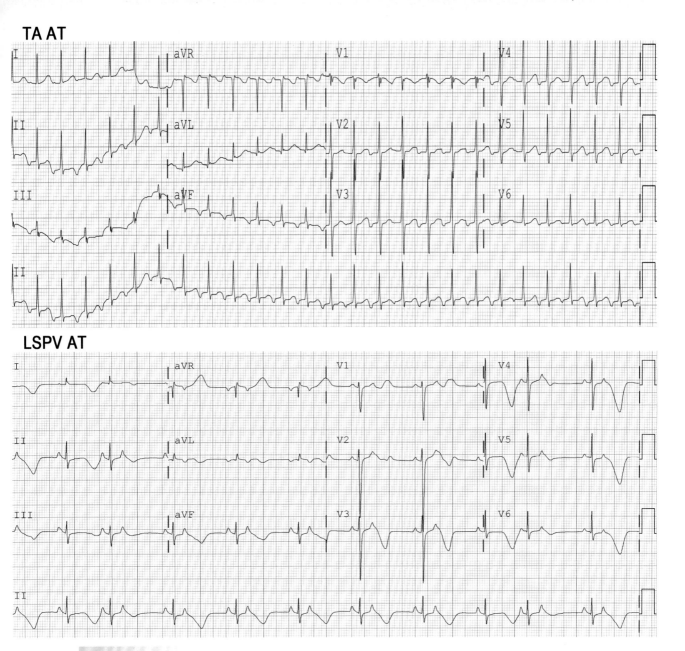

FIGURE 13-3 A 12-lead ECG of AT arising from the inferior tricuspid annulus (TA) (*top*) and LSPV (*bottom*) showing negative and positive precordial concordance, respectively. The LSPV tachycardia shows intermittent 4:2 exit Wenckebach block from the pulmonary vein causing relative bradycardia and QT prolongation.

ZONES OF TRANSITION

Gradual acceleration of tachycardia (warm-up phenomenon) occurs with automatic ATs. The morphology and atrial activation pattern of the first and subsequent P waves are identical because they are all driven by the same ectopic focus. Abrupt initiation by spontaneous atrial premature depolarizations occurs with triggered activity or reentry, in which case the first (initiating) and subsequent P waves can differ. Gradual deceleration of tachycardia (cool-down phenomenon) occurs with automatic ATs, while abrupt termination is observed with triggered activity and reentry. Because AT is not dependent on the AV node, a narrow complex tachycardia that repeatedly terminates spontaneously with AV block excludes AT.

PACING MANEUVERS FROM THE VENTRICLE ("AAV" RESPONSE)

While the response of AVNRT and ORT to entrainment from the ventricle is "AV" (or "AH"), it is "AAV" ("AAH") for AT (see Fig. 5-23).[18,19] Rarely, a macroreentrant AT can generate an "AV" response if 1) the AT circuit time > AVJ refractory period and 2) the recording atrial site is orthodromically captured during entrainment. (An antidromically captured site generates an "AAV" response.[20])

PACING MANEUVERS FROM THE ATRIUM (ABSENCE OF VA LINKING)

While both AVNRT and ORT show ventriculoatrial (VA) linking (ΔVA <10 ms) one beat after differential atrial overdrive pacing, AT does not (ΔVA >10 ms) (see Fig. 5-27).[21,22] Apparent VA linking, however, might occur if atrial overdrive pacing terminates AT, which is then reinitiated by typical AV nodal echoes (not by pacing per se) (Fig. 13-4).

MAPPING AND ABLATION

FOCAL ATRIAL TACHYCARDIA

The focal site of origin of AT can be identified by 1) activation mapping, 2) pacemapping, and 3) atrial overdrive pacing.[23–27] Creating three-dimensional electro-anatomic reconstructions of the atrium facilitates mapping within the atrial cavity and overcomes limitations of two-dimensional fluoroscopy.

Activation Mapping

Activation mapping identifies the earliest site of atrial activation relative to P-wave onset (pre–P wave) or reference atrial electrogram during tachycardia (Figs. 13-5 to 13-17). While variable, successful sites often show pre–P-wave values ≥20–30 ms. Successful electrograms can be fractionated (particularly from the crista terminalis where poor cell-to-cell coupling causes slow conduction), show a discrete high-frequency potential preceding local atrial activation with reversal during sinus rhythm (particularly from the musculature of the CS), or show a QS morphology on unipolar recordings (Figs. 13-7 and 13-12).[4,7,11,24,25] Because of close proximity to the phrenic nerve, high-output pacing should be performed prior to ablation of a crista tachycardia to ensure absence of phrenic nerve capture. In the presence of diaphragmatic stimulation, the phrenic nerve can be monitored during radiofrequency (RF) delivery by stimulating the superior right phrenic nerve with a catheter positioned in the right subclavian vein (as done during right-sided pulmonary vein cryoablation). Specific mention should be made when the earliest site of atrial activation is recorded at the His bundle region, in which case an NCC AT should be considered (Figs. 13-5 to 13-8). Mapping the NCC might identify the earliest site of atrial activation and allow safer ablation with a lower risk of causing AV block.[12–15]

Pacemapping

ATs give rise to specific P-wave morphologies and atrial activation patterns, which can be reproduced when pacing from its site of origin (Fig. 13-9).[26] Pacemapping is useful for brief episodes of AT that are difficult to sustain and not easily amenable to activation mapping.

Atrial Overdrive Pacing

While focal ATs cannot be entrained, atrial overdrive pacing at a rate slightly faster than tachycardia can be useful to localize its site of origin.[27] The difference between the post-pacing interval and tachycardia cycle length (PPI − TCL) is directly related to the distance between the pacing site and tachycardia focus. A pacing site demonstrating PPI − TCL <20 ms is a target for ablation (Fig. 13-18).

MACROREENTRANT ATRIAL TACHYCARDIA

Pacemapping

For macroreentrant AT, the P-wave morphology and corresponding atrial activation pattern reflect the exit site of the circuit. Pacing from the exit site or protected isthmus of slow conduction produces paced P-wave morphologies and atrial activation patterns identical to tachycardia (Fig. 13-19). A short stimulus-P (St-P) interval and perfect pacemap indicate exit site stimulation. A long St-P interval and perfect pacemap suggest stimulation from a region of slow conduction within the circuit (e.g., central isthmus, adjacent bystander site). However, functional barriers during tachycardia not present during sinus rhythm might generate imperfect pacemaps despite stimulation from a site within the circuit critical to tachycardia.

Entrainment Mapping

The target site for ablation is the critical isthmus of slow conduction identified by entrainment mapping or the creation of a line of block between two anatomic obstacles that transect the circuit.[28–30] Analogous to entrainment mapping of scar-related ventricular tachycardia, three criteria are used to define each site: 1) paced P-wave morphology (and atrial activation pattern) relative to tachycardia, 2) St-P − electrogram-P interval (egm-P), and 3) PPI − TCL.[28] Different entrainment sites are shown in Table 13-1 with the critical isthmus being the optimal target for ablation (Fig. 13-20). A three-dimensional color-coded electro-anatomic map based on entrainment mapping can help identify appropriate targets for ablation.[31]

Nonpropagated Extrastimulus

The critical isthmus of the macroreentrant circuit can also be identified by a nonpropagated extrastimulus terminating tachycardia.[32] Such a stimulus depolarizes the critical isthmus, rendering it refractory without propagating to the rest of the atrium (nonglobal capture).

UNUSUAL ELECTROPHYSIOLOGIC PHENOMENA

AT MIMICKING AVNRT NCC ATs with SP conduction can cause simultaneous atrial and ventricular activation ("A on V" tachycardia) and earliest atrial activation at the anteroseptum mimicking typical AVNRT (Fig. 13-4).[33] Differentiation requires evaluation of P-wave morphology, pacing maneuvers in the ventricle ("AAV" response), and/or pacing maneuvers in the atrium (absence of VA linking).

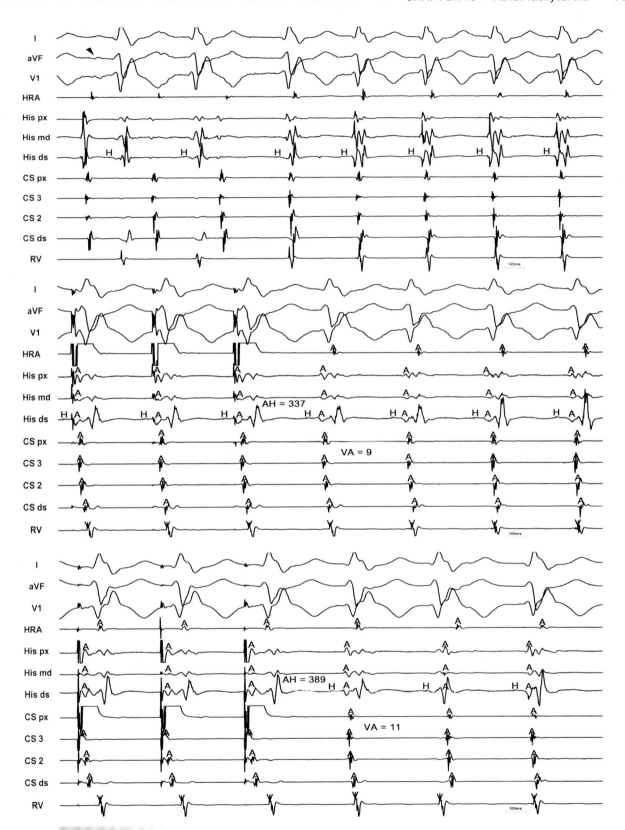

FIGURE 13-4 NCC AT mimicking typical AVNRT. *Top*: NCC AT with fast pathway (FP) Wenckebach transitioning to sustained SP conduction causing simultaneous AV activation. "A on V" tachycardia with atrial activation originating from the NCC (near the FP) mimics typical AVNRT. However, the P-wave morphology (biphasic [negative–positive] in lead II [*arrowhead*]) excludes AVNRT. *Middle and bottom*: Apparent VA linking. Despite different long AH intervals upon cessation of differential atrial pacing (high right atrium [HRA] and CS), the ΔVA = 2 ms because typical AV nodal echoes (not atrial pacing per se) reinitiates AT.

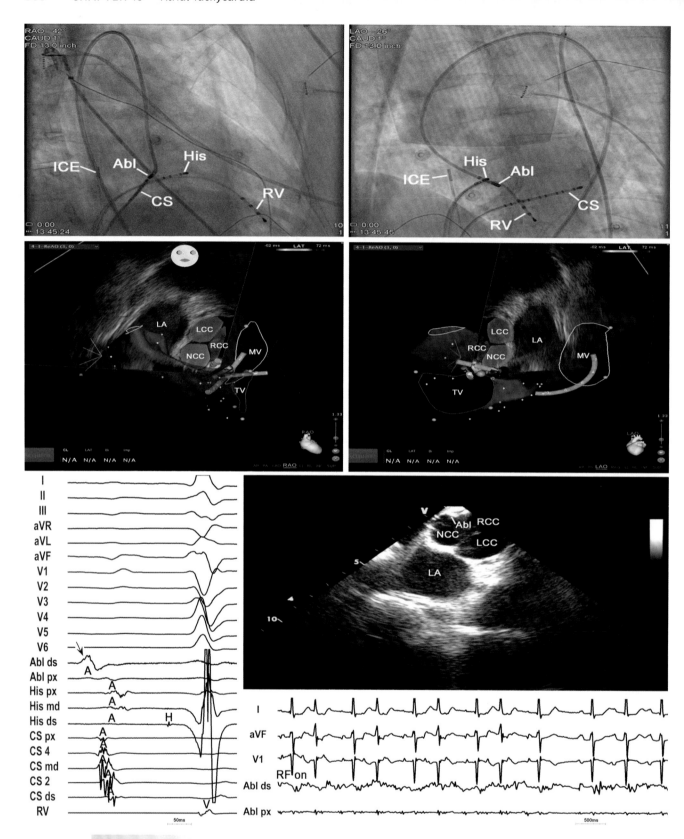

FIGURE 13-5 Ablation of NCC AT. The earliest site of atrial activation (*arrow*) precedes P-wave onset by 52 ms where application of RF energy (*red tag*) terminates tachycardia. Note that yellow tags denote the right-sided His bundle and the blue tag denotes the earliest site in right atrium.

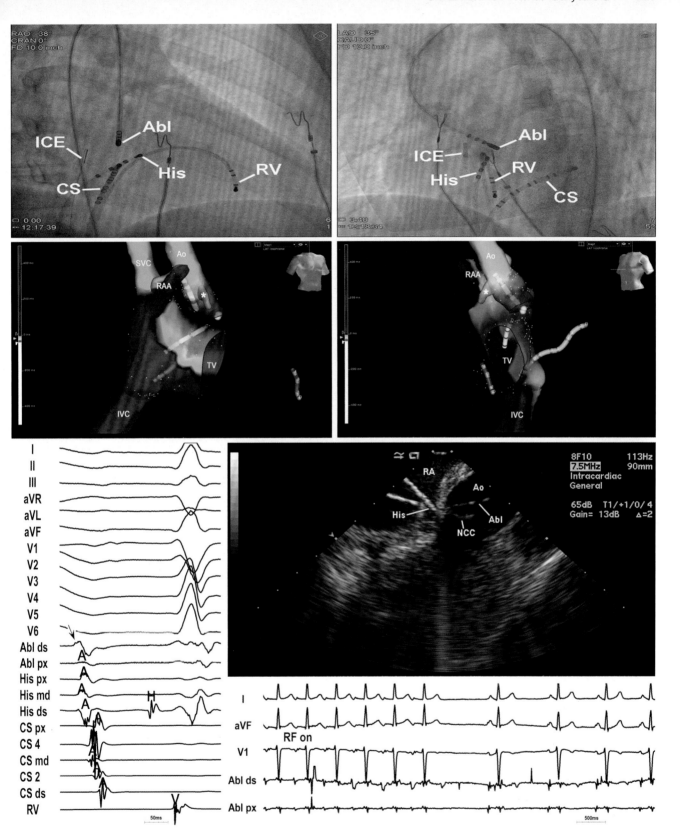

FIGURE 13-6 Ablation of NCC AT. The earliest site of atrial activation (*white, arrow*) precedes P-wave onset by 24 ms where application of RF energy terminates tachycardia in 1.9 sec. Note the proximity between the ablation catheter in the NCC and the His bundle on the other side of the septum. Note that yellow tags denote the left-sided His bundle and the asterisk denotes the right coronary artery.

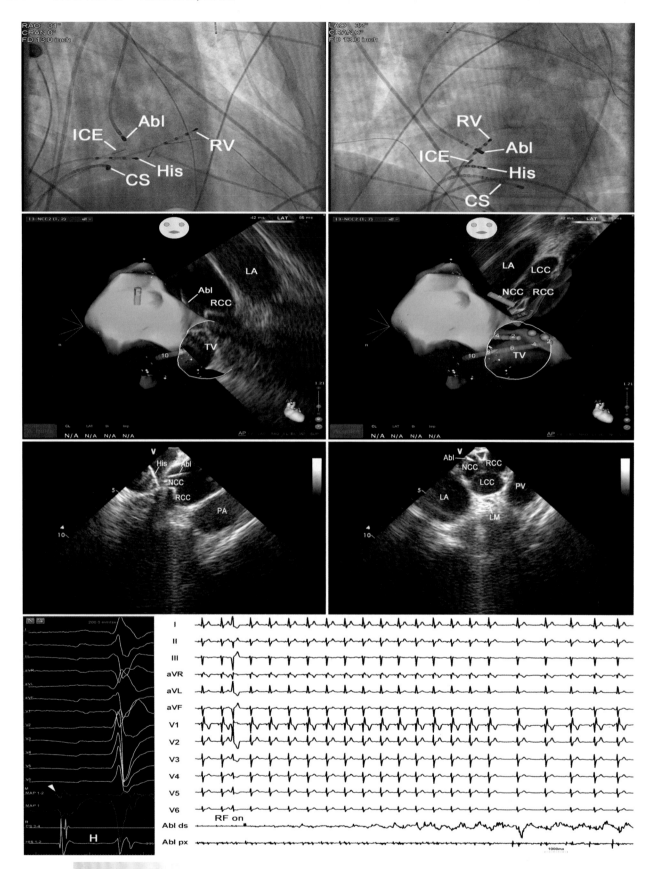

FIGURE 13-7 Ablation of NCC AT. The earliest site of atrial activation (*arrowhead*) precedes P-wave onset by 59 ms, and a unipolar QS signal is recorded. Application of RF energy terminates tachycardia in 11.6 sec. Note that the yellow tags denote the His bundle.

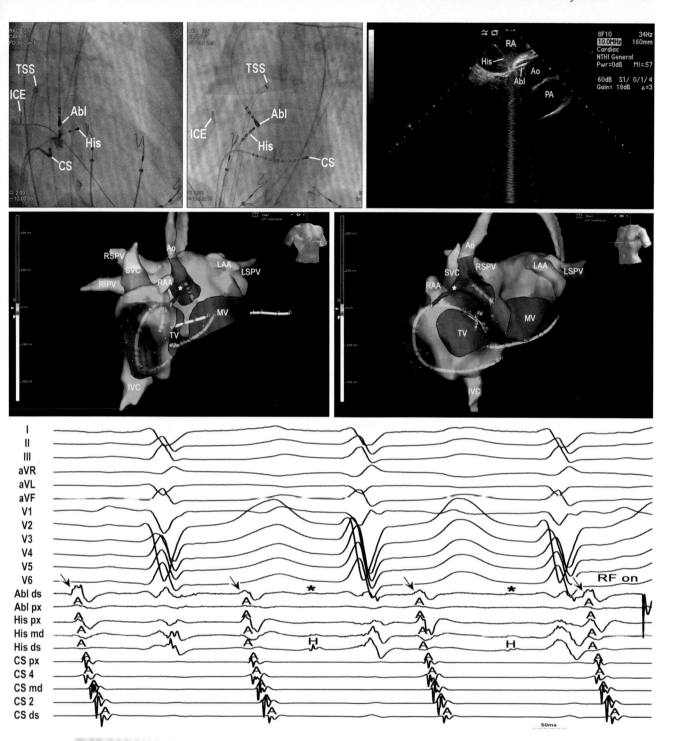

FIGURE 13-8 Ablation of NCC AT. The earliest site of atrial activation (*white, arrows*) precedes P-wave onset by 18 ms where application of RF energy terminated tachycardia. Note the very small, far-field His bundle electrograms (*black asterisk*) recorded on the ablation catheter and its close proximity to the His bundle catheter. Note that the white asterisk denotes the right coronary artery. TSS, Transeptal sheath.

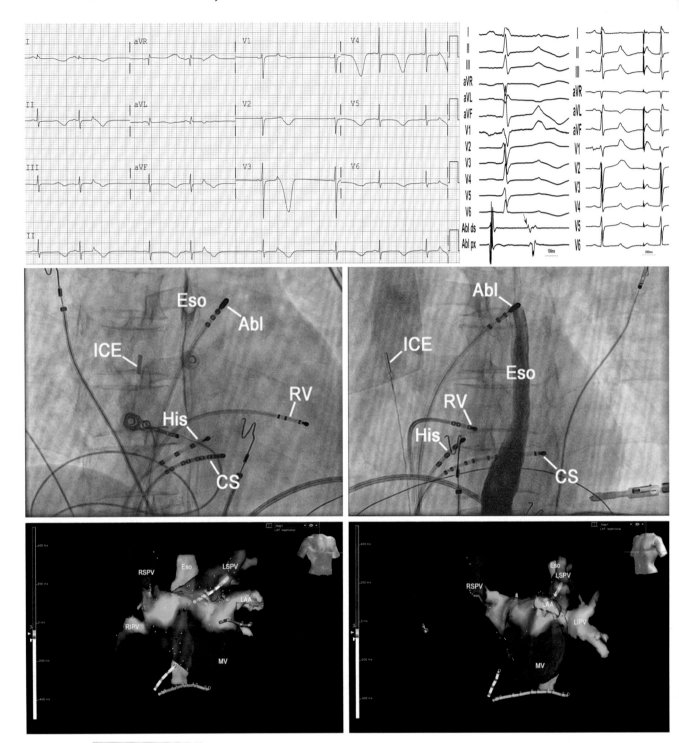

FIGURE 13-9 Ablation of LSPV AT. The earliest site of atrial activation (*arrow, white*) precedes P-wave onset by 41 ms where pacemaps matched clinical APCs and RF delivery abolished AT. Barium paste highlights the esophagus delineating its proximity to the ablation site.

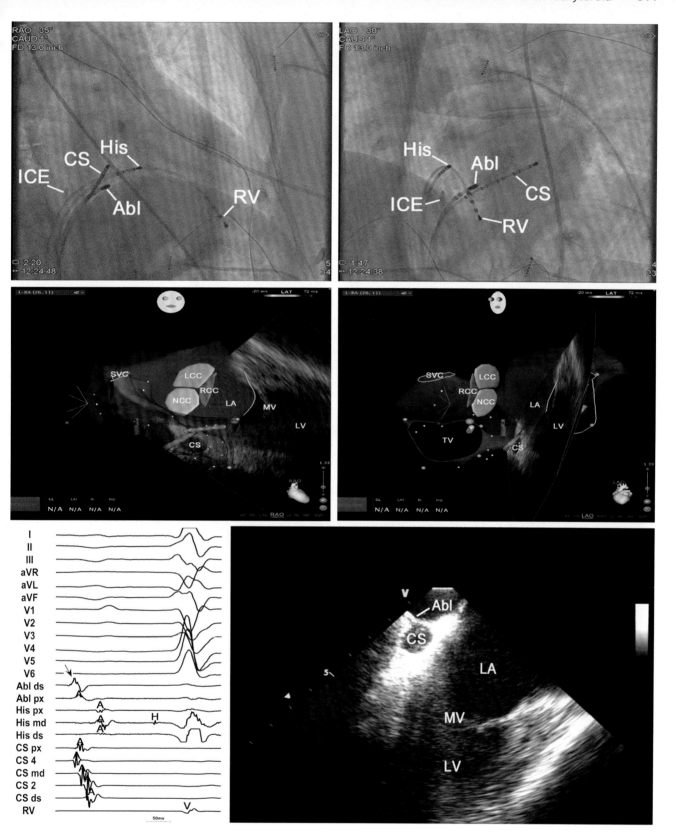

FIGURE 13-10 Ablation of CS AT. The earliest site of atrial activation (*red, arrow*) precedes P-wave onset by 24 ms where application of RF energy terminated tachycardia. Note that the yellow tag denotes the His bundle.

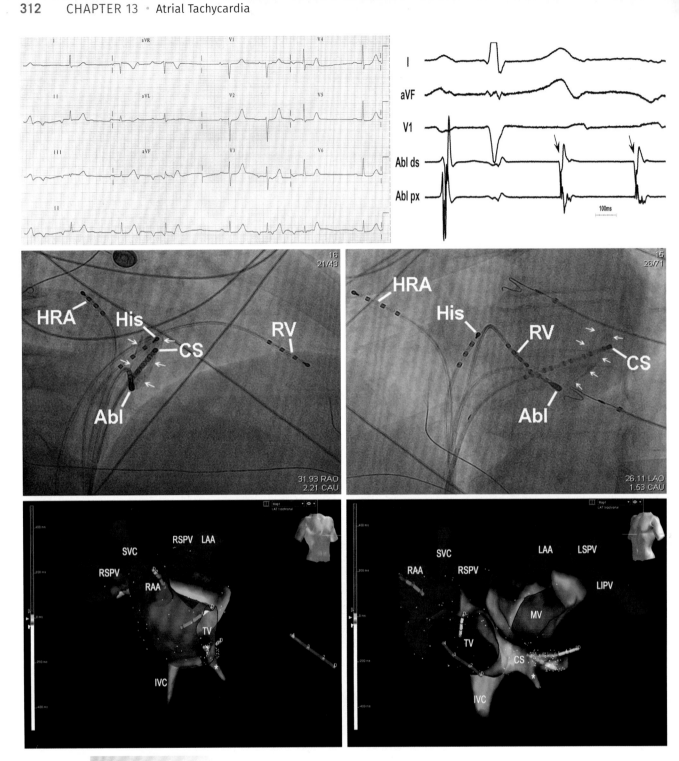

FIGURE 13-11 Ablation of CS AT. The successful ablation site records the earliest site of atrial activation (*black arrow, white*), which precedes P-wave onset by 24 ms. A venogram outlines the CS (*white arrows*).

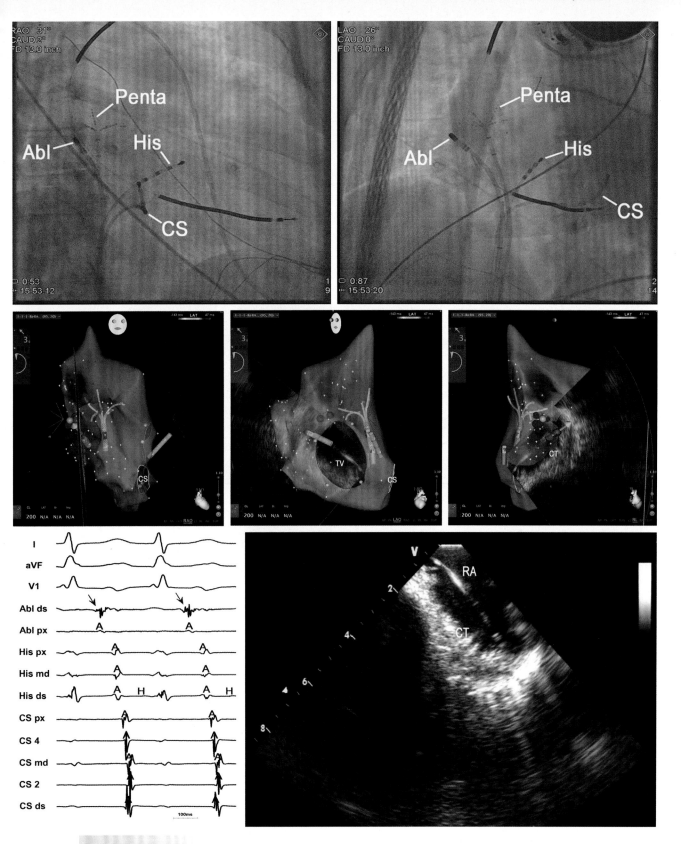

FIGURE 13-12 Ablation of "crista" tachycardia. The earliest site of atrial activation records a fractionated electrogram (*yellow tag, arrows*) that precedes P-wave onset by 39 ms but stimulates the right phrenic nerve during pacing (*blue tags*). RF delivery slightly inferiorly (*red tags*) where phrenic nerve stimulation did not occur successfully ablated AT. Penta, Pentaray catheter.

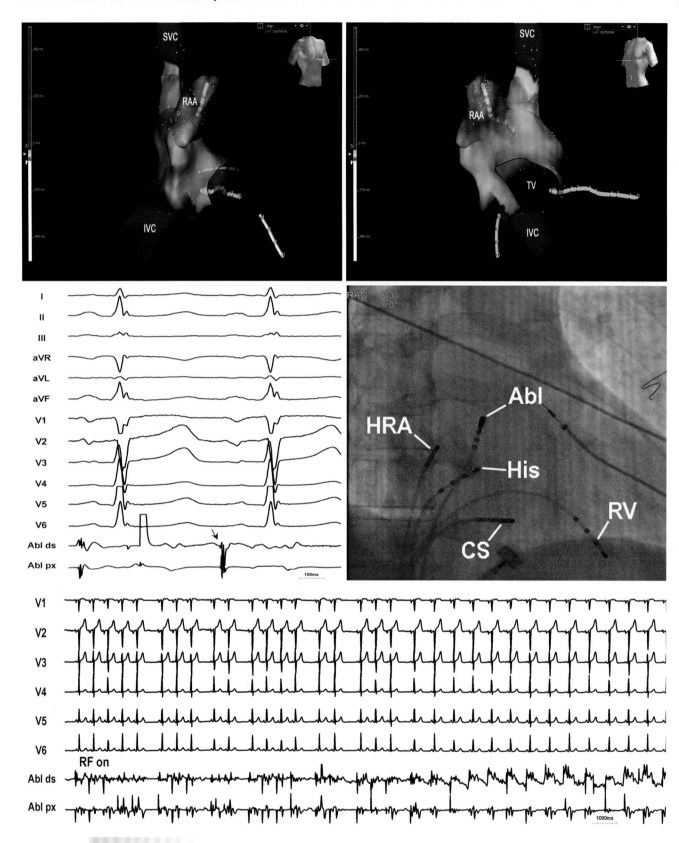

FIGURE 13-13 Ablation of right atrial appendage AT. The earliest site of atrial activation (*white, arrow*) precedes P-wave onset by 18 ms where application of RF energy terminated tachycardia in 3.4 sec. Note the slight difference in P-wave morphology between sinus rhythm (*left*) and AT (*right*).

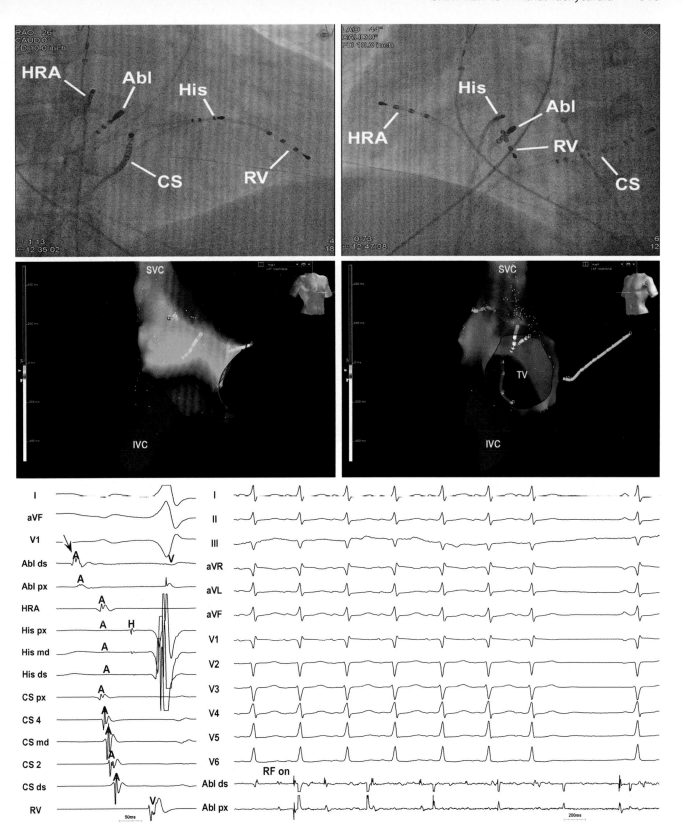

FIGURE 13-14 Ablation of anterior tricuspid annulus AT. The earliest site of atrial activation (*white, arrow*) precedes P-wave onset by 62 ms where application of RF energy terminated AT in 2.3 sec. A large atrial/small ventricular electrogram is recorded.

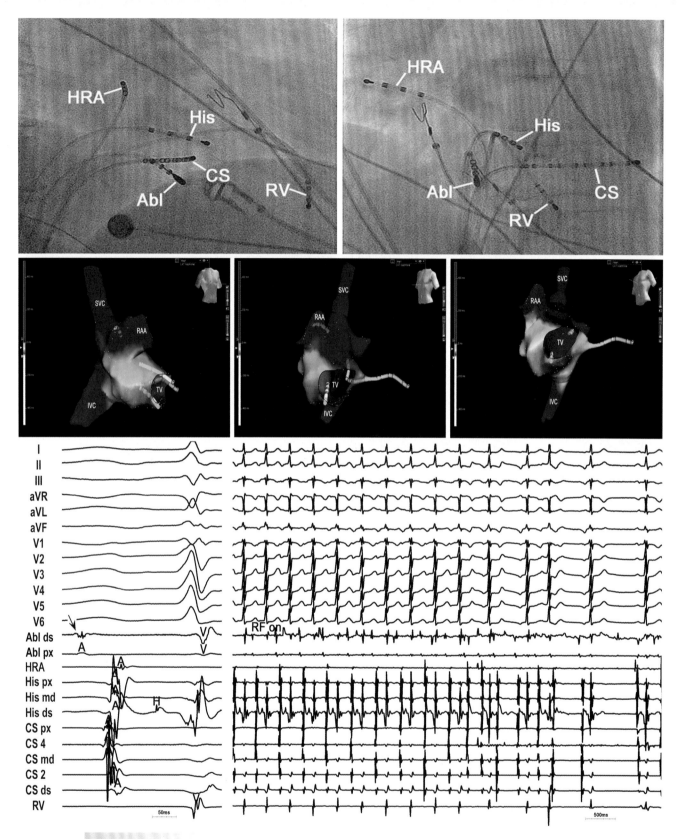

FIGURE 13-15 Ablation of inferior tricuspid annulus AT. The earliest site of atrial activation (*white, arrow*) precedes P-wave onset by 55 ms where application of RF energy slows and then terminates AT in 5.9 sec. Annular (atrial and ventricular) electrograms are recorded.

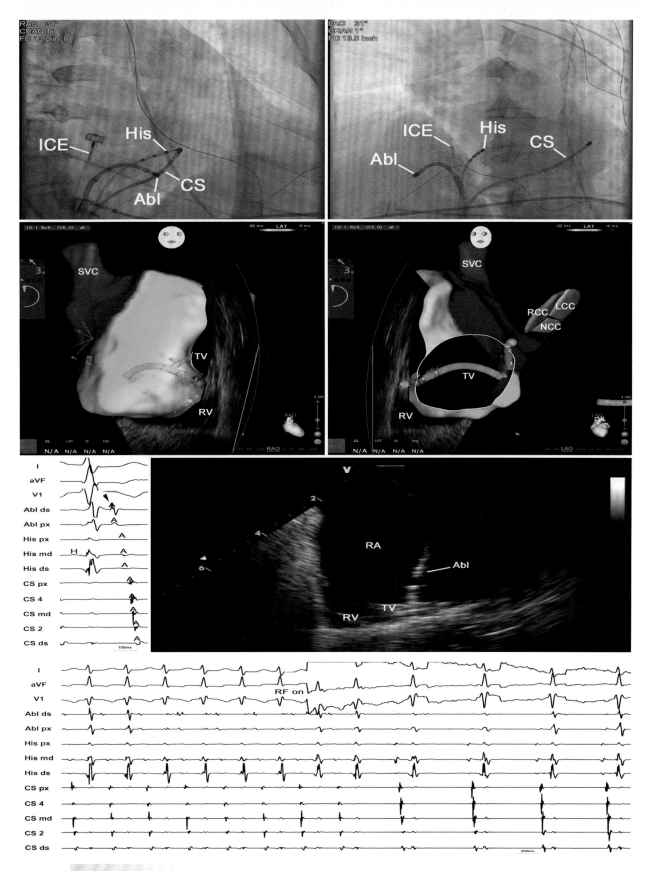

FIGURE 13-16 Ablation of lateral tricuspid annulus AT. Radiofrequency application to the earliest site of atrial activation (*red, arrowhead*) terminates AT in 0.74 sec. Annular (atrial and ventricular) electrograms are recorded.

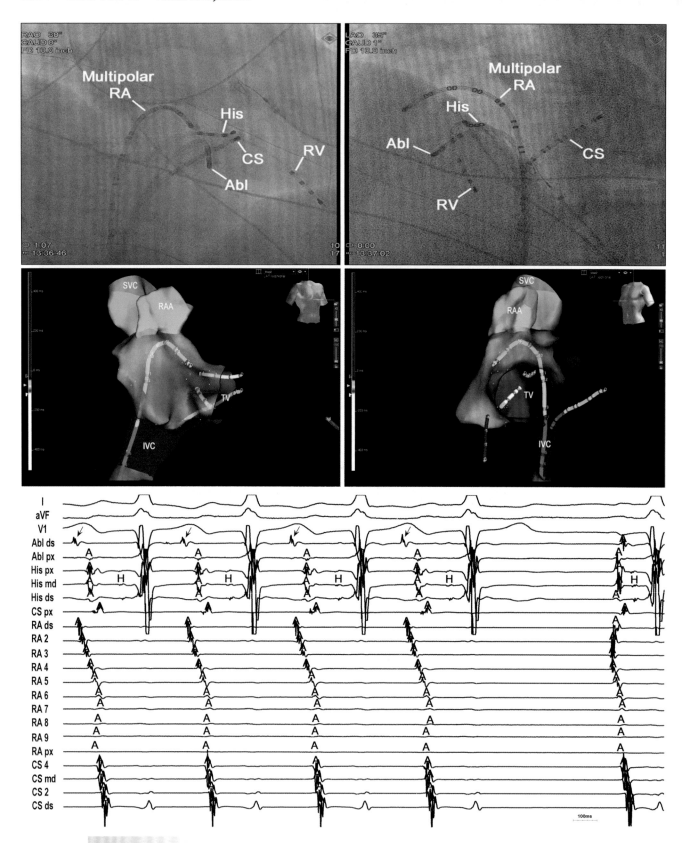

FIGURE 13-17 Ablation of lateral tricuspid annulus AT. Application of RF energy to the earliest site of atrial activation (*white, arrows*) terminates AT. Annular (atrial and ventricular) electrograms are recorded.

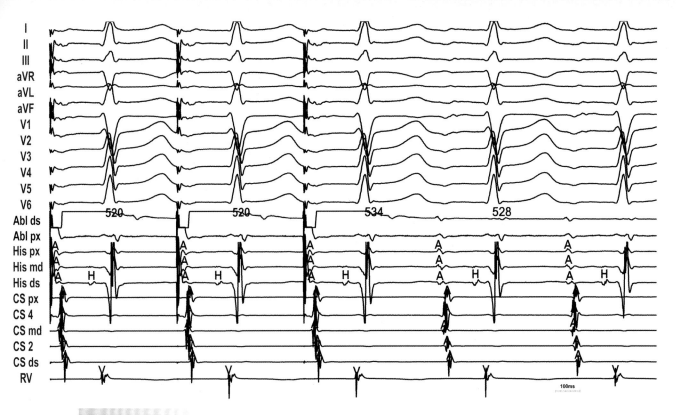

FIGURE 13-18 Post-pacing interval (PPI) after atrial overdrive pacing. At the successful ablation site of NCC AT, the paced activation sequence matches AT and PPI − TCL = 6 ms.

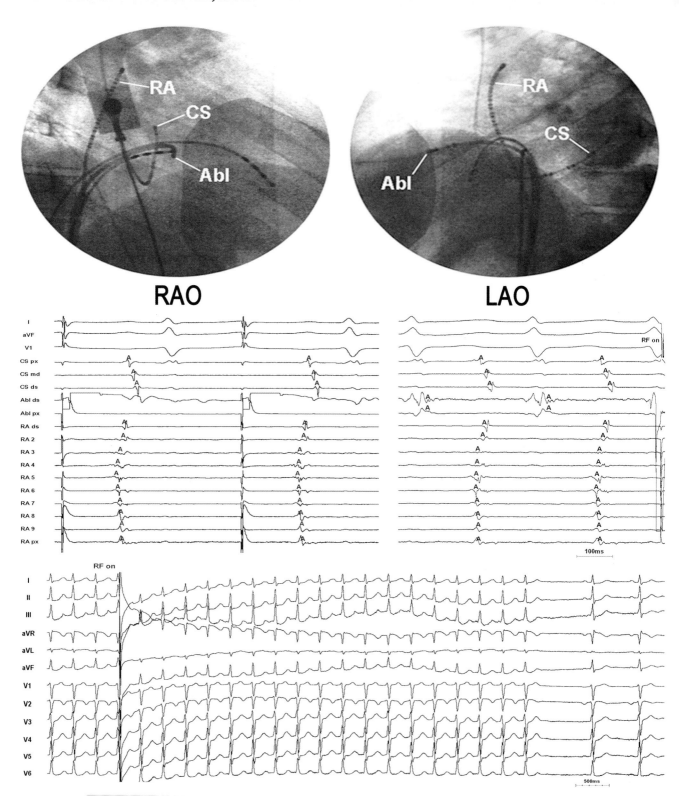

FIGURE 13-19 Paced (*left*) and activation (*right*) maps at the successful ablation site of a macroreentrant AT along the lateral tricuspid annulus. Paced and tachycardia atrial activation patterns are identical. Long St-P wave intervals match egm-P wave intervals, indicating an isthmus site (zone of slow conduction) within the circuit. Application of RF energy terminates tachycardia in 6.2 sec.

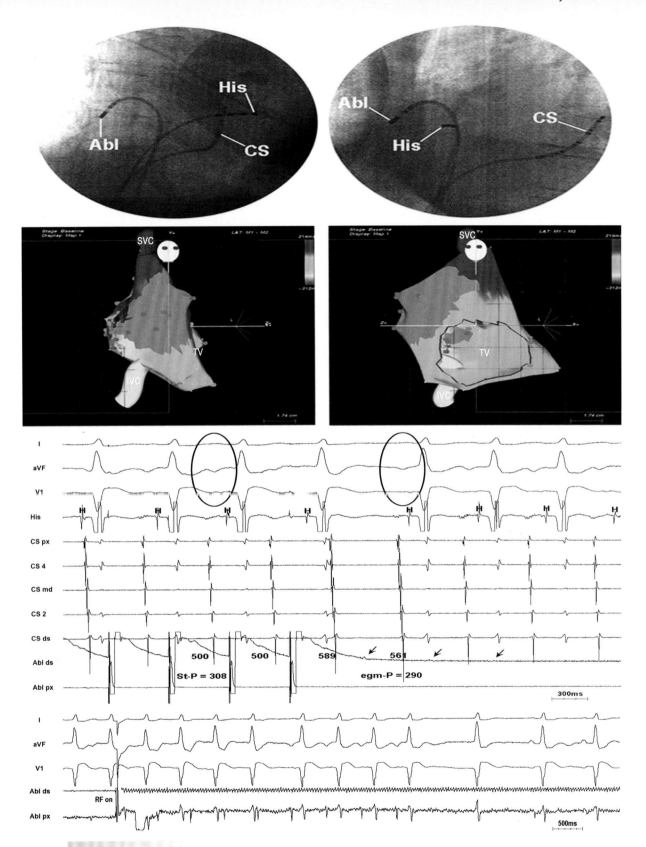

FIGURE 13-20 Central isthmus site (macroreentrant right AT). Paced and AT P waves (*encircled*) are identical (concealed fusion). The St-P wave interval (55% atrial tachycardia cycle length [ATCL]) − egm-P wave interval = 18 ms. The PPI − ATCL = 28 ms. Application of RF energy terminated tachycardia in 5.0 sec. Note that the gray area denotes a scar, the red tag denotes an ablation lesion, and the arrow denotes the mid-diastolic potential.

TABLE 13-1 Characteristics of macroreentrant AT circuit sites

Circuit site	Fusion type	St-P − egm-P	PPI − TCL
Exit	Concealed	≤30 ms (St-P <30% TCL)	≤30 ms
Central	Concealed	≤30 ms (St-P 30–60% TCL)	≤30 ms
Entrance	Concealed	≤30 ms (St-P >60% TCL)	≤30 ms
Outer loop	Manifest	>30 ms (except near Exit)	≤30 ms
Adjacent bystander	Concealed	>30 ms	>30 ms
Remote bystander	Manifest	>30 ms	>30 ms

REFERENCES

1. Roberts-Thomson KC, Kistler PM, Kalman JM. Focal atrial tachycardia I: clinical features, diagnosis, mechanisms, and anatomic location. Pacing Clin Electrophysiol 2006;29:643–652.
2. Kistler PM, Roberts-Thomson KC, Haqqani HM, et al. P-wave morphology in focal atrial tachycardia: development of an algorithm to predict the anatomic site of origin. J Am Coll Cardiol 2006;48:1010–1017.
3. Kistler PM, Kalman JM. Locating focal atrial tachycardias from P-wave morphology. Heart Rhythm 2005;2:561–564.
4. Roberts-Thomson KC, Kistler PM, Kalman JM. Focal atrial tachycardia II: management. Pacing Clin Electrophysiol 2006;29:769–778.
5. Teh AW, Kistler PM, Kalman JM. Using the 12-lead ECG to localize the origin of ventricular and atrial tachycardias: part 1. Focal atrial tachycardia. J Cardiovasc Electrophysiol 2009;20:706–709.
6. Tang CW, Scheinman MM, Van Hare GF, et al. Use of P wave configuration during atrial tachycardia to predict site of origin. J Am Coll Cardiol 1995;26:1315–1324.
7. Kalman JM, Olgin JE, Karch MR, Hamdan M, Lee RJ, Lesh MD. "Cristal tachycardias": origin of right atrial tachycardias from the crista terminalis identified by intracardiac echocardiography. J Am Coll Cardiol 1998;31:451–459.
8. Roberts-Thomson KC, Kistler PM, Haqqani HM, et al. Focal atrial tachycardias arising from the right atrial appendage: electrocardiographic and electrophysiologic characteristics and radiofrequency ablation. J Cardiovasc Electrophysiol 2007;18:367–372.
9. Morton JB, Sanders P, Das A, Vohra JK, Sparks PB, Kalman JM. Focal atrial tachycardia arising from the tricuspid annulus: electrophysiologic and electrocardiographic characteristics. J Cardiovasc Electrophysiol 2001;12:653–659.
10. Kistler PM, Fynn SP, Haqqani H, et al. Focal atrial tachycardia from the ostium of the coronary sinus: electrocardiographic and electrophysiological characterization and radiofrequency ablation. J Am Coll Cardiol 2005;45:1488–1493.
11. Badhwar N, Kalman JM, Sparks PB, et al. Atrial tachycardia arising from the coronary sinus musculature: electrophysiological characteristics and long-term outcomes of radiofrequency ablation. J Am Coll Cardiol 2005;46:1921–1930.
12. Ouyang F, Ma J, Ho SY, et al. Focal atrial tachycardia originating from the non-coronary aortic sinus: electrophysiological characteristics and catheter ablation. J Am Coll Cardiol 2006;48:122–131.
13. Liu X, Dong J, Ho SY, et al. Atrial tachycardia arising adjacent to noncoronary aortic sinus: distinctive atrial activation patterns and anatomic insights. J Am Coll Cardiol 2010;56:796–804.
14. Wang Z, Liu T, Shehata M, et al. Electrophysiological characteristics of focal atrial tachycardia surrounding the aortic coronary cusps. Circ Arrhythm Electrophysiol 2011;4:902–908.
15. Beukema RJ, Smit JJ, Adiyaman A, et al. Ablation of focal atrial tachycardia from the non-coronary aortic cusp: case series and review of the literature. Europace 2015;17:953–961.
16. Kistler PM, Sanders P, Hussin A, et al. Focal atrial tachycardia arising from the mitral annulus: electrocardiographic and electrophysiologic characterization. J Am Coll Cardiol 2003;41:2212–2219.
17. Kistler PM, Sanders P, Fynn SP, et al. Electrophysiological and electrocardiographic characteristics of focal atrial tachycardia originating from the pulmonary veins: acute and long-term outcomes of radiofrequency ablation. Circulation 2003;108:1968–1975.
18. Knight B, Zivin A, Souza J, et al. A technique for the rapid diagnosis of atrial tachycardia in the electrophysiology laboratory. J Am Coll Cardiol 1999;33:775–781.
19. Vijayaraman P, Lee BP, Kalahasty G, Wood MA, Ellenbogen KA. Reanalysis of the "pseudo A-A-V" response to ventricular entrainment of supraventricular tachycardia: importance of His-bundle timing. J Cardiovasc Electrophysiol 2006;17:25–28.
20. Jastrzebski M, Kukla P. The V-A-V response to ventricular entrainment during atrial tachycardia: what is the mechanism? J Cardiovasc Electrophysiol 2012;23:1266–1268.
21. Maruyama M, Kobayashi Y, Miyauchi Y, et al. The VA relationship after differential atrial overdrive pacing: a novel tool for the diagnosis of atrial tachycardia in the electrophysiologic laboratory. J Cardiovasc Electrophysiol 2007;18:1127–1133.
22. Sarkozy A, Richter S, Chierchia G, et al. A novel pacing manoeuvre to diagnose atrial tachycardia. Europace 2008;10:459–466.
23. Kay GN, Chong F, Epstein AE, Dailey SM, Plumb VJ. Radiofrequency ablation for treatment of primary atrial tachycardias. J Am Coll Cardiol 1993;21:901–909.
24. Lesh MD, Van Hare GF, Epstein LM, et al. Radiofrequency catheter ablation of atrial arrhythmias. Results and mechanisms. Circulation 1994;89:1074–1089.
25. Poty H, Saoudi N, Haissaguerre M, Daou A, Clementy J, Letac B. Radiofrequency catheter ablation of atrial tachycardias. Am Heart J 1996;131:481–489.
26. Tracy CM, Swartz JF, Fletcher RD, et al. Radiofrequency catheter ablation of ectopic atrial tachycardia using paced activation sequence mapping. J Am Coll Cardiol 1993;21:910–917.
27. Mohamed U, Skanes AC, Gula LJ, et al. A novel pacing maneuver to localize focal atrial tachycardia. J Cardiovasc Electrophysiol 2007;18:1–6.
28. Kalman JM, VanHare GF, Olgin JE, Saxon LA, Stark SI, Lesh MD. Ablation of 'incisional' reentrant atrial tachycardia complicating surgery for congenital heart disease. Use of entrainment to define a critical isthmus of conduction. Circulation 1996;93:502–512.
29. Chen S, Chiang C, Yang C, et al. Radiofrequency catheter ablation of sustained intra-atrial reentrant tachycardia in adult patients. Identification of electrophysiological characteristics and endocardial mapping techniques. Circulation 1993;88:578–587.
30. Triedman JK, Saul JP, Weindling SN, Walsh EP. Radiofrequency ablation of intra-atrial reentrant tachycardia after surgical palliation of congenital heart disease. Circulation 1995;91:707–714.
31. Esato M, Hindricks G, Sommer P, et al. Color-coded three-dimensional entrainment mapping for analysis and treatment of atrial macroreentrant tachycardia. Heart Rhythm 2009;6:349–358.
32. Scott LR, Hadian D, Olgin JE, Miller JM. Termination of reentrant atrial tachycardia by a nonpropagated extrastimulus. J Cardiovasc Electrophysiol 2001;12:388.
33. Barkagan M, Michowitz Y, Glick A, Tovia-Brodie O, Rosso R, Belhassen B. Atrial tachycardia originating in the vicinity of the noncoronary sinus of Valsalva: report of a series including the first case of ablation-related complete atrioventricular block. Pacing Clin Electrophysiol 2016;39:1165–1173.

Introduction

Atrial flutter is a macroreentrant atrial tachycardia that can be categorized by the location of its reentrant circuit and the protected isthmus of slow conduction. The most common type is counterclockwise (CCW) cavo-tricuspid isthmus (CTI)-dependent atrial flutter. The CTI is a protected isthmus of slow conduction between the tricuspid annulus and inferior vena cava (IVC) and the target site of ablation for CTI-dependent flutter.[1–4] CTI-dependent flutters revolve around the tricuspid annulus most commonly in a CCW ("typical") but also clockwise (CW) ("atypical") direction resulting in lateral to medial or medial to lateral activation of the CTI, respectively. Non–CTI-dependent flutters (also "atypical") occur in diseased atria and include 1) post-surgical right atrial flutters (e.g., incisional flutters around an old atriotomy or atrial septal defect) and 2) left atrial flutters (Fig. 14-1). Left atrial flutters are rare in patients with structurally normal atria and are seen after atrial fibrillation ablation (e.g., "gap" flutter through incomplete ablation lines, perimitral or roof flutter) or after mitral valve surgery. This chapter focuses on the diagnosis and ablation of CTI-dependent atrial flutter.

The purpose of this chapter is to:

1. Discuss the anatomy of the CTI.
2. Define the circuit and electrophysiologic features of CTI-dependent atrial flutter and the technique to demonstrate CTI dependency.
3. Discuss ablation of the CTI and mapping gaps along the ablation line.
4. Define procedural endpoints for successful ablation of the CTI.

ANATOMY OF THE CAVO-TRICUSPID ISTHMUS

The CTI is the region of right atrial tissue bounded posteriorly by the IVC and anteriorly by the tricuspid annulus forming a protected zone of slow conduction that plays a critical role in CTI-dependent flutter. The CTI can be divided into three sections: septal, central (6 o'clock on LAO view), and inferolateral isthmus.[5] The thicker paraseptal isthmus is bounded by the coronary sinus (CS) os and thick eustachian ridge and closer to the right inferior extension of the atrio-ventricular (AV) node and AV nodal artery. The inferolateral isthmus is the longest, contains pectinate muscles of the terminal crest, and is closest endocardially to the right coronary artery. The central isthmus is the shortest and thinnest but a potential site for pouch-like recesses. CTI ablation involves creation of a line of block (LOB) across the isthmus by a series of coalescing ablation lesions that connect the 1) tricuspid annulus to the IVC (posterior line transecting the central or inferolateral isthmus) or 2) tricuspid annulus to CS os—CS os to eustachian ridge/valve (septal line transecting the paraseptal isthmus with the eustachian ridge/valve serving as a LOB between the CS os and IVC).[2–4,6] Because the septal line is associated with a higher risk of AV block and traverses the thick muscular eustachian ridge making ablation difficult, a posterior line (particularly transecting the shorter, thinner central isthmus) is preferred as the initial target for ablation.[5,7]

CTI-DEPENDENT ATRIAL FLUTTER

CIRCUIT

The circuit for CCW CTI-dependent flutter is confined to the right atrium (RA) with lateral to medial conduction across the isthmus (Fig. 14-2). The CCW activation wavefront exits the medial end of the CTI near the CS os, ascends the interatrial septum, depolarizes the roof of the RA, and then descends along the anterolateral right atrial wall before depolarizing the lateral CTI. The left atrium is passively activated and not an integral

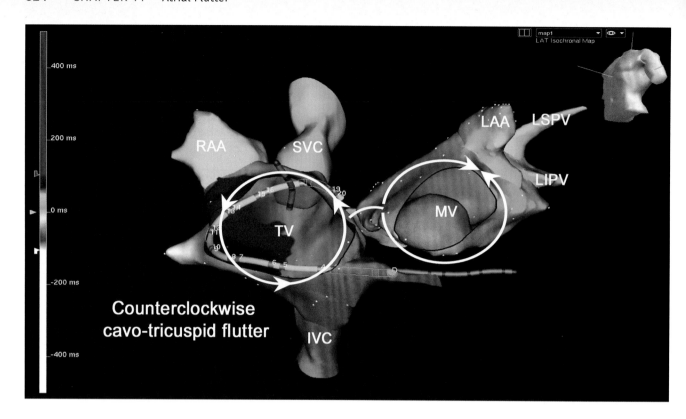

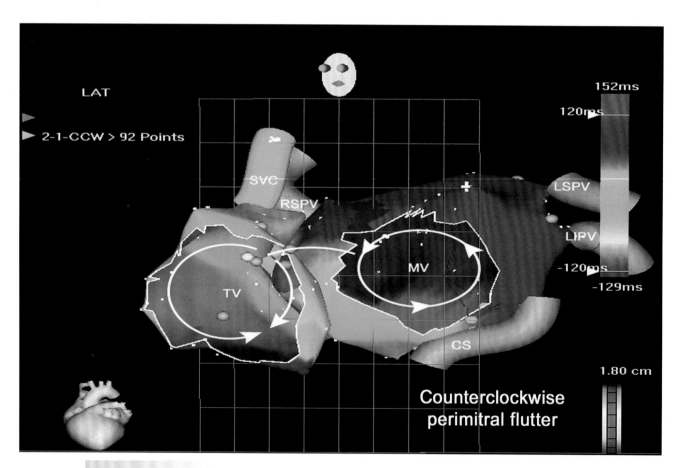

FIGURE 14-1 CCW CTI (*top*) and mitral isthmus (*bottom*) flutter. Note the "early meets late" pattern in the right and left atrium, respectively, with passive activation of the counterpart chamber.

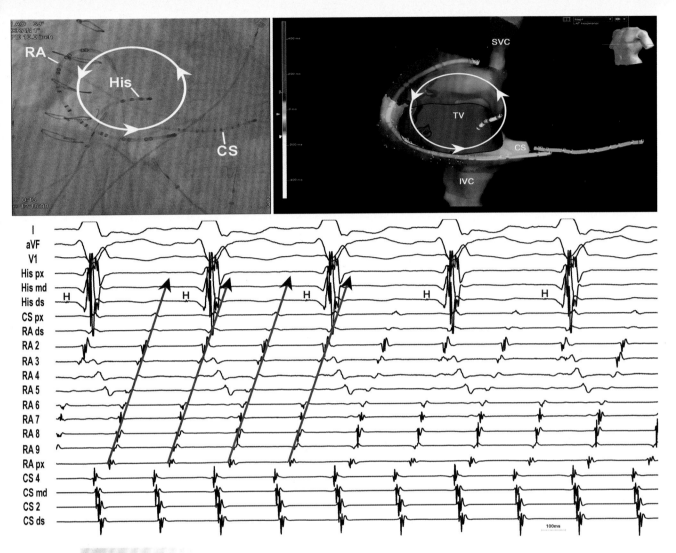

FIGURE 14-2 CCW CTI-dependent atrial flutter. Note the "early meets late" pattern (*white/purple* interface) with CCW activation around the tricuspid annulus.

part of the circuit. Several anatomic barriers prevent a short circuit of the reentrant pathway and include the 1) tricuspid annulus (anterior barrier); 2) IVC, eustachian ridge (medially), and crista terminalis (laterally) (posterior barriers); 3) and endocardial cavity of the RA.[6,8,9] The circuit for CW CTI-dependent atrial flutter is the reverse of its typical counterpart with medial to lateral activation of the CTI (Fig. 14-3).

ELECTROPHYSIOLOGIC FEATURES

12-Lead ECG

The classic CCW CTI-dependent atrial flutter is 1) positive in V1; 2) negative in II, III, aVF ("sawtooth" pattern); and 3) absent isoelectric line (except in V1) (V1/II discordance) (Fig. 14-4). The downslope, nadir, and upslope of the "sawtooth" flutter wave correspond to ascending activation of the interatrial septum, depolarization of the right atrial roof, and descending

activation of the anterolateral free wall, respectively. Location of the isthmus exit site at the posteroseptum near the CS os creates an anteriorly directed flutter vector and, therefore, slightly positive flutter waves in V1. Continuous activation of the RA that spans the entire flutter cycle length causes absence of an isoelectric interval between flutter waves. CW CTI-dependent atrial flutter is opposite of its CCW counterpart: 1) negative in V1 and 2) positive in II, III, and aVF (often with notching) (V1/II discordance) (Fig. 14-4). Atrial flutter showing V1/II concordance (e.g., positive in V1 and II) indicates a non–CTI-dependent flutter (e.g., left atrial flutter).

Electrophysiologic Study

Demonstrating CCW and CW activation around the tricuspid annulus during CTI-dependent flutter involves mapping the RA with multipolar recording catheters: anterolateral RA and CTI ("Halo" catheter), 2) CS os (posteroseptum), and 3) His

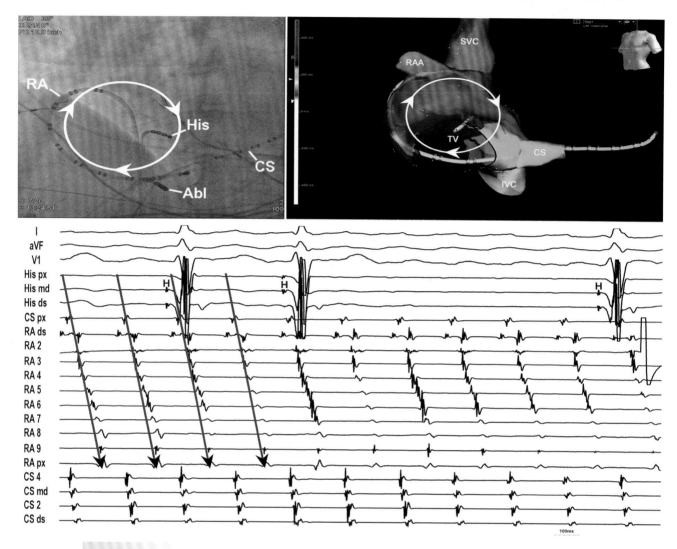

FIGURE 14-3 CW CTI-dependent atrial flutter. Note the "early meets late" pattern (*white/purple* interface) with CW activation around the tricuspid annulus.

bundle (anteroseptum) or a three-dimensional electro-anatomic mapping system. CCW CTI-dependent flutter is more readily induced by burst pacing than programmed extrastimulation, particularly from the smooth (medial) RA where pacing can induce medial to lateral block (unidirectional block) across the CTI (**Fig. 14-5**). Pacing from the trabeculated (lateral) RA induces CW CTI-dependent flutter.[10]

CTI DEPENDENCY

CTI dependency is determined by the response of atrial flutter to entrainment from the CTI (**Fig. 14-6**).[8,9] Delivery of pacing stimuli from the CTI at a cycle length 10–30 ms shorter than the flutter cycle length captures the atrium and penetrates its excitable gap, giving rise to orthodromic and antidromic wavefronts. The antidromic wavefront of the first stimulus (*n*) collides with tachycardia. Its orthodromic counterpart exits the isthmus, advances the atrium in the direction of tachycardia,

and collides with the antidromic wavefront of the next pacing stimulus (*n + 1*). Each *n* orthodromic wavefront collides with the *n + 1* antidromic wavefront until pacing stops. The last orthodromic wavefront has no antidromic wavefront with which to collide and completes one revolution around the circuit followed by continuation of atrial flutter. The post-pacing interval (PPI) (measured from the last pacing stimulus to the first atrial electrogram on the pacing catheter) equals the atrial flutter cycle length. The following criteria demonstrate CTI dependency with entrainment from the CTI: 1) concealed ECG fusion, 2) St-flutter wave = egm − flutter wave, and 3) PPI − atrial flutter cycle length ≤20 ms (**Fig. 14-6**). While surface ECG flutter morphology during entrainment and tachycardia are identical, intracardiac fusion occurs as a result of antidromic capture "upstream" to the pacing site. A PPI − atrial flutter cycle length >20 ms suggests a non–CTI-dependent flutter unless rate-dependent conduction delay within the circuit produces a long PPI (**Fig. 14-7**).[11]

Counterclockwise CTI Flutter

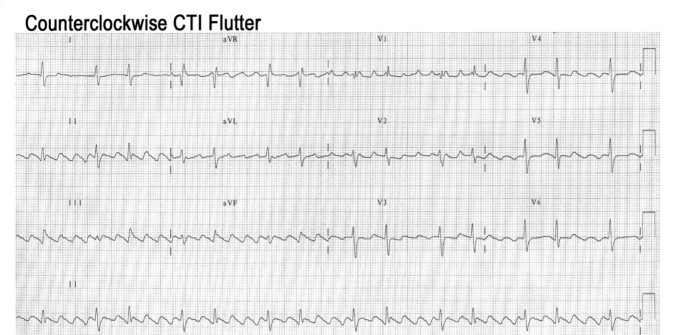

Clockwise CTI Flutter

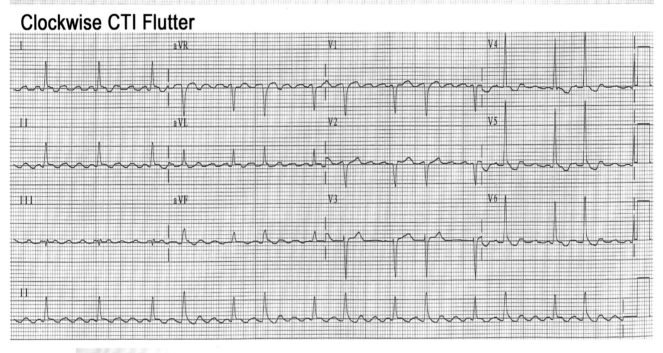

FIGURE 14-4 A 12-lead ECG of CCW and CW CTI-dependent atrial flutter. Note the discordant polarity of the atrial flutter waves in V1 and inferior leads. *Top*: Atrial flutter waves are positive in V1 and negative ("saw tooth") inferiorly. *Bottom*: Atrial flutter waves are negative in V1 and positive inferiorly. Both ECGs also show grouped QRS beating (alternating Wenckebach periodicity) due to two levels of AV block (upper level: 2:1; lower level: Wenckebach).

MAPPING AND ABLATION OF THE CTI

MAPPING

The CTI has a defined anatomic location, and ablation can be performed either during sinus rhythm (CS pacing) or atrial flutter.[12,13] Ongoing flutter, however, allows both entrainment

and termination to prove CTI dependency. The ablation catheter is positioned at the annular end of the CTI where small atrial and large ventricular electrograms are recorded. Radiofrequency (RF) energy is delivered in a point by point ("spot welding") or continuous ("drag") fashion as the catheter is pulled back across the floor of the CTI from annular to caval end. Effective lesions are indicated by voltage abatement and

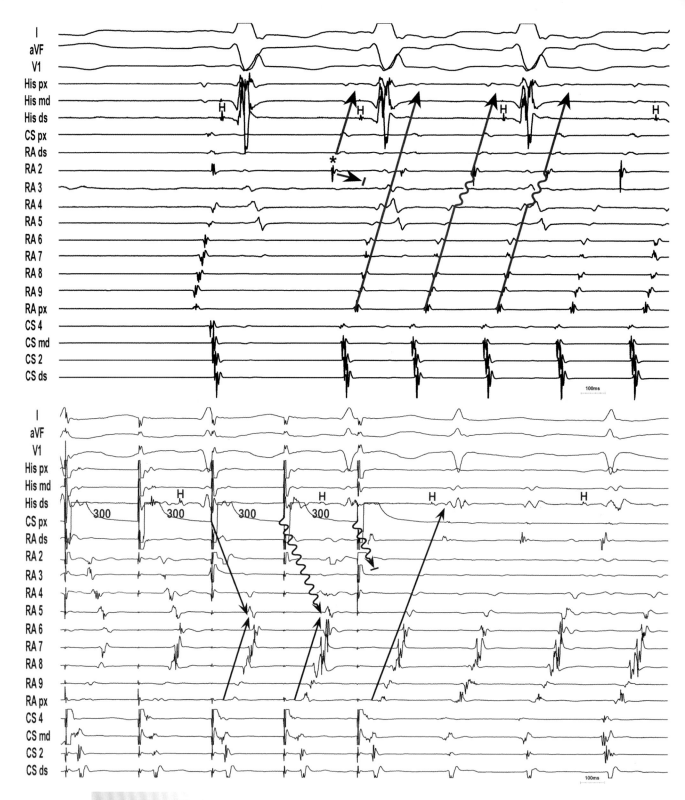

FIGURE 14-5 Induction of CCW CTI-dependent atrial flutter by an APC (*asterisk*) (*top*) and rapid atrial pacing (*bottom*). In both cases, medial to lateral CTI block ("unidirectional block") followed by CCW activation around the tricuspid annulus ("slow conduction") initiates macroreentry.

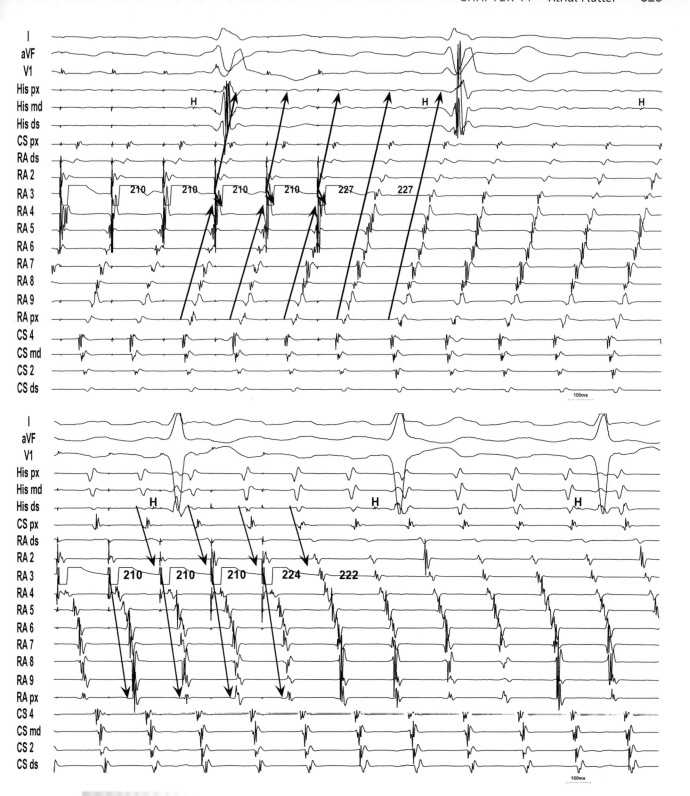

FIGURE 14-6 Entrainment of CCW (*top*) and CW (*bottom*) CTI-dependent atrial flutter from the CTI. In both cases, entrainment with concealed fusion and PPI ≈ TCL (<20 ms) indicate CTI dependency.

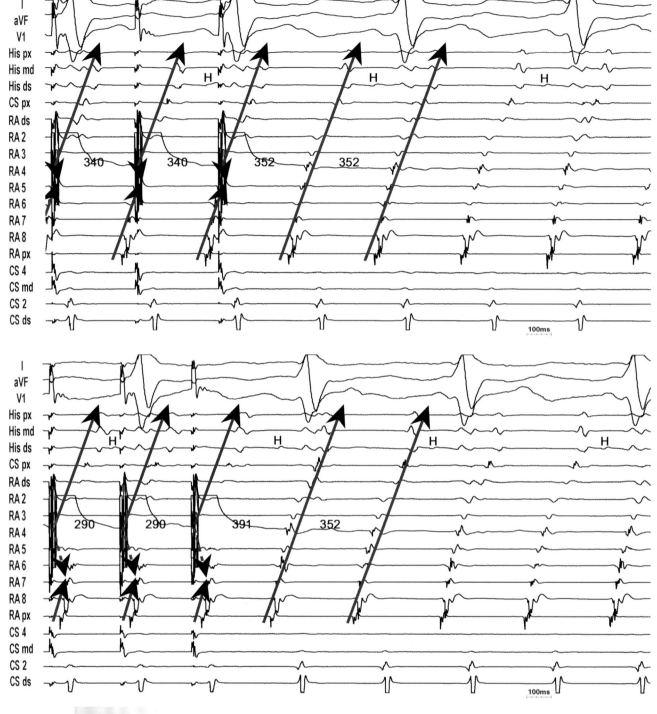

FIGURE 14-7 Entrainment of CCW CTI-dependent atrial flutter with progressive fusion and long PPI. *Top:* At a pacing cycle length of 340 ms, entrainment results in constant concealed fusion, the last orthodromically entrained electrograms occurring at the pacing cycle length (electrograms downstream to the point of orthodromic/antidromic collision [RA 4 and 5]), and PPI = TCL (first criteria of transient entrainment). A faster pacing cycle length of 290 ms results in progressive fusion (greater antidromic capture from the pacing site with the collision point shifted upstream [RA 6 and 7]) and PPI − TCL = 39 ms.

loss of sharp, high-frequency content (often accompanied by referred pain to the right shoulder). RAO fluoroscopy estimates the degree of posterior catheter movement along the CTI, while the LAO view reveals medial or lateral drift of the catheter from the ablation line.

During Atrial Flutter

Successful CTI ablation results in cycle length slowing and/or termination of CTI-dependent flutter. The last recorded atrial electrogram is immediately upstream to the ablation line (Figs. 14-8 to 14-11).

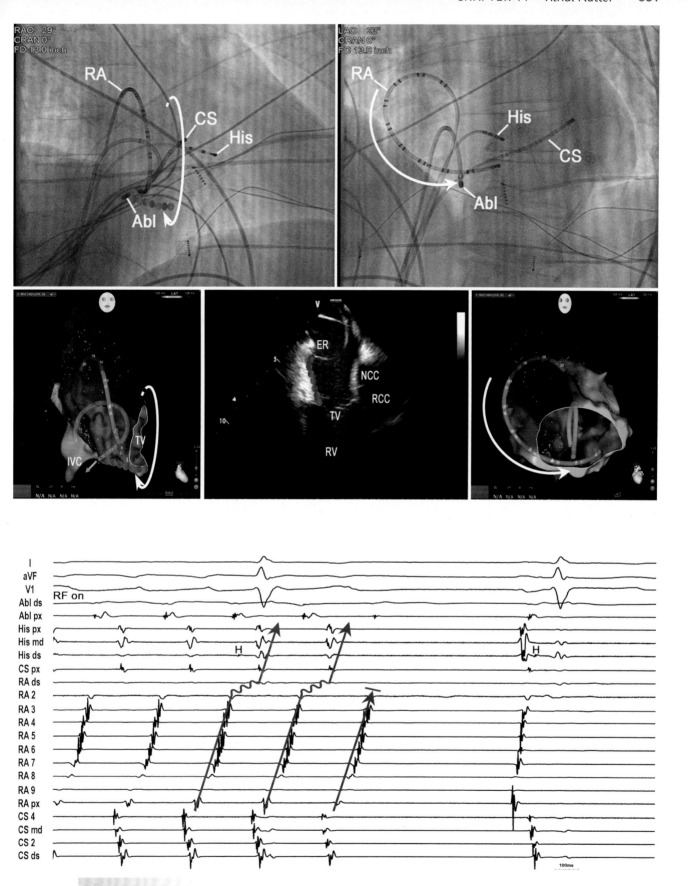

FIGURE 14-8 Termination of CCW CTI-dependent atrial flutter by ablation. Note the catheter inversion technique to target the thick posterior eustachian ridge. Red tags denote ablation lesions across the CTI.

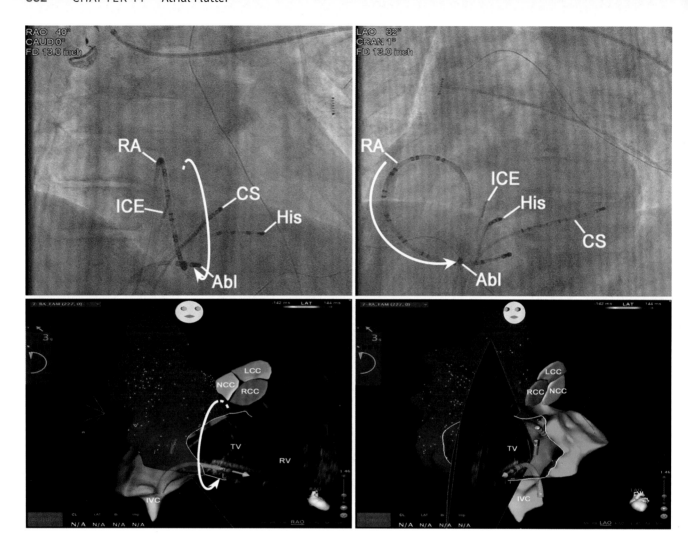

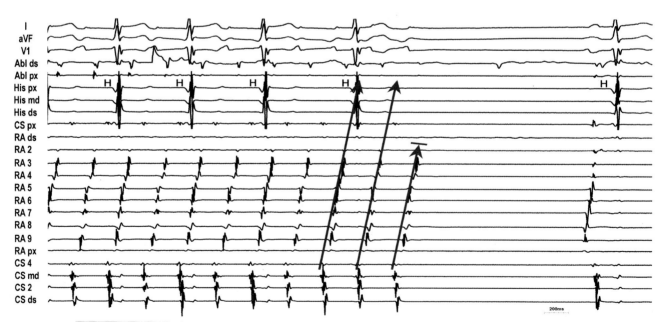

FIGURE 14-9 Termination of CCW CTI-dependent atrial flutter by ablation. Atrial flutter breaks in the CTI at the ablation line confirming isthmus dependency.

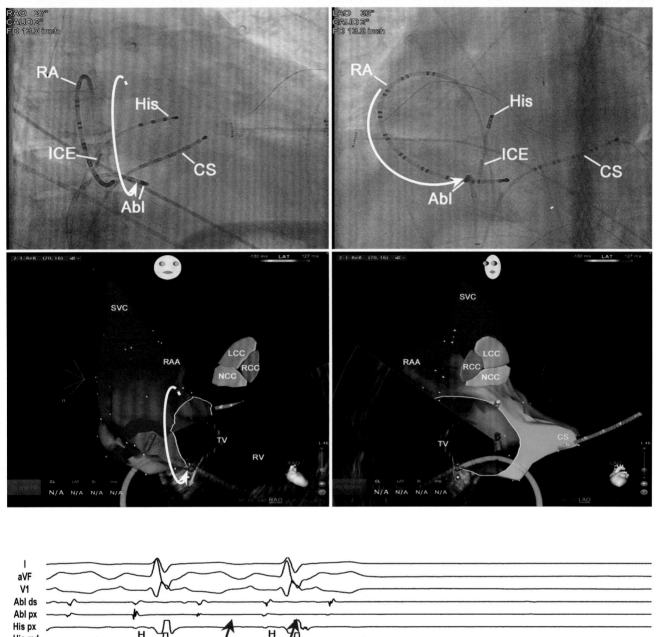

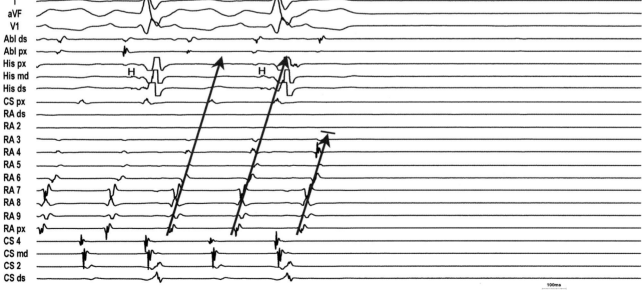

FIGURE 14-10 Termination of CCW CTI-dependent atrial flutter by ablation. Atrial flutter breaks in the CTI at the ablation line confirming isthmus dependency.

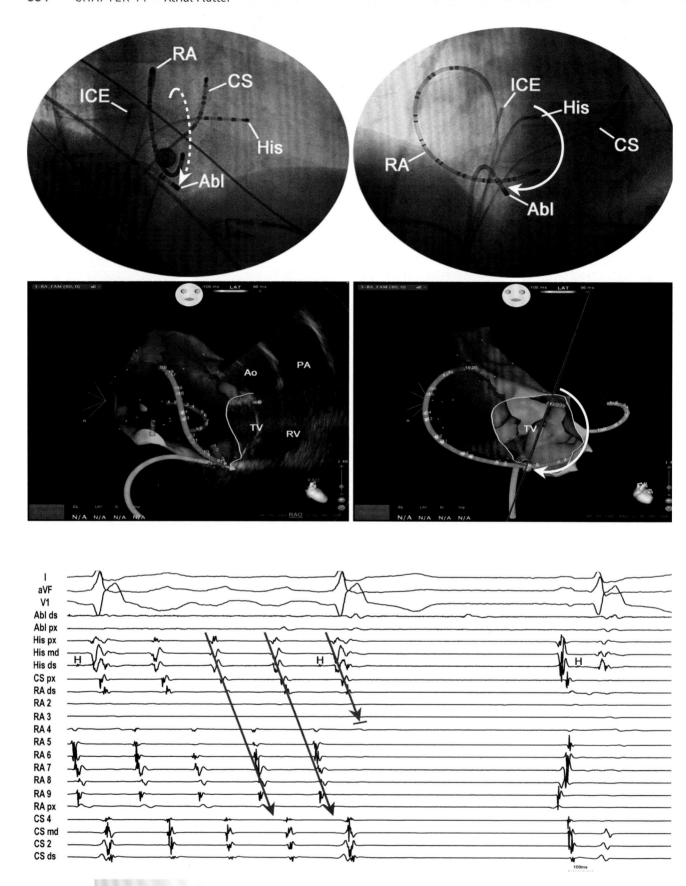

FIGURE 14-11 Termination of CW CTI-dependent atrial flutter by ablation. Atrial flutter breaks in the CTI at the ablation line confirming isthmus dependency.

During NSR

Pacing medial and lateral to the intended ablation line allows assessment of CTI conduction before and after ablation.

Pre-ablation

CS pacing can be substituted for direct stimulation of the CTI medial to the line. CS pacing generates two activation wavefronts (a CW wavefront that travels across the CTI and a CCW wavefront that travels up the interatrial septum), both of which collide along the anterolateral free wall of the RA creating a "chevron" pattern on Halo recordings (Fig. 14-12). Pacing lateral to the line also generates two activation wavefronts (a CW wavefront that travels up the anterolateral wall of the RA and a CCW wavefront that travels across the CTI), both of which collide along the anteroseptum of the RA causing atrial activation at the CS os to precede or coincide with that at the His bundle region (Fig. 14-13).

Post-ablation

During CS pacing, the CW wavefront fails to cross the ablation line so that most of the RA including the lateral CTI is activated by the CCW wavefront (Fig. 14-12). Similarly, the CCW wavefront during lateral pacing fails to cross the ablation line so that most of the RA including the medial CTI is activated by the CW wavefront resulting in atrial activation at the His bundle preceding that at the CS os (His-CS reversal) (Fig. 14-13). Collision of CW and CCW wavefronts at the ablation line when pacing on either side of the line generates a corridor of parallel, widely spaced double potentials (DPs) along its length. Rarely, CTI block can be rate dependent (Fig. 14-14). CW CTI block can also be confirmed by retrograde conduction over the AV node (atrio-ventricular nodal reentrant tachycardia [AVNRT] or ventricular pacing) or a posteroseptal AP (medial [septal] to the LOB) (Figs. 14-15 and 14-16).[14]

GAP MAPPING

Common anatomic sites for persistent gaps across the CTI are 1) anteriorly (vestibule of the tricuspid valve immediately posterior to the tricuspid annulus) and 2) posteriorly (cavo-atrial junction and eustachian ridge).[15,16] A gap along the ablation line can be mapped by identifying single or fractionated electrograms adjacent to sites along the line demonstrating narrowly spaced DPs (Figs. 14-17 and 14-18).[17] DPs indicate a line of local conduction block with activation on both sides of the line.[18,19] Narrowly spaced DPs result from activation on both sides of an incomplete line by a single wavefront that passes through the gap. The degree of DP separation is directly related to the distance from the gap. Closer recordings to the gap result in narrowing of DPs until a single or fractionated electrogram is recorded at the gap. A peculiar target for successful ablation is a site where a nonpropagated extrastimulus terminates atrial flutter. Such an extrastimulus depolarizes a critical portion of the circuit, rendering it refractory without propagating to the surrounding atrium (nonglobal capture).[20]

DIFFICULT CTI ABLATION

Strategies to overcome difficult CTI ablation include 1) using a long sheath (for stability) or irrigated ablation catheter (to deliver more power), 2) creating a line lateral to the initial line (avoiding the thicker septal CTI), 3) targeting sites with maximum voltage atrial electrograms ("muscle bundle" hypothesis), and 4) using intracardiac echocardiography (ICE) to identify anatomic abnormalities (thick eustachian ridge, pouch-like recess) to guide lesion deployment (Fig. 14-19).[21,22] A catheter inversion technique is particularly useful when a "vertical or right-angled" eustachian ridge makes ablation using a pullback approach difficult (Figs. 14-8 and 14-19).[23]

PROCEDURAL ENDPOINTS

Termination of CTI-dependent atrial flutter and inability to induce atrial flutter are unreliable endpoints for successful ablation. The goal of ablation is to create bidirectional block across the CTI.[13,17] Adenosine or isoproterenol can be used to unmask dormant CTI conduction after acutely successful ablation.[24–27]

WIDELY SPACED DOUBLE POTENTIALS

The gold standard demonstrating bidirectional conduction block across the CTI is recording a corridor of parallel, widely spaced (≥110 ms) DPs along the ablation line when pacing medial and lateral to the ablation line (Figs. 14-12 and 14-13).[17] The widely spaced DPs result from activation on both sides of the line by the CW and CCW wavefronts generated during pacing. In contrast to widely spaced DPs that represent complete block, narrowly spaced DPs (<90 ms) result from incomplete block and a gap in the ablation line that requires further ablation. These narrowly spaced DPs reflect activation on both sides of the line by a single wavefront that traverses the gap. For intermediate-spaced DPs (90–110 ms), the following clues suggest complete CTI block: 1) isoelectric interval between DPs, 2) negative second potential (DP_2) (reflecting reversal of electrogram polarity on the opposite side of the line), and 3) maximal variation between DPs <15 ms along the entire length of the line (parallel DPs).

ATRIAL ACTIVATION/ELECTROGRAM POLARITY REVERSAL

Before ablation, pacing one end of the CTI activates the opposite end by transisthmus conduction. After ablation, loss of transisthmus conduction results in reversal of atrial activation at the opposite end of the CTI line. This directional shift in CTI activation causes reversal in its atrial activation sequence and electrogram polarity.[28–30]

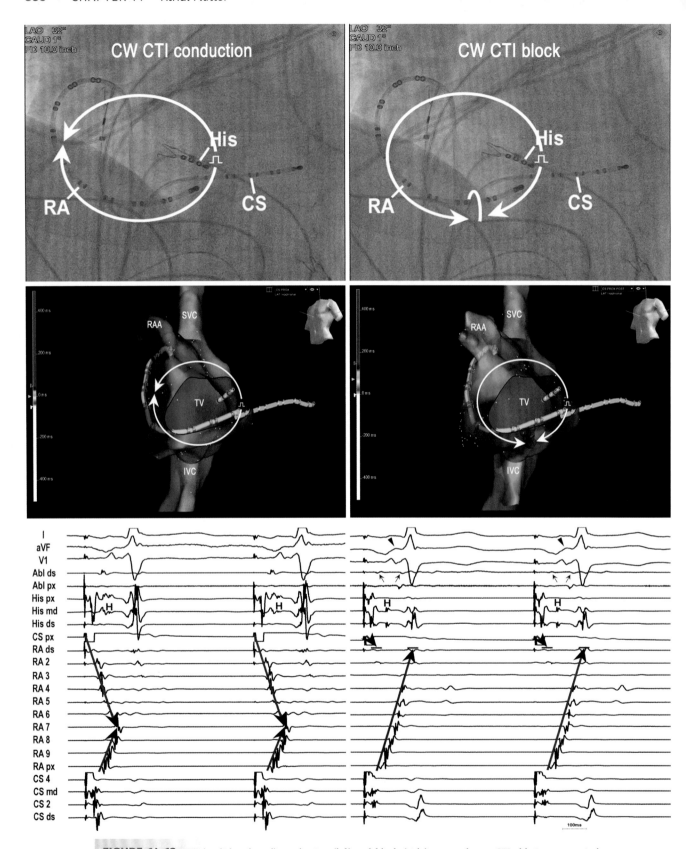

FIGURE 14-12 CW (medial to lateral) conduction (*left*) and block (*right*) pre- and post-CTI ablation, respectively. Before ablation, CS proximal pacing shows a "chevron" pattern on the "Halo" catheter with latest atrial activation along the anterolateral wall of the RA (RA 7, *purple*). After ablation, widely spaced DPs (*arrows*, 116 ms) are recorded along the ablation line with latest atrial activation now on the opposite side of the line. Note the positive terminal P-wave forces in lead II (*arrowheads*).

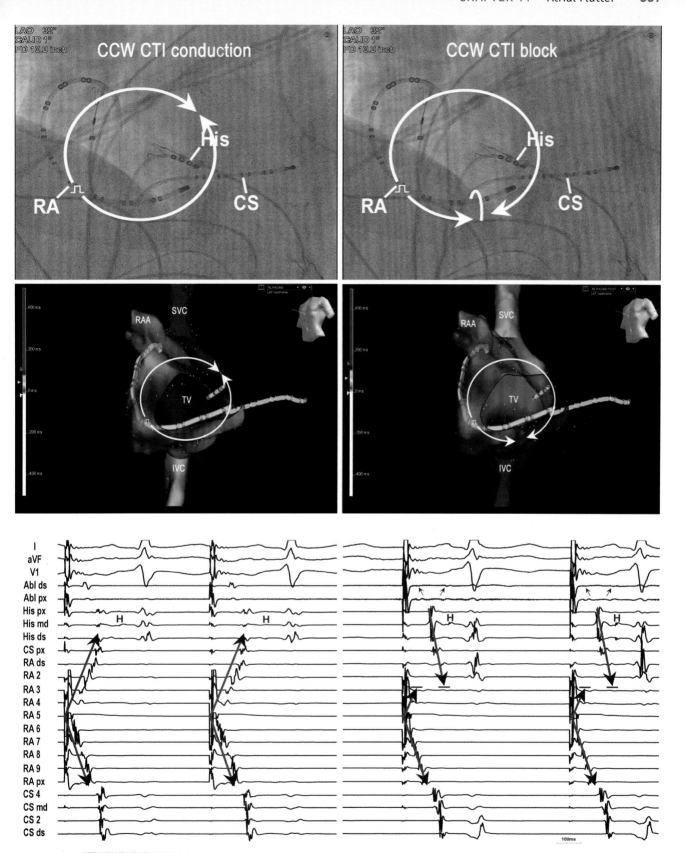

FIGURE 14-13 CCW (lateral to medial) conduction (*left*) and block (*right*) pre- and post-CTI ablation, respectively. Before ablation, RA 5 pacing shows latest atrial activation along the anteroseptal wall of the RA (His region, *purple*). After ablation, widely spaced DPs (*arrows*, 121 ms) are recorded along the line with latest atrial activation now on the opposite side of the line.

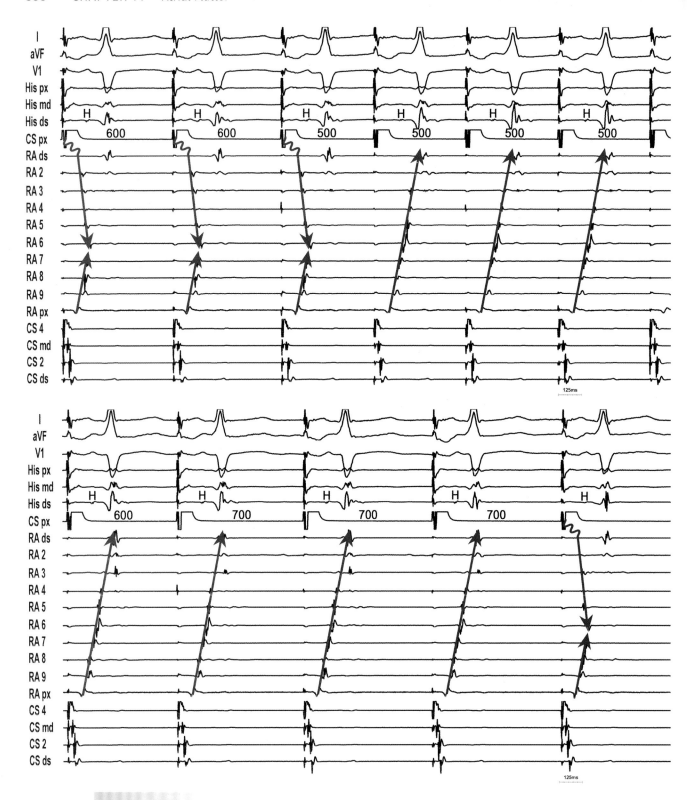

FIGURE 14-14 Rate-dependent CTI block with hysteresis. At a pacing cycle length of 600 ms, CW delay occurs across the CTI. Shortening the cycle length (500 ms) causes CTI block, which persists despite increasing the cycle length back to 600 ms until it is lengthened further to 700 ms.

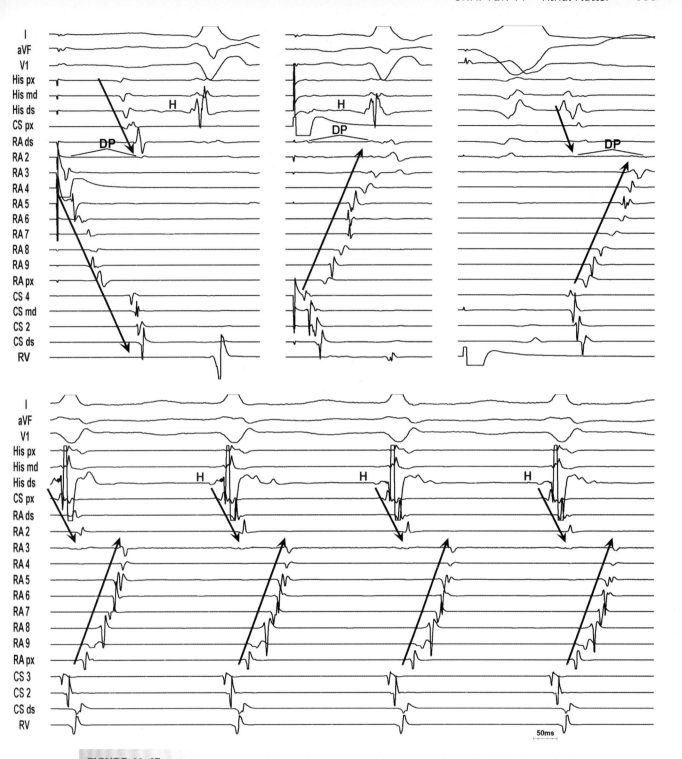

FIGURE 14-15 CTI block demonstrated by atrial pacing, ventricular pacing, and typical AVNRT. RA 4 and CS px pacing (*top left and middle*) demonstrate bidirectional block across the CTI. CW CTI block is also illustrated during ventricular pacing (*top right*) and typical AVNRT (*bottom*) with retrograde conduction over the fast pathway (FP). Widely spaced DPs (DP = 125 ms) are recorded along the ablation line (RA 2). AVNRT with CTI block simulates CCW CTI-dependent atrial flutter, except that right atrial activation only spans 37% of the tachycardia cycle length (TCL).

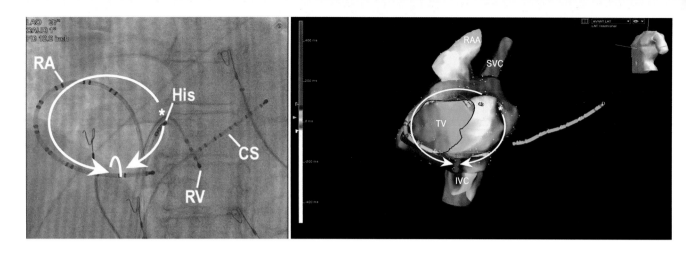

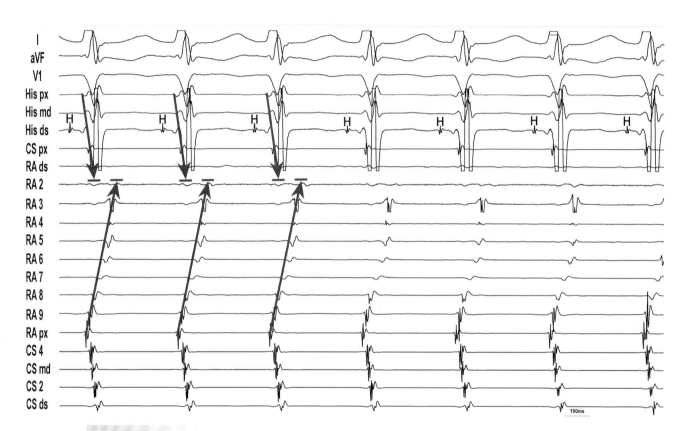

FIGURE 14-16 Typical AVNRT with CTI block. The earliest site of atrial activation (*white asterisk*) is at the fast pathway (FP) along the anteroseptal RA. Widely spaced DPs are recorded at the ablation line (*red tags*/RA 2) due to CW block across the CTI.

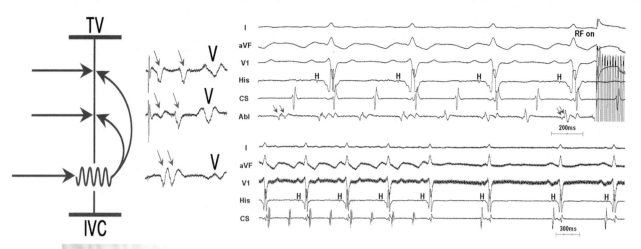

FIGURE 14-17 Gap mapping. Dragging the mapping catheter along the ablation line closer to the gap results in narrowing of DPs (*arrows*)—the second of which has higher voltage. Applications of RF energy terminate atrial flutter.

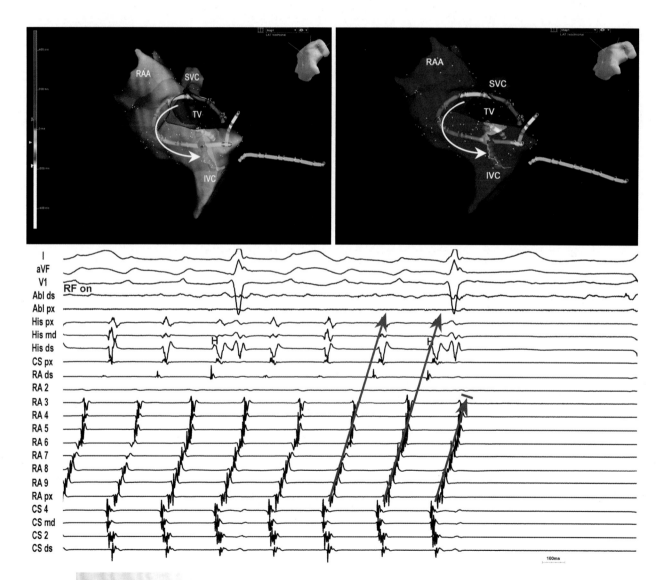

FIGURE 14-18 Gap mapping. After an initial CTI line, a gap at the distal ventricular end of the line allowed breakthrough across the CTI (*white* area on purple propagation map). Targeting the gap terminates atrial flutter.

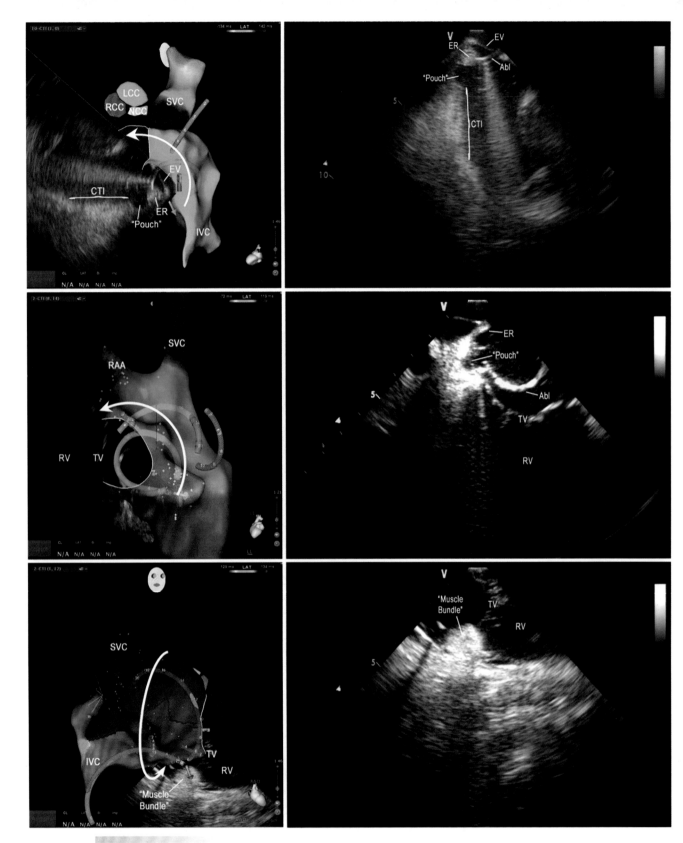

FIGURE 14-19 Complex CTI anatomy. *Top:* Sub-eustachian pouch and thick eustachian ridge. A catheter inversion technique and ICE imaging directing ablation to the thick, rounded, muscular ridge and around the pouch allowed termination of atrial flutter and bidirectional CTI block. *Middle:* Sub-eustachian pouch and thick, step-like, vertical ridge also successfully targeted with the catheter inversion technique. *Bottom:* A thick, rounded muscle bundle anteriorly at the tricuspid vestibule. Despite multiple RF applications, ablation directly on the muscle bundle caused only transient block. Durable CTI block required RF delivery lateral to the muscle bundle. ER, Eustachian ridge; EV, Eustachian valve.

POSITIVE TERMINAL P-WAVE FORCES

A surface ECG clue of CTI block is a positive terminal P-wave force in the inferior leads during medial and, in particular, lateral CTI pacing.[31] Before ablation, simultaneous CW and CCW wavefronts cause the RA to be activated in a caudo-cranial direction with CTI pacing. After CTI block, pacing one side of the line results in cranio-caudal activation of the opposite RA, generating late terminal positive P-wave forces in the inferior leads (Fig. 14-12). Positive terminal P-wave forces, however, does not differentiate significant CTI delay from block.

DIFFERENTIAL ATRIAL PACING

Differential atrial pacing is a useful maneuver to differentiate conduction delay from block across the CTI.[28,32] To evaluate CCW CTI block, the time between a pacing stimulus delivered immediately adjacent and lateral to the line (site A) and the recorded electrogram on the other side of the line (site D) is compared to the time between the pacing stimulus delivered lateral to site A (site B) and the electrogram recorded at site D. AD > BD indicates CCW CTI block, while AD < BD indicates CTI delay (Fig. 14-20). To evaluate CW CTI block, the time between the pacing stimulus immediately adjacent and medial to the line (site D) and the recorded electrogram at site A is compared to the time between the pacing stimulus medial to site D (site C) and the electrogram at site A. DA > CA indicates CW CTI block, while DA < CA indicates CTI delay (Fig. 14-21).

UNUSUAL ELECTROPHYSIOLOGIC PHENOMENA

DOUBLE WAVE REENTRY

Double wave reentry is a transient, accelerated form of CCW CTI-dependent atrial flutter induced by atrial extrastimulation during flutter. A critically timed extrastimulus blocks antidromically in the CTI and propagates orthodromically causing two macroreentrant wavefronts (double wave) within the same circuit. Double wave reentry occurs when atrial flutter has a sufficiently large excitable gap to accommodate two tachycardia wavelengths.[33]

LOWER LOOP REENTRY

Lower loop reentry is a subtype of CTI-dependent atrial flutter occurring when an inferior portion of the posterior barrier provided by the crista terminalis is incomplete. A lower loop develops that short circuits the larger macroreentrant loop. Lower loop reentry may occur simultaneously or alternate with CCW CTI-dependent atrial flutter.[34]

INTRA-ISTHMUS REENTRY

Intra-isthmus reentry is another subtype of CTI-dependent atrial flutter where the reentrant circuit is confined mostly to the septal side of the CTI around the CS ostium and a potential cause of flutter recurrence after prior CTI ablation.[35,36] It is diagnosed by entrainment mapping along the tricuspid annulus showing manifest fusion and long PPI–tachycardia cycle length (TCL) (>25 ms) around the annulus (including the lateral CTI), except at the medial CTI where concealed entrainment and PPI − TCL ≤25 ms occurs. Activation around the tricuspid annulus can show fusion ("focal pattern" with centrifugal spread) or CCW/CW activation ("pseudomacroreentrant pattern" with early meeting late) (CCW activation resulting from functional CTI block). Successful ablation electrograms are prolonged (∼35–70% TCL), fractionated signals.[35]

TRANSPLANT FLUTTER

After atrio-atrial orthotopic heart transplantation, atrial flutter can arise from remnant recipient but more commonly donor atrial tissue (recipient or donor flutter, respectively) (Fig. 14-22).[37–39] Suture lines at the atrial anastomosis form a barrier and electrically isolate recipient from donor atria (although intermittent conduction can occur through a gap in the line). The ventricles are driven by the donor atrium.

LONGITUDINAL DISSOCIATION OF THE CTI

The presence of two pathways in the CTI—a faster pathway (longer effective refractory period [ERP]) connecting to the proximal muscle sleeves of the CS and a slower pathway (shorter ERP) connecting to the middle CS—causes a change in CS activation when atrial flutter accelerates during entrainment (functional block in the faster pathway) or slows during RF delivery (ablation of the faster pathway).[40]

UNUSUAL ATRIO-VENTRICULAR CONDUCTION RATIOS

1:1 AV Conduction

Atrial flutter with 1:1 AV conduction is almost invariably associated with aberration and commonly mistaken for ventricular tachycardia (VT) (Fig. 14-23). It occurs in situations in which the atrial flutter cycle length > AV node/His bundle ERP: 1) use of Na channel blockers (which prolong atrial flutter cycle length and slow His-Purkinje conduction) without AV nodal blockade and 2) exercise-induced atrial flutter (where heightened sympathetic tone shortens AV node ERP). Other odd AV conduction ratios (e.g., 3:1) are uncommon and observed with antiarrhythmic drug therapy.

Alternating Wenckebach

Another unusual AV conduction pattern is alternating Wenckebach periodicity resulting from two levels of block (bi-level block) in the AV junction. Alternating Wenckebach with three consecutive nonconducted flutter waves between Wenckebach cycles results from 2:1 and Wenckebach block in the upper and lower levels, respectively. Reversal of the block pattern (Wenckebach in the upper level and 2:1 in the lower level) causes two consecutive nonconducted flutter waves between Wenckebach cycles (Figs. 14-4, 14-24 and 14-25).[41,42]

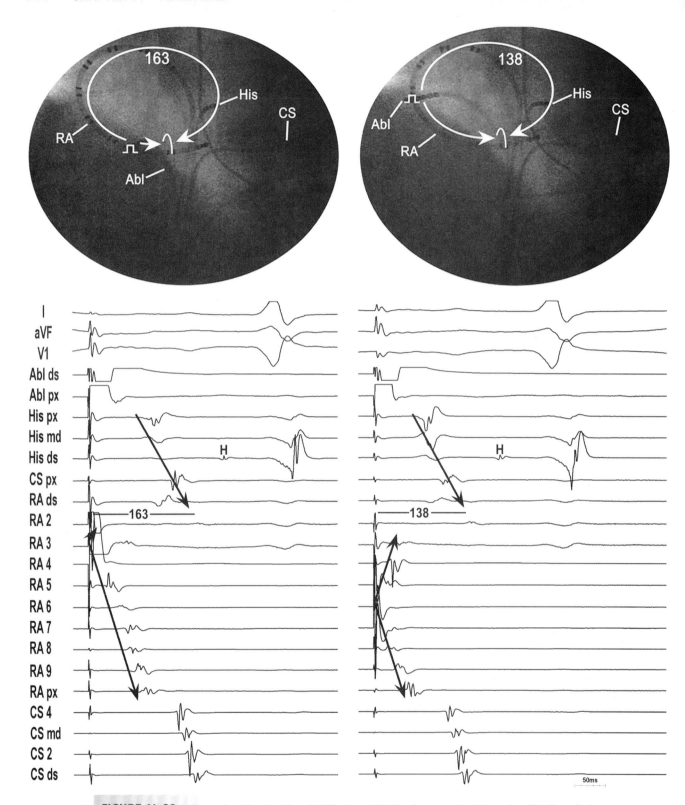

FIGURE 14-20 Differential atrial pacing (lateral CTI). Pacing (RA 3) adjacent to the ablation line (RA 2) resulted in a long conduction time to its opposite side (163 ms), which shortened when pacing more laterally (RA 6, 138 ms). These findings indicate CCW block across the CTI.

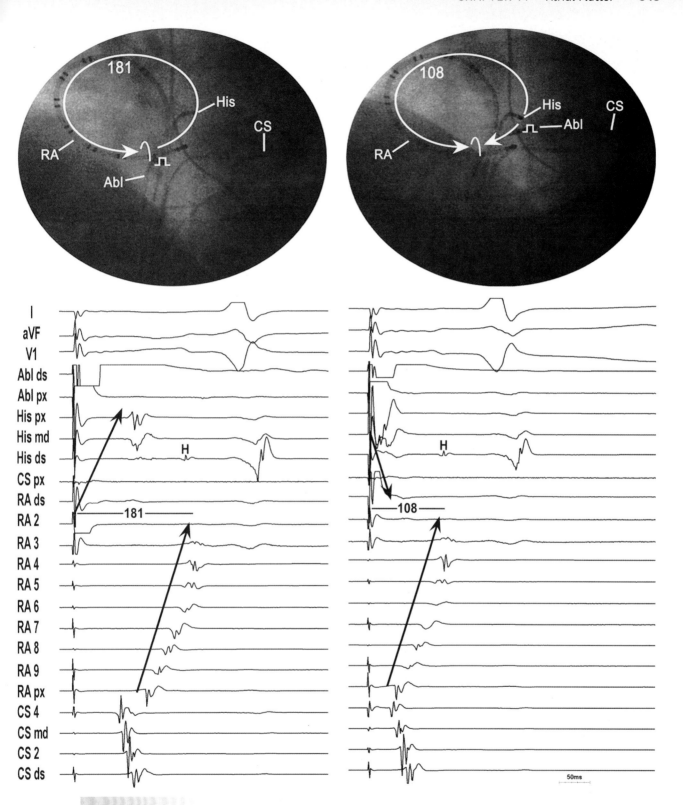

FIGURE 14-21 Differential atrial pacing (medial CTI). Pacing (RA 2) adjacent to the ablation line resulted in a long conduction time to its opposite side (181 ms), which shortened when pacing more laterally (His, 108 ms). These findings indicate CW block across the CTI.

NSR

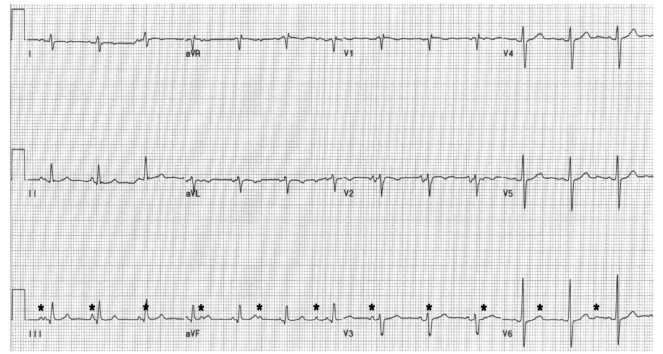

"Recipient flutter"

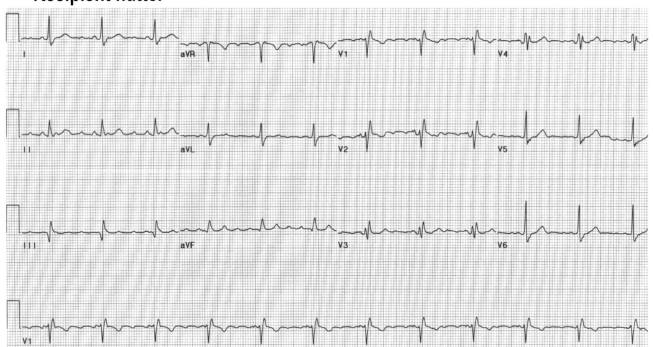

FIGURE 14-22 Transplant flutter. *Top:* Recipient (*asterisk*) and donor atrium are in sinus rhythm and dissociated from each other. Note that the donor sinus rate is faster due to vagal denervation. *Bottom:* The recipient atrium is in atrial flutter, while the donor atrium remains in sinus rhythm and drives the ventricle.

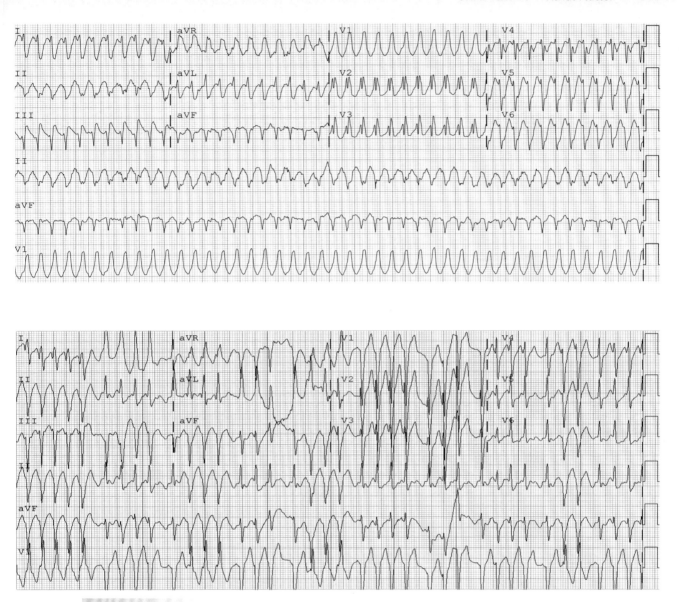

FIGURE 14-23 Atrial flutter with 1:1 AV conduction. *Top*: Rate-related right bundle branch block (RBBB) simulates monomorphic VT. *Bottom*: Rate-related RBBB and left bundle branch block (LBBB) simulates polymorphic VT.

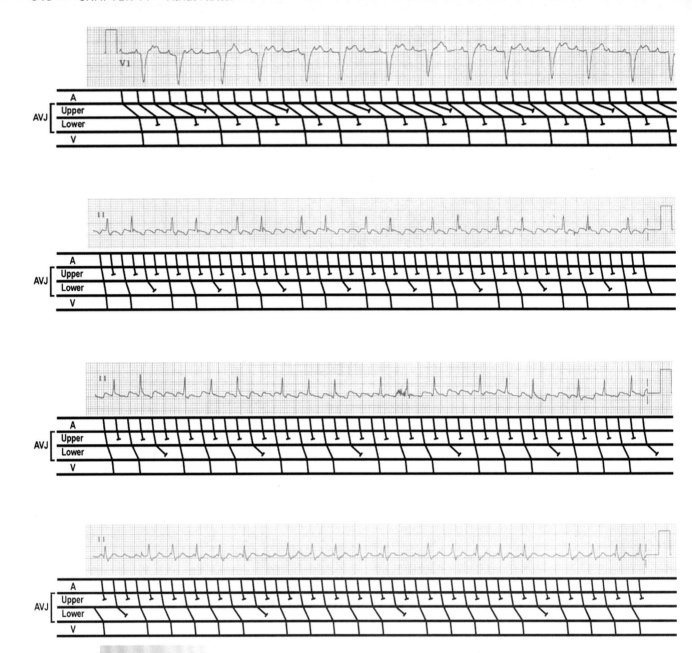

FIGURE 14-24 Alternating Wenckebach periodicity (two levels of block). *Top panel*: Upper level Wenckebach and lower level 2:1 block (two nonconducted flutter waves between Wenckebach cycles). *Lower three panels*: Upper level 2:1 block and lower level Wenckebach (three nonconducted flutter waves between Wenckebach cycles) resulting in bigeminal, trigeminal, and pentageminal AV conduction patterns.

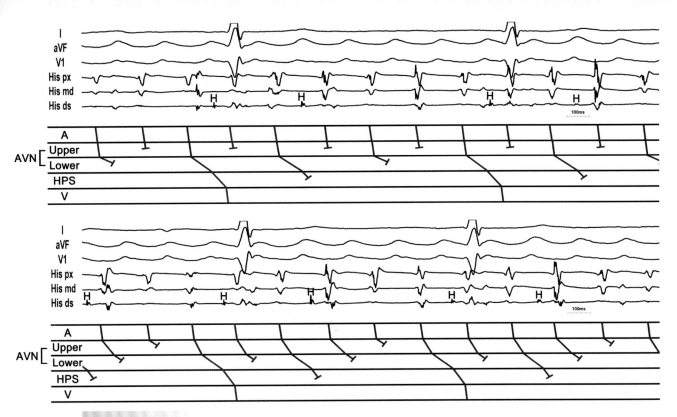

FIGURE 14-25 Alternating Wenckebach periodicity with infrahisian block (three levels of block). Within each Wenckebach cycle, flutter waves either conduct or block to the His bundle with AH prolongation preceding block (alternating Wenckebach), causing 6:2 and 5:2 atrio-His bundle conduction ratios. *Top:* Upper level 2:1 block and lower level Wenckebach in the AV node (three nonconducted flutter waves between Wenckebach cycles). *Bottom:* Upper level Wenckebach and lower level 2:1 block in the AV node (two nonconducted flutter waves between Wenckebach cycles). In both cases, a third layer of block occurs below the His bundle, causing 6:1 and 5:1 AV conduction ratios, respectively. (With a narrow QRS complex, block could be in the distal His bundle beyond the His bundle recording site.)

REFERENCES

1. Olshansky B, Okumura K, Hess PG, Waldo AL. Demonstration of an area of slow conduction in human atrial flutter. J Am Coll Cardiol 1990;16: 1639–1648.
2. Cosio FG, López-Gil M, Goicolea A, Arribas F, Barroso JL. Radiofrequency ablation of the inferior vena cava-tricuspid valve isthmus in common atrial flutter. Am J Cardiol 1993;71:705–709.
3. Feld GK, Fleck RP, Chen P, et al. Radiofrequency catheter ablation for the treatment of human type 1 atrial flutter. Identification of a critical zone in the reentrant circuit by endocardial mapping techniques. Circulation 1992;86: 1233–1240.
4. Schwartzman D, Callans DJ, Gottlieb CD, Dillon SM, Movsowitz C, Marchlinski FE. Conduction block in the inferior vena caval-tricuspid valve isthmus: association with outcome of radiofrequency ablation of type I atrial flutter. J Am Coll Cardiol 1996;28:1519–1531.
5. Cabrera JA, Sánchez-Quintana D, Farré J, Rubio JM, Ho SY. The inferior right atrial isthmus: further architectural insights for current and coming ablation technologies. J Cardiovasc Electrophysiol 2005;16:402–408.
6. Nakagawa H, Lazzara R, Khastgir T, et al. Role of the tricuspid annulus and the eustachian valve/ridge on atrial flutter. Relevance to catheter ablation of the septal isthmus and a new technique for rapid identification of ablation success. Circulation 1996;94:407–424.
7. Passman RS, Kadish AH, Dibs SR, Engelstein ED, Goldberger JJ. Radiofrequency ablation of atrial flutter: a randomized controlled trial of two anatomic approaches. Pacing Clin Electrophysiol 2004;27:83–88.
8. Kalman JM, Olgin JE, Saxon LA, Fisher WG, Lee RJ, Lesh MD. Activation and entrainment mapping defines the tricuspid annulus as the anterior barrier in typical atrial flutter. Circulation 1996;94:398–406.
9. Olgin JE, Kalman JM, Fitzpatrick AP, Lesh MD. Role of right atrial endocardial structures as barriers to conduction during human type I atrial flutter. Activation and entrainment mapping guided by intracardiac echocardiography. Circulation 1995;92:1839–1848.
10. Olgin JE, Kalman JM, Saxon LA, Lee RJ, Lesh MD. Mechanism of initiation of atrial flutter in humans: site of unidirectional block and direction of rotation. J Am Coll Cardiol 1997;29:376–384.
11. Vollmann D, Stevenson WG, Lüthje L, et al. Misleading long post-pacing interval after entrainment of typical atrial flutter from the cavotricuspid isthmus. J Am Coll Cardiol 2012;59:819–824.
12. Poty H, Saodi N, Nair M, Anselme F, Letac B. Radiofrequency catheter ablation of atrial flutter. Further insights into the various types of isthmus block: application to ablation during sinus rhythm. Circulation 1996;94:3204–3213.
13. Poty H, Saoudi N, Abdel Aziz AA, Nair M, Letac B. Radiofrequency catheter ablation of type 1 atrial flutter. Prediction of late success by electrophysiological criteria. Circulation 1995;92:1389–1392.
14. Vijayaraman P, Kok LC, Wood MA, Ellenbogen KA. Right ventricular pacing to assess transisthmus conduction in patients undergoing isthmus-dependent atrial flutter ablation: a new useful technique? Heart Rhythm 2006;3:268–272.
15. Shah D, Haïssaguerre MK, Jaïs P, Takahashi A, Hocini M, Clémenty J. High-density mapping activation through an incomplete isthmus ablation line. Circulation 1999;99:211–215.
16. Sra J, Bhatia A, Dhala A, et al. Electroanatomic mapping to identify breakthrough sites in recurrent typical human flutter. Pacing Clin Electrophysiol 2000;23:1479–1492.
17. Tada H, Oral H, Sticherling C, et al. Double potentials along the ablation line as a guide to radiofrequency ablation of typical atrial flutter. J Am Coll Cardiol 2001;38:750–755.
18. Cosio FG, Arribas F, Barbero JM, Kallmeyer C, Goicolea A. Validation of double-spike electrograms as markers of conduction delay or block in atrial flutter. Am J Cardiol 1988;61:775–780.
19. Shimizu A, Nozaki A, Rudy Y, Waldo AL. Characterization of double potentials in a functionally determined reentrant circuit: multiplexing studies during interruption of atrial flutter in the canine pericarditis model. J Am Coll Cardiol 1993;22:2022–2032.
20. Francisco GM, Sharma S, Dougherty A, Kantharia BK. Atrial tachyarrhythmia: what is the ideal site for successful ablation. J Cardiovasc Electrophysiol 2008;19:759–761.

21. Redfearn DP, Skanes AC, Gula LJ, Krahn AD, Yee R, Klein GJ. Cavotricuspid isthmus conduction is dependent on underlying anatomic bundle architecture: observations using a maximum voltage-guided ablation technique. J Cardiovasc Electrophysiol 2006;17:832–838.

22. Gami AS, Edwards WD, Lachman N, et al. Electrophysiological anatomy of typical atrial flutter: the posterior boundary and causes for difficulty with ablation. J Cardiovasc Electrophysiol 2010;21:144–149.

23. Sporton SC, Davies DW, Earley MJ, Markides V, Nathan AW, Schilling RJ. Catheter inversion: a technique to complete isthmus ablation and cure atrial flutter. Pacing Clin Electrophysiol 2004;27(Pt 1):775–778.

24. Vijayaraman P, Dandamudi G, Naperkowski A, Oren J, Storm R, Ellenbogen KA. Adenosine facilitates dormant conduction across cavotricuspid isthmus following catheter ablation. Heart Rhythm 2012;9:1785–1788.

25. Morales GX, Macle L, Khairy P, et al. Adenosine testing in atrial flutter ablation: unmasking of dormant conduction across the cavotricuspid isthmus and risk of recurrence. J Cardiovasc Electrophysiol 2013;24: 995–1001.

26. Morales G, Darrat YH, Lellouche N, et al. Use of adenosine to shorten the post ablation waiting period for cavotricuspid isthmus-dependent atrial flutter. J Cardiovasc Electrophysiol 2017;28:876–881.

27. Nabar A, Rodriguez LM, Timmermans C, Smeets J, Wellens HJ. Isoproterenol to evaluate resumption of conduction after right atrial isthmus ablation in type 1 atrial flutter. Circulation 1999;99:3286–3291.

28. Chen J, deChillou C, Basiouny T, et al. Cavotricuspid isthmus mapping to assess bidirectional block during common atrial flutter radiofrequency ablation. Circulation 1999;100:2507–2513.

29. Tada H, Oral H, Sticherling C, et al. Electrogram polarity and cavotricuspid isthmus block during ablation of typical atrial flutter. J Cardiovasc Electrophysiol 2001;12:393–399.

30. Yamabe H, Okumura K, Misumi I, et al. Role of bipolar electrogram polarity mapping in localizing recurrent conduction in the isthmus early and late after ablation of atrial flutter. J Am Coll Cardiol 1999;33:39–45.

31. Hamdan MH, Kalman J, Barron HV, Lesh MD. P-wave morphology during right atrial pacing before and after atrial flutter ablation—a new marker for success. Am J Cardiol 1997;79:1417–1420.

32. Shah D, Haïssaguerre M, Takahashi A, Jaïs P, Hocini M, Clémenty J. Differential pacing for distinguishing block from persistent conduction through an ablation line. Circulation 2000;102:1517–1522.

33. Cheng J. Acceleration of typical atrial flutter due to double-wave reentry induced by programmed electrical stimulation. Circulation 1998;97:1589–1596.

34. Cheng J, Cabeen WR Jr, Scheinman MM. Right atrial flutter due to lower loop reentry: mechanism and anatomic substrates. Circulation 1999;99:1700–1705.

35. Yang Y, Varma N, Badhwar N, et al. Prospective observations in the clinical and electrophysiological characteristics of intra-isthmus reentry. J Cardiovasc Electrophysiol 2010;21:1099–1106.

36. Yang Y, Varma N, Keung EC, Scheinman MM. Reentry within the cavotricuspid isthmus: an isthmus dependent circuit. Pacing Clin Electrophysiol 2005;28:808–818.

37. Heist EK, Doshi SK, Singh JP, et al. Catheter ablation of atrial flutter after orthotopic heart transplantation. J Cardiovasc Electrophysiol 2004;15:1366–1370.

38. Marine JE, Schuger CD, Bogun F, et al. Mechanism of atrial flutter occurring late after orthotopic heart transplantation with atrio-atrial anastomosis. Pacing Clin Electrophysiol 2005;28:412–420.

39. Aryana A, Heist EK, Ruskin JN, Singh JP. Masking of sinus rhythm by recipient atrial flutter in a patient with orthotopic heart transplant. J Cardiovasc Electrophysiol 2008;19:876–877.

40. Shen MJ, Knight BP, Kim SS. Fusion during entrainment at the cavotricuspid isthmus: what is the mechanism? Heart Rhythm 2018;15:787–789.

41. Amat-y-Leon F, Chuquimia R, Wu D, et al. Alternating Wenckebach periodicity: a common electrophysiological response. Am J Cardiol 1975;36:757–764.

42. Halpern MS, Nau GJ, Levi RJ, Elizari MV, Rosenbaum MB. Wenckebach periods of alternate beats. Clinical and experimental observations. Circulation 1973;48:41–49.

Atrial Fibrillation 15

Introduction

Atrial fibrillation is the most common arrhythmia and causes rapid, chaotic, and uncoordinated contraction of the atria. It can be classified by presentation as 1) paroxysmal ($\geq$2 episodes lasting <7 days), 2) persistent (sustained episode lasting >7 days or requiring pharmacologic or electrical cardioversion), and 3) permanent (unsuccessful or unattempted cardioversion).[1] Longstanding persistent atrial fibrillation is sustained atrial fibrillation lasting >1 year.

The purpose of this chapter is to:
1. Discuss the pathophysiology of atrial fibrillation.
2. Discuss the different catheter-based approaches for atrial fibrillation ablation.
3. Discuss ablation of post-atrial fibrillation ablation left atrial (LA) flutter/tachycardia.

PATHOPHYSIOLOGY

The onset and perpetuation of atrial fibrillation require both triggers and susceptible atrial substrate. The mechanisms of atrial fibrillation are categorized into 1) focal triggers, 2) arrhythmogenic substrate, and 3) modulating factors.

FOCAL TRIGGERS

Spontaneous and rapid firing from the muscular sleeves of the pulmonary veins (PVs) have been identified as the dominant source of triggers for atrial fibrillation (Fig. 15-1).[2,3] These muscular sleeves that extend for 1–3 cm into the PVs have a complex architecture whose longitudinal and spiral fiber orientation supports anisotropic conduction and localized reentry. The mechanisms underlying these focal discharges include reentry, automaticity, and triggered activity.[4,5] Non-PV triggers of atrial fibrillation (posterior LA; crista terminalis; interatrial septum; other thoracic veins such as superior vena cava [SVC], coronary sinus [CS], vein of Marshall) and supraventricular tachycardias (e.g., atrio-ventricular nodal reentrant tachycardia [AVNRT], orthodromic reciprocating tachycardia [ORT]) have also been reported (Fig. 15-2).[6–9] Sustained, rapid electrical discharges from arrhythmogenic PV foci not only trigger atrial fibrillation but also drive it (focal trigger, rotor, and venous wave hypotheses).[10] These focal discharges result in self-sustaining, high-frequency reentrant rotors, which when encountering tissue incapable of 1:1 conduction undergo spatial fragmentation and fibrillatory conduction.[11]

ARRHYTHMOGENIC SUBSTRATE

Profibrillatory conditions include inhomogeneity of atrial refractoriness (dispersion of refractoriness) and slow conduction occurring with atrial fibrosis, thereby promoting reentry within the atrium.[12] A certain number of wavelets is needed to sustain fibrillation, and therefore, a critical mass of atrial tissue is required (multiple wavelet hypothesis).[13] Each reentrant wavelet propagates randomly, collides with oncoming wavelets, or extinguishes spontaneously. Atrial fibrillation, itself, causes electrical and anatomical remodeling (tachycardia-mediated atrial myopathy) that begets more atrial fibrillation.

MODULATING FACTORS

The autonomic nervous system plays a critical role in the development of atrial fibrillation with increases in both sympathetic and parasympathetic tone preceding its onset.[14,15] Sympathetic stimulation increases automaticity and triggered activity. Stimulation of vagal ganglionic plexi triggers PV firing, shortens atrial refractory periods, and increases dispersion of atrial refractoriness. Four ganglionic plexi are preferentially located in the epicardial fat pads at the junction of the left superior pulmonary vein (LSPV) and atrial roof, postero-inferior junctions of the right and left inferior pulmonary vein (LIPVs), and the anterior border of the right superior PV (RSPV).

ATRIAL FIBRILLATION ABLATION

Prior to catheter ablation, surgical treatment of atrial fibrillation included the Cox-Maze operation, which was based on

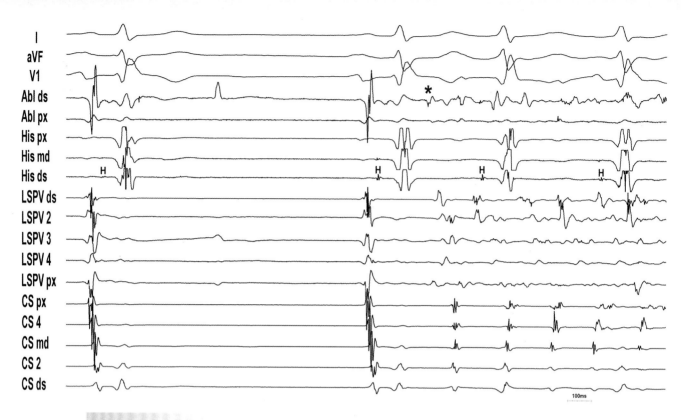

FIGURE 15-1 Spontaneous LSPV firing initiating atrial fibrillation. Early atrial activity (*asterisk*) recorded from the ablation catheter in the LSPV initiates atrial fibrillation.

the multiple wavelet hypothesis and decreased surface area by compartmentalizing the atrium through a series of strategically placed surgical incisions.[16–18] Attempt to replicate the surgery using a transvenous ablation catheter was only modestly successful, time-consuming, and associated with a high complication rate.[19] Attention turned to the PVs when it was demonstrated that ablation of focal PV triggers could eliminate atrial fibrillation.[2,3,20] Longitudinal- and spiral-oriented muscle sleeves spreading from the funnel-shaped antrum into the PVs facilitate anisotropic conduction and reentry. The occurrence of PV stenosis as a complication of this approach shifted the ablation target to the PV ostium (or antrum) with the idea that atrial fibrillation could not occur despite rapid PV firing if the PVs were electrically disconnected from the atrium.[21] Catheter-based strategies for atrial fibrillation include 1) PV isolation (PVI) and ablation of non-PV triggers, 2) substrate modification, and 3) vagal denervation. Pre-procedural (CT/MRI) and intraprocedural (intracardiac echocardiography [ICE], pulmonary venography) imaging facilitate an understanding of PV anatomy during ablation (**Figs. 15-3 and 15-4**).

FOCAL TRIGGERS

The cornerstone of atrial fibrillation ablation is PVI—either by radiofrequency (RF) or cryoablation.

Radiofrequency Ablation

Electrophysiologically guided PVI involves recording PV potentials from a circular mapping catheter (e.g., Lasso) situated at the ostium of the targeted vein and therefore generally requires two transeptal punctures unless a double or retained guide wire approach is used. To help avoid entrapment of the catheter in the mitral valve apparatus, the circular mapping catheter should be torqued clockwise (posteriorly) when exiting the transeptal sheath and positioned in the PV away from the more anterior mitral valve. The circular mapping catheter records fused electrograms consisting of a blunt LA (far-field) and high-frequency PV (near-field) potential. During left PV ablation, these electrograms overlap during sinus rhythm because of synchronous activation and best separated by distal CS pacing (**Fig. 15-5**). Two approaches to PVI include segmental ostial and wide area circumferential ablation (WACA)—the latter having a higher success rate.[22–27] Segmental ostial ablation successively targets the earliest breakthrough site of PV potentials around the circular mapping catheter until PV muscle conduction is eliminated or dissociated from the LA (**Fig. 15-6**).[22] WACA targets the antrum of the PVs (≥5 mm outside the PV ostium), debulking the atrium and causing PVI with contiguous focal lesions around the PVs individually, ipsilaterally, or entirely en bloc (**Fig. 15-7**).[23] Voltage abatement (≤0.05 mV) within encircled areas validate line continuity. Clues that the ablation catheter

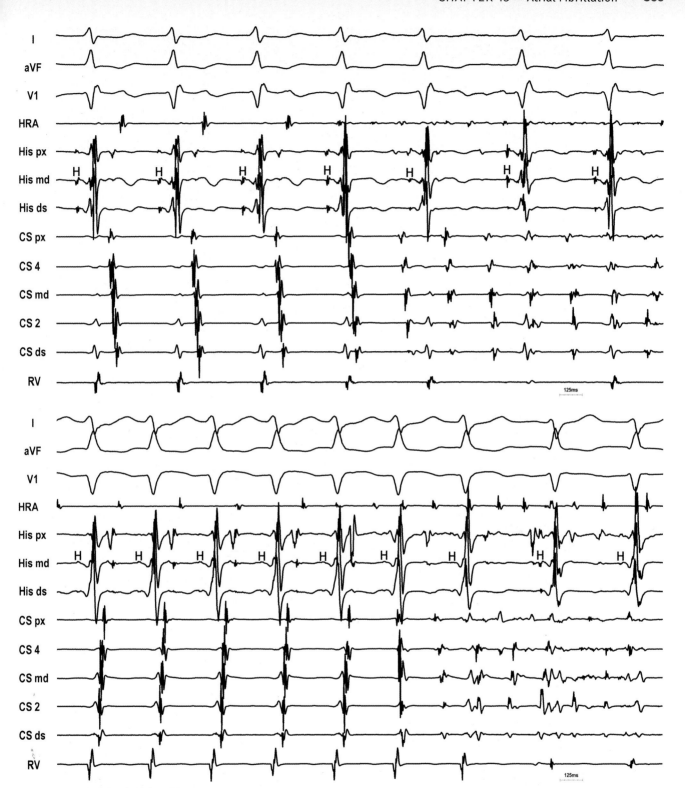

FIGURE 15-2 Degeneration of AVNRT (*top*) and ORT (*bottom*) to atrial fibrillation. ORT uses a left free wall accessory pathway (AP).

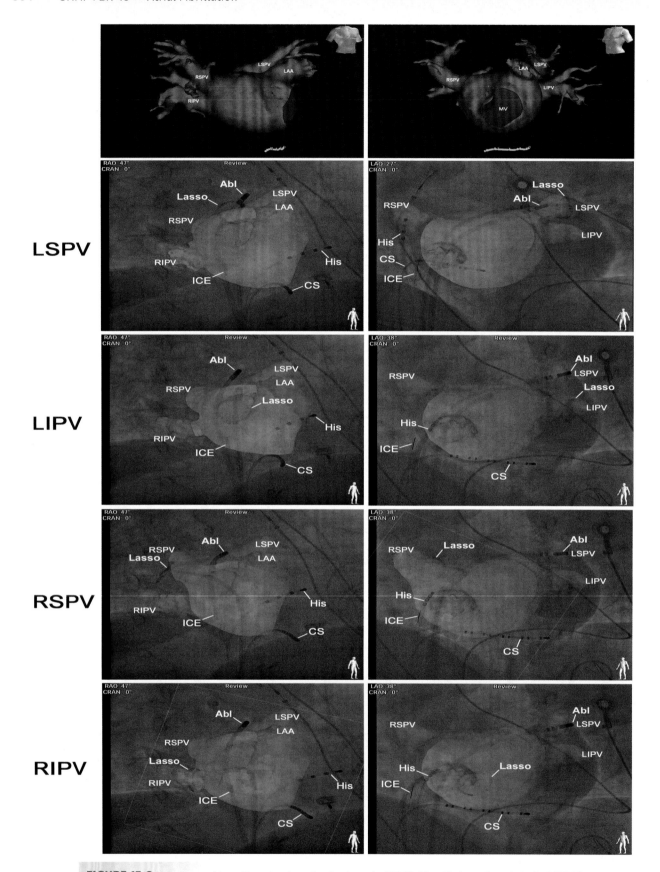

FIGURE 15-3   PV anatomy (three-dimensional rotational atriography [ATG]). The ablation catheter is in the LSPV. The circular mapping catheter (Lasso) is positioned in each of the four PVs. Note that the left-sided PV ostia are seen "en face" in the RAO view and "longitudinally" in the LAO view. The opposite is true for the right-sided PV ostia. The longitudinal views allow visualization fibril the catheters exiting the cardiac silhouette.

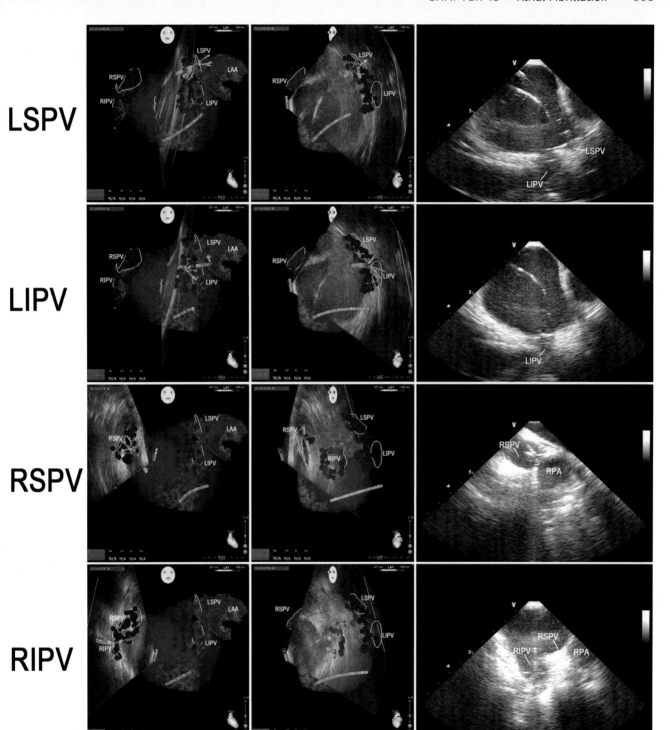

FIGURE 15-4 PV anatomy ICE. A PentaRay catheter is positioned in each of the four PVs. The red tags denote ablation lesions around the PV antra.

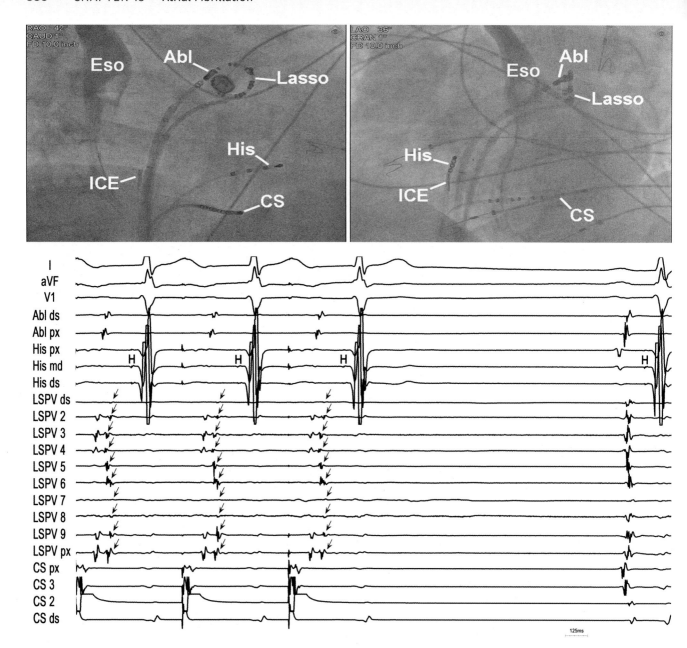

FIGURE 15-5 Separation of LSPV potentials from LA electrograms by CS pacing. CS pacing separates the high-frequency (near-field) LSPV potentials (*arrows*) from LA (far-field) electrograms, which otherwise overlap during sinus rhythm. Barium paste highlights the esophagus and its proximity to the ablation site.

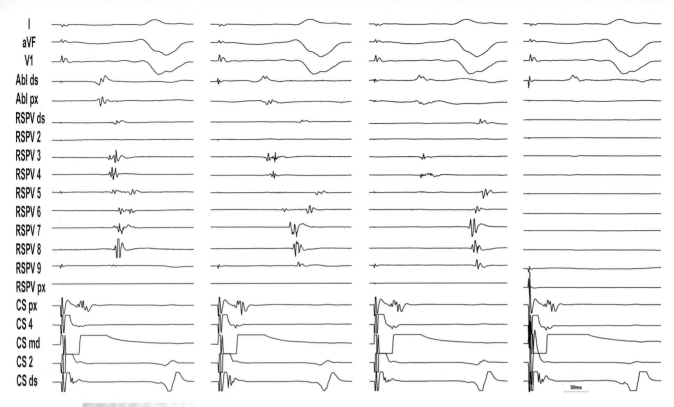

FIGURE 15-6 Segmental ostial ablation. Ablation circumferentially targeting the conducting fascicles around the RSPV incrementally changing activation on the circular mapping catheter until isolation is achieved.

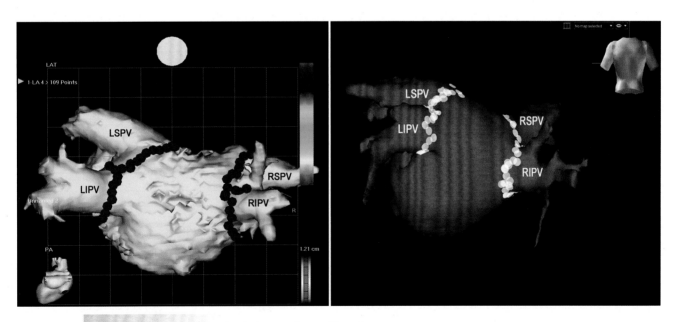

FIGURE 15-7 WACA. The red and white tags denote ablation lesions.

is in the PV where RF delivery should be avoided include 1) fluoroscopic demonstration of the catheter tip beyond the cardiac silhouette, 2) ICE imaging of catheter tip beyond the PV ostium, 3) loss of electrical signals, and 4) increase in catheter impedance (>140–150 ohms). The endpoint of PVI is entrance block (elimination or dissociation of PV potentials from the LA) and exit block (PV stimulation causes PV sleeve capture without conduction to the atrium) (**Figs. 15-8 to 15-12**).

Complications

Extensive ablation directed toward the thin LA wall can cause collateral damage to adjacent structures (esophagus, phrenic nerve). Techniques that might help avoid esophageal injury during ablation on the posterior wall include 1) limiting RF energy (e.g., 25 Watts or high power/short duration [50 Watts/2–5 sec]), 2) decreasing tissue contact pressure (avoiding perpendicular orientation of the catheter tip and posterior LA), 3) moving the tip of the ablation catheter during RF delivery (avoid time-dependent tissue heating), and 4) real-time esophageal monitoring during ablation (luminal esophageal temperature [LET] probe, ICE visualization, barium paste in the esophagus) (**Fig. 15-13**).[4,28] Techniques that might help avoid phrenic nerve injury, particularly with ablation near the RSPV, include 1) high-output pacing from the ablation site to ensure absence of phrenic nerve stimulation prior to RF delivery and 2) fluoroscopic monitoring or phrenic nerve pacing from the right subclavian vein to ensure continued right diaphragmatic function during ablation.[4]

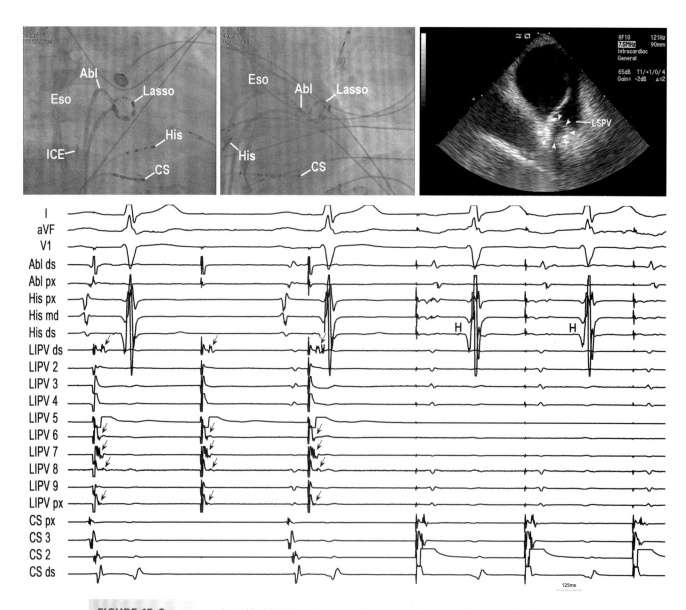

FIGURE 15-8 Entrance and exit block. LIPV pacing causes sleeve capture (*arrows*) without conduction to the atrium (exit block). CS pacing captures the atrium but fails to conduct into the LIPV (entrance block). White arrowheads denote circular mapping catheter (Lasso) on ICE.

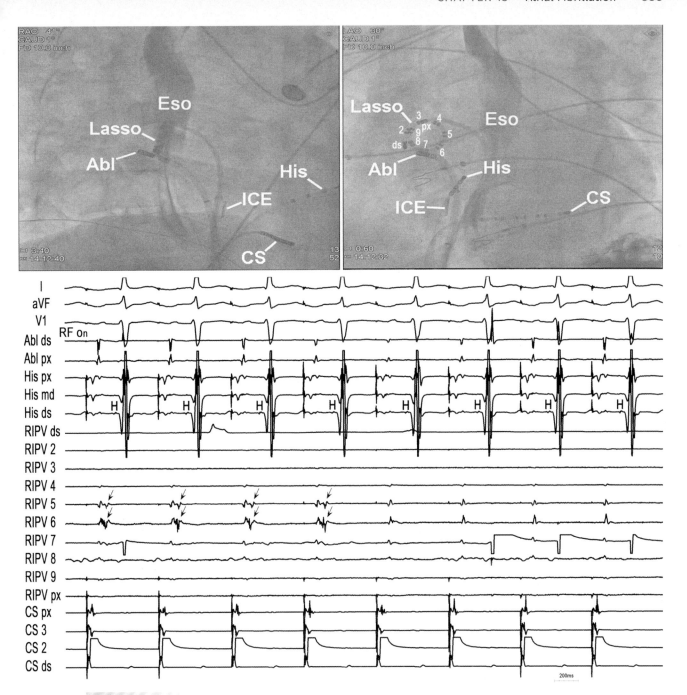

FIGURE 15-9 Entrance block. RF delivery to the inferior ostium of the RIPV (seventh Lasso dipole) causes abrupt loss of PV potentials (*arrows*). Barium paste highlights the esophagus and its proximity to the ablation site.

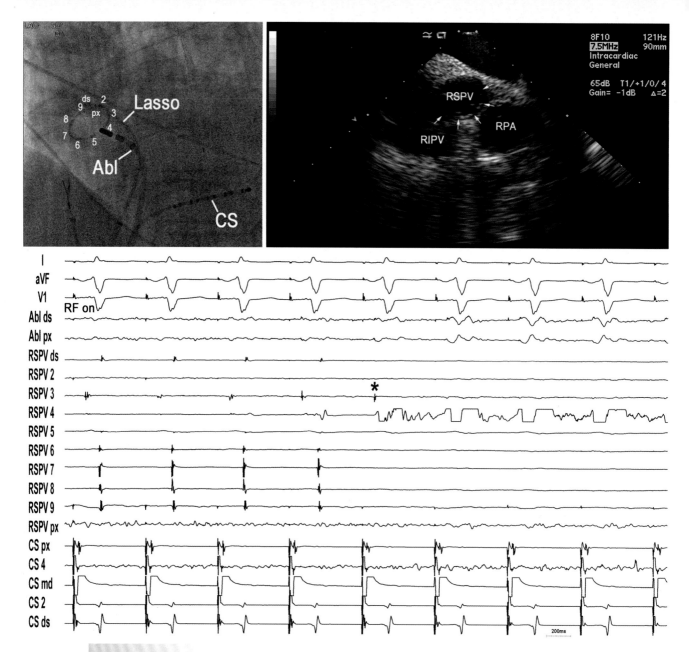

FIGURE 15-10 Entrance block. RF delivery to the RSPV (fourth Lasso dipole) causes abrupt loss (*asterisk*) of PV potentials. White arrows denote circular mapping catheter (Lasso) in RSPV.

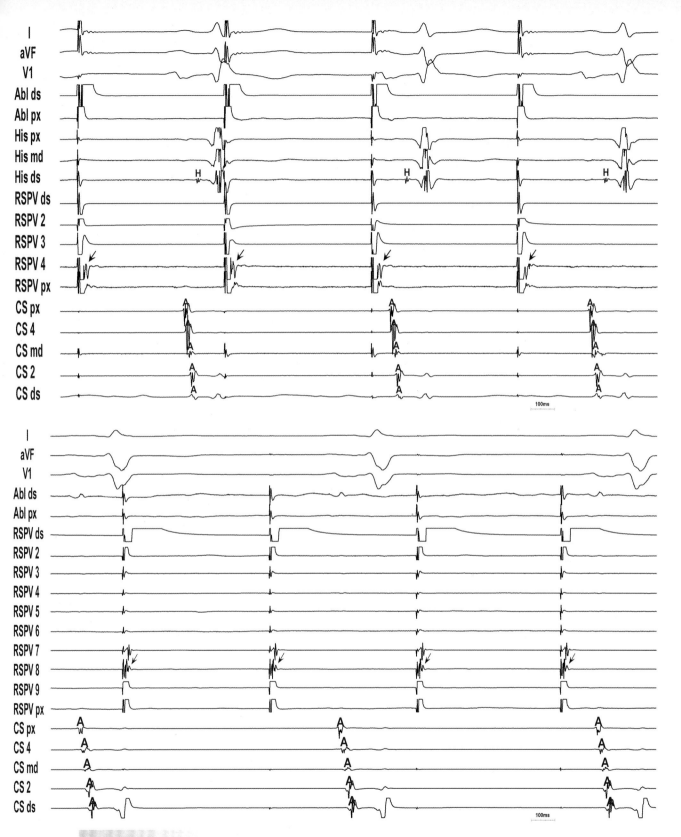

FIGURE 15-11 Entrance and exit block. In both cases, RSPV pacing causes sleeve capture (*arrows*) without conduction to the atrium (exit block), while sinus complexes fail to conduct into the vein (entrance block).

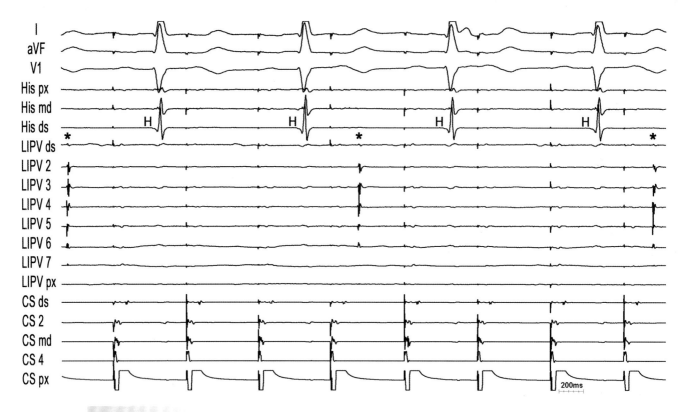

FIGURE 15-12 Spontaneous PV firing. CS pacing fails to conduct into the LIPV (entrance block), while spontaneous firing within the LIPV (*asterisks*) fails to conduct to the atrium (exit block).

Pulmonary Vein Potential Pitfalls

After PVI, adenosine or isoproterenol can unmask dormant PV conduction and/or non-PV triggers and, therefore, need for further ablation.[29–32] Far-field electrograms from neighboring electrically active structures (LA appendage [LAA] for LSPV and SVC for RSPV) can be misinterpreted as PV potentials resulting in unnecessary RF applications, particularly with widely spaced electrode pairs having a larger "antenna" (Figs. 15-14 and 15-15). Far-field electrograms can be differentiated from true PV potentials by 1) morphology, 2) distribution, and 3) pacing techniques. PV potentials demonstrate near-field characteristics (high frequency, sharp, narrow width) and are circumferentially distributed around the PV, while far-field electrograms (low frequency, dull, wider width) are segmentally distributed to sites overlying the electrically active neighboring structure. Pacing the neighboring structure (e.g., LAA) and capturing the electrogram (potential anticipation) confirms a far-field signal (Fig. 15-14).[33,34] (Conversely, when demonstrating exit block by pacing within the PV, it is also important not to far-field capture the electrically active neighboring structure and therefore atrium, which could be falsely interpreted as persistent conduction.)

Cryoablation

Rather than point-by-point focal RF ablation, cryoablation is an alternative PVI technique using a balloon catheter to occlude the PV and liquid nitrogen to freeze its antrum.[35–37] A circular mapping catheter inserted through the lumen of the cryoballoon allows monitoring of PV potentials while providing distal support, and therefore, only a single transseptal puncture is required. The transseptal puncture site should be low and anterior on the fossa ovalis allowing for a large turning radius of the cryocatheter to reach the posterior and superior PVs (particularly, the more difficult right inferior pulmonary vein [RIPV]). Keeping the cryoballoon coaxial to the vein with maintenance of forward pressure, advancing the sheath to the back hemisphere of the balloon for proximal support, and using the circular mapping catheter as a distal luminal supporting wire ("rail") in different vein branches (inferior for inferior veins/superior for superior veins) facilitate balloon occlusion of the targeted vein. Because the balloon heads superiorly toward the PV antrum, inferior leaks during initial attempts at vein occlusion are common (worst site of balloon-to-PV contact) and can be sealed by a 1) "pull down" technique (pulling the entire assembly down to prevent the balloon from "riding" upward) or 2) curving the cryosheath and pushing the assembly inferiorly downward toward the antrum ("hockey stick" sign—especially for RIPV). A large common or oval ostium can make complete occlusion difficult. Signs of PV occlusion are 1) difficult contrast injection with retention in the vein ("hang up"), 2) absence of leaks on color Doppler sweep, and 3) pulmonary venous pressure waveforms (transition from LA [venous A and V wave] to pulmonary

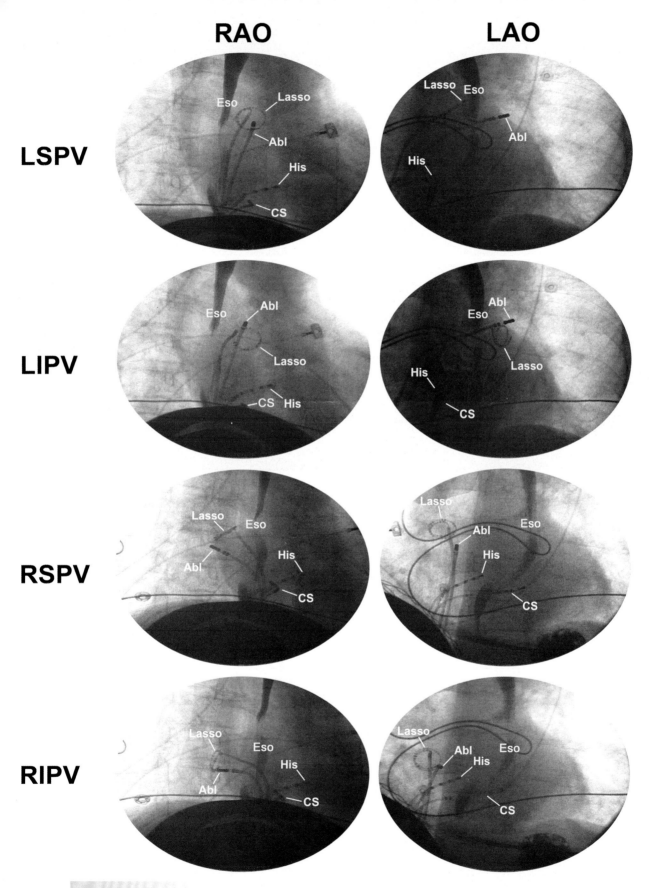

FIGURE 15-13 Barium esophagrams. Swallowed barium paste highlights the esophagus and its proximity to each of the four PVs and corresponding ablation sites.

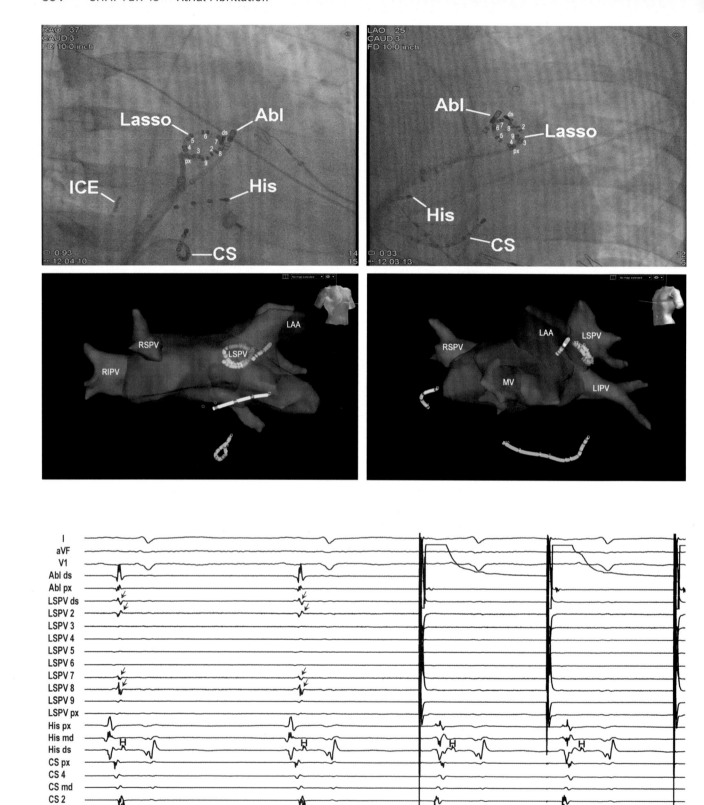

FIGURE 15-14 False PV potentials (far-field LAA). PV-like potentials (*arrows*) are recorded from the anterior LSPV (Lasso ds, 2, 7, 8) adjacent to the LAA (ablation catheter). Pacing from the LAA captures and "pulls in" these potentials (potential anticipation) indicating that they are not true PV potentials but far-field signals from the posterior LAA. Note their segmental (noncircumferential) distribution.

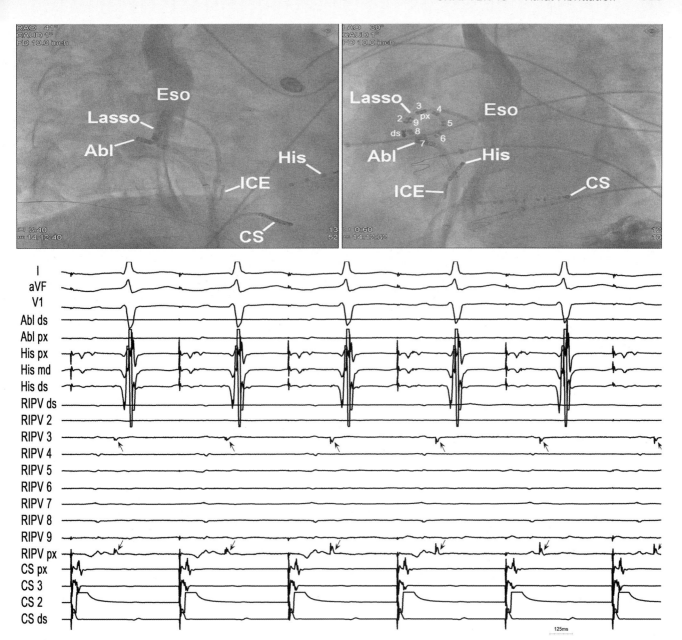

FIGURE 15-15 False PV potentials. "Ringing" on the circular mapping catheter between adjacent dipoles (third and px) creates pseudo-PV potentials (*arrows*) that can be mistaken for persistent PV conduction.

artery pressure [only higher pressure V wave]). Because of the different viscosities between contrast and saline, it is important to adequately flush any dye out of the lumen of the cryoballoon in order to accurately record pulmonary venous pressures (**Figs. 15-16 to 15-20**).[38] Optimal cryoablation endpoints include 1) nadir temperatures ($<-50°C$), 2) time to isolation (TTI) <60 sec, 3) freezing time ($-30°C$ by 30 sec, $-40°C$ by 60 sec) (rapid freezing with shorter freezing times correlates with effective cryoablation), and 4) rewarming time (interval thaw time to $0°C$ by ≥10 sec) (longer rewarming times indicate more therapeutic ice crystallization with tissue-ice bonding at $0°C$).[39–42] In contrast to the abrupt loss of PV potentials that signify entrance

block during RF ablation, cryoablation causes LA–PV delay prior to disappearance of PV potentials (**Fig. 15-21**).[43] (A distally positioned circular mapping catheter can be pulled back to the nose of the cryoballoon within 10 sec of the cryofreeze to record PV potential before the central lumen freezes.) Pacing from the circular mapping catheter can also show PV–LA delay prior to exit block. The dosing and duration of cryofreeze applications depends on how successful the cryoablation endpoints were achieved (e.g., 180 sec [TTI <90 sec] or 150 sec [TTI <30 sec]). After the freeze, the cryoballoon should not be manipulated until the temperature reaches $35°C$ during the thaw in order to avoid tissue tearing from cryoadherence.

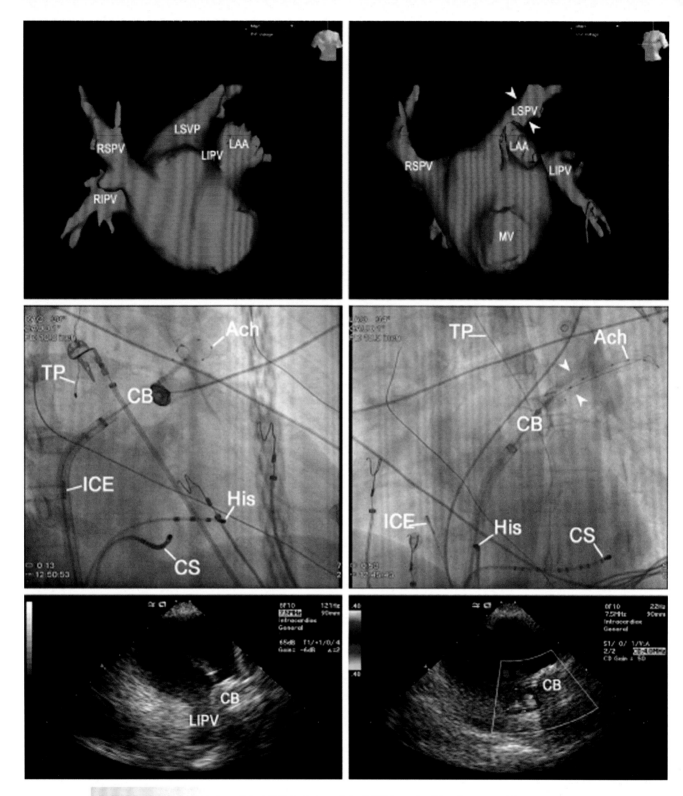

FIGURE 15-16 Cryoablation of the LSPV. Occlusion of the LSPV (*arrowheads*) is documented by contrast retention during dye injection. Color Doppler shows no visible leaks (the red color flow originates from the LIPV). ICE shows "golf ball on tee" appearance of the cryoballoon. *Abbreviations:* Ach, Achieve circular mapping catheter; CB, cryoballoon; TP, temperature probe in esophagus.

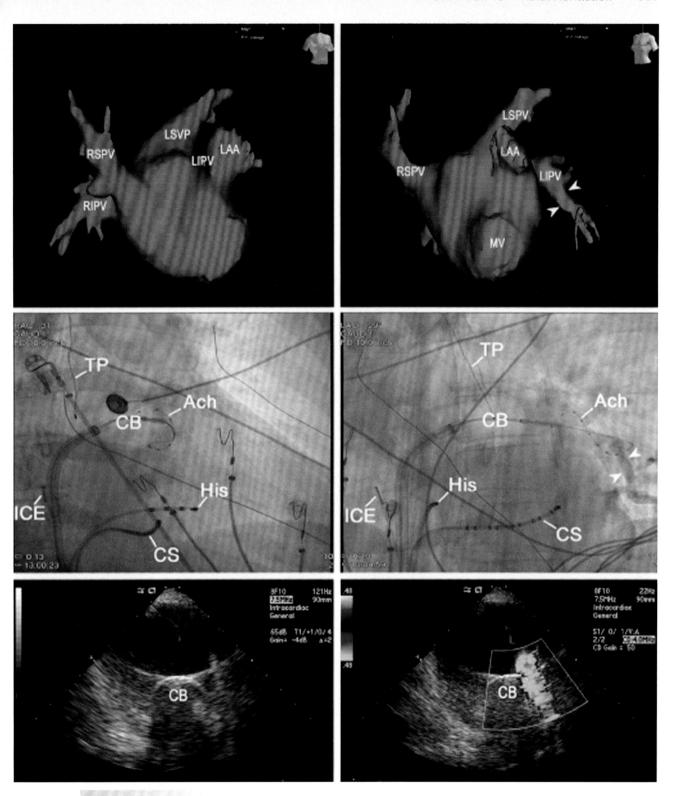

FIGURE 15-17 Cryoablation of the LIPV. Occlusion of the LIPV (*arrowheads*) is documented by contrast retention during dye injection. Color Doppler shows no visible leaks (the blue color flow originates from the LSPV). *Abbreviations:* Ach, Achieve circular mapping catheter; CB, cryoballoon; TP, temperature probe in esophagus.

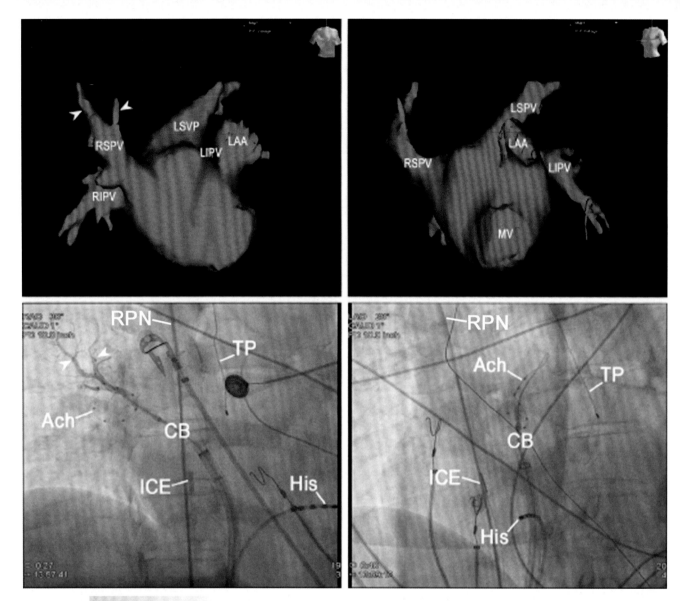

FIGURE 15-18 Cryoablation of the RSPV. Occlusion of the RSPV (*arrowheads*) is documented by contrast retention during dye injection. *Abbreviations*: Ach, Achieve circular mapping catheter; CB, cryoballoon; RPN, catheter to pace right phrenic nerve; TP, temperature probe in esophagus.

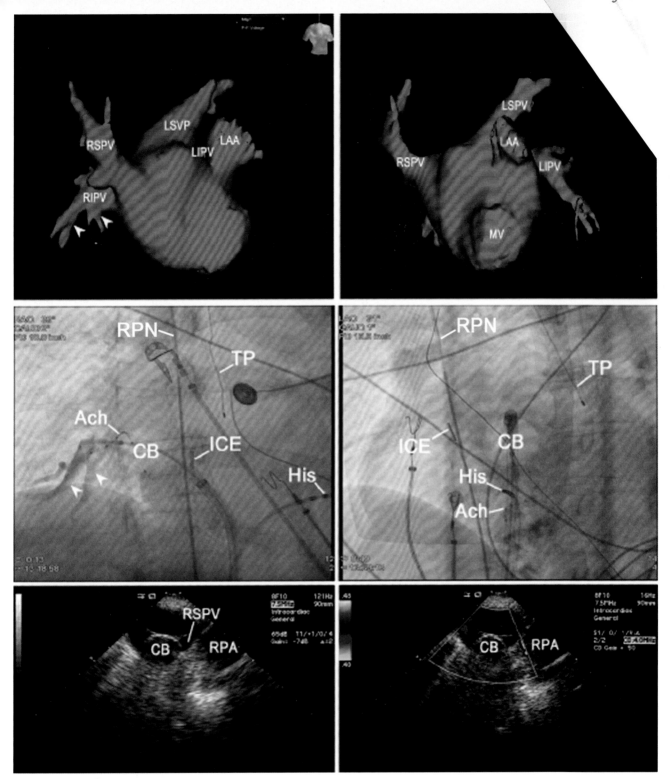

FIGURE 15-19 Cryoablation of the RIPV. Occlusion of the RIPV (*arrowheads*) is documented by contrast retention during dye injection. Color Doppler shows no visible leaks. *Abbreviations*: Ach, Achieve circular mapping catheter; CB, cryoballoon; RPN, catheter to pace right phrenic nerve; TP, temperature probe in esophagus.

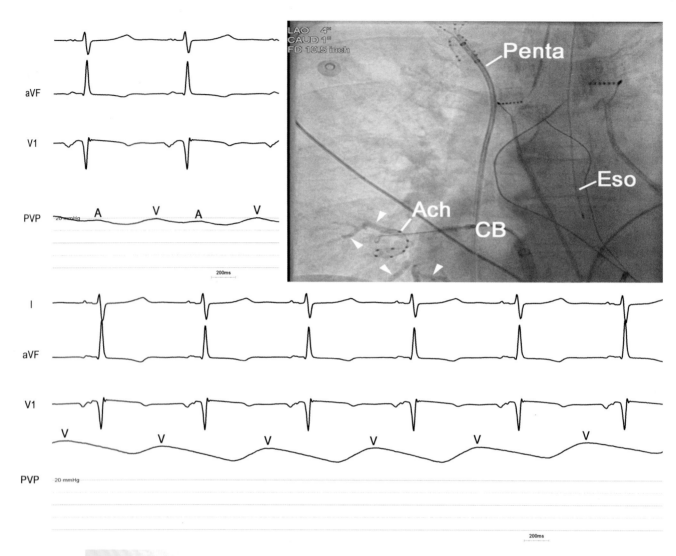

FIGURE 15-20 Pulmonary venous pressures. Before occlusion (*top left*), PVP waveforms show an A and V wave. Occlusion (*bottom*) causes a pulmonary artery waveform with a higher pressure V wave only. White arrowheads denote contrast retention during RIPV occlusion. *Abbreviations*: Ach, Acheive circular mapping catheter; CB, cryoballoon. Penta, Pentaray catheter to pace right phrenic nerve.

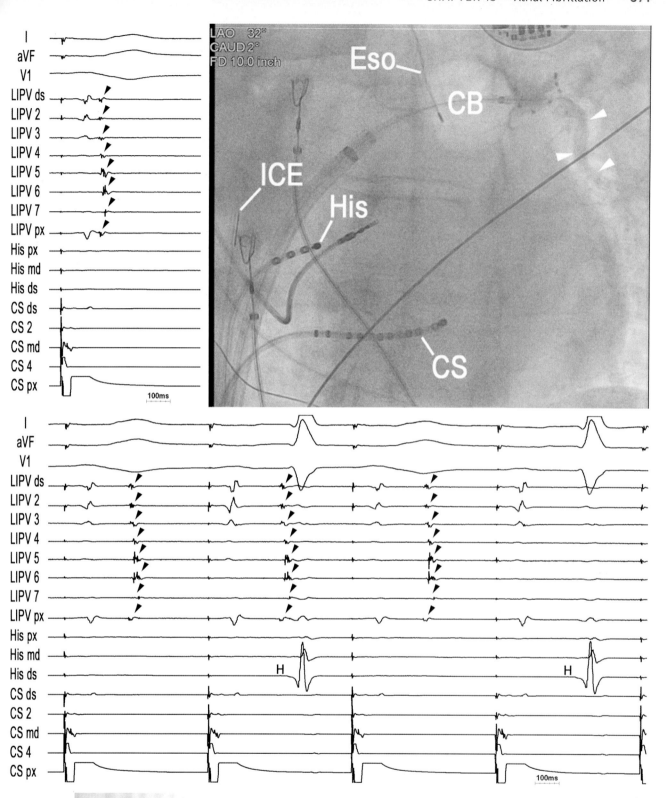

FIGURE 15-21 Entrance block (cryoablation). Occlusion of the LIPV (*white arrowheads*) is documented by contrast retention during dye injection. In contrast to abrupt loss of PV potentials by RF ablation, cryoablation causes progressive PV delay before block (*black arrowheads*). *Abbreviation:* CB, cryoballoon.

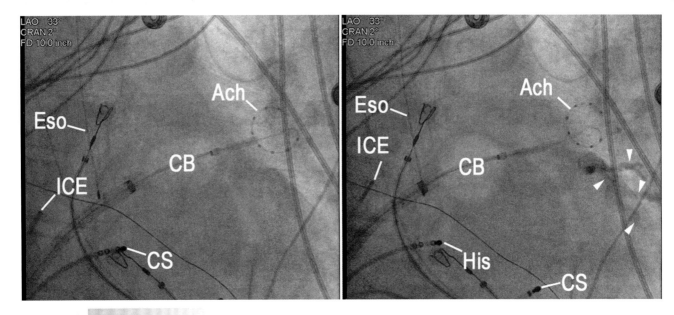

FIGURE 15-22 Deep-seated cryoballoon (CB). *Left:* "Marshmallow" appearance of the cryoballoon in the LSPV. *Right:* Rounded appearance of the cryoballoon pulled back to the antrum and occluding the LSPV (*arrowheads*). *Abbreviation:* Ach, Achieve circular mapping catheter.

Complications

Cryocomplications occur when the balloon is "deep seated" in the PV, resulting in 1) "marshmallow" appearance of the balloon, 2) ultracold temperatures <−55°C, or 3) rapid or precipitous drop in temperatures (−40°C within 30 sec) (**Fig. 15-22**). The proximal seal technique prevents deep seating of the cryoballoon by establishing initial vein occlusion, slowly pulling back the balloon to allow a slight amount of dye leakage, and then advancing the balloon simultaneous with freeze onset (because the initial injection of refrigerant causes balloon expansion). (This balloon expansion, however, can also cause a "pop out" phenomenon of a well-seated balloon in the PV antrum at the start of the freeze.)

Phrenic Nerve Injury

Cryoablation of the right-sided PVs can cause hypothermic injury and is related to the distance between the right phrenic nerve (hypothetical "vertical line" from catheter pacing phrenic nerve in right subclavian vein) and cryoballoon. The phrenic nerve is monitored by placing a catheter in the right subclavian vein (junction of SVC and right subclavian vein or alternatively anterolateral right atrium [RA]–SVC junction) and pacing the right phrenic nerve superior to the PV during the cryofreeze. Signs of phrenic nerve injury include 1) loss of diaphragmatic contraction with palpation, visualization (fluoroscopy/ICE), or auscultation (auditory cardiotocography) or 2) 35% decrease in diaphragmatic compound motor action potentials (CMAPs) (**Fig. 15-23**). CMAPs are measured using a modified lead I (or electrode catheter in the subdiaphragmatic hepatic veins) that overlies the right hemidiaphragm and provides the earliest detection of phrenic nerve injury.[44,45] During phrenic nerve stimulation, reduction of the CMAP by 35% predicts phrenic nerve injury. Use of the double stop technique allows immediate balloon deflation and more rapid tissue rewarming. The balloon, however, should not be moved until it is sufficiently rewarmed because of cryoadherence.

Atrio-esophageal Fistulas

Atrio-esophageal fistulas from cryoablation most commonly involves the LIPV.[46] It has been suggested that the "two-hit" phenomenon of esophageal ulceration aggravated by acid reflux contributes to fistula formation (and hence the use of prophylactic proton pump inhibitors). Interrupting cryoablation at LET = 15°C reduces the risk of esophageal injury.[47]

SUBSTRATE MODIFICATION

While PVI alone can treat paroxysmal or short duration persistent atrial fibrillation, it is often insufficient for longstanding persistent atrial fibrillation and adjunctive ablation is required.[48] Other methods to modify the arrhythmogenic substrate include 1) electrogram-based ablation (complex fractionated atrial electrogram [CFAE]), 2) linear lesions, and 3) mechanistic-based ablation. These techniques can terminate atrial fibrillation or convert it to atrial flutter/tachycardias (distillation of fibrillation to slower, mappable tachycardias).

Electrogram-Based Ablation

A hierarchical distribution of electrogram frequencies throughout the atria exists during atrial fibrillation with higher activation frequencies preferentially at the LA–PV junction. This distribution supports the rotor hypothesis with frequency gradients between small reentrant sources (rotors) and more distant sites.

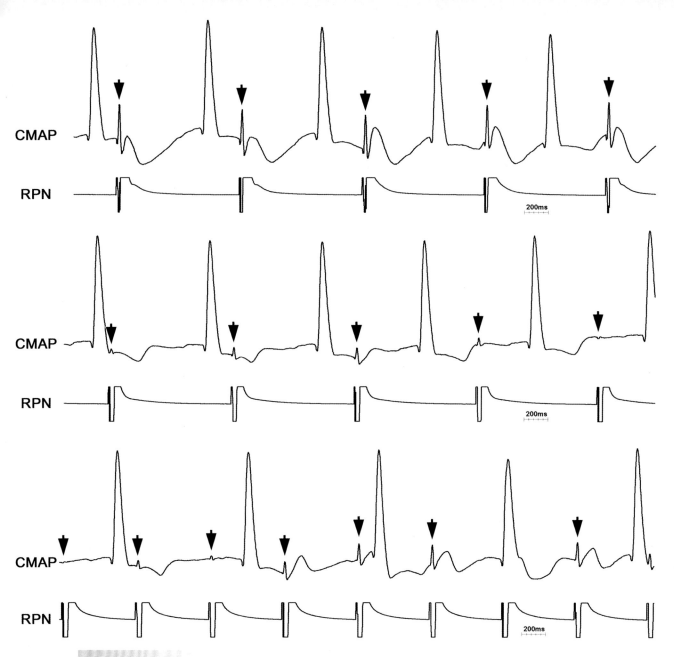

FIGURE 15-23 CMAPs. Cryoablation of the RSPV causes reduction and transient loss of the CMAP (*arrows*) followed by partial recovery. *Abbreviation:* RPN, catheter to pace right phrenic nerve.

Ablation strategies target regions with the highest dominant frequencies, CFAE, or electrograms demonstrating a local temporal gradient between two closely spaced dipoles (small reentrant circuit).[49–53] CFAEs are correlated with slow conduction and pivot points of wavelet reentry and defined as having 1) ≥2 deflections and/or perturbation of the baseline with continuous deflection from a prolonged activation complex or 2) atrial electrograms with a very short cycle length (≤120 ms)—both over a 10-sec recording period (**Fig. 15-24**). They tend to cluster around the PVs, interatrial septum, roof of the LA, left posteroseptal mitral annulus, and CS ostium.

Linear Lesions

LA ablation lines include a 1) mitral isthmus line (lateral mitral annulus to LIPV or anterior LA transection [anterior mitral annulus to roof line or encircled right PVs]), 2) roof line (between the two superior PVs), and 3) box isolation of low voltage (<0.5 mV) fibrotic areas.[54–56] Mitral isthmus block might require both endocardial and epicardial (CS) ablation. Bidirectional block across the ablation lines is demonstrated by 1) pacing on both sides of the line and recording a corridor of widely spaced double potentials with reversal of atrial activation on the other side of the line (activation detour) and

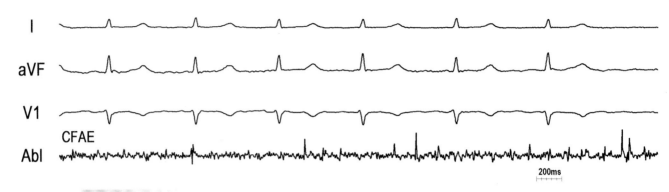

FIGURE 15-24 CFAEs. Continuous, high-frequency electrical activity is recorded on the ablation catheter.

2) differential atrial pacing. With clockwise mitral isthmus block, LAA pacing (lateral to the line) causes widely spaced double potentials (>150 ms) along the line and CS proximal to distal activation (reversal of activation). With roof block, LAA pacing (anterior to the line) causes widely spaced double potential along the line and ascending activation of the posterior wall (reversal of activation).

Mechanistic-Based Ablation

In contrast to an electrogram-based approach that lacks specificity (bystander site), a mechanistic approach is based on AF dynamics and targets patient-specific local sources (rotor cores and focal impulses) that drive and sustain atrial fibrillation: focal impulse and rotor modulation (FIRM).[57]

MODULATING FACTORS

Vagal Denervation

Parasympathetic stimulation reduces atrial refractory periods, increases dispersion of refractoriness, and induces atrial fibrillation. Vagal denervation is another adjunctive technique for atrial fibrillation ablation.[58] Application of RF energy to ganglionic plexi located near the PV ostia elicits vagal reflexes (sinus bradycardia [<40 bpm], asystole, AV block, or hypotension), and ablation is continued until the reflex is abolished (**Fig. 15-25**). Complete vagal denervation occurs when all vagal reflexes around the PV ostia are eliminated. High-frequency stimulation (50 ms cycle length, 12 V, 1–10 ms pulse width) can be used to map ganglionic plexi.

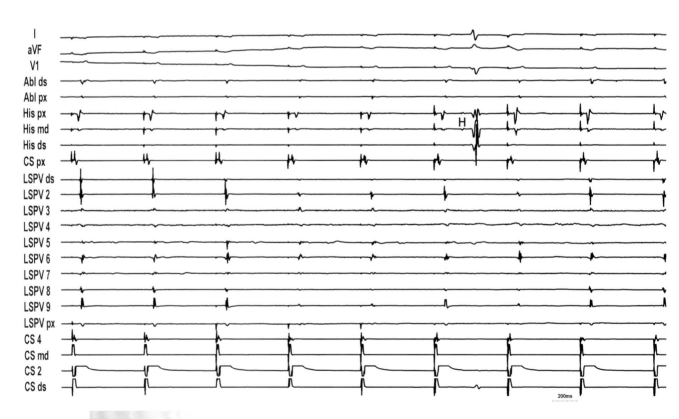

FIGURE 15-25 Vagal reflex. RF delivery to a ganglionic plexus induces high-grade AV block.

TAILORED APPROACH

Because of the heterogeneity of atrial fibrillation mechanisms, no single ablation strategy or standardized lesion set is uniformly effective. PVI alone may be sufficient to treat paroxysmal atrial fibrillation arising from a focal PV source and normal atria but is often insufficient for longstanding persistent atrial fibrillation.[59–62] In the latter case, additional substrate modification becomes necessary. The ideal approach individualizes the ablation strategy based on the clinical and electrophysiologic profiles of each patient.[63]

ENDPOINTS

The endpoints for atrial fibrillation ablation depend on the strategy employed and the type of atrial fibrillation. PVI requires entrance block into the PV (elimination or dissociation of PV potentials from the LA) and exit block from the PV (PV sleeve capture without conduction to the LA). Adenosine can be used to assess for PV reconnection; while isoproterenol can be given to trigger non-PV foci. Linear lines are validated by demonstrating bidirectional conduction block (pacing and recording on both side of the line) to prevent macroreentry involving gaps along the line. CFAE ablation and vagal denervation aim to eliminate all sites with CFAEs and vagal reflexes, respectively. While noninducibility of atrial fibrillation after ablation has been proposed as a useful endpoint for paroxysmal atrial fibrillation, it seems to be unnecessary or even not feasible for longstanding persistent atrial fibrillation.[64,65] For persistent atrial fibrillation, another endpoint is termination of atrial fibrillation by ablation. Despite these endpoints, recurrent atrial fibrillation can occur after ablation but often disappears within several months accompanying lesion maturation (3-month blanking period). The major factor for atrial fibrillation recurrence and the need for a repeat procedure is PV reconnection.[66]

POST-ABLATION LEFT ATRIAL FLUTTER/TACHYCARDIA

While LA flutter/tachycardia arising after ablation of atrial fibrillation might be a proarrhythmic result from previous ablation lines, it can also be considered an intermediate defragmentation step in the organization of atrial fibrillation before achieving durable sinus rhythm. Two general mechanisms of post-atrial fibrillation ablation LA flutter/tachycardia are 1) focal and 2) macroreentrant—and dependent upon the index ablation strategy employed. They are associated with the recurrence of atrial fibrillation and recovery of PV conduction.[67,68] Segmental ostial ablation can cause a focal atrial tachycardia often within or near recovered PVs where reisolation of the veins or targeting a critical reentrant isthmus is effective.[69–72] WACA is associated with macroreentrant LA flutters through ≥2 residual gaps in the ablation circle or a reentrant circuit imposed by linear constraining barriers: around ipsilateral PVs (roof-dependent flutter), the mitral annulus (perimitral flutter),

or within the CS.[73–76] A third proposed mechanism of post-atrial fibrillation ablation LA flutter/tachycardia is an intermediary between focal and macroreentry called localized reentry. With localized reentry, the majority (≥75%) of the tachycardia cycle length is recordable ("macroreentry") but confined to a small, well-circumscribed region (≤2 cm) from which centrifugal activation of the LA occurs ("focal").[77] Characteristic electrograms in the region are low amplitude, polyphasic signals showing a zone of slow conduction (conduction gradient between proximal and distal dipoles of the mapping catheter) and where PPI − TCL <30 ms.

LA flutter/tachycardias are mapped using both 1) activation ("pinging") and 2) entrainment mapping, often in combination with a three-dimensional electro-anatomic mapping system.[77–83]

CS atrial activation sequences help differentiate clockwise perimitral/lateral LA (left-sided PV, LAA) tachycardias (CS ds to px activation) from counterclockwise perimitral/septal LA (right-sided PV)/RA tachycardias (CS px to ds activation).[84] Quick entrainment demonstrating PPI − TCL >30 ms from two opposite atrial segments rules out macroreentrant LA tachycardia: septal and lateral LA (horizontal LA axis) for perimitral reentry and posterior and anterior LA (longitudinal LA axis) for roof-dependent reentry.

Focal tachycardia shows 1) more cycle length variability (>15%), 2) centrifugal activation pattern (<75% cycle length recorded), 3) and PPI ≤30 ms at its point source (single atrial segment). Isoelectric intervals separating tachycardia/flutter P waves also suggest a focal mechanism (e.g., small circuit reentry). After atrial fibrillation ablation, the two most common macroreentrant LA flutter/tachycardias are perimitral reentry and roof-dependent flutter. Macroreentrant tachycardias show 1) less cycle length variability (<15%), 2) "early meets late" activation pattern (>75% cycle length recorded), and 3) PPI − TCL ≤30 ms in two opposite atrial segments. The presence of constant intracardiac fusion (orthodromic/antidromic collision) during transient entrainment also indicates macroreentry (first criteria of transient entrainment).[85] A color-coded three-dimensional entrainment map identifies areas critical for the reentrant circuit and helps determine the strategy for lesion deployment.[86] Entrainment mapping differentiates sites integral to tachycardia (PPI − TCL ≤30 ms) from a bystander (PPI − TCL >30 ms) but is difficult when tachycardia changes or cycle lengths vary (multiloop tachycardias).[87] It is important to entrain from the cavo-tricuspid isthmus (CTI) and demonstrate that tachycardia is not CTI dependent with an atypical flutter morphology resulting from extensive LA ablation. For macroreentrant atrial flutter, ablation targets a critical isthmus (broad fractionated "gap potential") or creating a line of block transecting the narrowest part of the circuit between regions of scar or anatomic obstacles (line connecting the two superior PVs at the most cranial aspect of the LA for roof-dependent atrial flutter) (Fig. 15-26). Termination of atrial flutter by a nonpropagated extrastimulus (nonglobal capture) is a rare finding identifying a critical isthmus and is also an important target site for ablation.[88]

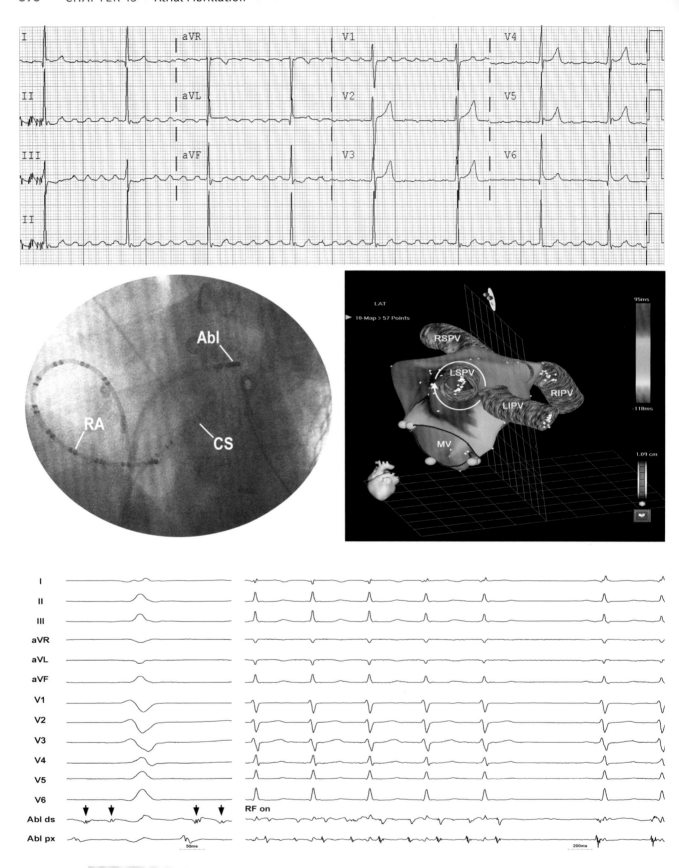

FIGURE 15-26 LA flutter/tachycardia after atrial fibrillation ablation. LA flutter (positive in lead V1 and II [V1/II concordance]) revolves around the LSPV. A prolonged double potential or "gap potential" (*arrows*) is recorded at the successful ablation site.

REFERENCES

1. Fuster V, Rydén LE, Cannom DS, et al. ACC/AHA/ESC 2006 guidelines for the management of patients with atrial fibrillation—executive summary: a report of the American College of Cardiology/American Heart Association Task Force on Practice Guidelines and the European Society of Cardiology Committee for Practice Guidelines (Writing Committee to Revise the 2001 Guidelines for the Management of Patients With Atrial Fibrillation). J Am Coll Cardiol 2006;48:854–906.

2. Haïssaguerre M, Jaïs P, Shah DC, et al. Spontaneous initiation of atrial fibrillation by ectopic beats originating in the pulmonary veins. N Engl J Med 1998;339:659–666.

3. Jaïs P, Haïssaguerre M, Shah DC, et al. A focal source of atrial fibrillation treated by discrete radiofrequency ablation. Circulation 1997;95:572–576.

4. Calkins H, Brugada J, Packer DL, et al. HRS/EHRA/ECAS expert consensus statement on catheter and surgical ablation of atrial fibrillation: recommendations for personnel, policy, procedures and follow-up. A report of the Heart Rhythm Society (HRS) Task Force on catheter and surgical ablation of atrial fibrillation. Heart Rhythm 2007;4:816–861.

5. Natale A, Raviele A, Arentz T, et al. Venice chart international consensus document on atrial fibrillation ablation. J Cardiovasc Electrophysiol 2007;18:560–580.

6. Lin W, Tai C, Hsieh M, et al. Catheter ablation of paroxysmal atrial fibrillation initiated by non-pulmonary vein ectopy. Circulation 2003;107:3176–3183.

7. Lee S, Tai C, Hsieh M, et al. Predictors of non-pulmonary vein ectopic beats initiating paroxysmal atrial fibrillation: implication for catheter ablation. J Am Coll Cardiol 2005;46:1054–1059.

8. Tsai C, Tai C, Hsieh M, et al. Initiation of atrial fibrillation by ectopic beats originating from the superior vena cava: electrophysiological characteristics and results of radiofrequency ablation. Circulation 2000;102:67–74.

9. Sauer WH, Alonso C, Zado E, et al. Atrioventricular nodal reentrant tachycardia in patients referred for atrial fibrillation ablation: response to ablation that incorporates slow-pathway modification. Circulation 2006;114:191–195.

10. Haïssaguerre M, Sanders P, Hocini M, Jaïs P, Clémenty J. Pulmonary veins in the substrate for atrial fibrillation: the "venous wave" hypothesis. J Am Coll Cardiol 2004;43:2290–2292.

11. Jalife J, Berenfeld O, Mansour M. Mother rotors and fibrillatory conduction: a mechanism of atrial fibrillation. Cardiovasc Res 2002;54:204–216.

12. Moe GK, Abildskov JA. Atrial fibrillation as a self-sustaining arrhythmia independent of focal discharge. Am Heart J 1959;58:59–70.

13. West TC, Landa JF. Minimal mass required for induction of a sustained arrhythmia in isolated atrial segments. Am J Physiol 1962;202:232–236.

14. Bettoni M, Zimmermann M. Autonomic tone variations before the onset of paroxysmal atrial fibrillation. Circulation 2002;105:2753–2759.

15. Zhou J, Scherlag B, Edwards J, Jackman W, Lazzara R, Po S. Gradients of atrial refractoriness and inducibility of atrial fibrillation due to stimulation of ganglionated plexi. J Cardiovasc Electrophysiol 2007;18:83–90.

16. Cox JL, Canavan TE, Schuessler RB, et al. The surgical treatment of atrial fibrillation. II. Intraoperative electrophysiologic mapping and description of the electrophysiologic basis of atrial flutter and atrial fibrillation. J Thorac Cardiovasc Surg 1991;101:406–426.

17. Cox JL, Schuessler RB, D'Agostino HJ Jr, et al. The surgical treatment of atrial fibrillation. III. Development of a definitive surgical procedure. J Thorac Cardiovasc Surg 1991;101:569–583.

18. Cox JL. The surgical treatment of atrial fibrillation. IV. Surgical technique. J Thorac Cardiovasc Surg 1991;101:584–592.

19. Swartz JF, Pellerseis G, Silvers J, Patten L, Cervantez D. A catheter-based curative approach to atrial fibrillation in humans [abstract]. Circulation 1994;90:I-335.

20. Haïssaguerre M, Jaïs P, Shah DC, et al. Electrophysiological end point for catheter ablation of atrial fibrillation initiated from multiple pulmonary venous foci. Circulation 2000;101:1409–1417.

21. Haïssaguerre M, Shah DC, Jaïs P, et al. Electrophysiological breakthroughs from the left atrium to the pulmonary veins. Circulation 2000;102: 2463–2465.

22. Oral H, Knight BP, Ozaydin M, et al. Segmental ostial ablation to isolate the pulmonary veins during atrial fibrillation: feasibility and mechanistic insights. Circulation 2002;106:1256–1262.

23. Pappone C, Rosanio S, Oreto G, et al. Circumferential radiofrequency ablation of pulmonary vein ostia: a new anatomic approach for curing atrial fibrillation. Circulation 2000;102:2619–2628.

24. Lemola K, Oral H, Chugh A, et al. Pulmonary vein isolation as an end point for left atrial circumferential ablation of atrial fibrillation. J Am Coll Cardiol 2005;46:1060–1066.

25. Ouyang F, Bänsch D, Ernst S, et al. Complete isolation of left atrium surrounding the pulmonary veins: new insights from the double-Lasso technique in paroxysmal atrial fibrillation. Circulation 2004;110:2090–2096.

26. Oral H, Scharf C, Chugh A, et al. Catheter ablation for paroxysmal atrial fibrillation: segmental pulmonary vein ostial ablation versus left atrial ablation. Circulation 2003;108:2355–2360.

27. Proietti R, Santangeli P, Di Biase L, et al. Comparative effectiveness of wide antral versus ostial pulmonary vein isolation: a systematic review and meta-analysis. Circ Arrhythm Electrophysiol 2014;7:39–45.

28. Bunch TJ, Day JD. Novel ablative approach for atrial fibrillation to decrease risk of esophageal injury. Heart Rhythm 2008;5:624–627.

29. Arentz T, Macle L, Kalusche D, et al. "Dormant" pulmonary vein conduction revealed by adenosine after ostial radiofrequency catheter ablation. J Cardiovasc Electrophysiol 2004;15:1041–1047.

30. Datino T, Macle L, Qi XY, et al. Mechanisms by which adenosine restores conduction in dormant canine pulmonary veins. Circulation 2010;121: 963–972.

31. Macle L, Khairy P, Weerasooriya R, et al; for the ADVICE trial investigators. Adenosine-guided pulmonary vein isolation for the treatment of paroxysmal atrial fibrillation: an international, multicentre, randomised superiority trial. Lancet 2015;386:672–679.

32. Elayi CS, Di Biase L, Bai R, et al. Administration of isoproterenol and adenosine to guide supplemental ablation after pulmonary vein antrum isolation. J Cardiovasc Electrophysiol 2013;24:1199–1206.

33. Shah D, Haïssaguerre M, Jaïs P, et al. Left atrial appendage activity masquerading as pulmonary vein potentials. Circulation 2002;105:2821–2825.

34. Shah D. Electrophysiological evaluation of pulmonary vein isolation. Europace 2009;11:1423–1433.

35. Packer DL, Kowal RC, Wheelan KR, et al. Cryoballoon ablation of pulmonary veins for paroxysmal atrial fibrillation: first results of the North American Arctic Front (STOP AF) pivotal trial. J Am Coll Cardiol 2013;61:1713–1723.

36. Kuck KH, Brugada J, Fürnkranz A, et al; for FIRE AND ICE Investigators. Cryoballoon or radiofrequency ablation for paroxysmal atrial fibrillation. N Engl J Med 2016;374:2235–2245.

37. Su W, Kowal R, Kowalski M, et al. Best practice guide for cryoballoon ablation in atrial fibrillation: the compilation experience of more than 3000 procedures. Heart Rhythm 2015;12:1658–1666.

38. Siklódy CH, Minners J, Allgeier M, et al. Pressure-guided cryoballoon isolation of the pulmonary veins for the treatment of paroxysmal atrial fibrillation. J Cardiovasc Electrophysiol 2010;21:120–125.

39. Su W, Aryana A, Passman R, et al. Cryoballoon best practices II: practical guide to procedural monitoring and dosing during atrial fibrillation ablation from the perspective of experienced users. Heart Rhythm 2018;15:1348–1355.

40. Fürnkranz A, Köster I, Chun K, et al. Cryoballoon temperature predicts acute pulmonary vein isolation. Heart Rhythm 2011;8:821–825.

41. Ghosh J, Martin A, Keech AC, et al. Balloon warming time is the strongest predictor of late pulmonary vein electrical reconnection following cryoballoon ablation for atrial fibrillation. Heart Rhythm 2013;10:1311–1317.

42. Aryana A, Mugnai G, Singh SM, et al. Procedural and biophysical indicators of durable pulmonary vein isolation during cryoballoon ablation of atrial fibrillation. Heart Rhythm 2016;13:424–432.

43. Andrade JG, Dubuc M, Collet D, Khairy P, Macle L. Pulmonary vein signal interpretation during cryoballoon ablation for atrial fibrillation. Heart Rhythm 2015;12:1387–1394.

44. Franceschi F, Koutbi L, Mancini J, Attarian S, Prevôt S, Deharo JC. Novel electromyographic monitoring technique for prevention of right phrenic nerve palsy during cryoballoon ablation. Circ Arrhythm Electrophysiol 2013;6:1109–1114.

45. Lakhani M, Saiful F, Parikh V, Goyal N, Bekheit S, Kowalski M. Recordings of diaphragmatic electromyograms during cryoballoon ablation for atrial fibrillation accurately predict phrenic nerve injury. Heart Rhythm 2014;11: 369–374.

46. John RM, Kapur S, Ellenbogen KA, Koneru JN. Atrioesophageal fistula formation with cryoballoon ablation is most commonly related to the left inferior pulmonary vein. Heart Rhythm 2017;14:184–189.

47. Fürnkranz A, Bordignon S, Böhmig M, et al. Reduced incidence of esophageal lesions by luminal esophageal temperature-guided second-generation cryoballoon ablation. Heart Rhythm 2015;12:268–274.

48. Kottkamp H, Bender R, Berg J. Catheter ablation of atrial fibrillation: how to modify the substrate? J Am Coll Cardiol 2015;65:196–206.

49. Sanders P, Berenfeld O, Hocini M, et al. Spectral analysis identifies sites of high-frequency activity maintaining atrial fibrillation in humans. Circulation 2005;112:789–797.

50. Nademanee K, McKenzie J, Kosar E, et al. A new approach for catheter ablation of atrial fibrillation: mapping of the electrophysiologic substrate. J Am Coll Cardiol 2004;43:2044–2053.

51. Nademanee K, Schwab M, Porath J, Abbo A. How to perform electrogram-guided atrial fibrillation ablation. Heart Rhythm 2006;3:981–984.

52. Wright M, Haïssaguerre M, Knecht S, et al. State of the art: catheter ablation of atrial fibrillation. J Cardiovasc Electrophysiol 2008;19:583–592.

53. O'Neill MD, Jaïs P, Hocini M, et al. Catheter ablation for atrial fibrillation. Circulation 2007;116:1515–1523.

54. Jaïs P, Hocini M, O'Neill MD, et al. How to perform linear lesions. Heart Rhythm 2007;4:803–809.

55. Jaïs P, Hocini M, Hsu LF, et al. Technique and results of linear ablation at the mitral isthmus. Circulation 2004;110:2996–3002.

56. Hocini M, Jaïs P, Sanders P, et al. Techniques, evaluation, and consequences of linear block at the left atrial roof in paroxysmal atrial fibrillation: a prospective randomized study. Circulation 2005;112:3688–3696.

57. Narayan SM, Krummen DE, Shivkumar K, Clopton P, Rappel WJ, Miller JM. Treatment of atrial fibrillation by the ablation of localized sources: CONFIRM (CONventional ablation for atrial fibrillation with or without Focal Impulse and Rotor Modulation) trial. J Am Coll Cardiol 2012;60:628–636.

58. Pappone C, Santinelli V, Manguso F, et al. Pulmonary vein denervation enhances long-term benefit after circumferential ablation for paroxysmal atrial fibrillation. Circulation 2004;109:327–334.

59. Oral H, Knight BP, Tada H, et al. Pulmonary vein isolation for paroxysmal and persistent atrial fibrillation. Circulation 2002;105:1077–1081.

60. Haïssaguerre M, Sanders P, Hocini M, et al. Catheter ablation of long-lasting persistent atrial fibrillation: critical structures for termination. J Cardiovasc Electrophysiol 2005;16:1125–1137.

61. Haïssaguerre M, Hocini M, Sanders P, et al. Catheter ablation of long-lasting persistent atrial fibrillation: clinical outcome and mechanisms of subsequent arrhythmias. J Cardiovasc Electrophysiol 2005;16:1138–1147.

62. Hocini M, Sanders P, Jaïs P, et al. Techniques for curative treatment of atrial fibrillation. J Cardiovasc Electrophysiol 2004;15:1467–1471.

63. Oral H, Chugh A, Good E, et al. A tailored approach to catheter ablation of paroxysmal atrial fibrillation. Circulation 2006;113:1824–1831.

64. Oral H, Chugh A, Lemola K, et al. Noninducibility of atrial fibrillation as an end point of left atrial circumferential ablation for paroxysmal atrial fibrillation: a randomized study. Circulation 2004;110:2797–2801.

65. Oral H, Pappone C, Chugh A, et al. Circumferential pulmonary-vein ablation for chronic atrial fibrillation. N Engl J Med 2006;354:934–941.

66. Verma A, Kilicaslan F, Pisano E, et al. Response of atrial fibrillation to pulmonary vein antrum isolation is directly related to resumption and delay of pulmonary vein conduction. Circulation 2005;112:627–635.

67. Kobza R, Hindricks G, Tanner H, et al. Late recurrent arrhythmias after ablation of atrial fibrillation: incidence, mechanisms, and treatment. Heart Rhythm 2004;1:676–683.

68. Ouyang F, Antz M, Ernst S, et al. Recovered pulmonary vein conduction as a dominant factor for recurrent atrial tachyarrhythmias after complete circular isolation of the pulmonary veins: lessons from double Lasso technique. Circulation 2005;111:127–135.

69. Oral H, Knight BP, Morady F. Left atrial flutter after segmental ostial radiofrequency catheter ablation for pulmonary vein isolation. Pacing Clin Electrophysiol 2003;26:1417–1419.

70. Gerstenfeld EP, Callans DJ, Dixit S, et al. Mechanisms of organized left atrial tachycardias occurring after pulmonary vein isolation. Circulation 2004;110:1351–1357.

71. Cummings JE, Schweikert R, Saliba W, et al. Left atrial flutter following pulmonary vein antrum isolation with radiofrequency energy: linear lesions or repeat isolation. J Cardiovasc Electrophysiol 2005;16:293–297.

72. Villacastín J, Pérez-Castellano N, Moreno J, González R. Left atrial flutter after radiofrequency catheter ablation of focal atrial fibrillation. J Cardiovasc Electrophysiol 2003;14:417–421.

73. Mesas CE, Pappone C, Lang CC, et al. Left atrial tachycardia after circumferential pulmonary vein ablation for atrial fibrillation: electroanatomic characterization and treatment. J Am Coll Cardiol 2004;44:1071–1079.

74. Chae S, Oral H, Good E, et al. Atrial tachycardia after circumferential pulmonary vein ablation of atrial fibrillation: mechanistic insights, results of catheter ablation, and risk factors for recurrence. J Am Coll Cardiol 2007;50:1781–1787.

75. Chugh A, Oral H, Lemola K, et al. Prevalence, mechanisms, and clinical significance of macroreentrant atrial tachycardia during and following left atrial ablation for atrial fibrillation. Heart Rhythm 2005;2:464–471.

76. Chugh A, Oral H, Good E, et al. Catheter ablation of atypical atrial flutter and atrial tachycardia within the coronary sinus after left atrial ablation for atrial fibrillation. J Am Coll Cardiol 2005;46:83–91.

77. Jaïs P, Matsuo S, Knecht S, et al. A deductive mapping strategy for atrial tachycardia following atrial fibrillation ablation: importance of localized reentry. J Cardiovasc Electrophysiol 2009;20:480–491.

78. Jaïs P, Shah DC, Haïssaguerre M, et al. Mapping and ablation of left atrial flutters. Circulation 2000;101:2928–2934.

79. Ouyang F, Ernst S, Vogtmann T, et al. Characterization of reentrant circuits in left atrial macroreentrant tachycardia: critical isthmus block can prevent atrial tachycardia recurrence. Circulation 2002;105:1934–1942.

80. Weerasooriya R, Jaïs P, Wright M, et al. Catheter ablation of atrial tachycardia following atrial fibrillation ablation. J Cardiovasc Electrophysiol 2009;20:833–838.

81. Morady F, Oral H, Chugh A. Diagnosis and ablation of atypical atrial tachycardia and flutter complicating atrial fibrillation ablation. Heart Rhythm 2009;6:S29–S32.

82. Gerstenfeld EP, Marchlinski FE. Mapping and ablation of left atrial tachycardias occurring after atrial fibrillation ablation. Heart Rhythm 2007;4:S65–S72.

83. Miyazaki H, Stevenson WG, Stephenson K, Soejima K, Epstein LM. Entrainment mapping for rapid distinction of left and right atrial tachycardias. Heart Rhythm 2006;3:516–523.

84. Pascale P, Shah AJ, Roten L, et al. Pattern and timing of the coronary sinus activation to guide rapid diagnosis of atrial tachycardia after atrial fibrillation ablation. Circ Arrhythm Electrophysiol 2013;6:481–490.

85. Barbhaiya C, Kumar S, Ng J, et al. Overdrive pacing from downstream sites on multielectrode catheters to rapidly detect fusion and to diagnose macroreentrant atrial arrhythmias. Circulation 2014;129:2503–2510.

86. Esato M, Hindricks G, Sommer P, et al. Color-coded three-dimensional entrainment mapping for analysis and treatment of atrial macroreentrant tachycardia. Heart Rhythm 2009;6:349–358.

87. Colombowala IK, Massumi A, Rasekh A, et al. Variability in post-pacing intervals predicts global atrial activation pattern during tachycardia. J Cardiovasc Electrophysiol 2008;19:142–147.

88. Lim K, Knight BP. Pace termination of left atrial flutter after ablation for atrial fibrillation: what is the mechanism? Heart Rhythm 2008;5:1619–1620.

Sinus Node and Atrio-ventricular Junction Modification/Ablation

16

Introduction

Inappropriate sinus tachycardia (IAST) is an uncommon entity that can cause debilitating symptoms and even a tachycardia-mediated cardiomyopathy.[1-3] Generally, it is a diagnosis of exclusion following negative evaluation for secondary causes. Proposed mechanisms include 1) increased automaticity from an intrinsic defect in the sino-atrial node (SAN) and/or 2) sympathovagal imbalance.[2] Catheter modification of the SAN provides an option for symptomatic, drug-refractory IAST.

The atrio-ventricular (AV) node provides electrical continuity between the atrium and ventricle and serves as a filter to prevent rapid ventricular rates during atrial fibrillation. However, short AV nodal functional refractory periods can result in rapid ventricular rates that might necessitate modification or ablation followed by permanent pacemaker implantation to achieve rate control.[4-7]

The purpose of this chapter is to:

1. Describe the anatomy of the sinus and AV node–His bundle axis.
2. Discuss the technique of sinus node modification.
3. Discuss different approaches of AV node modification/ablation.

SINO-ATRIAL NODE AND AV NODE–HIS BUNDLE AXIS

The SAN is a crescent-shaped epicardial structure (mean length = 13.5 mm) situated along the superolateral right atrium (RA) near its junction with the superior vena cava (SVC) and with its long axis running parallel along the sulcus terminalis (terminal groove).[8] Because sinus nodal cells located cranially discharge at faster rates than caudal cells, the superior SAN is the initial target site for ablation during sinus node modification.

The compact AV node is a subendocardial structure located along the right interatrial septum posterior and inferior to the His bundle. The His bundle lies at the apex of the triangle of Koch, which is defined by the 1) ostium of the coronary sinus, 2) septal leaflet of the tricuspid valve, and 3) tendon of Todaro. The His bundle penetrates the crest of the interventricular septum where it can be recorded on both sides of the interventricular septum providing right- and left-sided approaches to AV junction ablation.

SINO-ATRIAL NODE MODIFICATION

The initial target site during SAN modification is the superior SAN identified by mapping the earliest site of atrial activation during sinus tachycardia (**Figs. 16-1 and 16-2**).[9-13] Delivery of radiofrequency (RF) energy can cause initial acceleration of sinus tachycardia. Because of the close proximity between the right phrenic nerve and SAN, it is important to test for phrenic nerve capture by high-output pacing in order to avoid diaphragm paralysis during ablation. In the presence of diaphragmatic capture, the phrenic nerve can be monitored during RF delivery by pacing the right phrenic nerve with a catheter placed in the right subclavian vein (as done during right-sided pulmonary vein cryoablation). With ablation of the superior SAN, the earliest site of atrial activation shifts caudally along the SAN, resulting both in a reduction in sinus rate and P-wave amplitude in the inferior leads. Ablation lesions are progressively delivered caudally along the sinus node until the sinus rate is 1) reduced by 25% or below 90 bpm (baseline), 2) reduced 25%

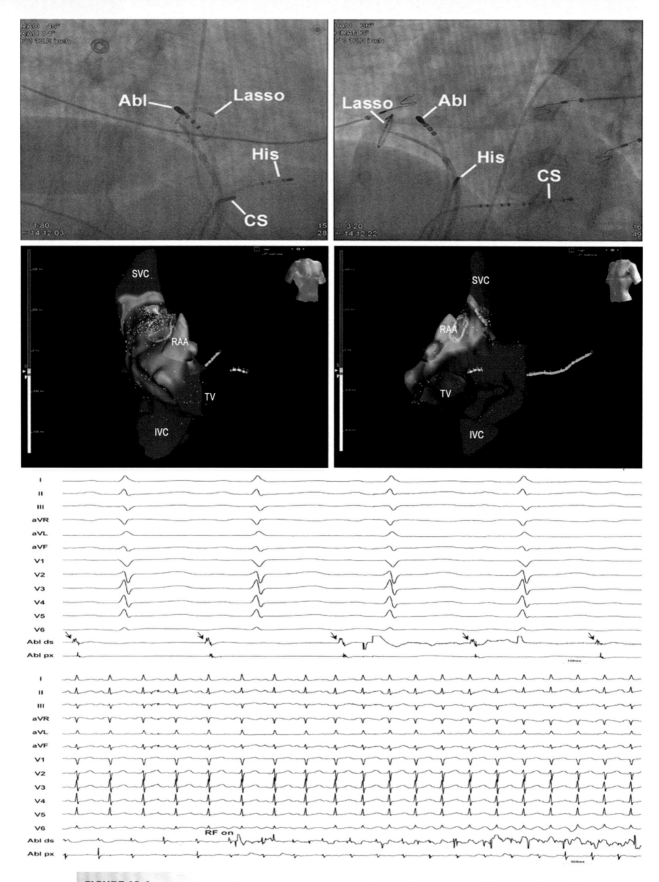

FIGURE 16-1 SAN modification. During sinus tachycardia, the earliest site of atrial activation (*white, arrows*) is recorded from the superior SAN at the cavo-atrial junction. Delivery of RF energy causes transient acceleration of sinus tachycardia.

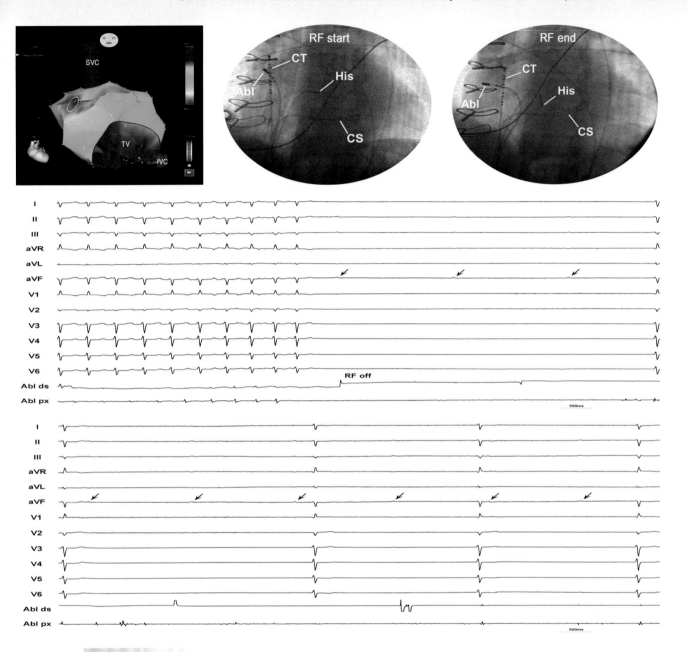

FIGURE 16-2 SAN modification (transplanted heart). During donor IAST, the earliest site of atrial activation was along the anterolateral RA near the cavo-atrial junction (*red*). RF energy was delivered cranio-caudally along the SAN causing transient sinus arrest and a junctional escape rhythm. Note the slower recipient sinus rate (*arrows*) that persists unperturbed and fails to conduct to the ventricle (recipient–donor suture line) giving the appearance of AV block.

or below 120 bpm (isoproterenol), and 3) accompanied by flattening of the inferior P-wave amplitude indicating a caudal shift in the SAN focus.[10,11,13,14] Ablation can be facilitated by intracardiac echocardiography targeting the superior crista terminalis (the internal counterpart of the sulcus terminalis) and irrigated ablation catheters (because of the epicardial location of the SAN and the thick terminal crest separating the SAN from the endocardial cavity).[8,14,15] In difficult cases, success might be achieved by targeting the arcuate ridge (band of myocardium

connecting the superior crista terminalis to the septum near the superior limbus) or an epicardial approach.[16,17]

ATRIO-VENTRICULAR JUNCTION MODIFICATION/ABLATION

The ideal goal of AV junction modification or ablation is to control the ventricular rate or promote biventricular pacing without causing complete pacemaker dependency. Endpoints, therefore, can be either 1) total AV junction ablation with development of third-degree AV block and a nodal escape rhythm or 2) reduction in the ventricular rate in atrial fibrillation (<120 bpm on isoproterenol) without causing complete AV block.[6]

RIGHT-SIDED APPROACH

Direct Compact AV Node Ablation

The target site for AVJ modification is the compact AV node where ablation allows emergence of a stable nodal escape rhythm that avoids pacemaker dependency. Targeting the more distal His bundle increases the chance of causing a slow and unpredictable ventricular escape rhythm. After advancing the ablation catheter into the right ventricle, it is pulled back to the tricuspid annulus and aligned along the anteroseptum with clockwise torque to locate the His bundle potential. From this site, the catheter is pulled back slowly further until it records a large atrial signal and small far-field (low-amplitude/low-frequency) His bundle electrogram (**Figs. 16-3 to 16-5**) and/or is posteroinferior to the His bundle (**Figs. 16-6 and 16-7**). Delivery of RF energy to this site causes rapid junctional tachycardia preceding AV block. When a recordable His bundle electrogram is difficult to identify, high-output pacing that generates a narrow paced QRS complex helps locate the His bundle.[18]

Electrical Isolation of the AV Node

An alternative ablation strategy is a stepwise approach that attempts to electrically isolate or disconnect the AV node from the atrial myocardium, thereby preserving nodal automaticity.[19-23] The slow pathway of the AV node along the posteroseptum is targeted because of its shorter refractory period. Slow pathway ablation alone, however, is generally insufficient to achieve a durable desired endpoint. RF energy is then applied to progressively more anterior and superior sites along the mid- and anteroseptum (the latter targeting the fast pathway of the AV node above the tendon of Todaro) until adequate rate control is achieved (**Figs. 16-8 and 16-9**).

LEFT-SIDED APPROACH

When AV junction ablation is unsuccessful from the right side, the His bundle can be targeted beneath the commissure of the noncoronary cusp (NCC)/right coronary cusp (RCC) as it penetrates the crest of the interventricular septum (**Fig. 16-10**).[24-26] The left-sided His bundle potential can be validated by comparing its timing to a right-sided His bundle electrogram or demonstrating His bundle capture with high-output pacing. Alternatively, when underlying bundle branch block is present, the conducting bundle branch or fascicle can be targeted.[27] Because of their more distal location, however, left-sided His bundle or fascicular ablation results in ventricular escape rhythms that are unpredictable and easily suppressed by ventricular pacing.

UNUSUAL ELECTROPHYSIOLOGIC PHENOMENA

IAST IN THE TRANSPLANTED HEART

IAST has rarely been described in a transplanted heart (**Figs. 16-2 and 16-11**).[3] Because the donor allograft is denervated, development of IAST supports an intrinsic defect in SAN cells rather than sympathovagal imbalance as its mechanism.

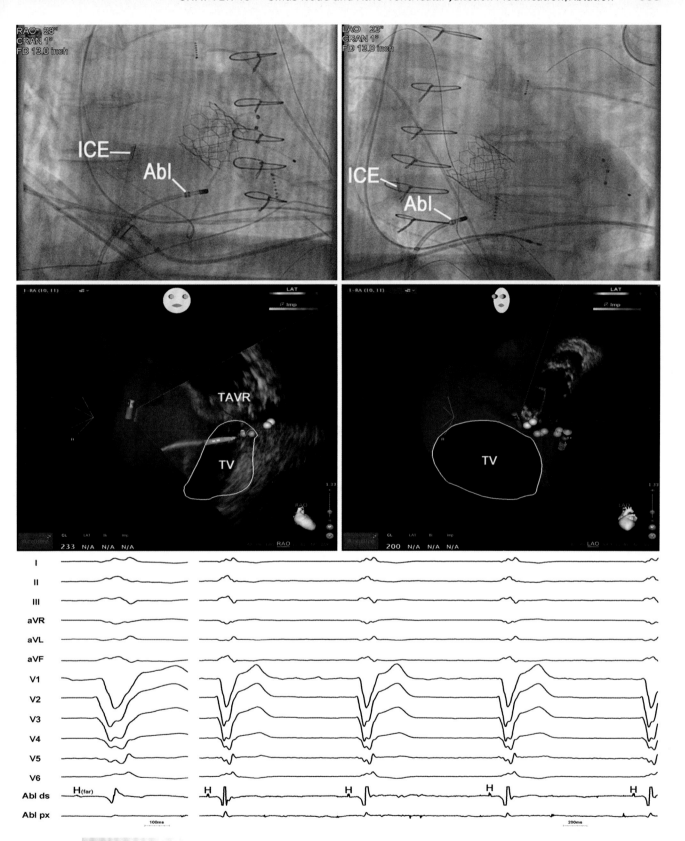

FIGURE 16-3 AV node modification. The compact AV node posteroinferior to the His (*yellow tags*) and right bundle (*white tags*) is targeted where a small far-field (low-amplitude/low-frequency) His bundle electrogram is recorded. RF energy caused complete AV block and stable junctional escape rhythm. A true, sharp, near-field His bundle potential is recorded during the junctional escape rhythm. Note the proximity of the transaortic valve replacement (TAVR) to the His bundle.

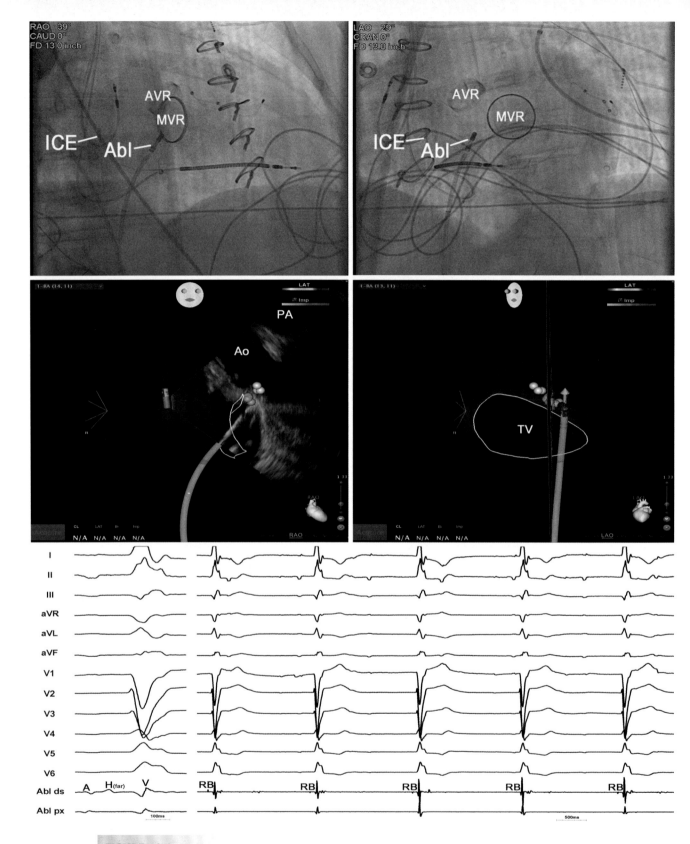

FIGURE 16-4 AV node modification. The compact AV node posteroinferior to the His (*yellow tags*) and right bundle (*white tags*) is targeted where a small far-field (low-amplitude/low-frequency) His bundle electrogram is recorded. RF delivery caused complete AV block and a stable junctional rhythm.

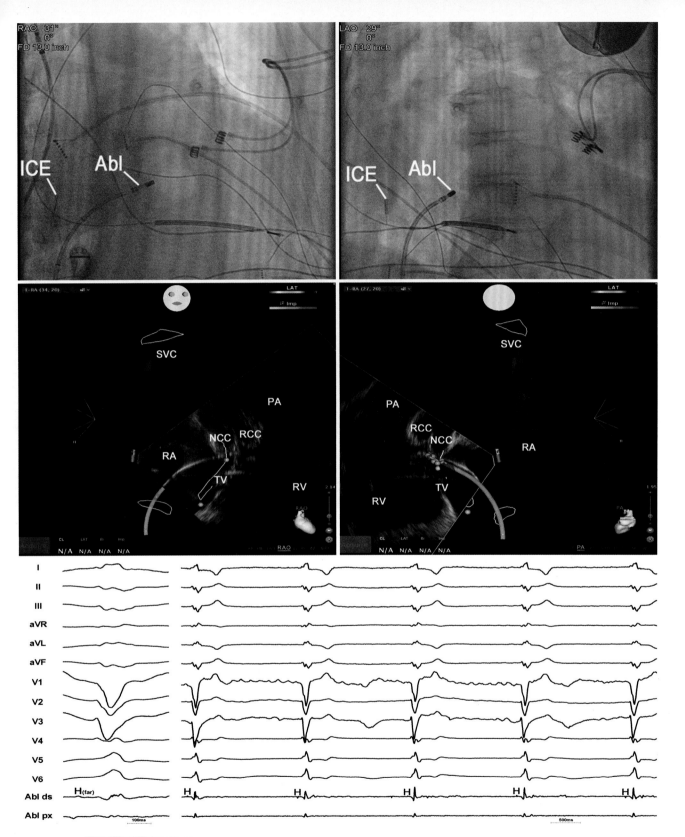

FIGURE 16-5 AV node modification. The compact AV node posteroinferior to the His bundle (*yellow tags*) is targeted where a small far-field (low-amplitude/low-frequency) His bundle electrogram is recorded. RF delivery caused complete AV block and a stable junctional escape rhythm. A sharp, near-field His bundle potential is recorded during the escape rhythm.

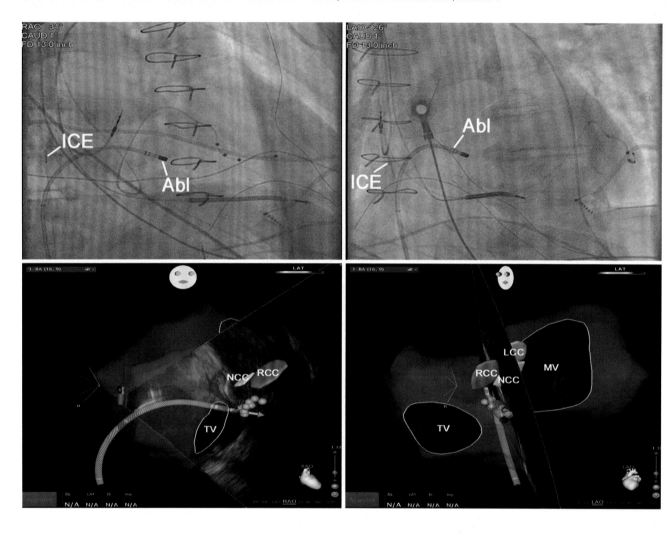

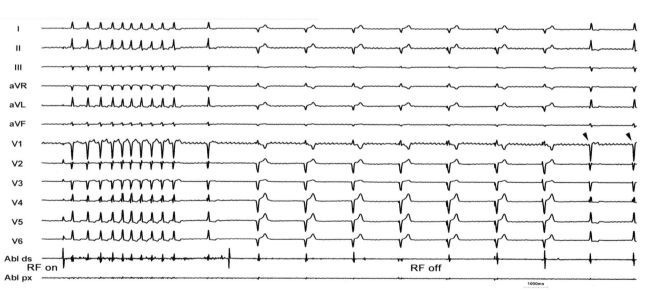

FIGURE 16-6 AV node modification. The compact AV node posteroinferior to the His bundle (*yellow tags*) is targeted. RF delivery causes rapid junctional tachycardia followed by complete AV block and transient biventricular pacing. With discontinuation of RF energy, a junctional escape rhythm (*arrowhead*) emerges.

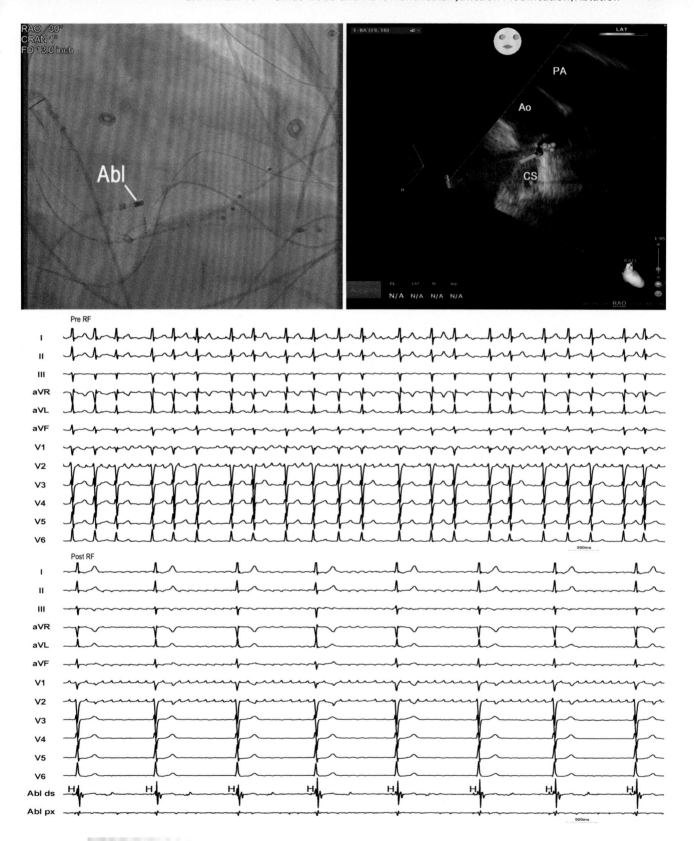

FIGURE 16-7 AV node modification. The compact AV node posteroinferior to the His bundle (*yellow tags*) is targeted. Before ablation, the ventricular rate in atrial fibrillation is rapid. After ablation, complete AV block with a junctional escape rhythm is present.

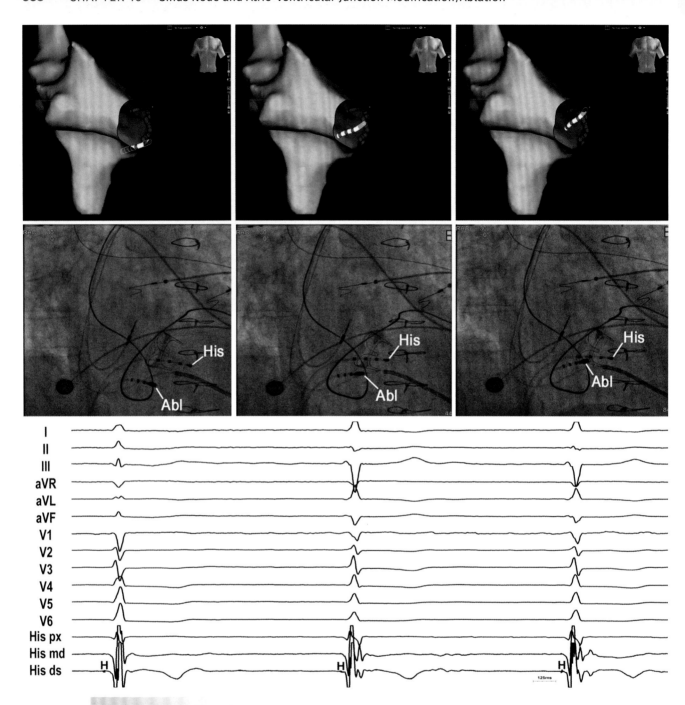

FIGURE 16-8 AV node modification. The atrio-nodal inputs along the interatrial septum are targeted (electrical isolation of the AV node). RF lesions (*red tags*) are delivered from postero- to midseptum, which slowed the ventricular rate during atrial fibrillation.

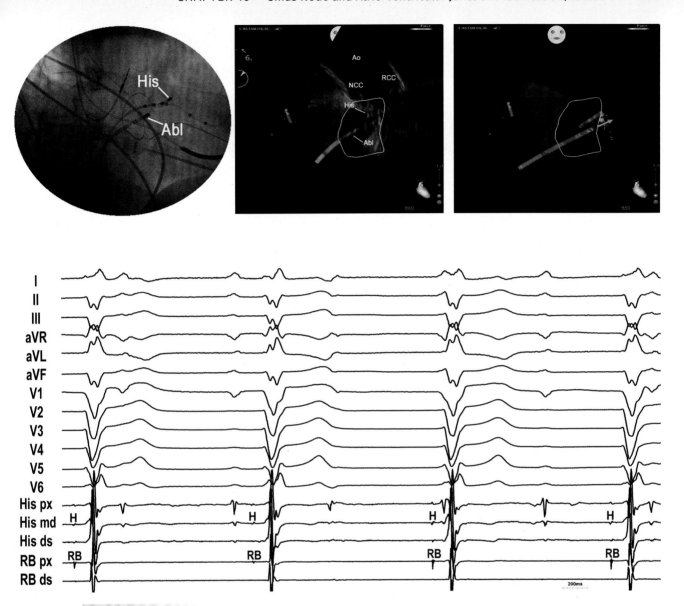

FIGURE 16-9 AV node modification. The atrio-nodal inputs along the interatrial septum are targeted (electrical isolation of the AV node). RF lesions (*red tags*) are delivered from postero- to midseptum (just beneath the His bundle [*yellow tags*]) until complete AV block and a junctional escape rhythm (with underlying left bundle branch block [LBBB]) occurs.

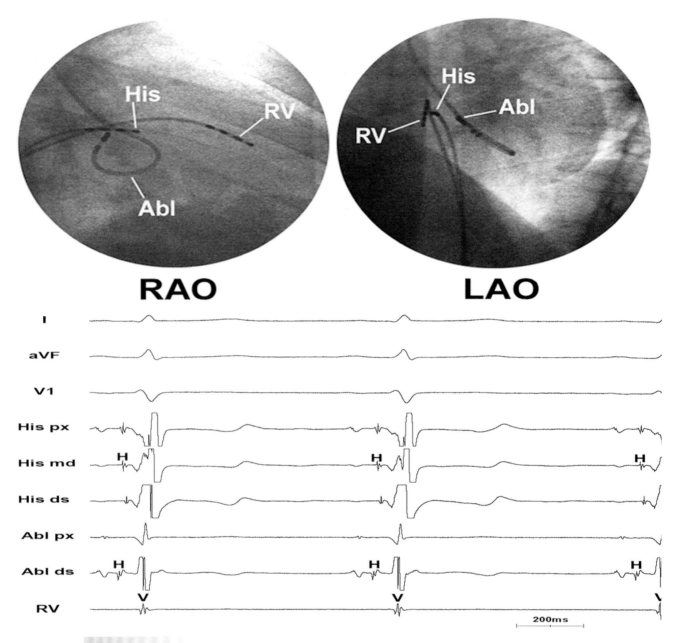

FIGURE 16-10 Transaortic approach to AV junction ablation. The ablation catheter is prolapsed retrogradely across the aortic valve and positioned beneath the NCC/RCC commissure opposite the right-sided His bundle catheter where a left-sided His bundle potential is recorded.

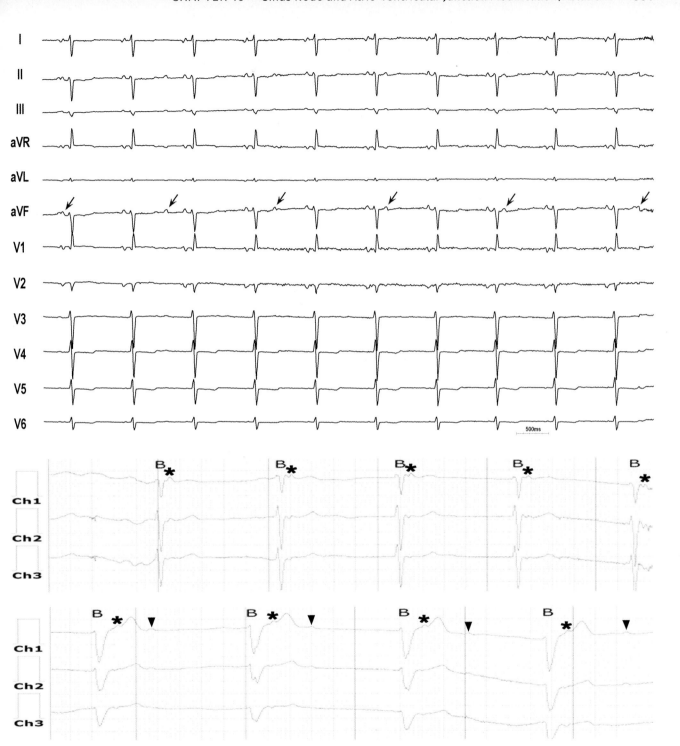

FIGURE 16-11 Transient donor SAN dysfunction post IAST ablation (transplanted heart). *Top*: Donor sinus rhythm coexisting with slower recipient sinus rhythm (a form of iatrogenic atrial parasystole [*arrows*]). *Bottom*: Sinus arrest with junctional (*middle*)/ventricular (*bottom*) escape rhythms and JA/VA conduction (*asterisk*), respectively. Note the recipient sinus rhythm (*arrowheads*) occurring independently.

REFERENCES

1. Bauernfeind RA, Amat-Y-Leon F, Dhingra RC, Kehoe R, Wyndham C, Rosen KM. Chronic nonparoxysmal sinus tachycardia in otherwise healthy persons. Ann Intern Med 1979;91:702–710.

2. Olshansky B, Sullivan R. Inappropriate sinus tachycardia. J Am Coll Cardiol 2013;61:793–801.

3. Ho RT, Ortman M, Mather PJ, Rubin S. Inappropriate sinus tachycardia in a transplanted heart—further insights into pathogenesis. Heart Rhythm 2011;8:781–783.

4. Scheinman MM, Morady F, Hess DS, Gonzalez R. Catheter-induced ablation of the atrioventricular junction to control refractory supraventricular arrhythmias. JAMA 1982;248:851–855.

5. Scheinman M, Morady F, Hess D, Gonzalez R. Transvenous catheter technique for induction of damage to the atrioventricular junction in man [abstract]. Am J Cardiol 1982;49:1013.

6. Williamson BD, Man KC, Daoud E, Niebauer M, Strickberger SA, Morady F. Radiofrequency catheter modification of atrioventricular conduction to control the ventricular rate during atrial fibrillation. N Engl J Med 1994;331:910–917.

7. Feld GK, Fleck RP, Fujimura O, Prothro DL, Bahnson TD, Ibarra M. Control of rapid ventricular response by radiofrequency catheter modification of the atrioventricular node in patients with medically refractory atrial fibrillation. Circulation 1994;90:2299–2307.

8. Sánchez-Quintana D, Cabrera JA, Farré J, Climent V, Anderson RH, Ho SY. Sinus node revisited in the era of electroanatomical mapping and catheter ablation. Heart 2005;91:189–194.

9. Lee RJ, Kalman JM, Fitzpatrick AP, et al. Radiofrequency catheter modification of the sinus node for "inappropriate" sinus tachycardia. Circulation 1995;92:2919–2928.

10. Man KC, Knight B, Tse HF, et al. Radiofrequency catheter ablation of inappropriate sinus tachycardia guided by activation mapping. J Am Coll Cardiol 2000;35:451–457.

11. Marrouche NF, Beheiry S, Tomassoni G, et al. Three-dimensional nonfluoroscopic mapping and ablation of inappropriate sinus tachycardia. Procedural strategies and long-term outcome. J Am Coll Cardiol 2002;39:1046–1054.

12. Mantovan R, Thiene G, Calzolari V, Basso C. Sinus node ablation for inappropriate sinus tachycardia. J Cardiovasc Electrophysiol 2005;16:804–806.

13. Gianni C, Di Biase L, Mohanty S, et al. Catheter ablation of inappropriate sinus tachycardia. J Interv Card Electrophysiol 2016;46:63–69.

14. Lin D, Garcia F, Jacobson J, et al. Use of noncontact mapping and saline-cooled ablation catheter for sinus node modification in medically refractory inappropriate sinus tachycardia. Pacing Clin Electrophysiol. 2007;30:236–242.

15. Kalman JM, Lee RJ, Fisher WG, et al. Radiofrequency catheter modification of sinus pacemaker function guided by intracardiac echocardiography. Circulation 1995;92:3070–3081.

16. Killu AM, Syed FF, Wu P, Asirvatham SJ. Refractory inappropriate sinus tachycardia successfully treated with radiofrequency ablation at the arcuate ridge. Heart Rhythm 2012;9:1324–1327.

17. Jacobson JT, Kraus A, Lee R, Goldberger JJ. Epicardial/endocardial sinus node ablation after failed endocardial ablation for the treatment of inappropriate sinus tachycardia. J Cardiovasc Electrophysiol 2014;25:236–241.

18. Kanjwal K, Grubb BP. Utility of high-output His pacing during difficult AV node ablation. An underutilized strategy. Pacing Clin Electrophysiol 2016;39:616–619.

19. Della Bella P, Carbucicchio C, Tondo C, Riva S. Modulation of atrioventricular conduction by ablation of the "slow" atrioventricular node pathway in patients with drug-refractory atrial fibrillation or flutter. J Am Coll Cardiol 1995;25:39–46.

20. Fleck RP, Chen PS, Boyce K, Ross R, Dittrich HC, Feld GK. Radiofrequency modification of atrioventricular conduction by selective ablation of the low posterior septal right atrium in a patient with atrial fibrillation and a rapid ventricular response. Pacing Clin Electrophysiol 1993;16:377–381.

21. Stabile G, Turco P, De Simone A, Coltorti F, De Matteis C. Radiofrequency modification of the atrioventricular node in patients with chronic atrial fibrillation: comparison between anterior and posterior approaches. J Cardiovasc Electrophysiol 1998;9:709–717.

22. Duckeck W, Engelstein ED, Kuch KH. Radiofrequency current therapy in atrial tachyarrhythmias: modulation versus ablation of atrioventricular nodal conduction. Pacing Clin Electrophysiol 1993;16:629–636.

23. Chhabra S, Greenspon AJ, Pavri BB, Frisch DR, Ho RT. Electrical isolation of atrioventricular node: a new technique of atrioventricular junction ablation to preserve a nodal escape rhythm. Heart Rhythm 2012;9:S169.

24. Sousa J, el-Atassi R, Rosenheck S, Calkins H, Langberg J, Morady F. Radiofrequency catheter ablation of the atrioventricular junction from the left ventricle. Circulation 1991;84:567–571.

25. Kalbfleisch SJ, Williamson B, Man KC, et al. A randomized comparison of the right- and left-sided approaches to ablation of the atrioventricular junction. Am J Cardiol 1993;72:1406–1410.

26. Fenrich AL Jr, Friedman RA, Cecchin FC, Kearney D. Left-sided atrioventricular nodal ablation using the transseptal approach: clinico-histolopathologic correlation. J Cardiovasc Electrophysiol 1998;9:757–760.

27. Sunthorn H, Hasija P, Burri H, Shah D. Unsuccessful AV nodal ablation in atrial fibrillation: an alternative method to achieve complete heart block. Pacing Clin Electrophysiol 2005;28:1247–1249.

Wide Complex Tachycardias

17

Introduction

The major differential diagnoses of a regular wide complex tachycardia (WCT) are 1) ventricular tachycardia (VT), 2) supraventricular tachycardia (SVT) with aberration or bundle branch block (BBB), and 3) preexcited tachycardia. Hyperkalemia- and pacemaker-mediated tachycardia, however, should be excluded (Fig. 17-1). The clinical history provides valuable clues for diagnosis. A WCT in the setting of a prior myocardial infarction, congestive heart failure, or recent angina pectoris has a high likelihood of being VT (Fig. 17-2).[1] A WCT in the presence of a type Ic antiarrhythmic drug for paroxysmal atrial fibrillation should raise suspicion of "drug flutter" with 1:1 atrio-ventricular (AV) conduction and rate-related aberration (Fig. 17-3).

The purpose of this chapter is to:
1. Differentiate VT from SVT with aberration by the 12-lead ECG.
2. Differentiate VT from preexcited tachycardia by the 12-lead ECG.
3. Diagnose WCT by intracardiac recordings, pacing, and vagal maneuvers.

12-LEAD ECG

BASELINE

The sinus rhythm ECG provides important information about the substrate to develop WCT including the 1) morphology of underlying BBB or aberrantly conducted QRS complexes, 2) morphology of spontaneous PVCs, 3) infarction patterns, 4) preexcitation, and the 5) status of AV conduction. A WCT whose QRS morphology is identical to underlying BBB suggests an SVT, except for the possibility of His-Purkinje type VT (e.g., bundle branch reentrant tachycardia [BBRT], interfascicular VT (see Figs. 21-2 and 21-15).[2] Conversely, a WCT whose QRS morphology is different or even narrower than underlying BBB or identical to spontaneous PVCs argues for VT.[3] A WCT in the setting of pathologic Q waves or preexcitation suggests VT or preexcited tachycardia, respectively. A WCT in the presence of AV block also favors VT because of inability for SVT to conduct rapidly to the ventricle.

VT VERSUS SVT WITH BBB

ECG clues differentiating VT from SVT with BBB include analysis of 1) QRS morphology, 2) QRS intrinsicoid deflection and width, 3) frontal QRS axis, 4) AV relationship, and 5) zones of transition.

QRS Morphology

WCTs are categorized either into right bundle branch block (RBBB) (terminal QRS positivity in V1) or left bundle branch block (LBBB) (terminal QRS negativity in V1) tachycardias. Bundle branch morphology itself is determined by the site of earliest ventricular activation. Because true aberrant conduction causes specific QRS morphology patterns, any deviation from the "typical aberration" suggests VT.

Morphologic features of LBBB tachycardias favoring VT over SVT with BBB include 1) initial r wave >30 ms in V1 or V2, 2) onset of the r wave to the nadir of the S wave in V1 or V2 >60 ms, 3) notching on the downstroke of the S wave in V1 or V2, and 4) q wave in V6 (Kindwall-Josephson criteria) (Fig. 17-4).[4] The first three criteria reflect the intrinsicoid deflection, which is narrow and rapid for aberration but slow and wide for VT (see below). LBBB alters normal left to right septal activation, causing loss of septal q waves in V6. Therefore, the presence of q waves in V6 during LBBB tachycardia favors VT.

Typical LBBB Tachycardias

WCT with typical LBBB morphology are a unique group and include 1) SVT with LBBB, 2) antidromic tachycardia using an atrio-fascicular or nodo-fascicular accessory pathway (AP) (whose distal insertion is in the right bundle), and 3) typical (counterclockwise) BBRT (whose exit site is from the right bundle) (see Figs. 11-20 and 21-10).[5]

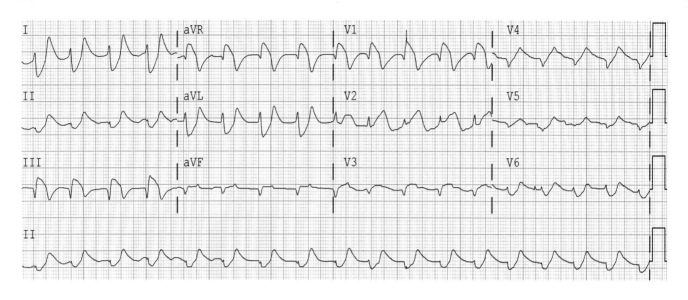

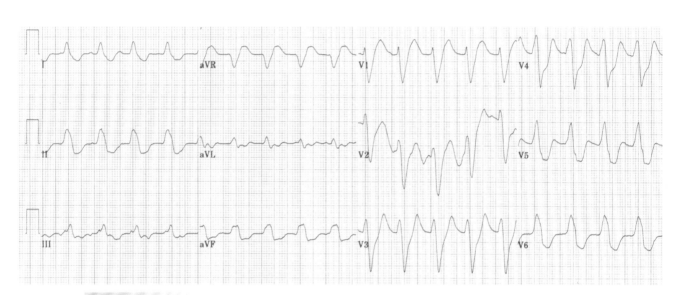

FIGURE 17-1 Hyperkalemia. Hyperkalemia mimics VT with RBBB (*top*) and LBBB (*bottom*) morphology. P waves are not visible because high potassium levels affect atrial depolarization. Note the "M" type pattern in lead I and V4, respectively, reflecting QRS widening/T wave peaking. Initial QRS forces are relatively rapid, while terminal forces are slurred and delayed because the His-Purkinje system is more resistant to hyperkalemia than ventricular muscle. Note also in the top ECG that hyperkalemia can cause ST segment elevation mimicking acute myocardial infarction ("dialyzable current of injury") or Brugada syndrome ("Brugada phenocopy").

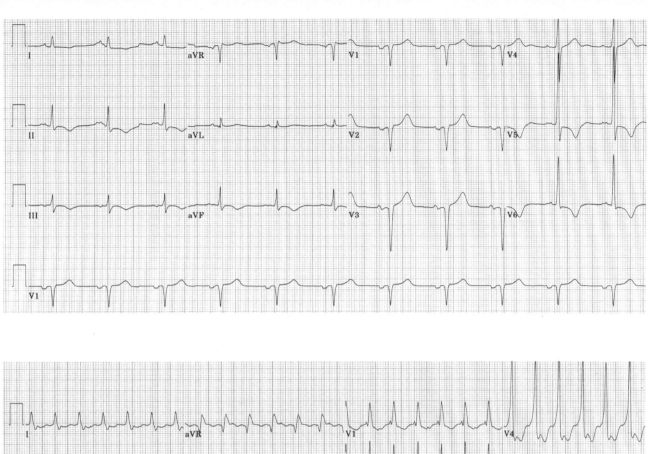

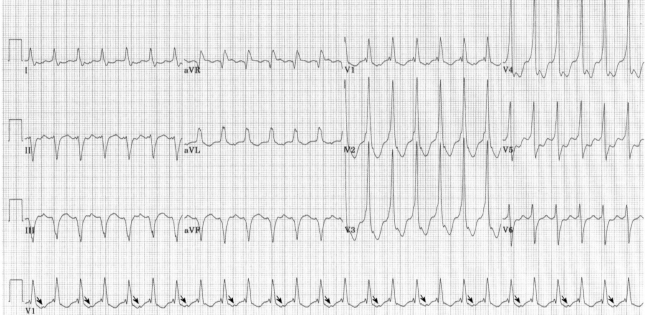

FIGURE 17-2 VT in the setting of an old myocardial infarction. *Top:* NSR with an old anterior infarct. *Bottom:* Relatively narrow, triphasic (rsR′)/left superior QRS complexes suggest origin near the LPF. 2:1 VA block (*arrows*) and initial aVR q wave >40 ms indicate VT.

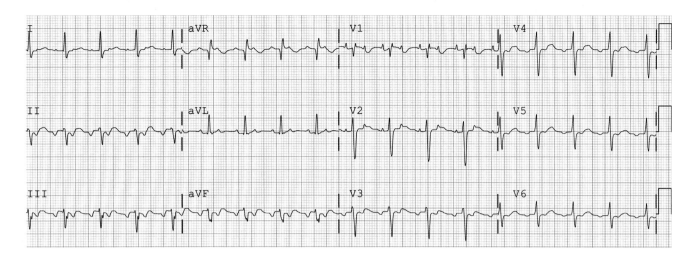

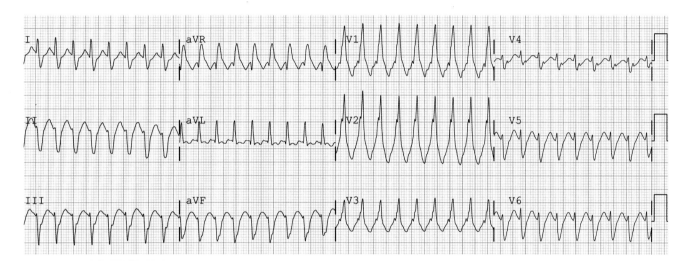

FIGURE 17-3 Atrial flutter with 1:1 AV conduction. The ventricular rate during 1:1 conduction (*bottom*) is exactly twice that during 2:1 conduction (*top*) resulting in RBBB aberration. The initial aVR q wave <40 ms.

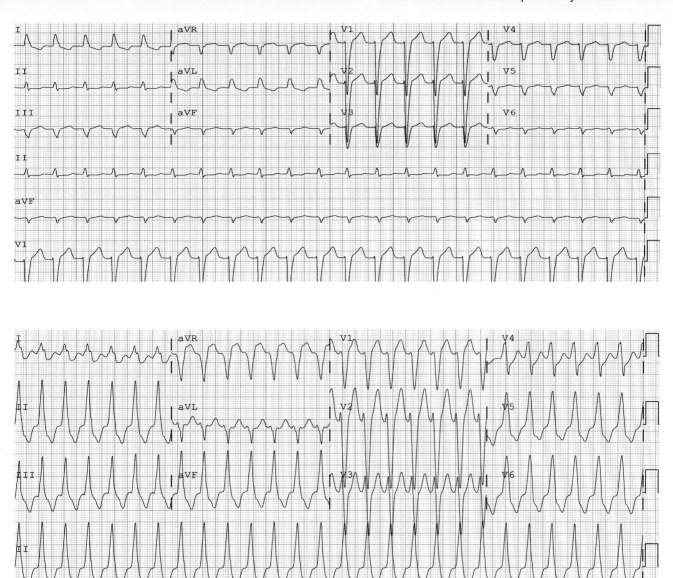

FIGURE 17-4 LBBB tachycardias. *Top:* Typical AVNRT with LBBB. The initial V1 r wave <30 ms and aVR Vi/Vt >1. *Bottom:* RVOT VT. The initial V1 r wave >30 ms and aVR Vi/Vt <1. The intrinsicoid deflection is narrower and more rapid during aberration.

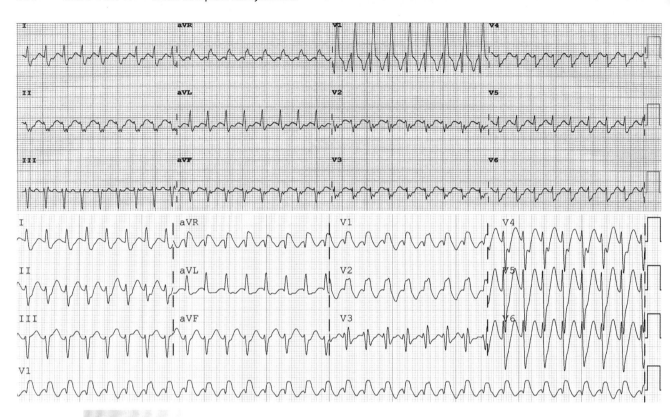

FIGURE 17-5 RBBB tachycardias. *Top*: ORT with RBBB. The aVR q wave <40 ms. *Bottom*: Idiopathic LV VT. Idiopathic LV VT mimics SVT with RBBB/LAFB because of origin near the LPF; however, the aVR q wave >40 ms.

Morphologic features of RBBB tachycardias favoring VT over SVT with BBB include 1) monophasic R, biphasic Rr′ (R > r′), and qR patterns in V1 and 2) R/S ratio <1 in V6 (Wellens criteria) (Fig. 17-5).[6] In contrast, right bundle branch aberration produces a triphasic rsR′ complex in V1 (the initial r wave reflects normal [left to right] depolarization of the interventricular septum and the R′ represents late activation of the right ventricle [RV]) and R/S ratio >1 in V6.

Typical RBBB Tachycardias
WCT with typical RBBB morphology include 1) SVT with RBBB, 2) idiopathic left ventricular (LV) VT (because it arises from/near the left posterior fascicle [LPF]), and 3) interfascicular reentrant tachycardia [IFRT]) (because macroreentry involves the LPF and left anterior fascicle [LAF]).

Absence of an RS complex in all the precordial leads is a specific morphology pattern that also favors VT (Brugada criteria).[7] It encompasses positive and negative concordance (precordial QRS complexes all positive or negative, respectively) and precordial qR patterns (q waves reflect prior infarction that are preserved during VT) (Fig. 17-6).

Concordance
Negative QRS concordance indicates tachycardia origin from the ventricular apex and strongly favors VT. However, SVT with LBBB can rarely show negative concordance due to laterodorsal rotation of the heart (Fig. 17-7).[8–10] Positive QRS concordance indicates tachycardia origin from the ventricular base and can be seen with VT or preexcited tachycardia using a left-sided AP

(the ventricular insertion of most typical left-sided APs is at the basal mitral annulus) (Fig. 17-8; see also Fig. 18-7).

QRS Width and Intrinsicoid
The width of initial forces (intrinsicoid deflection or R/S interval [onset of R wave to nadir of S wave]) and the QRS width itself are a function of conduction velocity or slew rate (dV/dt). The His-Purkinje system is the most rapidly conducting electrical structure in the heart.[11] Initial, rapid His-Purkinje conduction is preserved during BBB resulting in narrower intrinsicoid deflections and QRS widths than during VT (pure muscle-to-muscle conduction). An R/S interval in any precordial lead >100 ms indicates VT (Brugada criteria).[6] For RBBB and LBBB tachycardias, QRS durations >140 ms and >160 ms, respectively, also favor VT.[12] However, antiarrhythmic drugs (e.g., Classic Na channel blockers causing "drug flutter" with 1:1 AV conduction) slow His-Purkinje/myocardial conduction causing SVT with BBB to mimic VT (false-positive VT).

QRS Axis
While left anterior and posterior fascicular blocks produce left superior and right inferior axis deviation, no hemiblock pattern causes extreme right axis (right superior) deviation. Therefore, WCT with a right superior ("northwest") axis argues for VT. The combination of LBBB and LPFB is rare, and therefore, LBBB tachycardia with right axis deviation also suggests VT. Conversely, RBBB morphology with normal axis is uncommon during VT, and therefore, RBBB tachycardia with normal axis favors SVT.

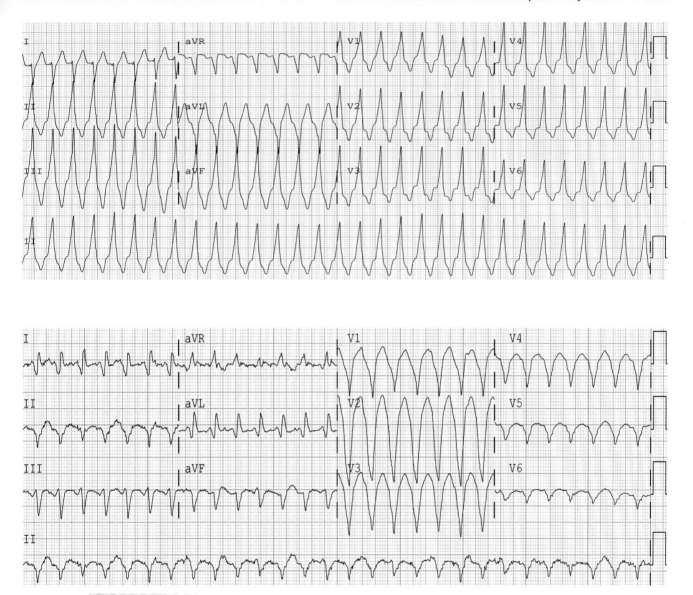

FIGURE 17-6 Concordance. *Top*: VT with positive concordance. The aVR Vi/Vt <1. *Bottom*: VT with negative concordance. Apical origin of VT causes a dominant R wave in aVR.

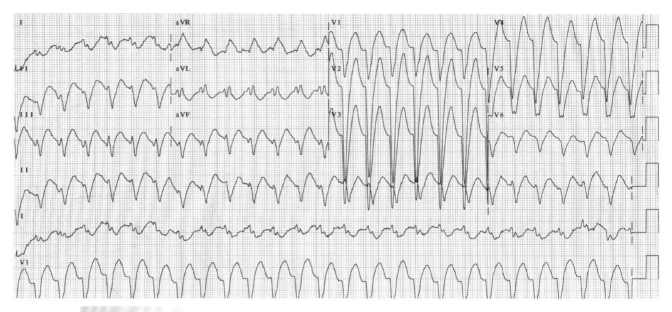

FIGURE 17-7 Negative concordance (SVT with LBBB). The V1 r wave is tiny (30 ms), and the aVR q wave <40 ms.

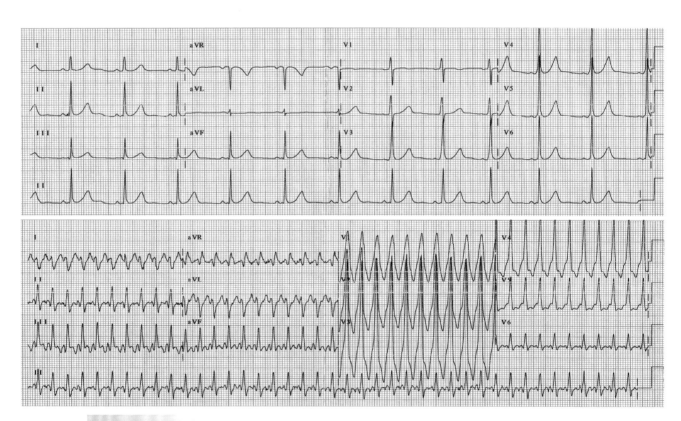

FIGURE 17-8 Preexcited tachycardia. *Top*: NSR with minimal preexcitation (left free wall AP). *Bottom*: Antidromic tachycardia. Note positive precordial concordance due to insertion of the AP at the base of the mitral annulus.

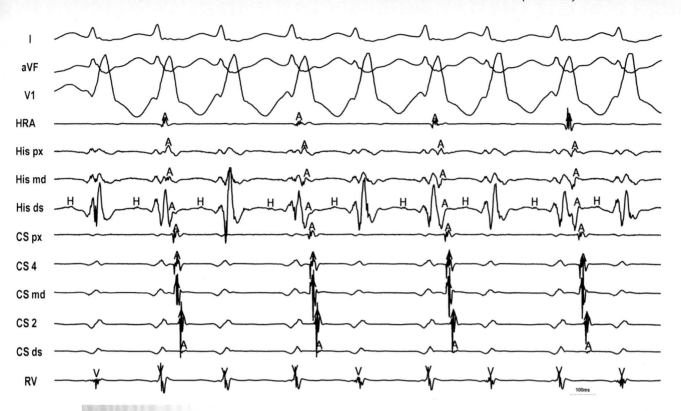

FIGURE 17-9 SVT with RBBB and AV dissociation (orthodromic nodo-fascicular reentrant tachycardia [NFRT]). His bundle potentials precede each QRS complex with normal HV intervals. A His refractory VPD delays the His bundle indicating presence of a nodo-fascicular accessory pathway (NF AP) (see Fig. 11-11).

Atrio-Ventricular Relationship

Both AV dissociation and <1:1 AV association (A rate < V rate) strongly indicate VT. However, there are four SVTs with AV dissociation 1) atrio-ventricular nodal reentrant tachycardia (AVNRT) with upper common final pathway block, 2) junctional tachycardia with JA block, 3) nodo-fascicular reentrant tachycardia with nodo-atrial block, and 4) intrahisian reentry with His-atrio block (**Fig. 17-9**).[13] Because these four SVTs are rare and need to be associated with either aberration or preexcitation to cause WCT, a WCT with AV dissociation is most likely VT. Manifestations of AV dissociation include 1) P waves marching through QRS complexes, 2) capture complexes, 3) fusion beats, and 4) early return of a sinus beat following tachycardia termination (less than the sinus cycle length) (**Fig. 17-10**).[14] Capture and fusion complexes are generally seen with slow VT when sinus impulses can penetrate the His-Purkinje system during the diastolic period. Fusion complexes (Dressler beats), however, are not specific to VT and are also observed during SVT with BBB when a PVC ipsilateral to BBB occurs. Similar to AV dissociation, the presence of AV association <1 (A rate < V rate) strongly supports VT (**Fig. 17-11**). AV association >1 (A rate > V rate) favors SVT. A 1:1 AV relationship can occur either with SVT and 1:1 AV conduction or VT and 1:1 VA conduction. During 1:1 conduction, non-retrograde P-wave morphologies and oscillations in PP cycle length that precede and predict changes in RR interval

favor SVT.[15] In contrast, oscillations in RR interval that precede and predict changes in PP interval are less useful and observed with both SVT (e.g., orthodromic reciprocating tachycardia [ORT]) and VT. Vagal maneuvers (adenosine or carotid sinus massage) can induce AV block that either unmasks an atrial tachyarrhythmia or terminates SVT, although adenosine can also terminate VT (cAMP-mediated triggered right ventricular outflow tract [RVOT] VT).[16,17] Vagal maneuvers can induce VA block, and persistence of WCT with VA block (appearance of AV dissociation) indicates VT.

Zones of Transition

During initiation of WCT, the absence of a P wave or presence of a foreshortened PR interval preceding the first beat of tachycardia supports VT. Tachycardia initiation after long coupling intervals ("short–long" sequence) that would exceed bundle branch refractoriness also favors VT. (In contrast, "long–short" sequences are less helpful and occur with both aberration and VT.)[18] Reproducible induction by atrial premature depolarizations (APDs) favors SVT. Analogous to spontaneous termination of narrow complex tachycardia (NCT) with AV block excludes atrial tachycardia (AT), spontaneous termination of WCT with VA block excludes VT (**Fig. 17-12**). Transition of NCT to WCT of the same rate (parity of rate) suggests SVT with aberration or bystander preexcitation (and excludes antidromic tachycardia) but might occur with a rare

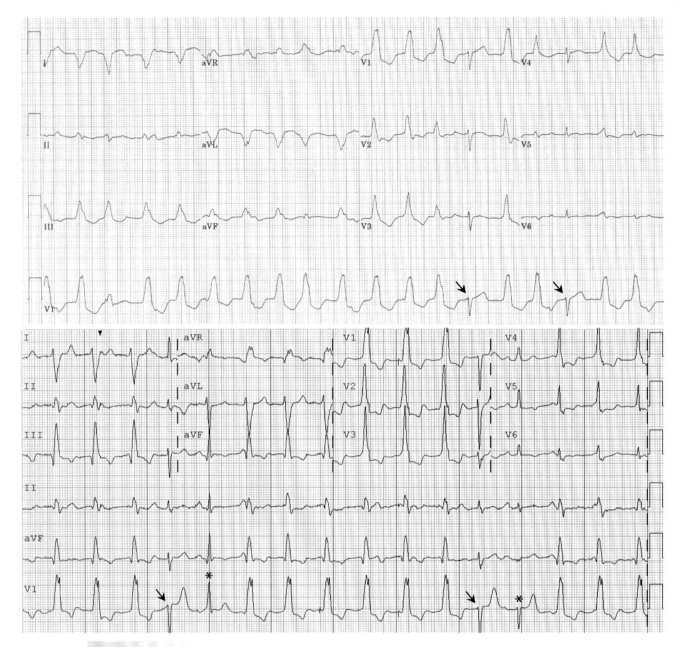

FIGURE 17-10 Capture and fusion complexes. Slow RBBB VT allows captures (*arrows*) and fusion (*asterisk*) complexes. The V1 monophasic R wave indicates ventricular origin.

double tachycardia where SVT induces VT of the same rate (parity of rate).

Algorithms

While summation of individual ECG clues can differentiate VT from SVT with aberration, specific four-step decision tree algorithms (Brugada, Miller) have been developed to facilitate diagnosis.[7,19] These algorithms use individual criteria with high VT specificity and grouped criteria to increase VT sensitivity. aVR is a unique endocavitary lead because its vector looks into the barrel of the LV, thereby generating an initial narrow, negative QRS complex (qR [RBBB], QS [LBBB]) during SVT

due to initial rapid His-Purkinje activation, regardless of BBB type. Analogous to the V1 Kindwall-Josephson criteria for LBBB tachycardias, the following aVR features therefore favor VT: 1) presence of initial dominant R wave (VT arising from the apical or inferior region heading toward aVR), 2) width of initial r or q wave >40 ms, 3) notching on the initial downstroke of a predominantly negative QRS complex, 4) ventricular activation-velocity ratio (Vi/Vt) ≤1 (degree of vertical excursion of the initial 40 ms of the QRS complex [Vi] less than the vertical excursion of the terminal 40 ms [Vt])—these latter three indices reflecting initial slow muscle-to-muscle conduction (intrinsicoid deflection) during VT.

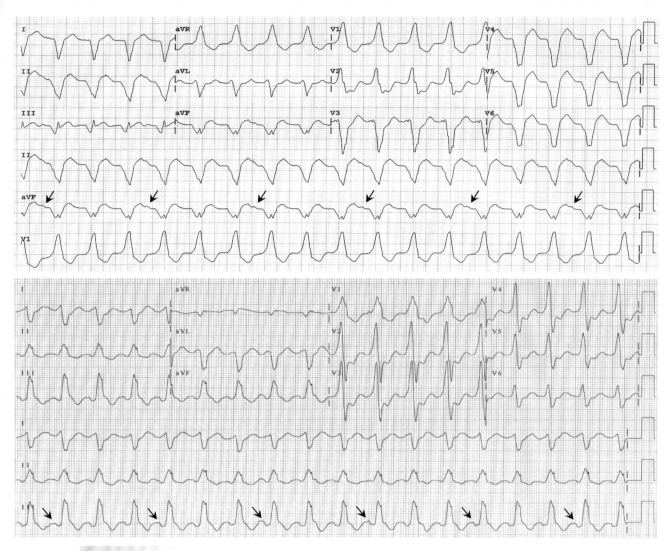

FIGURE 17-11 VT with 3:1 VA conduction. The V1 monophasic R wave (and northwest frontal axis [*top*]) indicates VT. Arrows denote P waves.

VT VERSUS PREEXCITED TACHYCARDIA

QRS complexes during VT and preexcited tachycardia are both produced by muscle-to-muscle conduction and are therefore difficult to distinguish morphologically. The following ECG clues support VT 1) predominantly negative QRS complexes in V4–V6, 2) QR complex in ≥1 lead (V2–V6), and 3) V rate > A rate.[20] Predominantly negative QRS complexes in V4–V6 indicate an apical origin of tachycardia where APs generally do not exist. QR complexes indicate the presence of scar and also suggest VT. Because the AV ratio during preexcited tachycardias is ≥1, V rate > A rate (AV dissociation or < 1:1 AV association) supports VT.

ELECTROPHYSIOLOGIC STUDY

Diagnosis of WCT during electrophysiologic study is established by 1) His bundle potentials and corresponding HV intervals, 2) AV relationship, and 3) response to pacing maneuvers.

HIS BUNDLE ELECTROGRAM/HV INTERVAL

Absence of His bundle potentials preceding QRS complexes or His bundle potentials occurring after QRS onset ("negative HV" intervals) excludes SVT with aberration and indicates either VT or preexcited tachycardia (**Figs. 17-13 to 17-16**). Foreshortened HV intervals (positive but short HV intervals) exclude SVT with aberration and antidromic tachycardia and can occur during VT (rapid, retrograde activation of the His bundle preceding QRS onset) or bystander preexcited tachycardia (e.g., preexcited AVNRT) (**Fig. 17-17; see also Figs. 18-3 and 18-4**). Normal or prolonged HV intervals occur during SVT with aberration and BBRT (**Figs. 17-18 and 17-19**).

AV RELATIONSHIP

While P waves can be difficult to identify on the surface ECG, intracardiac recordings provide better determination of the AV relationship (dissociation, association [<, =, or >1]) and atrial activation pattern particularly when the AV ratio is 1:1 (e.g., midline, eccentric).

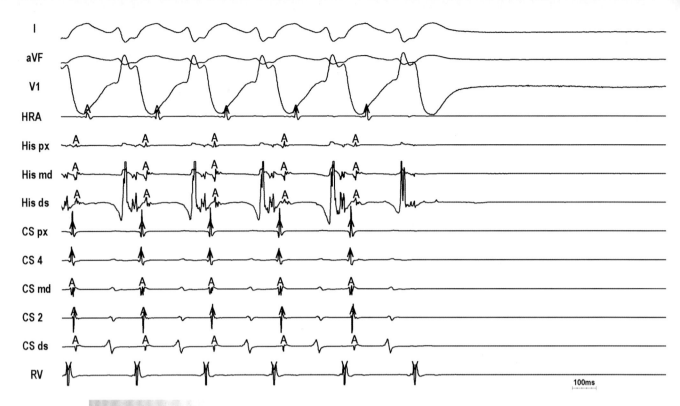

FIGURE 17-12 Preexcited tachycardia. Absence of His bundle potentials preceding each QRS complex excludes SVT with RBBB. Spontaneous termination with VA block excludes VT. These findings indicate a preexcited tachycardia—in this case, antidromic tachycardia using a left free wall AP. Note early ventricular activation along the lateral mitral annulus (CS ds).

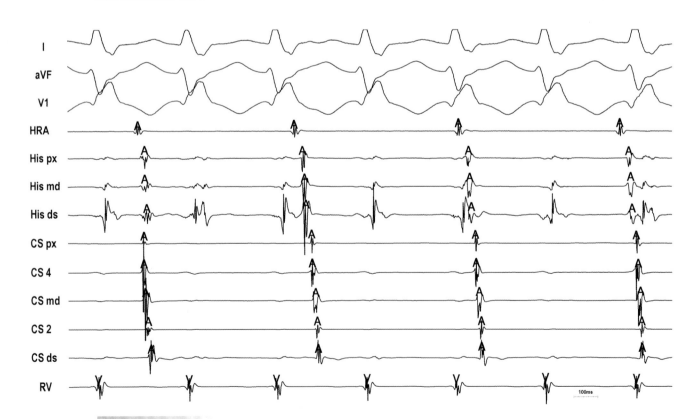

FIGURE 17-13 Idiopathic LV VT. Absence of His bundle potentials preceding each QRS complex excludes SVT with RBBB. AV dissociation excludes preexcited tachycardia.

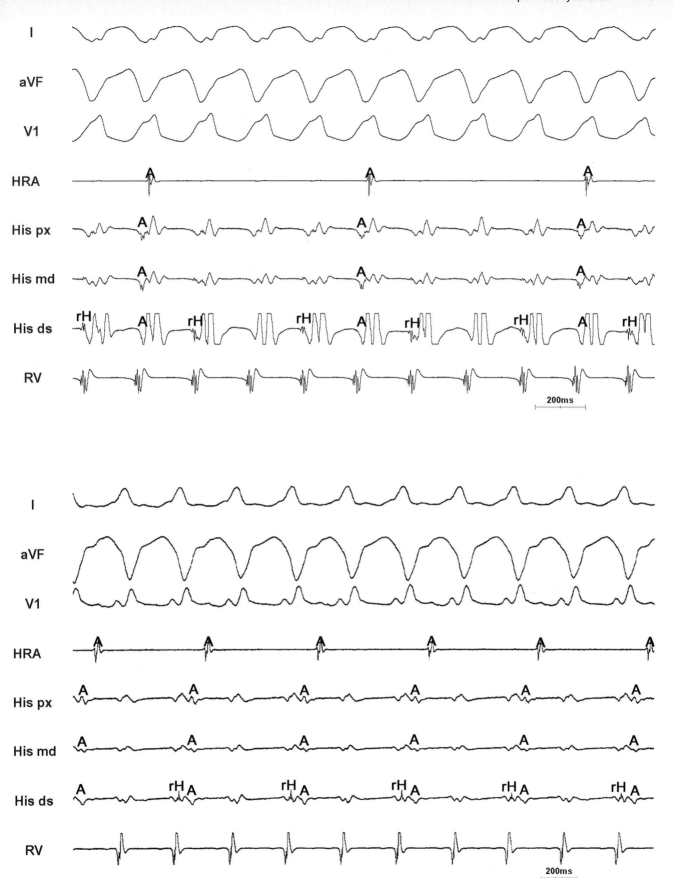

FIGURE 17-14 VT with 2:1 VH and 4:1 (*top*)/2:1 (*bottom*) VA conduction.

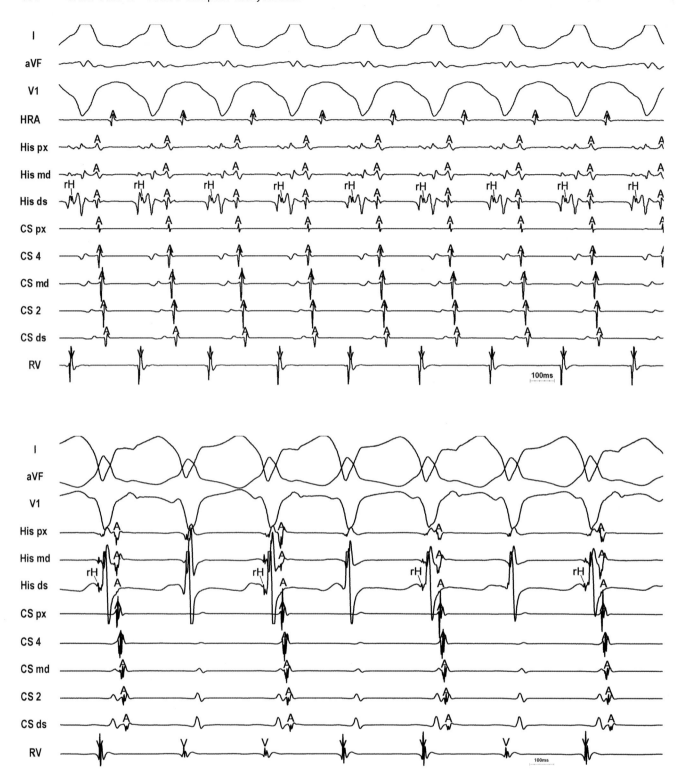

FIGURE 17-15 LBBB tachycardias. Absence of His bundle potentials preceding each QRS complex excludes SVT with LBBB. *Top*: Antidromic tachycardia using a right free wall AP. Retrograde His bundle potentials occur 56 ms after QRS onset (short VH tachycardia). *Bottom*: RVOT VT with 2:1 VH/VA conduction.

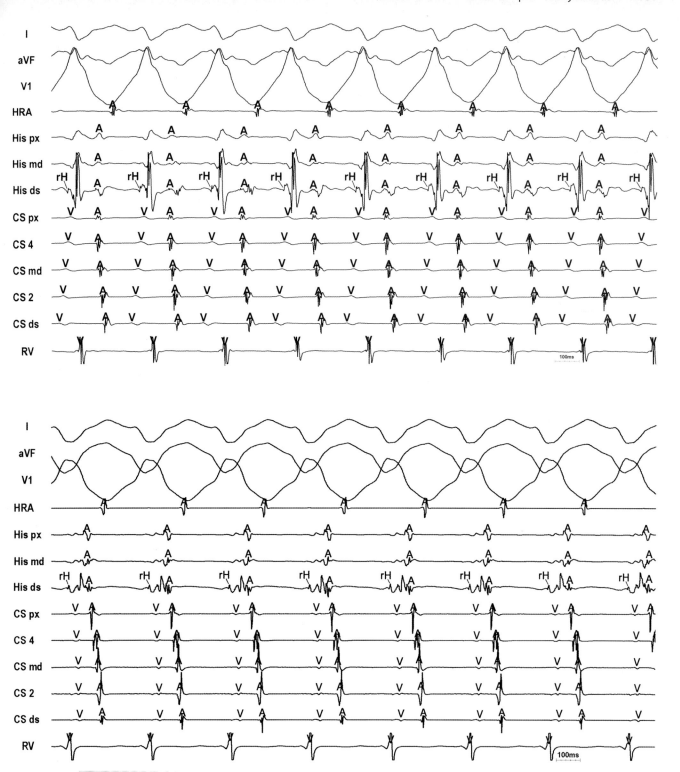

FIGURE 17-16 RBBB tachycardias. Absence of His bundle potentials preceding each QRS complex excludes SVT with RBBB. *Top*: Antidromic tachycardia using a left free wall AP. Retrograde His bundle potentials occur 52 ms after QRS onset (short VH tachycardia). Ventricular activation is early along the lateral mitral annulus (CS ds). *Bottom*: VT with 1:1 VH/ VA conduction. Ventricular activation is late along the mitral annulus (and later than RV due to LV inferoapical origin).

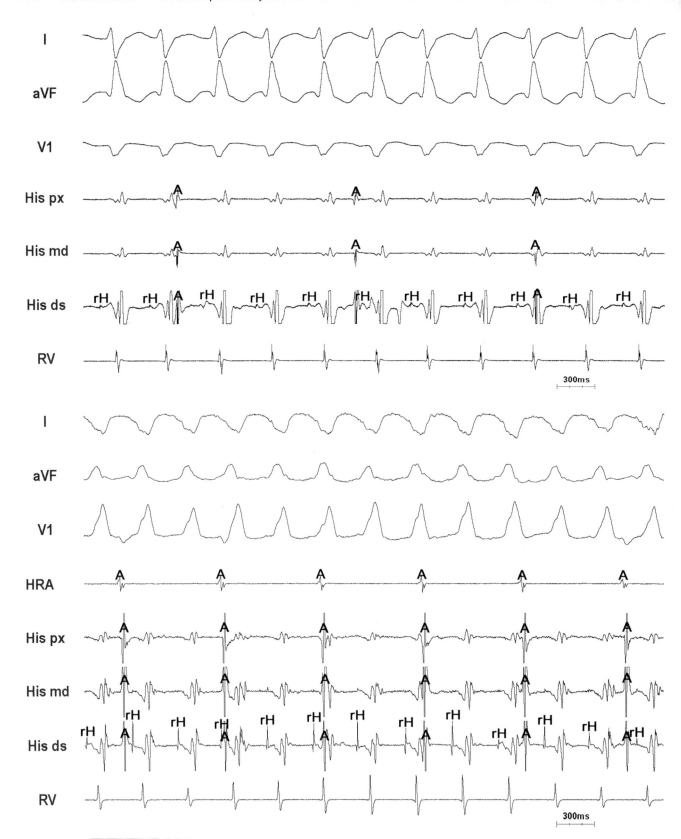

FIGURE 17-17 VT with 1:1 VH conduction and AV dissociation. Retrograde activation of the His bundle precedes antegrade activation of the ventricle resulting in positive but short HV intervals. Both foreshortened HV intervals and AV dissociation indicate VT.

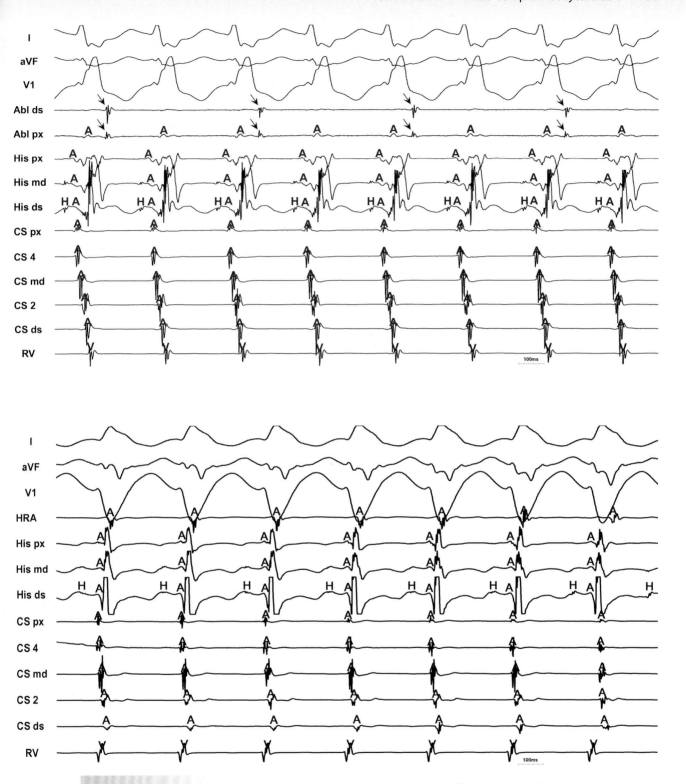

FIGURE 17-18 SVT with RBBB (*top*) and LBBB (*bottom*) (typical AVNRT). His bundle potentials precede each QRS complex with normal HV intervals. Atrial activation is midline and simultaneous with the ventricle. In the top tracing, the ablation catheter is positioned at the RA-SVC junction. Note the 2:1 block to the SVC (*arrows*).

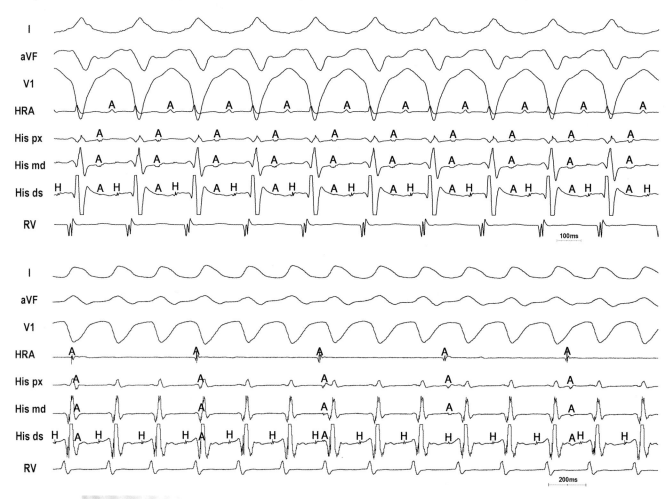

FIGURE 17-19 Typical LBBB tachycardias. *Top*: ORT with LBBB. His bundle potentials precede each QRS with normal HV intervals. *Bottom*: BBRT. His bundle potentials precede each QRS complex (HV = 58 ms) with AV dissociation.

PACING MANEUVERS

During NSR

Abrupt onset rapid pacing from the atrium can 1) unmask minimal (e.g., left free wall AP) or latent (e.g., atrio-fascicular or nodo-fascicular AP) preexcitation, 2) induce aberration, and 3) test the integrity of the conduction system. Identical aberrant and tachycardia QRS morphologies favor SVT or His-Purkinje type VT (BBRT, IFRT). Poor AV conduction and inability to support 1:1 conduction at the tachycardia rate argues for VT. Conversely, poor or absent VA conduction in a patient with a WCT and 1:1 AV relationship supports SVT (particularly, AT).

During WCT

While diagnosis of NCT is facilitated by pacing maneuvers from the ventricle, WCT diagnosis is established by pacing maneuvers from the atrium (inverse rule). During WCT, atrial pacing that penetrates the His-Purkinje system and narrows the QRS complex (capture or fusion beats) supports VT (**Fig. 17-20**). Atrial pacing that accelerates the ventricle to the pacing rate without

change in QRS morphology can be observed with 1) SVT with BBB, 2) preexcited tachycardia, and 3) His-Purkinje type VT (e.g., BBRT, IFRT) (**see Fig. 18-19**).[21] An early-coupled APD that terminates WCT with AV block excludes VT (analogous to an early-coupled ventricular premature depolarization [VPD] that terminates NCT with VA block excludes AT) (**Fig. 17-21**). An AVJ-refractory APD that advances or delays the ventricle indicates the presence of an AP and a preexcited tachycardia. An AVJ-refractory APD that resets WCT (advances or delays the ventricle *and* subsequent atrium) or terminates WCT with AV block excludes preexcited AVNRT/preexcited focal AT/VT and is virtually diagnostic of antidromic reciprocating tachycardia.[22] (Analogous to a His refractory VPD resetting or terminating NCT with VA block excludes AVNRT (unless a bystander nodo-fascicular/nodo-ventricular AP is present)/AT and indicates ORT (**see Figs. 18-14 to 18-16**)).

For typical LBBB tachycardias, entrainment from the RV can differentiate AVNRT with LBBB (post-pacing interval [PPI] − tachycardia cycle length [TCL] >115 ms) from typical BBRT (PPI − TCL <30) (**see Fig. 21-11**).[23,24]

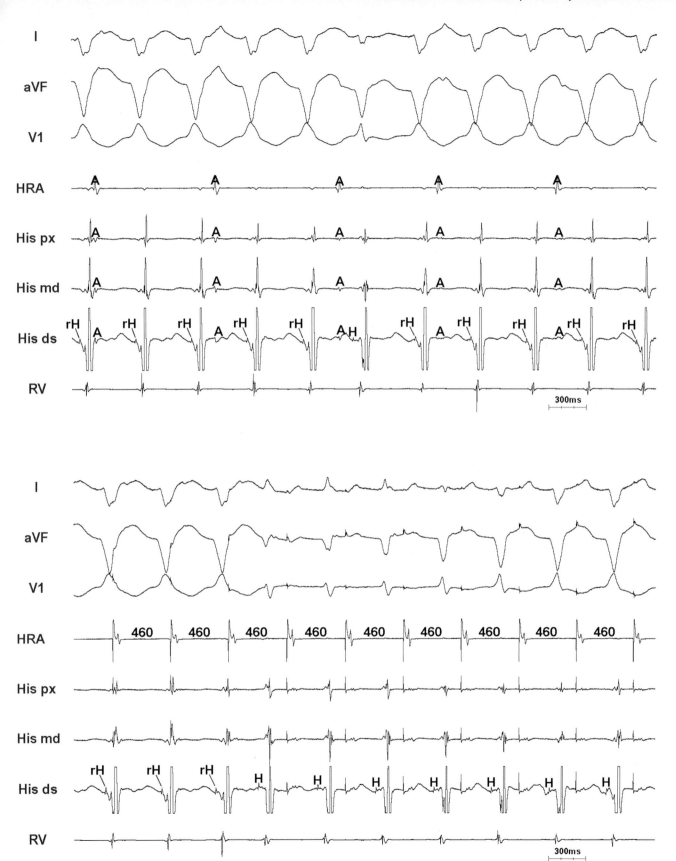

FIGURE 17-20 Fusion complexes. During VT, the His bundle is retrogradely activated (rH) and AV dissociation is present. A sinus beat (*top*) and atrial pacing (*bottom*) capture the His bundle antegradely (H) and fuse with VT.

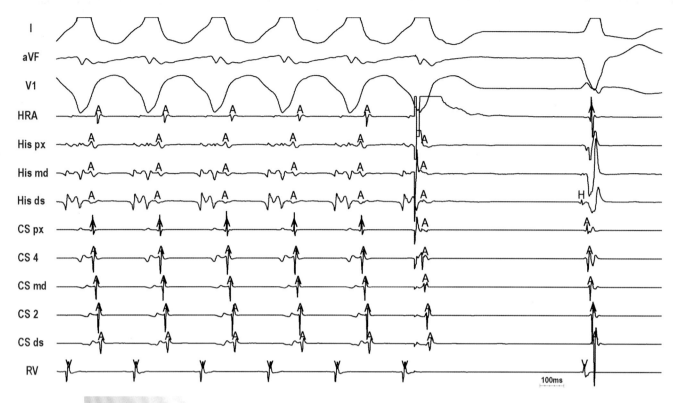

FIGURE 17-21 Termination of a WCT by an early APD with AV block. Absence of His bundle potentials preceding each QRS complex excludes SVT with LBBB. Termination by an early APD with AV block excludes VT. These findings indicate a preexcited tachycardia—in this case, antidromic tachycardia using a right free wall AP.

REFERENCES

1. Baerman JM, Morady F, DiCarlo LA Jr, de Buitleir M. Differentiation of ventricular tachycardia from supraventricular tachycardia with aberration: value of the clinical history. Ann Emerg Med 1987;16:40–43.
2. Guo H, Hecker S, Lévy S, Olshansky B. Ventricular tachycardia with QRS configuration similar to that in sinus rhythm and a myocardial origin: differential diagnosis with bundle branch reentry. Europace 2001;3:115–123.
3. Miller JM, Hsia HH, Rothman SA, Buxton AE. Ventricular tachycardia versus supraventricular tachycardia with aberration: electrocardiographic distinctions. In: Zipes DP, Jalife J, eds. Cardiac Electrophysiology: From Cell to Bedside. 3rd ed. Philadelphia, PA: WB Saunders, 2000:696–705.
4. Kindwall KE, Brown J, Josephson ME. Electrocardiographic criteria for ventricular tachycardia in wide complex left bundle branch morphology tachycardias. Am J Cardiol 1988;61:1279–1283.
5. Fedgchin B, Pavri BB, Greenspon AJ, Ho RT. Unique self-perpetuating cycle of atrioventricular block and phase IV bundle branch block in a patient with bundle branch reentrant tachycardia. Heart Rhythm 2004;1(4):493–496.
6. Wellens H, Bär F, Lie KI. The value of the electrocardiogram in the differential diagnosis of a tachycardia with a widened QRS complex. Am J Med 1978;64:27–33.
7. Antunes E, Brugada J, Steurer G, Andries E, Brugada P. The differential diagnosis of a regular tachycardia with a wide QRS complex on the 12-lead ECG: ventricular tachycardia, supraventricular tachycardia with aberrant intraventricular conduction, and supraventricular tachycardia with anterograde conduction over an accessory pathway. Pacing Clin Electrophysiol 1994;17:1515–1524.
8. Volders P, Timmermans C, Rodriguez LM, van Pol P, Wellens H. Wide QRS complex tachycardia with negative precordial concordance: always a ventricular origin? J Cardiovasc Electrophysiol 2003;14:109–111.
9. Rhee K, Nam G. Negative precordial concordance: is it a supraventricular tachycardia or ventricular tachycardia? Heart Rhythm 2009;6:133–134.
10. Kappos KG, Andrikopoulos GK, Tzeis SE, Manolis AS. Wide-QRS-complex tachycardia with a negative concordance pattern in the precordial leads: are the ECG criteria always reliable? Pacing Clin Electrophysiol 2006;29: 63–66.
11. Bayes de Luna A. Clinical Electrocardiography. A Textbook. Mount Kisco, NY: Futura, 1993:3–37.
12. Akhtar M, Shenasa M, Jazayeri M, Caceres J, Tchou PJ. Wide QRS complex tachycardia: reappraisal of a common clinical problem. Ann Intern Med 1988;109:905–912.
13. Lau EW. Infraatrial supraventricular tachycardias: mechanisms, diagnosis, and management. Pacing Clin Electrophysiol 2008;31:490–498.
14. Dressler W, Roesler H. The occurrence in paroxysmal ventricular tachycardia of ventricular complexes transitional in shape to sinoauricular beats; a diagnostic aid. Am Heart J 1952;44:485–493.
15. Jongnarangsin K, Pumprueg S, Prasertwitayakij N, et al. Utility of tachycardia cycle length variability in discriminating atrial tachycardia from ventricular tachycardia. Heart Rhythm 2010;7:225–228.
16. Camm AJ, Garratt C. Adenosine and supraventricular tachycardia. New Engl J Med 1991;325:1621–1629.
17. Lerman BB, Belardinelli L, West GA, Berne RM, DiMarco JP. Adenosine-sensitive ventricular tachycardia: evidence suggesting cyclic AMP-mediated triggered activity. Circulation 1986;74:270–280.
18. Gouaux JL, Ashman R. Auricular fibrillation with aberration simulating ventricular paroxysmal tachycardia. Am Heart J 1947;34:366–373.
19. Vereckei A, Duray G, Szénási G, Altemose GT, Miller JM. New algorithm using only lead aVR for differential diagnosis of wide QRS complex tachycardia. Heart Rhythm 2008;5:89–98.
20. Steurer G, Gürsoy S, Frey B, et al. The differential diagnosis on the electrocardiogram between ventricular tachycardia and preexcited tachycardia. Clin Cardiol 1994;17:306–308.
21. Merino JL, Peinado R, Fernández-Lozano I, Sobrino N, Sobrino J. Transient entrainment of bundle-branch reentry by atrial and ventricular stimulation: elucidation of the tachycardia mechanism through analysis of the surface ECG. Circulation 1999;100:1784–1790.
22. Sternick EB, Lokhandwala Y, Timmermans C, et al. Atrial premature beats during decrementally conducting antidromic tachycardia. Circ Arrhythm Electrophysiol 2013;6:357–363.
23. Michaud GF, Tada H, Chough S, et al. Differentiation of atypical atrioventricular node re-entrant from orthodromic reciprocating tachycardia using a septal accessory pathway by the response to ventricular pacing. J Am Coll Cardiol 2001;38:1163–1167.
24. Merino JL, Peinado R, Fernandez-Lozano I, et al. Bundle-branch reentry and the postpacing interval after entrainment by right ventricular apex stimulation: a new approach to elucidate the mechanism of wide-QRS-complex tachycardia with atrioventricular dissociation. Circulation 2001;103:1102–1108.

Preexcited Tachycardias

18

Introduction

Preexcited tachycardias refer collectively to tachycardias associated with antegrade conduction over an accessory pathway (AP). The AP can either 1) be a passive bystander serving a subsidiary role to the tachycardia mechanism (bystander preexcitation) or 2) be an integral part of the tachycardia mechanism (antidromic reciprocating tachycardia [ART]).

The purpose of this chapter is to:

1. Discuss the electrophysiologic features of bystander preexcited tachycardias.
2. Discuss the electrophysiologic features of ART and methods to differentiate ART from preexcited tachycardia atrio-ventricular nodal reentrant tachycardia (AVNRT).

BYSTANDER PREEXCITED TACHYCARDIAS

ATRIAL FIBRILLATION

The most common bystander preexcited tachycardia is pre-excited atrial fibrillation. Atrial fibrillation with bystander conduction over an AP produces an irregular, wide-complex tachycardia with variable QRS morphologies representing different degrees of fusion over the His-Purkinje system and AP (**Fig. 18-1**). The shortest preexcited RR interval is a measure of functional refractoriness of the AP, and a value <250 ms identifies an AP capable of causing rapid ventricular rates that could potentially degenerate into ventricular fibrillation.[1]

ATRIAL FLUTTER/TACHYCARDIA

Atrial flutter/tachycardia with 1:1 bystander conduction over an AP produces a regular, wide-complex tachycardia. The presence of 2:1 AP conduction excludes ART (**Fig. 18-2**).

ATRIO-VENTRICULAR NODAL REENTRANT TACHYCARDIA

AVNRT with bystander conduction over an AP results in a regular, wide-complex tachycardia. Preexcited QRS complexes represent fusion between His-Purkinje and AP conduction. During typical (slow–fast) AVNRT following fast pathway (FP) activation of the atrium, antegrade AP conduction competes with slow pathway (SP)–His-Purkinje activation, and therefore, QRS complex might appear maximally preexcited and mimic ART. During atypical (fast–slow) AVNRT following SP activation of the atrium, antegrade AP conduction completes with FP–His-Purkinje activation and

QRS complex might appear less preexcited which excludes ART. Loss of AP conduction normalizes QRS complexes without affecting tachycardia.[2]

Electrophysiologic Features

The characteristic electrophysiologic features of preexcited AVNRT are 1) regular, wide-complex tachycardia; 2) foreshortened (positive) or negative HV intervals; 3) antegrade His–right bundle (RB) activation sequence; and 4) concentric atrial activation pattern (**Fig. 18-3**).[3,4] QRS complexes represent fusion between His-Purkinje and AP conduction but might appear fully preexcited. Absence of maximal preexcitation excludes ART. When His bundle potentials are visible, HV intervals are short (positive) or negative and inversely related to the degree of preexcitation. The His-Purkinje system is activated antegradely, giving rise to an antegrade His-RB activation sequence (unless the AP inserts into the RB [e.g., atrio-fascicular/nodo-fascicular AP] in which case retrograde RB activation could occur nearly simultaneously with antegrade His bundle activation). The atrial activation pattern is midline and earliest at the His bundle region (typical [slow–fast] AVNRT) or coronary sinus os region (atypical [fast–slow] AVNRT) unless retrograde conduction occurs over left atrio-nodal inputs.

Zones of Transition

Induction of preexcited AVNRT (similar to its non-preexcited counterpart) requires that a premature impulse fall into the tachycardia window defined as the difference in refractory periods between the FP and SP of the atrio-ventricular (AV) node. The impulse 1) fails to conduct over one pathway (unidirectional block) and 2) conducts exclusively over the counterpart pathway with sufficient delay (slow conduction) to allow

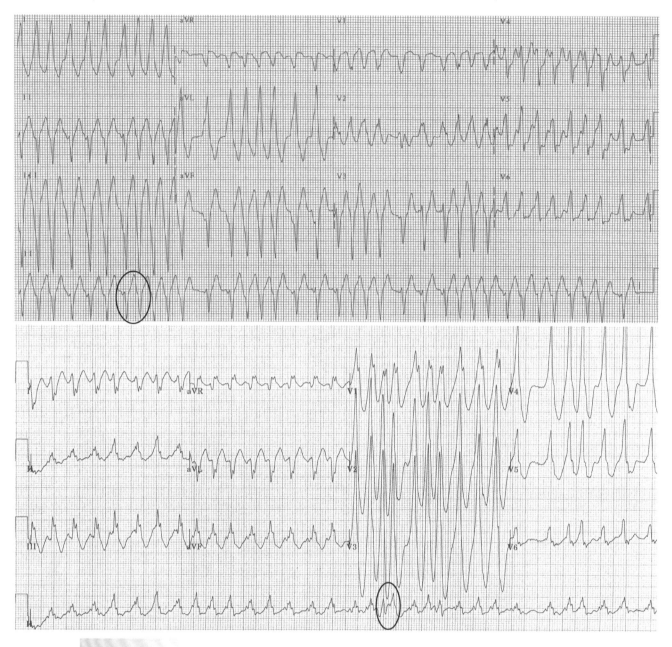

FIGURE 18-1 Preexcited atrial fibrillation. *Top:* Right posteroseptal AP. The shortest preexcited RR measures ~230 ms (*circled*). *Bottom:* Left free wall AP. The shortest preexcited RR intervals measure ~160 ms (*circled*).

the previously blocked pathway to recover excitability, conduct retrogradely, and initiate tachycardia. Oscillations in cycle length at tachycardia onset can reveal variable preexcitation, which excludes ART (**Figs. 18-3 and 18-4**). Block in either the FP or SP but not AP terminates tachycardia. Because the AP is a bystander, tachycardia persists despite loss of preexcitation (Fig 18-5).

Pacing Maneuvers

Both preexcited AVNRT and ART are regular, wide-complex preexcited tachycardias that can appear similar but differentiated by pacing maneuvers in the atrium (inverse rule).

AVJ-Refractory APD

During preexcited AVNRT, a critically timed atrial extrastimulus delivered near the atrial insertion site of the AP when the septal atrium is refractory ("committed") advances or delays the ventricle over the AP but does not reset or terminate tachycardia (failure to affect the subsequent atrium).[5] (The AVJ-refractory atrial premature depolarization [APD] that advances the ventricle over the AP is equivalent to delivery of a late-coupled ventricular premature depolarization (VPD) from the ventricular insertion site of the AP, which would fail to affect AVNRT because AVNRT has a large preexcitation index (> 100 ms)).[6] Moreover, advancement of the ventricle over

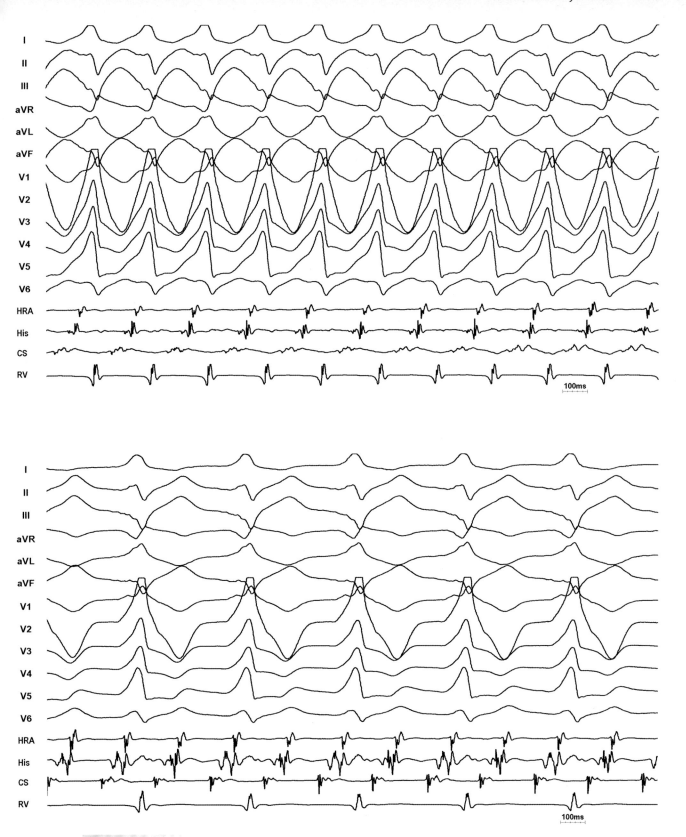

FIGURE 18-2 Preexcited atrial flutter with 1:1 (*top*) and 2:1 (*bottom*) conduction over a left posterior AP.

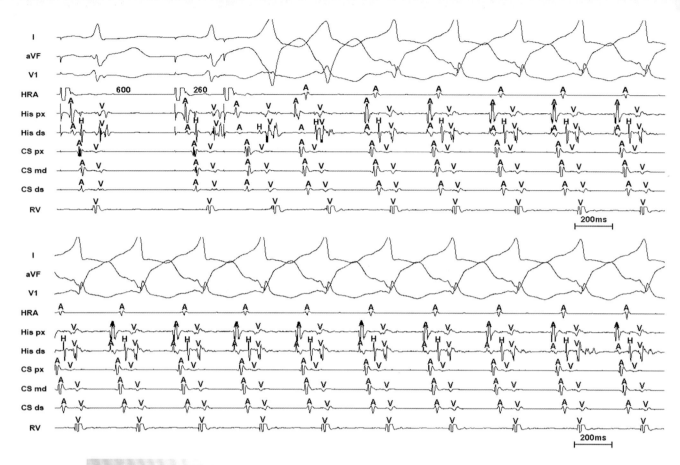

FIGURE 18-3 Preexcited AVNRT. Programmed atrial extrastimulation induces an atypical (fast–superior slow) AVNRT with bystander conduction over a left posteroseptal AP (earliest ventricular activation at CS px). His bundle potentials precede QRS onset with short HV intervals (HV = 8 ms). Absence of maximal preexcitation excludes ART.

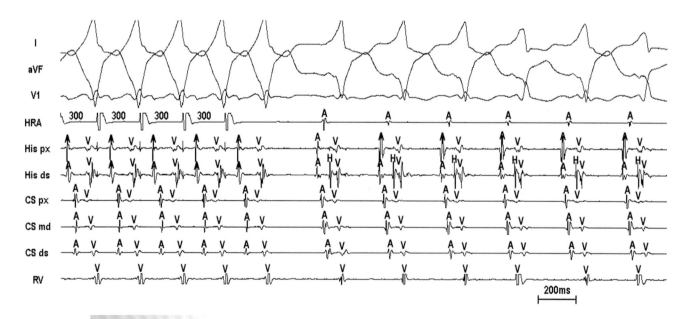

FIGURE 18-4 Preexcited AVNRT. Burst atrial pacing induces an atypical (fast–superior slow) AVNRT with bystander conduction over a left posteroseptal AP (earliest ventricular activation at CS px). Greater preexcitation during atrial pacing and variable preexcitation during tachycardia exclude ART. Preexcited QRS complexes represent fusion between His-Purkinje and AP conduction.

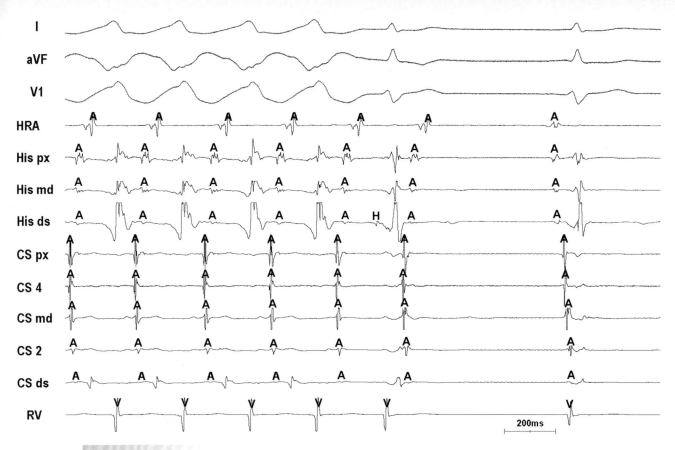

FIGURE 18-5 Preexcited AVNRT. Preexcited tachycardia persists for one beat despite loss of preexcitation excluding ART. It terminates with AV block excluding preexcited atrial tachycardia (AT). Loss of preexcitation reveals a short VA interval (65 ms) and earliest atrial activation at CS 4 (left atrio-nodal input). A subsequent junctional escape complex coincides with a sinus beat.

the AP might show a greater degree preexcitation indicating that QRS complexes during tachycardia are not maximally preexcited further excluding ART. (In contrast, during ART, an AVJ-refractory APD 1) advances or delays the ventricle over the AP *and* 2) resets tachycardia [advances or delays the subsequent atrium], indicating that both the ventricle and atrium are integral components of the circuit (obligatory 1:1 AV/VA relationship, see below).)

Rapid Atrial Pacing (Maximal Preexcitation)

During sinus rhythm, rapid atrial pacing near the AP at the shortest cycle length maintaining 1:1 AP conduction provides a morphology template of maximal preexcitation.[2] A preexcited tachycardia without maximal preexcitation excludes ART (Fig. 18-4).

Rapid Ventricular Pacing/Entrainment (ΔHA Value/PPI)

During AVNRT, the HA interval reflects simultaneous activation of the His bundle and atrium over the AV node (pseudo-interval), but during right ventricular (RV) entrainment (or pacing at the tachycardia cycle length [TCL]), it represents sequential activation over the AV node (true interval). Therefore, the $HA_{(preexcited\ AVNRT)} < HA_{(RV\ pacing)}$.[7] In contrast, during

both ART and RV entrainment (or pacing at TCL), the HA interval reflects sequential activation of the His bundle and atrium over the AV node. Therefore, the $HA_{(ART)} = HA_{(RV\ pacing)}$.[7] During entrainment of preexcited AVNRT from the ventricle, the post-pacing interval (PPI) is long similar to its non-preexcited counterpart.[8]

ANTIDROMIC REENTRANT TACHYCARDIA

MECHANISM

In contrast to bystander preexcitation, the AP during ART is an integral component of the tachycardia mechanism. During typical (true) ART, the antegrade and retrograde limbs of the circuit are the AP and His-Purkinje–AV node axis, respectively, both of which demonstrate short refractory periods.[9] Atypical ART uses two APs for antegrade and retrograde conduction ("pathway to pathway" tachycardia) with or without fusion (antegrade or retrograde) over the AV node.[10,11] (Alternatively, atypical ART with antegrade fusion over the AV node might be considered orthodromic reciprocating tachycardia [ORT] with antegrade bystander AP conduction depending on whether the AV node or antegrade AP forms the dominant antegrade limb of the circuit.)

Except for ART using a nodo-fascicular/nodo-ventricular AP, ART requires participation of both atria and ventricles and obligates a 1:1 AV relationship. Because of the close anatomic proximity between septal APs and the AV node–His-Purkinje axis as well as the limitations imposed by tissue refractoriness, ART is rare with septal APs (<4 cm from the AV node (concept of "distance delay")) unless slow conduction occurs over the AP or AV node (SP).[10,12] Therefore, presumed ART in the setting of a septal AP (particularly, posteroseptal) should raise suspicion of another pathway or an alternative diagnosis.[10]

ELECTROPHYSIOLOGIC FEATURES

The characteristic electrophysiologic features of ART are 1) regular, wide-complex tachycardia; 2) fixed, maximal preexcitation; 3) negative HV intervals; 4) retrograde RB or left bundle (LB)-His activation sequence (short and long VH interval tachycardias); 5) obligatory 1:1 AV relationship (except for nodo-fascicular/nodo-ventricular APs); and 6) concentric atrial activation pattern (unless another AP is used) (**Figs. 18-6 and 18-7**).[9–11] Antegrade AP conduction is unfused, and therefore, QRS complexes are fixed and maximally preexcited. Absence of constant, maximal preexcitation excludes ART. A very short VH interval (<30 ms) should raise suspicion for a atrio- or nodo-fascicular AP. Because atrio- or nodo-fascicular APs insert into the RB close to the His bundle, the VH interval (pseudo-interval) is shorter than for AV APs (true interval; AP far from the His bundle). Inclusion of the bundle branch ipsilateral or contralateral to the AP as a part of the retrograde limb of the circuit results in short or long VH tachycardias, respectively, with bundle branch preceding His bundle potentials. Retrograde conduction over the AV node produces a midline atrial activation pattern earliest at the His bundle region (FP) or coronary sinus os (SP) unless left atrio-nodal inputs are used.

AV Relationship

Except for ART using a nodo-fascicular/nodo-ventricular AP, ART requires participation of both atria and ventricles (obligatory 1:1 AV relationship).[11] Absence of 1:1 AV association excludes ART using an AV AP. Retrograde AV node delay and block causes tachycardia slowing and termination, respectively (**Figs. 18-8 and 18-9**).

Bundle Branch Block

Similar to ORT, ART uses the shortest circuit capable of sustained reentry and incorporates the bundle branch ipsilateral to the AP as an integral part of the circuit. Retrograde block in the ipsilateral bundle branch forces conduction across the interventricular septum and retrogradely over the contralateral bundle enlarging the circuit.[9,11,13–15] Ipsilateral bundle branch block (BBB) causes an increase in the 1) VH interval (conversion from short to long VH tachycardia) and generally the 2) VA interval and 3) TCL ("reverse Coumel's sign") (**Figs. 18-10; see also Fig. 11-20**). The increase in the VA interval and TCL occurs at the expense of an increase in the VH interval, provided that an equivalent decrease in the HA or AV intervals does not occur. Changes in TCL resulting from changes in the VH interval demonstrate dependence of tachycardia upon His-Purkinje conduction, which among preexcited tachycardias is unique to ART.

ZONES OF TRANSITION

ART is generally easier to induce with atrial as opposed to ventricular stimulation (**Figs. 18-11 and 18-12**).[9] Atrial pacing stimuli fall into the tachycardia window defined as the difference in antegrade refractory periods between the AV node and the AP. The initiating impulse blocks in the AV node–His-Purkinje axis (unidirectional block) and conducts exclusively over the AP producing a maximally preexcited QRS complex. Sufficient delay over the AP (slow conduction) allows the His-Purkinje–AV node axis to recover excitability, conduct retrogradely, and initiate tachycardia. Retrograde BBB ipsilateral to the AP facilitates tachycardia initiation by incorporating transeptal conduction into the circuit and thereby providing additional time for the His bundle–AV node to recover excitability. During ventricular stimulation, the initiating impulse blocks retrogradely in the AP and conducts exclusively over the His-Purkinje–AV node. Sufficient delay in the His-Purkinje system (e.g., "VH jump") and/or AV node allows subsequent antegrade conduction over the AP and initiation of ART (**Fig. 18-13**). Antidromic reentrant tachycardia terminates with block in the AP or AV node (typical ART) (**Figs. 18-9 and 18-12**). Therefore, persistence of tachycardia despite loss of preexcitation excludes ART.

PACING MANEUVERS

AVJ-Refractory APD

During ART, AVJ-refractory APDs delivered near the AP 1) advance or delay the ventricle over the AP *and* 2) advance or delay the subsequent atrium (reset tachycardia) (obligatory 1:1 AV relationship) (**Figs. 18-14 and 18-15**). (In contrast, during preexcited AVNRT, AVJ-refractory APDs that advance or delay the ventricle over the AP fail to affect the subsequent atrium and reset tachycardia.)[9,11,16,17] AVJ-refractory APDs terminating a preexcited tachycardia without reaching the ventricle (AV block) is virtually pathognomonic of ART and excludes preexcited AVNRT, preexcited focal AT, and VT (**Fig. 18-16**). Early-coupled (non–AVJ-refractory) APDs are less helpful for differentiating preexcited tachycardias, but termination with AV block excludes ventricular tachycardia (VT) (**Figs. 18-17 and 18-18**).

Rapid Atrial Pacing (Maximal Preexcitation)

During sinus rhythm, rapid atrial pacing near the AP at the shortest cycle length maintaining 1:1 AP conduction provides a morphology template of maximal preexcitation that matches ART (**Fig. 18-19**).[11]

Rapid Ventricular Pacing/ Entrainment (ΔHA Value/PPI)

During true ART and RV entrainment (or pacing at TCL), the HA interval reflects sequential activation of the His bundle and atrium over the AV node. Therefore, the $HA_{(ART)} = HA_{(RV\ pacing)}$ (**Figs. 18-20 and 18-21**).[7] During entrainment of ART from the ventricle, the PPI is short similar to its ORT counterpart (**Fig. 18-21**).[8]

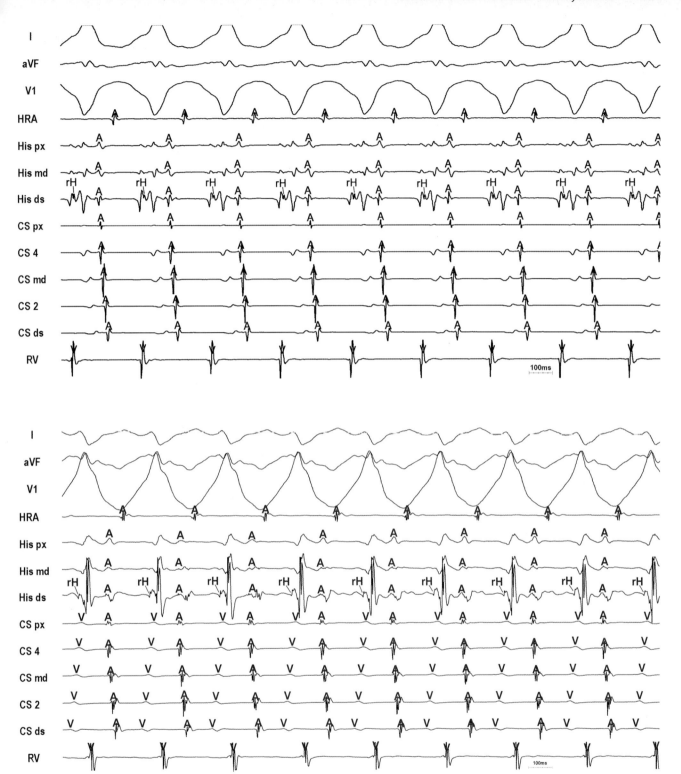

FIGURE 18-6 Antidromic tachycardia. Antegrade conduction occurs over a right free wall (*top*) and left free wall (*bottom*) AP with retrograde conduction over the FP. The VH interval is short (56 and 52 ms, respectively) due to retrograde conduction over the RB and LB (ipsilateral to the AP), respectively.

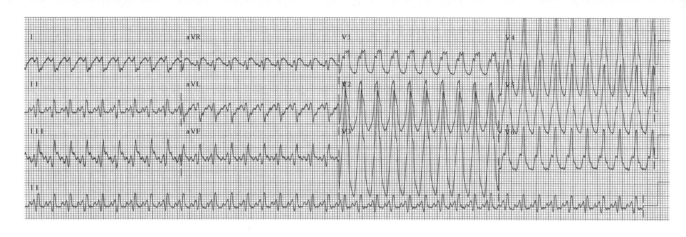

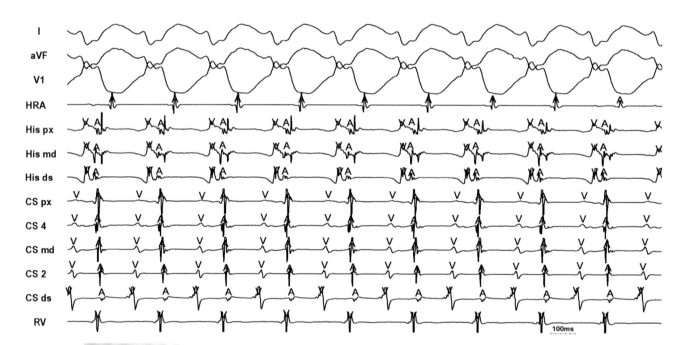

FIGURE 18-7 Antidromic tachycardia. Antegrade conduction occurs over a left free wall AP with retrograde conduction over the FP. Preexcited QRS complexes show positive precordial concordance. Note early ventricular activation along the lateral mitral annulus (CS ds).

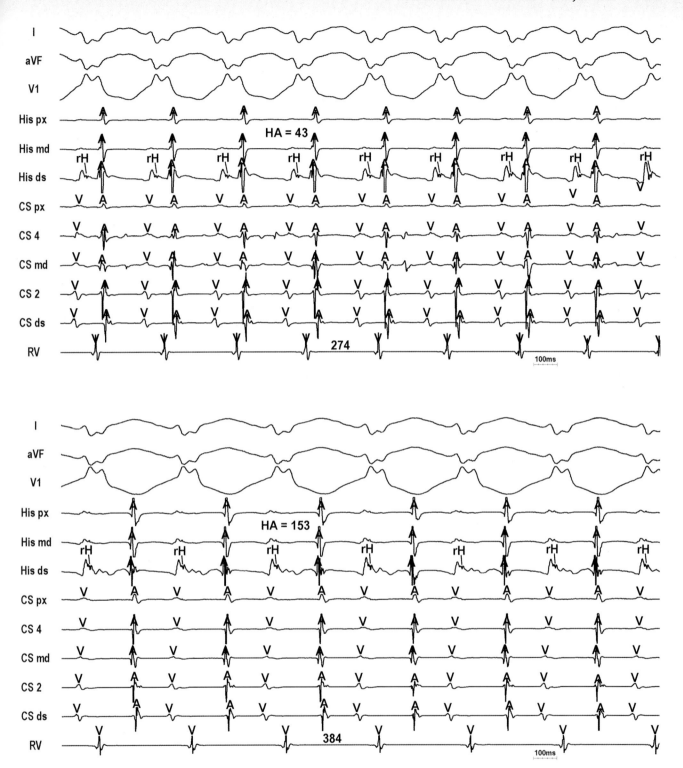

FIGURE 18-8 Antidromic tachycardia (cycle length dependency on the AV node). QRS complexes are maximally preexcited over a left free wall AP (early ventricular activation along the lateral mitral annulus [CS ds]). The VH interval = 89 ms. TCL is shorter (274 ms versus 384 ms) when retrograde FP conduction is faster (HA = 43 ms versus 153 ms).

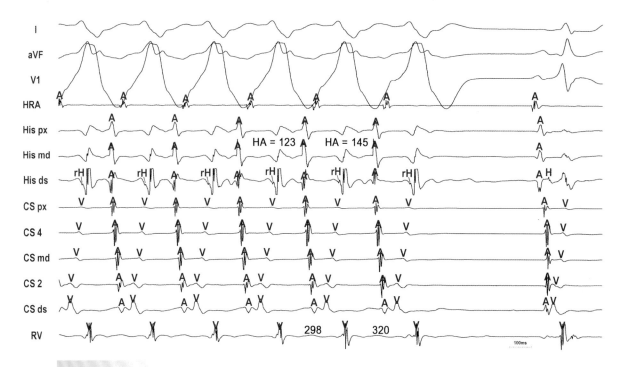

FIGURE 18-9 Termination of ART in the AV node. QRS complexes are maximally preexcited over a left free wall AP (early ventricular activation at CS ds). The VH interval is short (69 ms), indicating retrograde conduction over the LB (ipsilateral to the AP). Retrograde FP Wenckebach causes cycle length slowing and termination indicating AV nodal dependency and excluding VT. The subsequent sinus beat shows preexcitation.

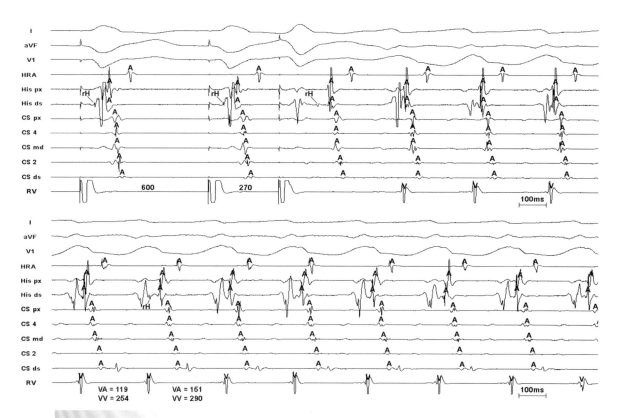

FIGURE 18-10 Induction of ART. *Top.* A single ventricular extrastimulus induces a "VH jump" and corresponding increasing in the VA interval indicating retrograde conduction over the FP. Sufficient VA prolongation (slow conduction) allows antegrade conduction over a left posterolateral AP and initiation of ART. *Bottom.* Transient retrograde left bundle branch block (LBBB) causes an increase in the VH and VA intervals and momentary slowing of tachycardia ("reverse Coumel's law").

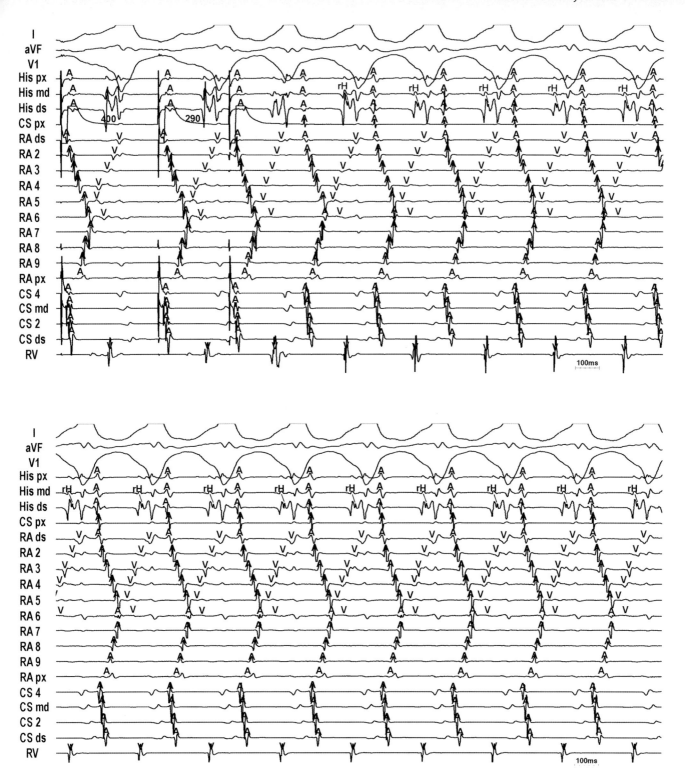

FIGURE 18-11 Induction of ART. A single atrial extrastimulus blocks in the AV node (unidirectional block) and conducts over a right free wall AP (earliest ventricular activation along the lateral tricuspid annulus [RA 5]) with sufficient delay to initiate ART. The VH interval is short (56 ms) due to retrograde conduction over the RB (ipsilateral to the AP).

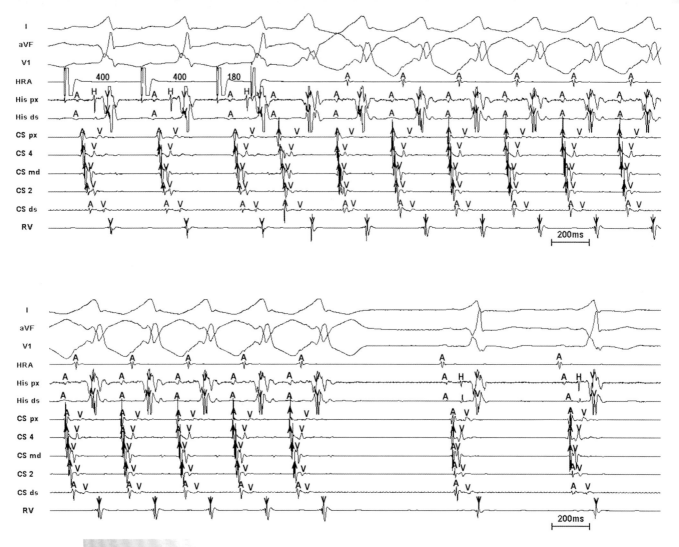

FIGURE 18-12 Induction of ART. *Top.* A single atrial extrastimulus blocks in the AV node (unidirectional block) and conducts over a left posterior AP (earliest ventricular activation at CS md) with sufficient delay to induce ART. *Bottom.* Tachycardia terminates spontaneously with retrograde block in the FP (VA block) excluding VT. Subsequent sinus beats show preexcitation.

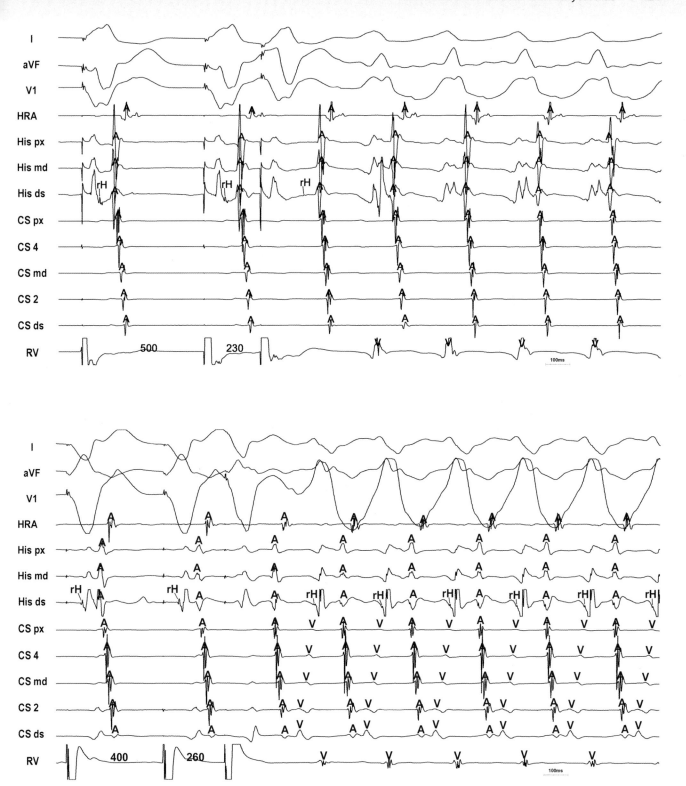

FIGURE 18-13 Induction of ART. *Top*: A single ventricular extrastimulus induces a "VH jump" and equivalent increase in the VA interval indicating retrograde conduction over the FP. Sufficient VA prolongation (slow conduction) allows antegrade conduction over a left free wall AP and initiation of ART. *Bottom*: A single ventricular extrastimulus also induces ART using a left free wall AP (earliest ventricular activation at CS ds). The VH interval is short (69 ms) due to retrograde conduction over the LB (ipsilateral to the AP).

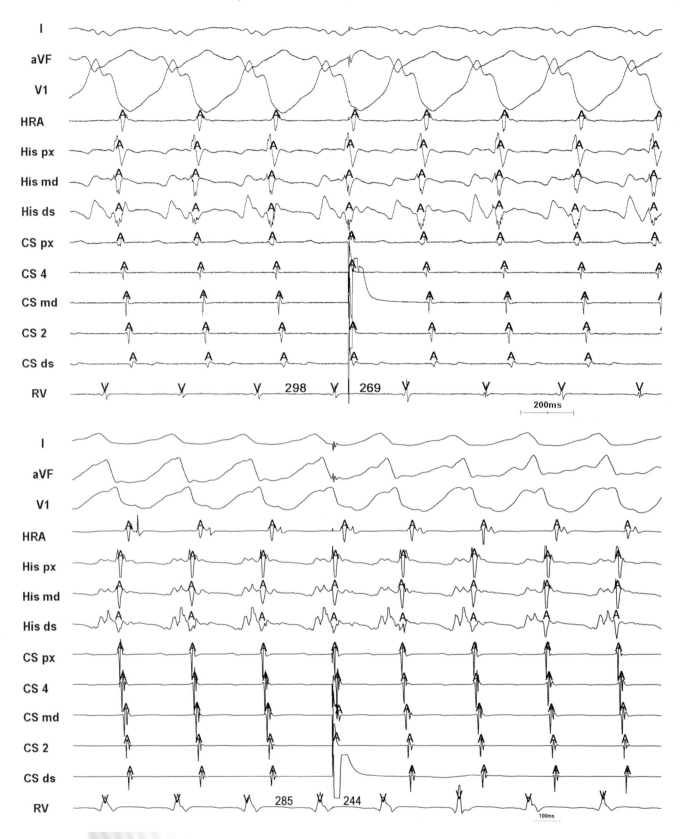

FIGURE 18-14 Resetting of ART by AVJ-refractory APDs. In both cases, the AVJ-refractory APD 1) advances the ventricle (proving presence of an AP) and 2) resets tachycardia (proving AP participation in tachycardia). The advanced ventricle is the equivalent to delivery of late-coupled VPDs ("preexcitation index" ≤29 and 41 ms, respectively—not sufficiently early to affect a preexcited AVNRT).

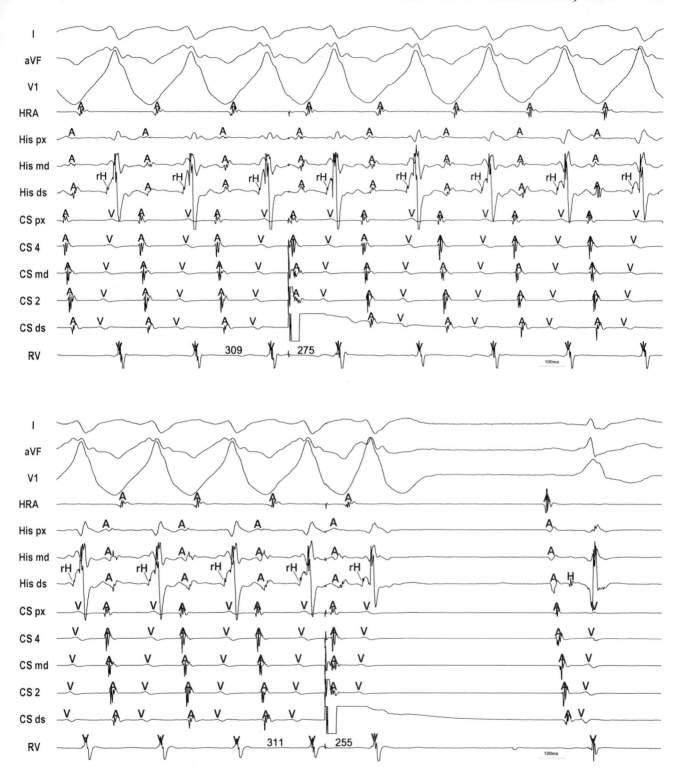

FIGURE 18-15 Resetting and termination of ART by AVJ-refractory APDs. *Top:* An AVJ-refractory APD advances the ventricle by 34 ms (proving presence of a left free wall AP) and subsequent atrium (resetting tachycardia) (proving AP participation in tachycardia). The advanced ventricle is the equivalent to delivery of a late-coupled VPD ("preexcitation index" ≤34 ms)—not sufficiently early to affect a preexcited AVNRT. *Bottom:* An earlier AVJ-refractory APD advances the ventricle by 56 ms but fails to conduct retrogradely over the AV node terminating tachycardia.

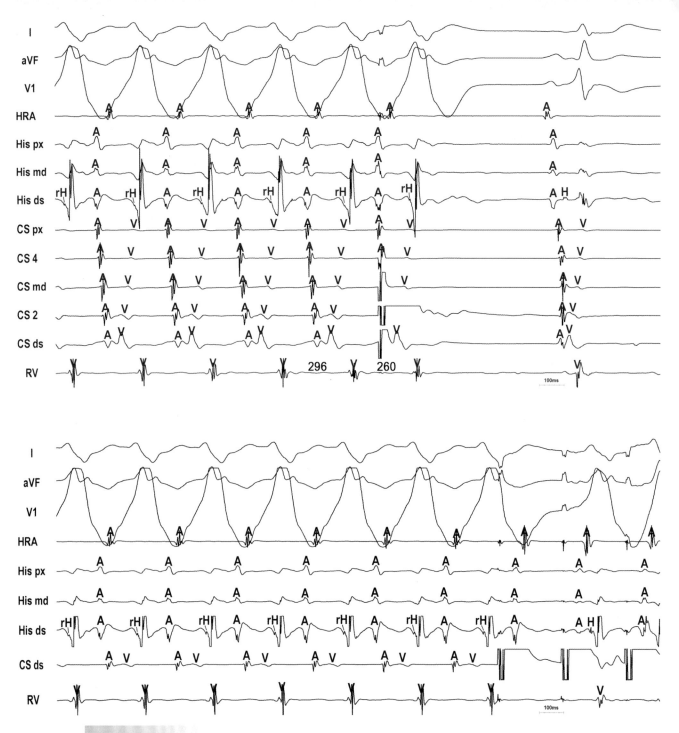

FIGURE 18-16 Termination of ART by AVJ-refractory APDs. *Top*: An AVJ-refractory APD advances the ventricle by 36 ms (proving presence of an AP) but fails to conduct retrogradely over the AV node terminating tachycardia. *Bottom*: During atrial overdrive pacing from the lateral mitral annulus (CS ds), the first stimulus is AVJ-refractory and terminates tachycardia with AV block excluding preexcited AVNRT, preexcited focal AT, and VT. Subsequent atrial paced complexes conduct with ventricular preexcitation.

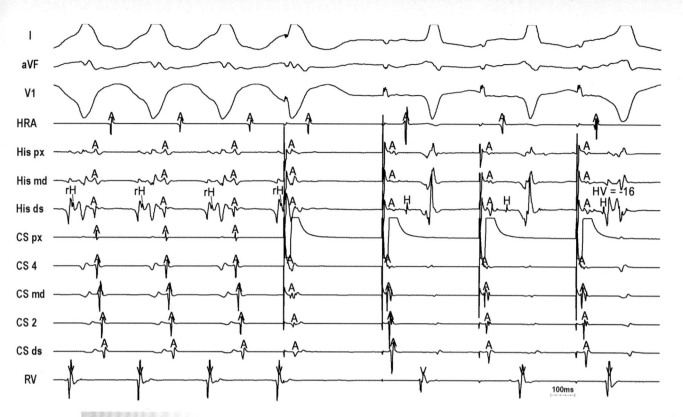

FIGURE 18-17 Termination of ART by an early-coupled APD. During atrial pacing, the first stimulus is early (non–AVJ refractory) but terminates tachycardia with AV block excluding VT. Subsequent atrial paced complexes conduct with progressive ventricular preexcitation.

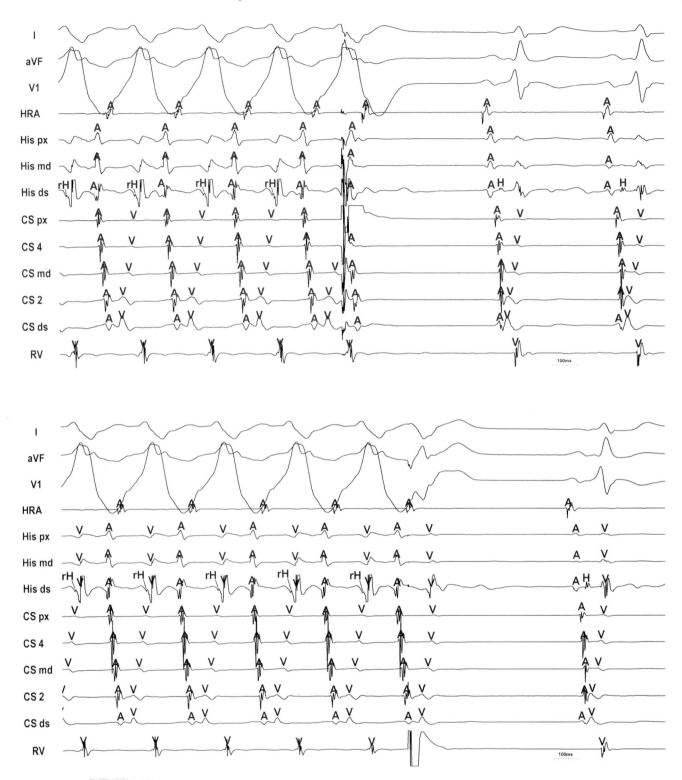

FIGURE 18-18 Termination of ART by early-coupled APDs and VPDs. *Top*: An early (non–AVJ refractory) APD terminates tachycardia with AV block excluding VT. *Bottom*: An early-coupled RV VPD fuses with tachycardia arising from the LV (left free wall AP), encroaches on retrograde His bundle/AV node refractoriness, and terminates tachycardia with VA block.

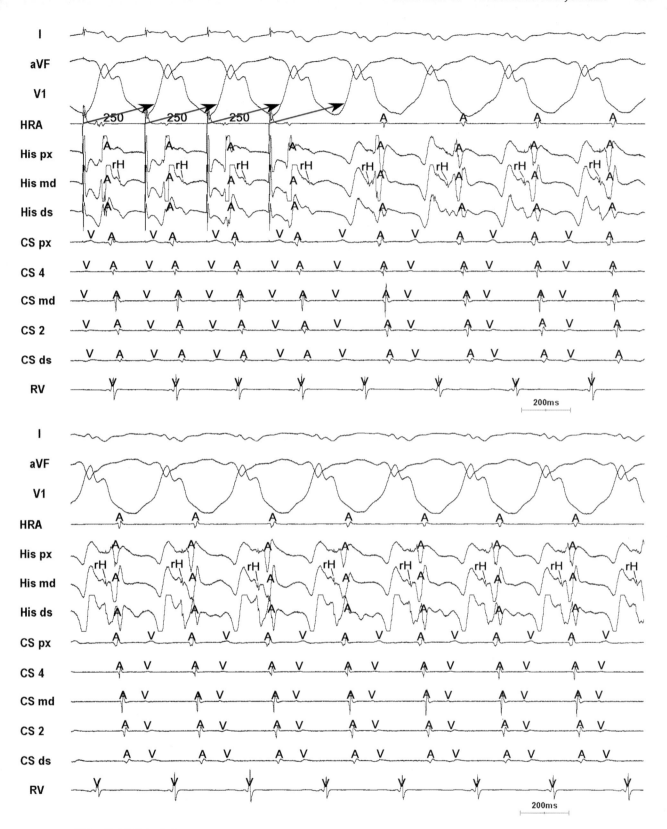

FIGURE 18-19 Maximal preexcitation. Rapid atrial pacing induces ART over a left posterior AP. Paced and tachycardia QRS complexes are identical and maximally preexcited. During pacing, progressive increase in the stimulus-delta (St-delta) interval is accompanied by parallel increases in the stimulus-His (St-H) interval (fixed VH interval) indicating retrograde activation of the His bundle (rH). Antegrade block in the AV node ("unidirectional block") and long St-delta and VH interval (122 ms) ("slow conduction")—the latter due to retrograde left bundle branch block (LBBB) (ipsilateral to the AP) with retrograde conduction over the right bundle—facilitates ART induction.

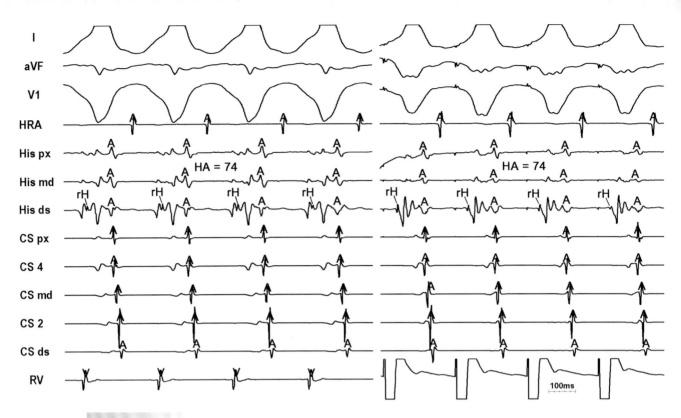

FIGURE 18-20 ΔHA value (antidromic tachycardia). The HA intervals for ART and ventricular pacing at the TCL are identical (ΔHA = 0 ms) because both represent sequential activation of the His bundle and atrium over the AV node.

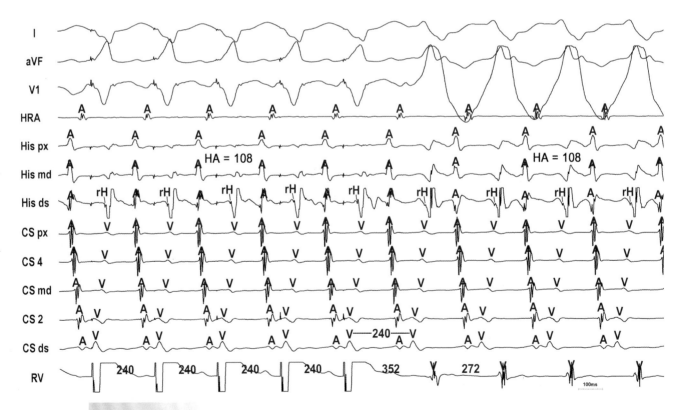

FIGURE 18-21 Entrainment of ART from the ventricle. Entrainment results in constant QRS fusion between RV pacing and LV activation over a free wall AP with the last orthodromically captured ventricular electrograms (CS ds to px) returning at the pacing cycle length (240 ms) (first criteria of transient entrainment). The PPI–TCL is short (80 ms). The ΔHA = 0 ms. These findings exclude preexcited AVNRT.

REFERENCES

1. Klein GJ, Bashore TM, Sellers TD, Pritchett EL, Smith WM, Gallagher JJ. Ventricular fibrillation in the Wolff-Parkinson-White syndrome. N Engl J Med 1979;301:1080–1085.

2. Glikson M, Belhassen B, Eldar M. Atypical AV nodal reentry with bystander accessory pathway: an unusual mechanism of preexcited tachycardia. Pacing Clin Electrophysiol 1999;22:390–392.

3. Bhatia A, Sra J, Akhtar M. Preexcitation syndromes. Curr Probl Cardiol 2016;41:99–137.

4. Ellenbogen KA, Ramirez NM, Packer DL, et al. Accessory nodoventricular (Mahaim) fibers: a clinical review. Pacing Clin Electrophysiol 1986;9:868–884.

5. Carmo A, Melo SL, Scanavacca MI, Sosa E. Wide complex tachycardia: an unusual presentation. Heart Rhythm 2012;9:996–997.

6. Miles W, Yee R, Klein G, Zipes D, Prystowsky E. The preexcitation index: an aid in determining the mechanism of supraventricular tachycardia and localizing accessory pathways. Circulation 1986;74:493–500.

7. Hurwitz JL, Miller JM, Josephson ME. The value of the HA interval in diagnosing preexcited tachycardias due to AV nodal reentry. J Am Coll Cardiol 1991;17:323A.

8. Michaud GF, Tada H, Chough S, et al. Differentiation of atypical atrioventricular node re-entrant tachycardia from orthodromic reciprocating tachycardia using a septal accessory pathway by the response to ventricular pacing. J Am Coll Cardiol 2001;38:1163–1167.

9. Packer DL, Gallagher JJ, Prystowsky EN. Physiological substrate for antidromic reciprocating tachycardia. Prerequisite characteristics of the accessory pathway and atrioventricular conduction system. Circulation 1992;85:574–588.

10. Bardy GH, Packer DL, German LD, Gallagher JJ. Preexcited reciprocating tachycardia in patient with Wolff-Parkinson-White syndrome: incidence and mechanism. Circulation 1984;70:377–391.

11. Atié J, Brugada P, Brugada J, et al. Clinical and electrophysiologic characteristics of patients with antidromic circus movement tachycardia in the Wolff-Parkinson-White syndrome. Am J Cardiol 1990;66:1082–1091.

12. Man DC, Sarter BH, Coyne RF, et al. Antidromic reciprocating tachycardia in patients with paraseptal accessory pathways: importance of critical delay in the reentry circuit. Pacing Clin Electrophysiol 1999;22:386–389.

13. Kuck KH, Brugada P, Wellens HJ. Observations on the antidromic type of circus movement tachycardia in the Wolff-Parkinson-White syndrome. J Am Coll Cardiol 1983;2:1003–1010.

14. Sternick EB, Scarpelli RB, Gerken LM, Wellens HJ. Wide QRS tachycardia with sudden rate acceleration: what is the mechanism? Heart Rhythm 2009;6:1670–1673.

15. Guttigoli A, Mittal S, Stein KM, Lerman BB. Wide-complex tachycardia with an abrupt change in cycle length: what is the mechanism? J Cardiovasc Electrophysiol 2003;14:781–783.

16. Sternick EB, Lokhandwala Y, Timmermans C, et al. Atrial premature beats during decrementally conducting antidromic tachycardia. Circ Arrhythm Electrophysiol 2013;6:357–363.

17. Gentlesk PJ, Sauer WH, Peele ME, Eckart RE. Spontaneous premature atrial depolarization proving the mechanism of a wide complex tachycardia. Pacing Clin Electrophysiol 2008;31:1625–1627.

19 Idiopathic Ventricular Tachycardia and Fibrillation

Introduction

Idiopathic ventricular tachycardia (VT) and ventricular fibrillation (VF) can occur in the absence of structural heart disease. Two anatomic sites showing a predilection for idiopathic VT are the 1) outflow tracts (most common) and 2) papillary muscles, although other sites (e.g., valve annuli) have also been described. Idiopathic left ventricular (LV) VT (verapamil-sensitive VT) is a specific form of VT arising from/near the left-sided fascicles (most commonly the left posterior fascicle). Idiopathic VF is triggered by short-coupled PVCs (<300 ms) often near the Purkinje system that can be targeted for ablation.

The purpose of this chapter is to:

1. Discuss the mechanism, electrophysiologic features, and ablation of outflow tract and papillary muscle VT.
2. Discuss the mechanism, electrophysiologic features, and ablation of idiopathic LV tachycardia.
3. Discuss the mechanism and ablation of idiopathic VF.

OUTFLOW TRACT TACHYCARDIAS

MECHANISM

Exercise-induced, adrenergically mediated right ventricular outflow tract (RVOT) VT serves as the mechanistic paradigm for outflow tract tachycardias. Its initiation by atrial and ventricular stimulation, facilitation by isoproterenol, and suppression by adenosine and propranolol suggest a focal mechanism dependent on catecholamine-sensitive, cAMP-mediated delayed afterdepolarizations and triggered activity.[1,2] Isoproterenol (via beta receptor agonism and guanosine stimulatory proteins) activates adenyl cyclase, which promotes conversion of ATP to cAMP. This leads to a cascade of downstream events: protein kinase A phosphorylation of the L-type Ca^+ channel, ryanodine receptor activation, and Ca^+ release from the sarcoplasmic reticulum. Intracellular calcium overload (Ca^+ induced Ca^+ release and Ca^+ sparks) induces delayed afterdepolarizations and triggered activity. VT can be suppressed by adenosine and vagal maneuvers (via A1 and M2 receptor agonism and guanosine inhibitory proteins) or beta blockers (via beta receptor antagonism)—all of which inhibit adenyl cyclase and cAMP formation or by L-type Ca^+ channel blockers.

OUTFLOW TRACT ANATOMY

Right Ventricular Outflow Tract

In the embryologic heart, partitioning of the bulbus cordis and truncus arteriosus separates the pulmonary infundibulum (conus arteriosus), valve, and trunk from the aortic vestibule, valve, and aorta. Because of the spiral orientation of the aorticopulmonary septum, the RVOT wraps anteriorly and leftward around the aortic root (Fig. 19-1).[3,4] Despite its name, therefore, the crescent-shaped RVOT is actually positioned leftward and anterior to the left ventricular outflow tract (LVOT). The most anterior portion of the outflow tract is the RVOT free wall, while the most leftward portion is the junction between the RVOT anteroseptum and free wall. The posteroseptum of the RVOT lies directly anterior to the right coronary cusp (RCC) of the aortic valve travelling anteriorly and leftward to meet the anteroseptum. The pulmonic valve sits anterior, leftward and 5–10 mm superior (cephalo-caudal separation) to the aortic valve. Underneath the pulmonary valve at the anteroseptum of the RVOT is the most common site for VT. VT can also arise above the valves from the pulmonary sinus cusps because of myocardial sleeves extending superiorly into the valve leaflets. The left pulmonary cusp is the most inferior, while the right and anterior cusps are situated more superiorly. The left atrial appendage is close to the anterior pulmonary artery and a possible source of far-field left atrial electrograms.

Left Ventricular Outflow Tract

The centrally positioned aortic valve sits posterior, rightward, and inferior to the pulmonic valve and whose cusp also contain arrhythmogenic myocardial sleeves. The posterior or noncoronary cusp (NCC) of the aortic valve is the most posterior leaflet; abuts the right and left atrium; and is a potential source of atrial

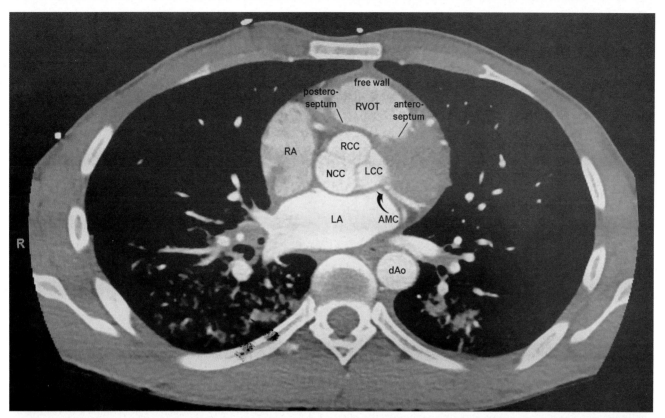

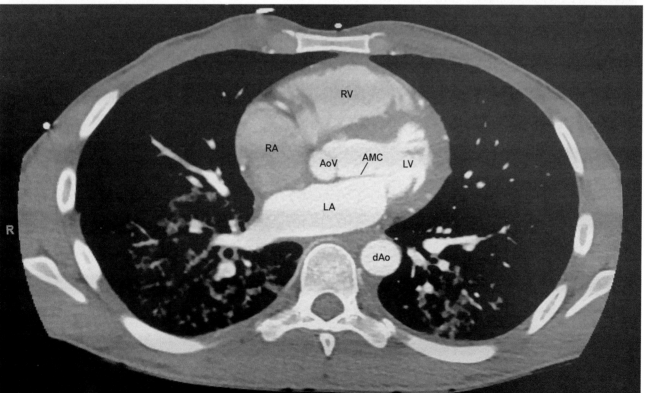

FIGURE 19-1 Anatomy of the outflow tracts. The RVOT wraps around the aortic root. Its free wall is the most anterior structure producing VT with a late (≥V4) precordial QRS transition. The RVOT septum sits posterior to the free wall generating VT with an earlier (V3) precordial transition. Note that the RVOT anteroseptum is the most leftward structure so that VT arising from this site is negative in lead I. Travelling more posteriorly, the RCC sits behind the RVOT posteroseptum followed by the LCC and AMC resulting in VT with progressive earlier (≤V2) precordial transition.

tachycardia (AT), accessory pathways, and only rarely VT. The commissure between the NCC/RCC lies opposite the commissure separating the septal/anterior leaflets of the tricuspid valve where the membranous portion of the interventricular septum and penetrating His bundle are located—the latter being recorded beneath the aortic valve. Both the RCC and left coronary cusp (LCC) are anterior to the NCC and potential sources of VT. The RCC directly abuts the posteroseptum of the pulmonary infundibulum posteriorly beneath the pulmonic valve. Close proximity of the right atrial appendage to the RCC can give rise to far-field atrial electrograms at this site. The LCC is posterior, leftward, and superior to the RCC and abuts the pulmonary trunk above the pulmonary valve, and therefore, the left main coronary artery travels close to the posterior pulmonary trunk. VT can also arise from the aortic vestibule beneath the valve. The aorto-mitral continuity (region between the LCC/NCC commissure and anterior leaflet of the mitral valve) is generally devoid of myocardial tissue but when present can be a source of accessory pathways and VT. The posterior-superior process of the LV or "AV septum" is the region where the right atrium abuts the LV (because of the apical displacement of the tricuspid valve relative to the mitral valve).

The epicardial region of the LVOT is the LV summit and a potential source of VT. The great cardiac vein (GCV) travels epicardially near the LCC at the base of the heart, crosses the left circumflex (LCx) coronary artery, and runs alongside the left anterior descending (LAD) coronary artery to become the anterior interventricular vein. (The intersection of the GCV, LCx, and LAD forms the triangle of Brocq and Mouchet.[5])

12-LEAD ECG

RVOT VT

RVOT ectopy can present with different levels of arrhythmia expression (isolated PVCs, salvos of nonsustained VT, or sustained VT) that can be considered a continuum of a single mechanism (cAMP-mediated triggered activity).[6] The characteristic electrocardiographic features of RVOT tachycardia include 1) left bundle branch block (LBBB) morphology and 2) inferior axis (**Figs. 19-2 and 19-3**). Electrocardiographic clues to identify the RVOT VT site of origin are its 1) precordial QRS transition, 2) frontal axis (particularly, QRS vector in lead I), 3) QRS width, and 4) presence/absence of notching in the inferior leads.[7–12] Because the RVOT free wall is the most anterior part of the outflow tract, RVOT free wall VT shows 1) LBBB morphology with possibly an absent r wave in V1 (because V1 is an anteriorly and rightward-directed vector) and late (at or beyond V4) precordial transition; 2) short, broad QRS complexes (because of sequential right ventricular [RV] to LV activation); and 3) notching in the inferior leads. RVOT septal VT shows 1) LBBB morphology, which may show a small r wave in V1 (because the RV septum is posterior to the free wall) and earlier (V3) precordial transition; 2) narrower QRS complexes (because of simultaneous RV/LV activation); and 3) tall, smooth QRS contours. A common site for RVOT VT is the anteroseptum just beneath the pulmonic valve at its junction with the free wall—the most leftward part of the outflow tract. At this site, QRS complexes

in lead I (a horizontally leftward-directed vector) are therefore negative. As the VT origin moves from anterior (left) to posterior (right) either along the septum or the free wall, lead I QRS complexes transition from negative to positive.[7] Similar to aortic sinus cusps, the pulmonary sinus cusps have also been identified as an important source of RVOT VT.[13,14] Mapping within the pulmonary cusps might require a supportive long sheath with a reverse U-shaped curve of the ablation tip by prolapsing it retrogradely across the pulmonic valve from the RV. A trileaflet view of the pulmonary valve from the right atrial appendage allows delineation of the three pulmonary cusps that might facilitate VT localization (**see Fig. 3-19**). VT arising from the pulmonary artery have higher inferior R wave amplitudes and greater aVL/aVR Q wave ratios than their subvalvular RVOT counterpart because of the more superior and leftward location of the pulmonary artery.[15–17]

RVOT versus LVOT VT

From anterior to posterior, outflow tract sites for VT include 1) RV free wall, 2) RV posteroseptum, 3) RCC, 4) LCC, and 5) aorto-mitral continuity (region between the LCC/NCC commissure and anterior leaflet of the mitral valve). The RCC directly abuts the posteroseptum of the RVOT, and therefore, PVCs arising from these two sites are difficult to differentiate by ECG (LBBB morphology, V3 precordial lead transition).[18–20] By using the normally conducted QRS complex to control for influences of cardiac rotation on precordial transition, the V2 transition ratio (V2 r/rs [VT]/ V2 r/rs [NSR]) is one method to differential left- from right-sided outflow tract VT. A V2 transition ratio >0.6 suggests LVOT origin.[18]

LVOT VT

Early (≤V2) precordial transition with inferior axis indicates LVOT origin.[21–35] The absence/presence of an s wave in V5 or V6 might differentiate a supravalvular/subvalvular site, respectively.[24,32] Site-specific QRS morphologies include 1) RCC: LBBB morphology with small, broad r wave in V2; 2) RCC–LCC commissure: LBBB QS (notching on the downstroke) or qrS morphology; 3) LCC: V1 M or W pattern with precordial transition ≤V2; and 4) AMC: V1 qR pattern (**Figs. 19-4 and 19-5**).[25] (These ECG signatures, however, are based on pacemapping techniques, which have inherent limitations [preferential conduction within the LVOT, far-field capture] in reproducing true VT morphologies.) For RCC–LCC commissure VT, the V1 qrS complex represents initial posterior activation of the aortic root and LVOT (q wave) followed by anterior activation of the interventricular septum and RVOT (r wave) and then late activation of the LV (S wave).[27,32] For AMC VT, V1 morphologies can transition from anterior AMC (rS [broad r] or qR) to mid-AMC (prominent R wave)—the latter showing positive concordance except for a large S wave in V2 ("rebound transition").[35] Rarely, VT can arise from the NCC.[36] Epicardial VTs are broader and show slurring of the initial portion of the QRS complex (pseudo delta wave) with maximal deflection index (onset of r wave to nadir of S wave in any precordial lead/total QRS duration >55%) or a precordial break pattern (V2 R wave less than V1 and V3 R wave).[37,38]

RVOT AS

RVOT PS

RVOT FW

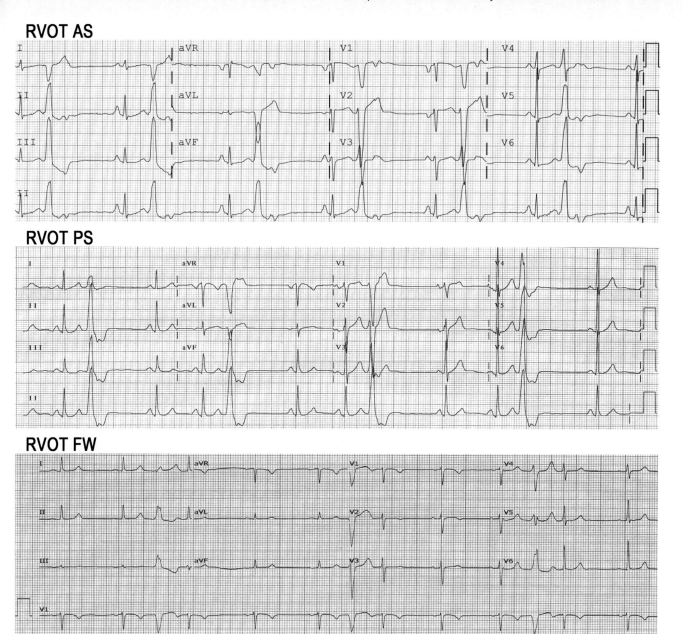

FIGURE 19-2 RVOT PVCs. All manifest LBBB morphology. The RVOT anteroseptal (AS) PVC shows a tall/smooth contour with V3–V4 transition and right inferior axis (negative QRS in lead I). The RVOT posteroseptal (PS) PVC shows a tall/smooth contour with V2–V3 transition and left inferior axis (positive QRS in lead I). The RVOT free wall (FW) PVC shows a short/broad contour with inferior notching and V5 transition. An r wave in V1 is absent.

RVOT AS

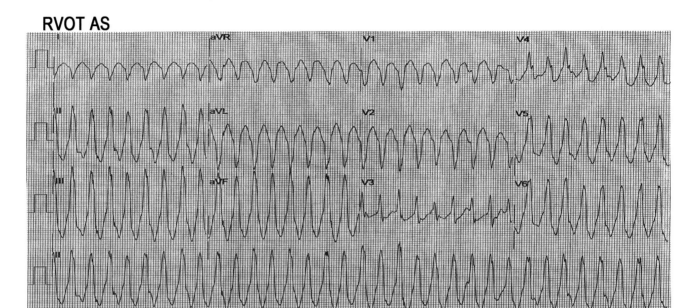

RVOT FW

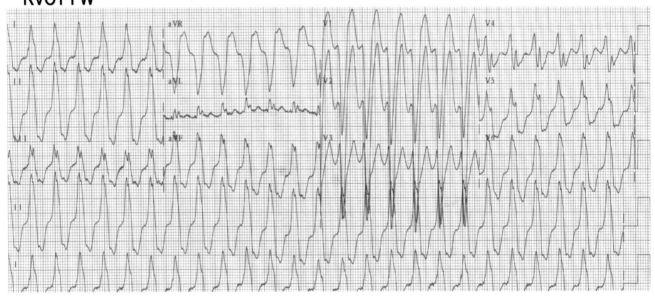

FIGURE 19-3 RVOT VT. Both manifest LBBB morphology. RVOT anteroseptal (AS) VT shows a tall/smooth contour, V2–V3 transition, and right inferior axis (negative QRS in lead I). RVOT free wall (FW) VT shows broad QRS complexes with inferior notching and V4 transition.

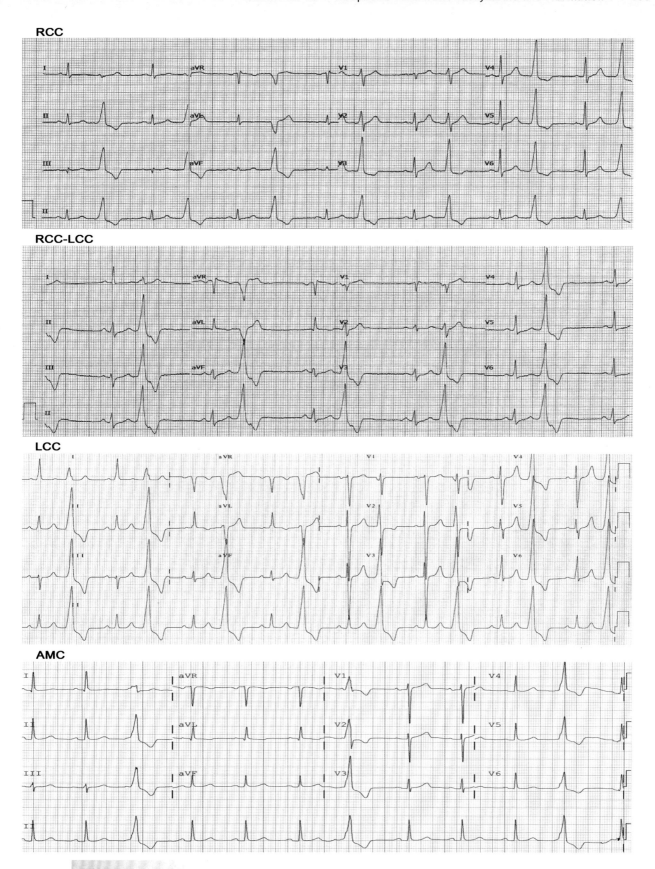

FIGURE 19-4 LVOT PVCs. The RCC PVC shows an LBBB morphology but broad r wave in V2. The RCC–LCC PVC has a distinctive V1 QS complex with notching on its downstroke. The LCC PVC shows a "W" type pattern. The AMC PVC manifests RBBB morphology with positive precordial concordance except for a "rebound transition" pattern (S wave in V2 but not V1 or V3).

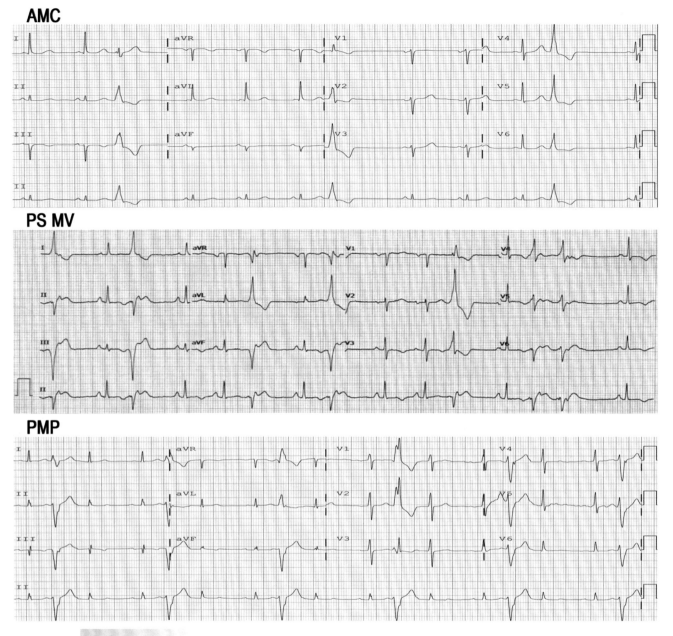

FIGURE 19-5 Different RBBB PVCs. The AMC PVC shows a V1 qR pattern with positive precordial concordance except for a "rebound transition" pattern (small S wave in V2). The posteroseptal (PS) mitral valve (MV) PVC shows V1 rSR' morphology and left superior axis. The posteromedial papillary muscle (PMP) PVCs are interpolated and show atypical qR pattern and left superior axis.

MAPPING AND ABLATION

When mapping and ablation is performed in the RVOT, it is important to be aware that the wall of the RVOT is thin and the left main coronary artery runs close to the posterior pulmonary trunk above the pulmonary valve. Because of the close anatomic proximity of the RVOT posteroseptum and RCC, the ECG morphology of VT arising from these two sites is similar and differentiating RVOT versus LVOT site of origin can be difficult. The following suggest an LVOT origin: PVC onset − RV apex electrogram (QRS − RVA) ≥49 ms, diffuse breakout pattern along the RVOT posteroseptum, and only

transient VT suppression with ablation along the RVOT posteroseptum.[39] The small, confined space of the LVOT and aortic cusps can make catheter manipulation and torqueing relatively difficult, while their close proximity to sensitive structures (His bundle and coronary artery ostium [~1.5 cm above the nadir of the cusps]) makes ablation in this region potentially dangerous. A properly positioned His bundle catheter provides the location of both the penetrating His bundle and aortic root. The location of the coronary artery ostia should be identified prior to ablation (aortic root or selective coronary artery angiography or intracardiac echocardiography [ICE] imaging), and radiofrequency (RF) delivery should be avoided within 5 mm of the coronary artery.

Activation Mapping

The focal origin of tachycardia allows activation mapping by identifying the earliest site of near-field bipolar ventricular activation (near-field earliest electrogram determination) and/or local unipolar "QS" configuration relative to PVC onset (RVOT: **Figs. 19-6 to 19-10**; LVOT: **Figs. 19-11 to 19-21**). Successful electrograms often precede QRS onset by 30–50 ms, although there is no degree of electrogram prematurity predictive of success.[11,12] For supravalvular VT (aortic cusps, pulmonary artery), two-component electrograms can be seen: sharp "spike" potentials (near-field) followed by low-frequency ventricular electrogram (far-field) preceding VT QRS complexes with their reversal (far-field/near-field) during sinus rhythm (analogous to pulmonary vein sleeve potentials) (**Figs. 19-8, 19-9, 19-12, and 19-13**).[15,16] With PA mapping, a far-field atrial electrogram (left atrial appendage) can be recorded.

Pacemapping

Pacemapping provides an alternative mapping approach, particularly when ventricular ectopy is minimal or induction of tachycardia is difficult. Pacing from the site of origin can yield an accurate 12-lead ECG match between paced and tachycardia QRS complexes (RVOT: **Figs. 19-6, 19-8, and 19-10**; LVOT: **Figs. 19-11, 19-13, and 19-16 to 19-18**). Pacemapping, particularly from the supravalvular sites, however, have several limitations: 1) Because of their close proximity and preferential conduction from RCC to RVOT posteroseptum, the excellent and even best pacemaps of a LBBB morphology RCC VT can sometimes be produced from the RVOT; 2) because of the close proximity to conducting fascicles, high-output LVOT pacing can recruit these fascicles, causing poor pacemaps (large virtual electrode); 3) pacemapping from the RCC–LCC commissure can sometimes be associated with long St-QRS intervals and QRS alternans; and 4) pacemapping from the PA can be difficult due to lack of ventricular capture or even left atrial appendage capture.[15,16,27,31]

PAPILLARY MUSCLE VT

The papillary muscles are another important source of idiopathic VT (**Figs. 19-5 and 19-22 to Fig. 19-24**). These includes the posteromedial and anterolateral papillary muscles of the LV and the septal and anterior papillary–moderator band complex of the RV.[40-45] VT tends to be more common from the LV posteromedial than anterolateral papillary muscle, has wider QRS duration (>160 ms) compared to left fascicular VT, and exhibits multiple morphologies (multiple exit sites due to the complex architecture of the papillary muscle). Because of its thickness, a source deep in the papillary muscle can be difficult to ablate. LV anterolateral papillary muscle VT shows RBBB/inferior axis, while posteromedial papillary muscle VT has RBBB/superior axis.[40-42,44] VT originating from the moderator band–anterior papillary muscle complex shows 1) LBBB morphology, 2) late precordial transition (>V4), and 3) left superior axis (see below).[45]

OTHER VT

VT can also arise from other structures within the ventricle including the tricuspid and mitral annuli (**Figs. 19-25 and 19-26**).[46]

IDIOPATHIC LEFT VENTRICULAR TACHYCARDIA

MECHANISM

Idiopathic LV tachycardia is a verapamil-sensitive tachycardia often arising from the mid postero-inferior portion of the LV septum.[47-50] The ability to entrain tachycardia and suppression by verapamil supports a reentrant mechanism using a calcium-dependent zone of slow conduction. Initiation by rapid atrial pacing also suggests that the reentrant circuit is close to the left posterior fascicle (**Fig. 19-27**).[47]

12-LEAD ECG

The characteristic ECG features of idiopathic LV tachycardia are a 1) RBBB (rSR') morphology and 2) left superior axis (**Fig. 19-27**).[48] Origin of tachycardia from or near the left posterior fascicle generates QRS complexes that mimic typical RBBB/LAFB. Idiopathic LV VT arising from the left anterior fascicle produces VT with a RBBB/LPFB pattern, while upper septal VT can generate narrow QRS complex VT.[51]

MAPPING AND ABLATION

Activation Mapping

Origin of tachycardia from the left posterior fascicle is supported by recording Purkinje potentials at successful ablation sites along the septum of the LV.[51-56] Target criteria include sites demonstrating 1) earliest Purkinje potentials relative to QRS onset along the posteroapical septum, 2) late diastolic potentials preceding Purkinje potentials along the basal portion of the LV septum, or 3) fragmented antegrade Purkinje potentials along the LV septum slightly inferior to the left posterior fascicle (**Fig. 19-28**). Late diastolic potentials might represent the entrance to the zone of slow conduction.

Pacemapping

Pacemapping can be performed at sites along the LV septum where Purkinje potentials are recorded during sinus rhythm. However, local capture of the Purkinje network can cause different pacing sites to yield similar pacemaps.[52]

IDIOPATHIC VENTRICULAR FIBRILLATION

Idiopathic VF is a syndrome characterized by recurrent episodes of VF triggered by short-coupled (<300 ms) PVCs falling into the vulnerable phase of the ventricle with or without early repolarization (**Figs. 19-29 and 19-30**).[57-63] Dominant triggers have been shown to arise from the Purkinje system, papillary

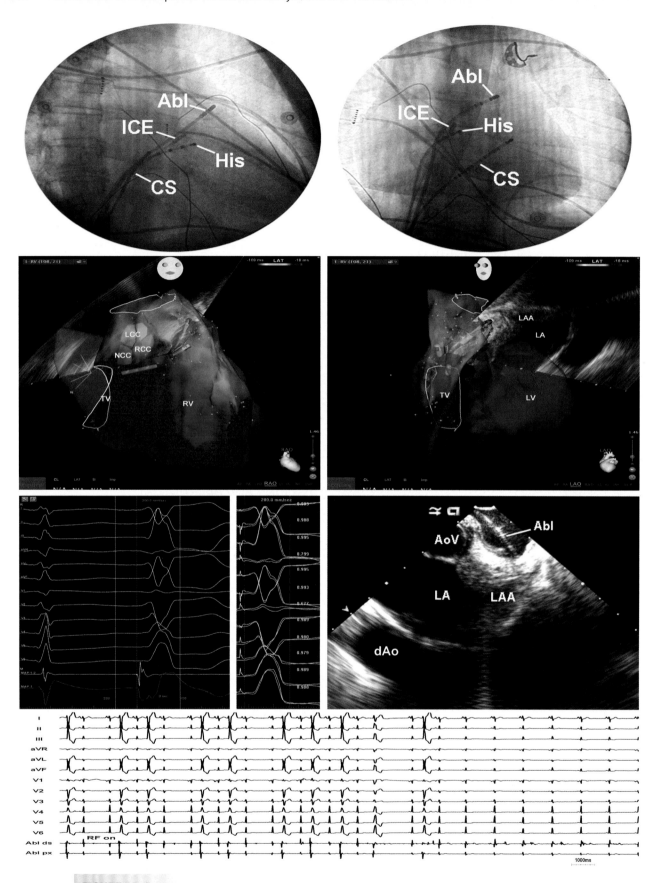

FIGURE 19-6 RVOT anteroseptal PVC. At the successful ablation site (*red tag*), the bipolar electrogram precedes PVC onset by 29 ms, unipolar signal is "QS," and the pacemap score is 95%. Application of RF energy causes disappearance of PVCs in 5.2 sec.

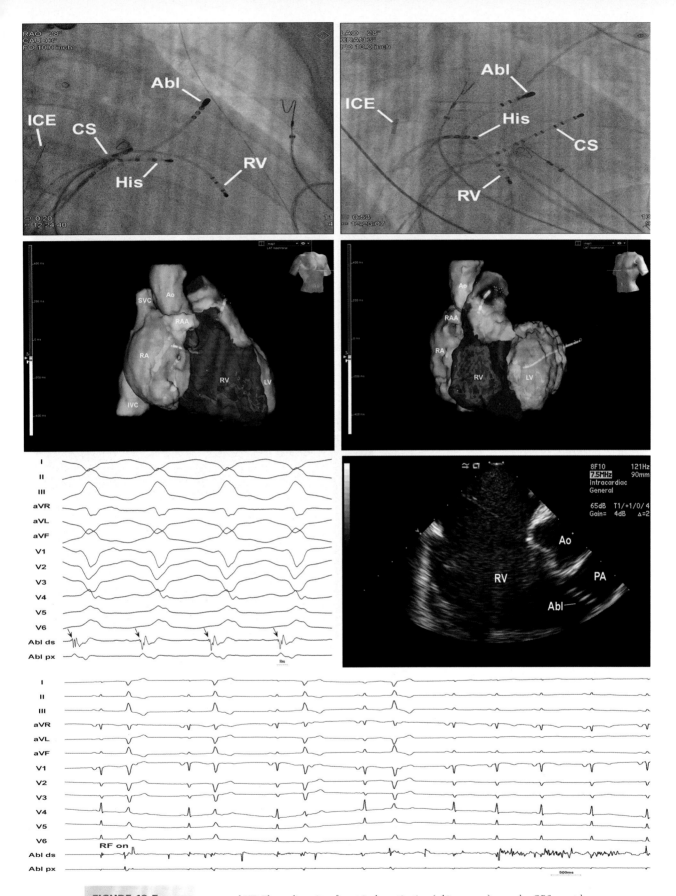

FIGURE 19-7 RVOT anteroseptal VT. The earliest site of ventricular activation (*white, arrows*) precedes QRS onset by 30 ms where application of RF energy causes disappearance of PVCs in 5.1 sec.

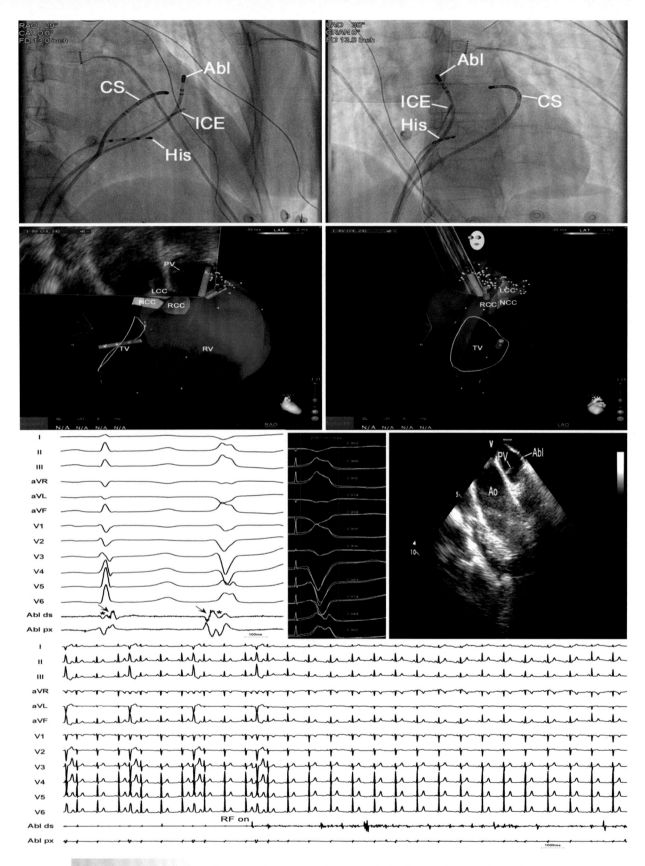

FIGURE 19-8 RVOT free wall PVC. At the successful ablation site (*red tag*) along the RVOT free wall (level of the pulmonary valve [PV]), a two-component electrogram is seen: near-field (*arrows*) and far-field (*asterisk*) potentials. The near-field potential precedes PVC onset by 26 ms followed by the far-field potential with both potential timing and polarity reversal during sinus rhythm. The pacemap score is 99%. Application of RF energy causes immediate disappearance of the PVCs.

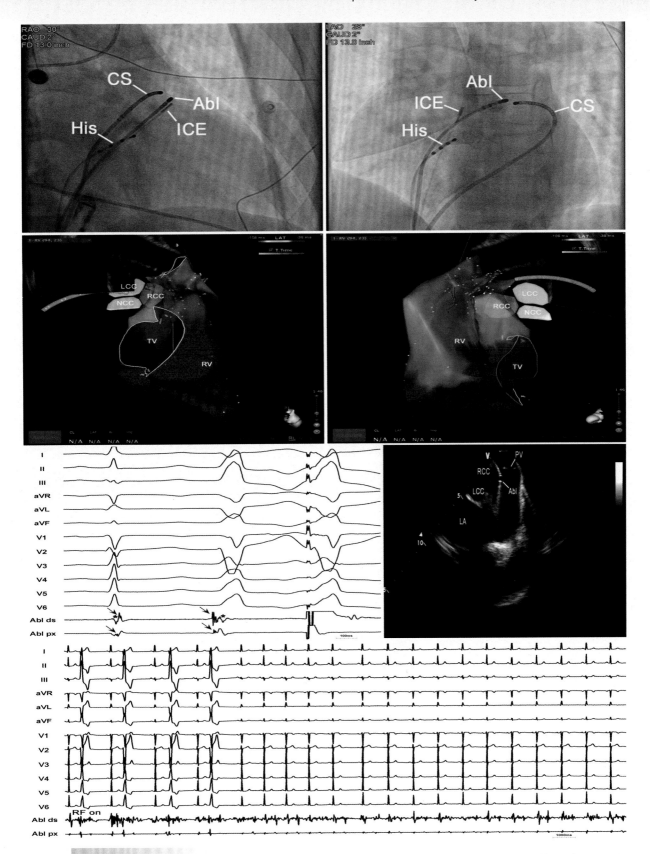

FIGURE 19-9 Pulmonary artery PVC. At the successful ablation site (*red tag*) in the pulmonary artery (above the pulmonic valve [PV]), a two-component electrogram is seen: sharp, "spike" near-field (*arrows*) and low-frequency far-field (*asterisk*) potentials. The near-field potential precedes PVC onset by 35 ms followed by the far-field potential with potential timing reversal during sinus rhythm. The pacemap matches PVC morphology. Application of RF energy causes disappearance of the PVCs.

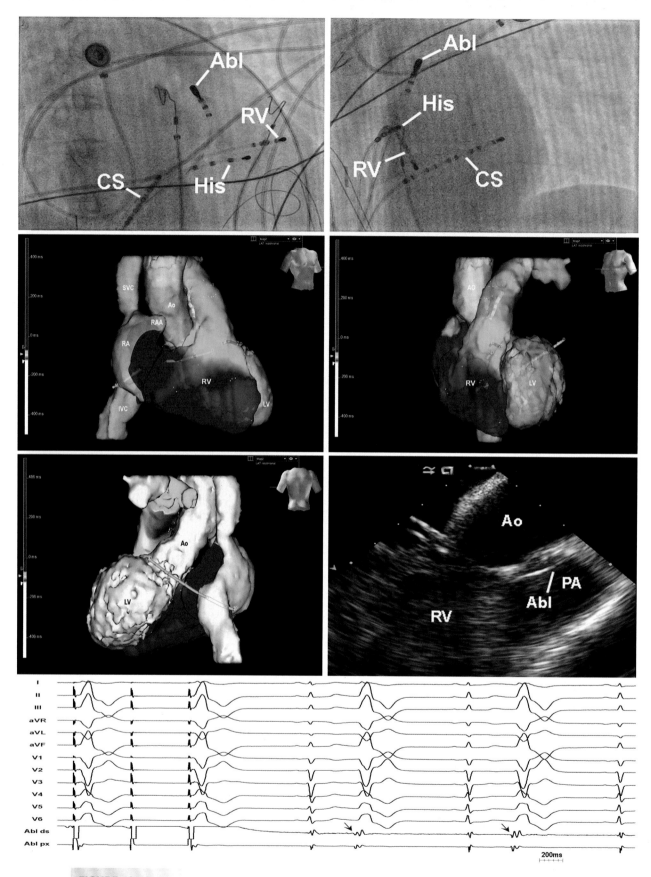

FIGURE 19-10 Pulmonary artery PVC. The earliest site of activation (*white, arrows*) is in the pulmonary artery where local bipolar electrograms precede PVC onset by 27 ms and was associated with an excellent pacemap despite a high capture threshold.

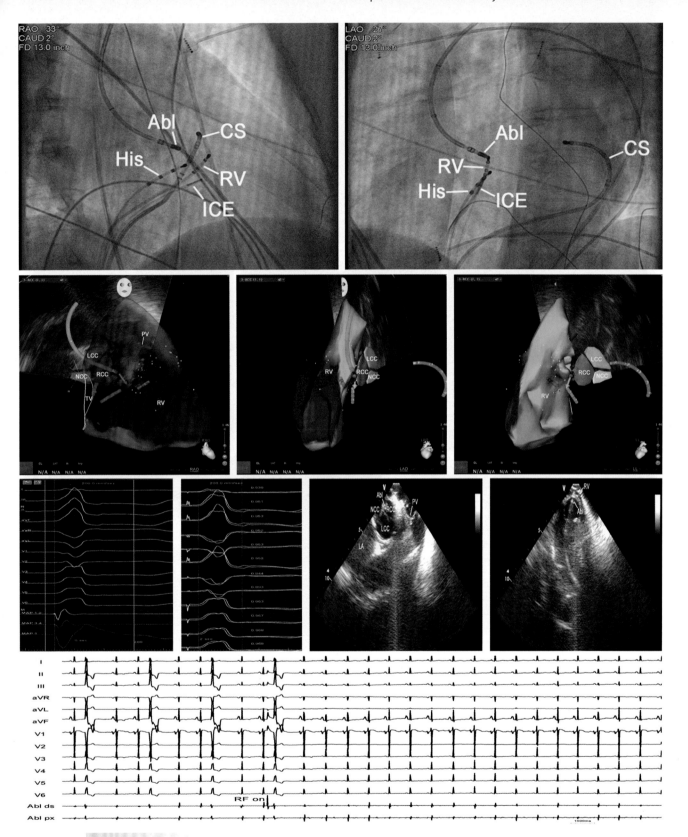

FIGURE 19-11 RCC PVC. At the successful ablation site, the bipolar electrogram precedes PVC onset by only 11 ms, but the unipolar electrogram shows a QS signal, and the pacemap score is 94%. Application of RF energy causes disappearance of the PVCs. Note earliest activation in the RV (*red*) is along the RVOT posteroseptum directly opposite the RCC.

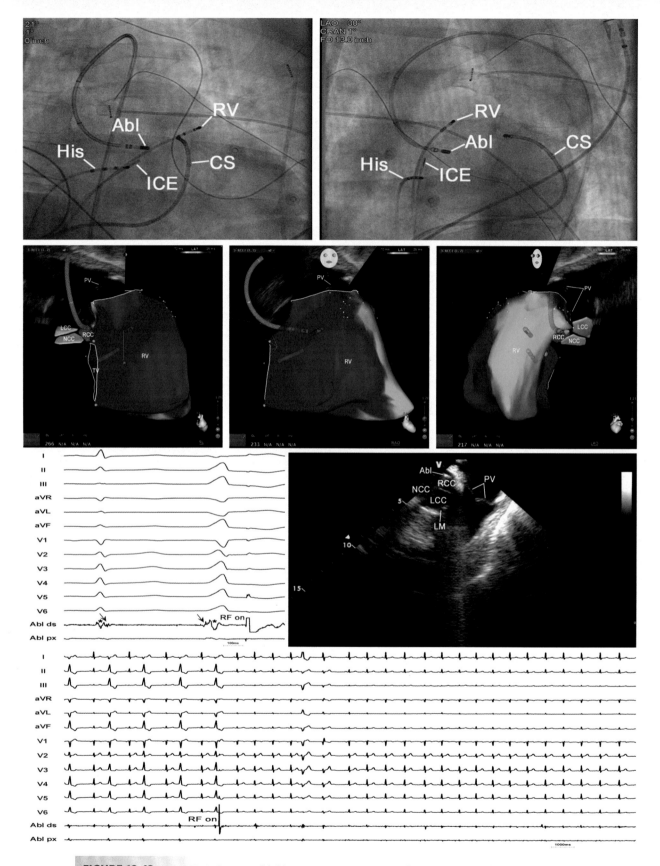

FIGURE 19-12 RCC PVC. At the successful ablation site, a two-component electrogram is seen: sharp, "spike" near-field (*arrows*) and low-frequency far-field (*asterisk*) potentials. The near-field potential precedes PVC onset by 30 ms followed by the far-field potential with potential timing reversal during sinus rhythm. Application of RF energy causes immediate disappearance of the PVCs.

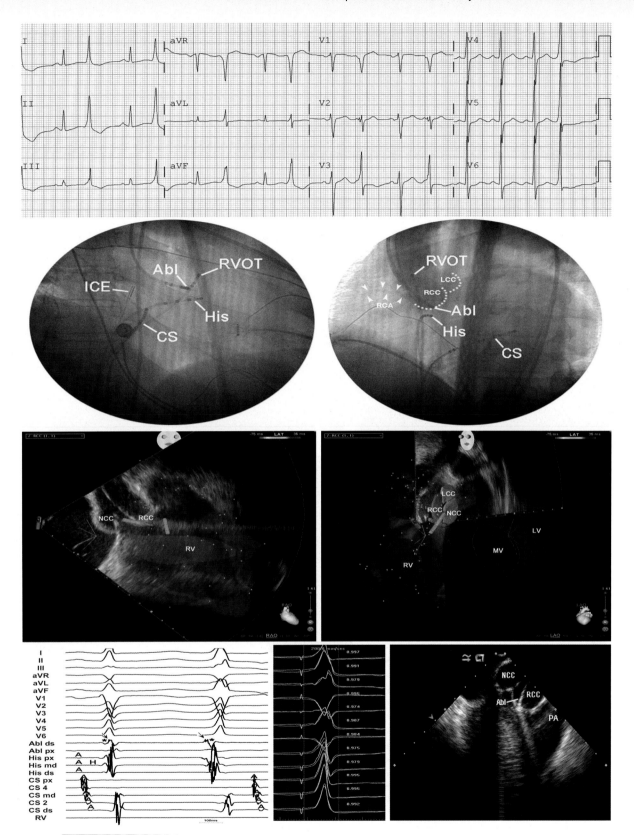

FIGURE 19-13 RCC PVC. The PVCs show an LBBB/left inferior axis and a V2–V3 precordial transition and are narrow. At the successful site (*red tag*), a two-component electrogram is seen: sharp, "spike" near-field (*arrows*) and low-frequency far-field (*asterisk*) potentials. The near-field potential precedes PVC onset by 22 ms followed by the far-field potential with potential timing reversal during sinus rhythm. The pacemap score is 99%. (Pacemapping from the adjacent RVOT posteroseptum generated a score of 95% and later precordial transition: The V2 R was not sufficiently tall, indicating the need for a more posterior [RCC] location.) Note also the location of the successful ablation site in the RCC relative to the right coronary artery (RCA).

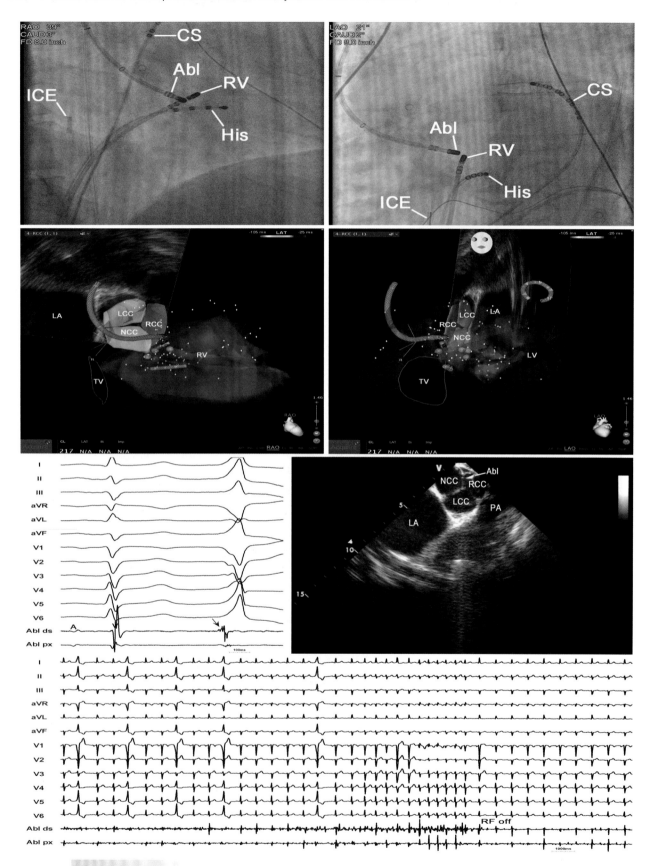

FIGURE 19-14 RCC–NCC PVC. At the successful ablation site, the bipolar electrogram is fractionated and precedes PVC onset by 15 ms (*arrow*). During sinus rhythm, it records a small atrial electrogram but no His bundle potential. Twenty four seconds into RF energy, however, junctional tachycardia occurred requiring RF discontinuation after which PVCs permanently disappeared. Yellow tags denote left-sided His bundle potentials

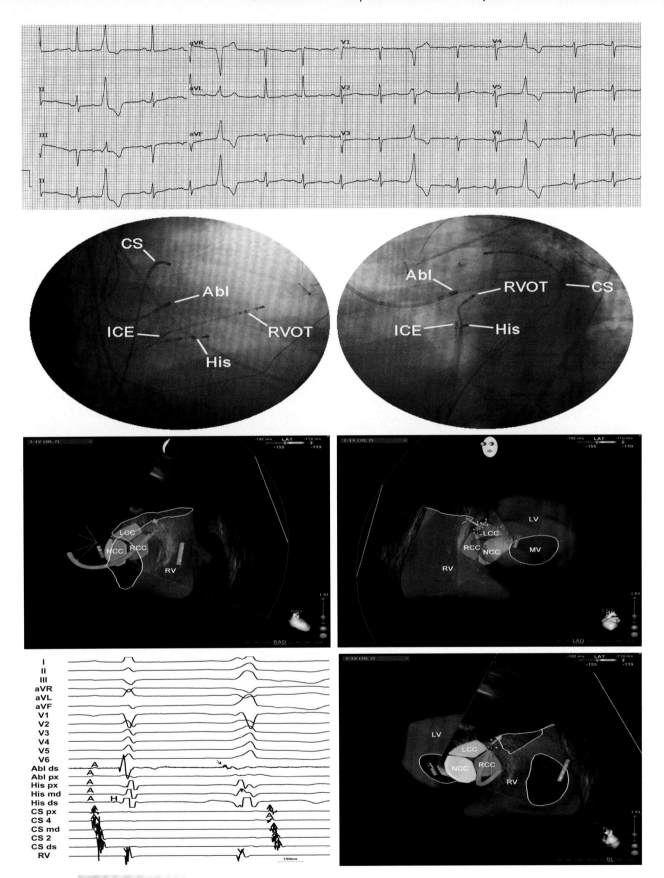

FIGURE 19-15 RCC–LCC PVC. The PVCs show a V1 QS morphology with distinctive notching of its downstroke. At the successful ablation site beneath the RCC–LCC commissure (aortic vestibule), the bipolar electrogram is fractionated and precedes PVC onset by 41 ms (*arrow*).

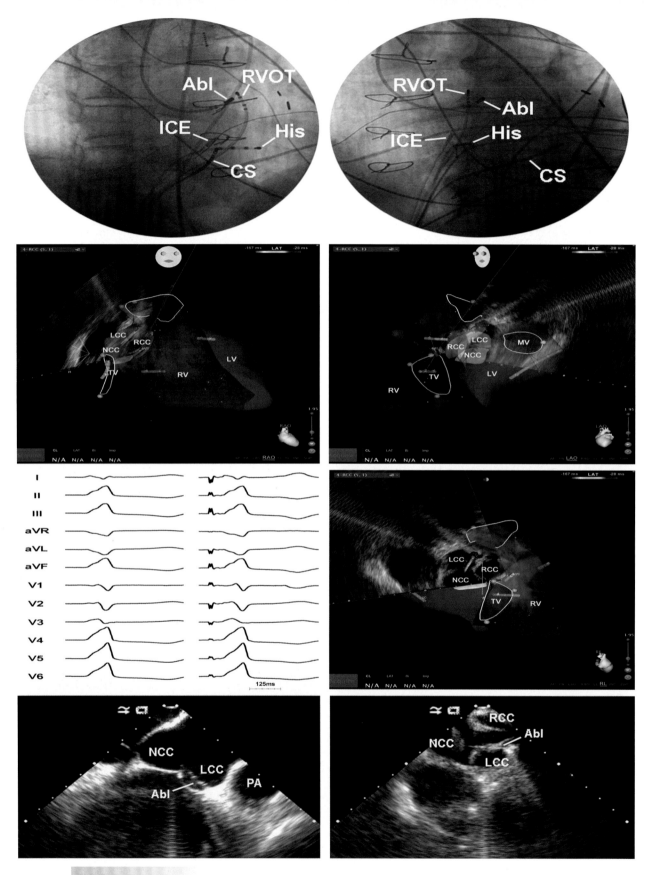

FIGURE 19-16 LCC–RCC PVC. The PVCs show a V1 qrS morphology. At the successful ablation site (*red tags*), the bipolar electrogram preceded PVC onset by 30 ms (not shown). The pacemap matches the PVC morphology with a slightly prolonged St-QRS interval.

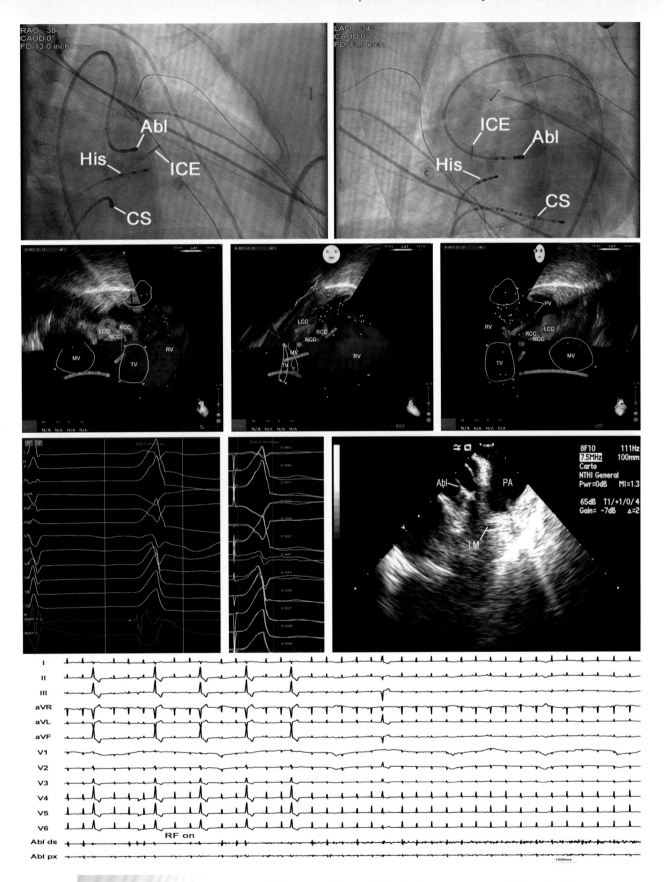

FIGURE 19-17 LCC PVC. At the successful ablation site (*red tag*), the bipolar electrogram precedes PVC onset by 28 ms, the unipolar electrogram is "QS," and the pacemap score is 99%. Application of RF energy causes disappearance of PVCs in 6.4 sec.

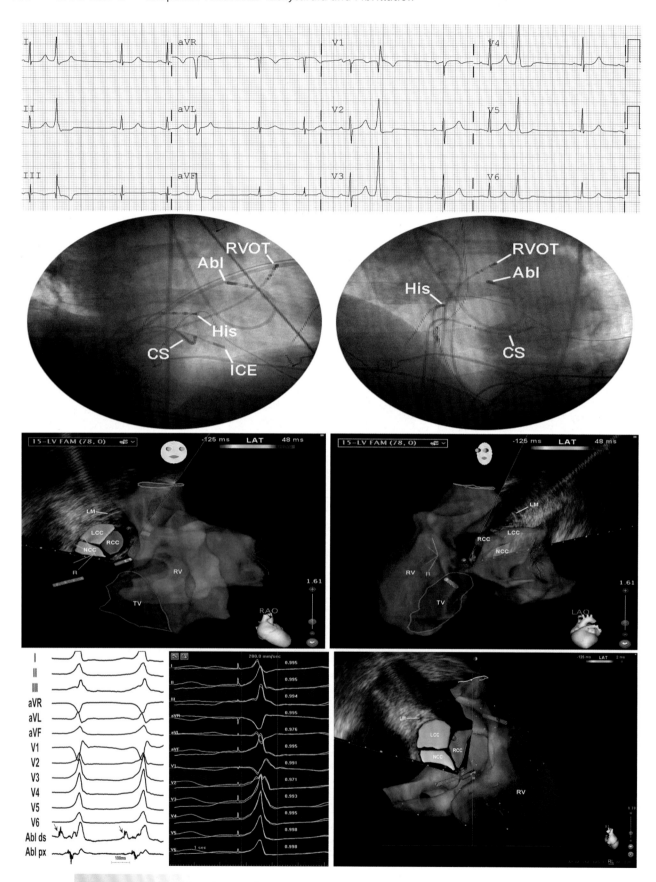

FIGURE 19-18 LCC PVC. The PVCs show a V1 qR morphology. At the successful ablation site (*red tag*) beneath the LCC (aortic vestibule), the bipolar electrogram shows presystolic potentials (*arrows*) preceding PVC onset by 52 ms with a pacemap score of 99%.

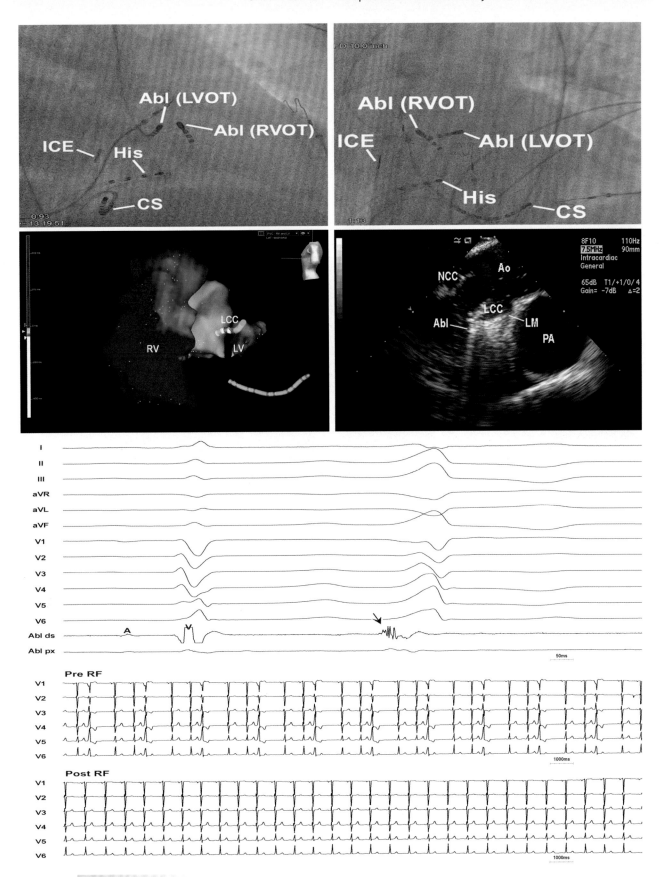

FIGURE 19-19 LCC PVC. At the successful ablation site beneath the LCC (aortic vestibule) (*white*), the bipolar electrogram is a highly fractionated signal preceding PVC onset by 23 ms (*arrow*). Application of RF energy causes permanent disappearance of the PVCs.

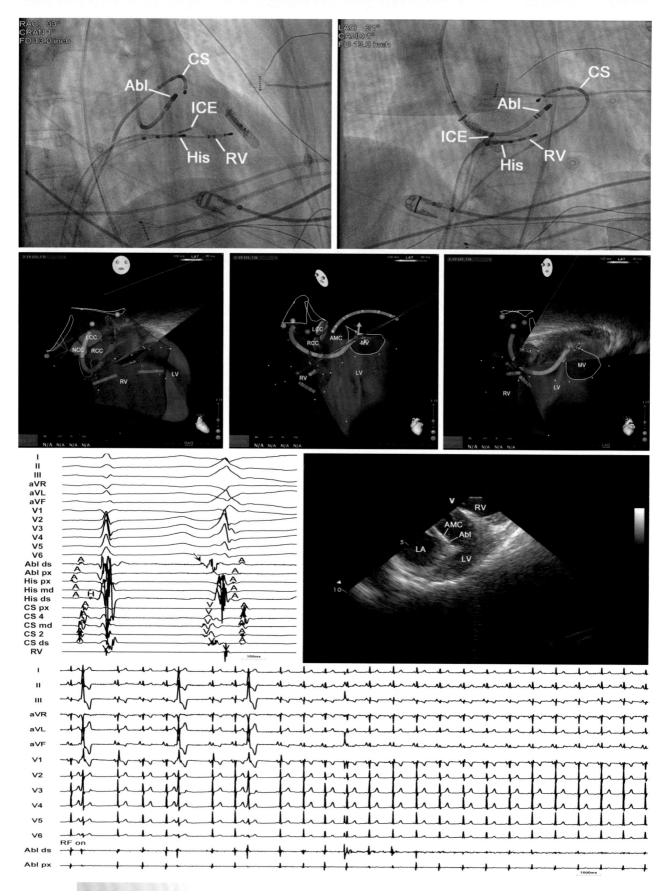

FIGURE 19-20 Aorto-mitral continuity (AMC) PVC. At the successful ablation site, the bipolar electrogram precedes PVC onset by 35 ms (*arrow*). A small vatrial electrogram is recorded. Application of RF energy causes disappearance of the PVCs.

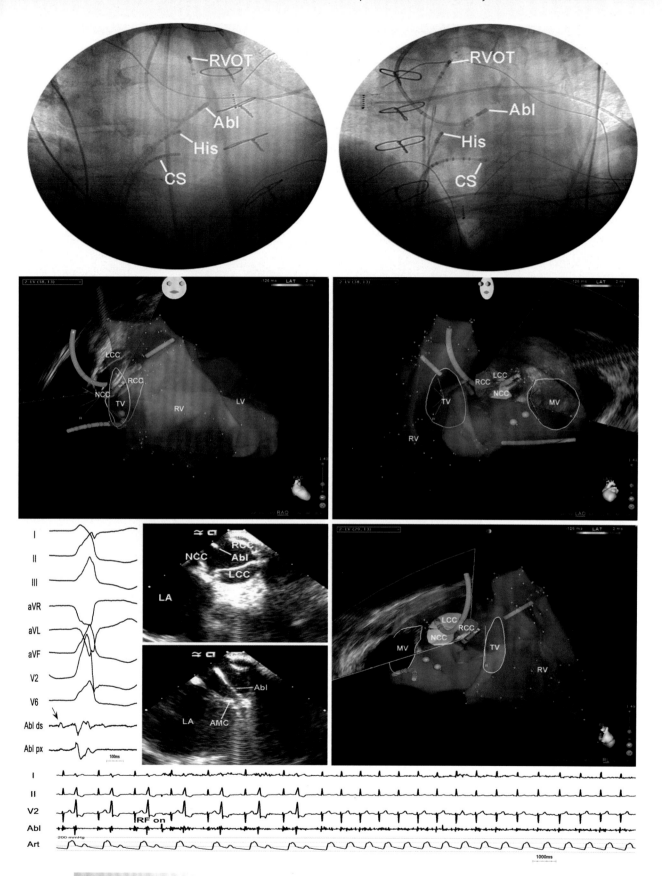

FIGURE 19-21 Aorto-mitral continuity (AMC) PVC. At the successful ablation site (*red tags*), the bipolar electrogram shows an early, presystolic potential (pre-PVC onset × 80 ms) (*arrow*). Application of RF energy causes disappearance of the PVCs in 6.7 sec.

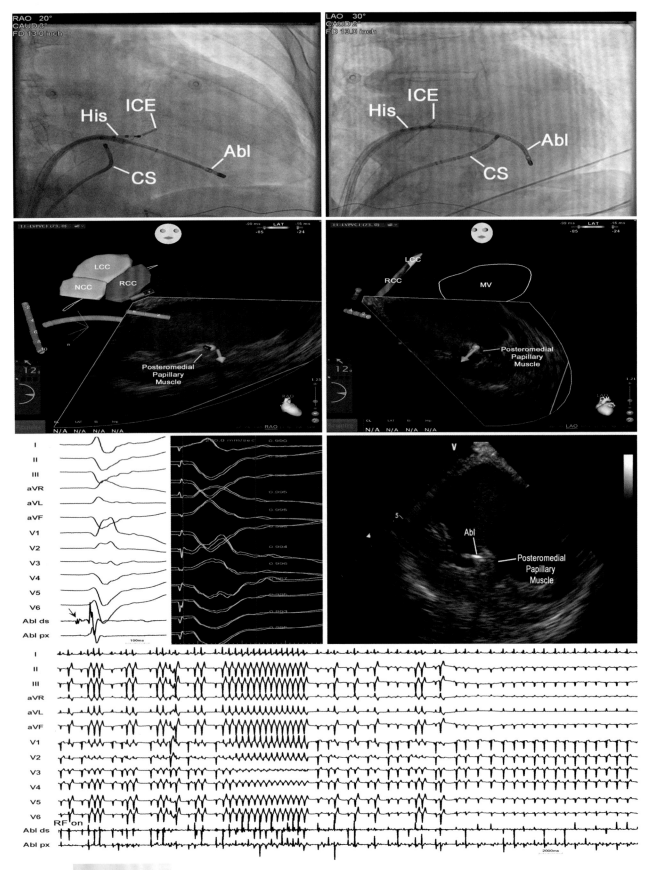

FIGURE 19-22 Posteromedial papillary muscle (PMP) PVC. At the successful ablation site, the bipolar electrogram shows an early, presystolic potential preceding PVC onset × 48 ms (*arrow*). The pacemap score is 99%. Application of RF energy causes a flurry of VT followed by quiescence.

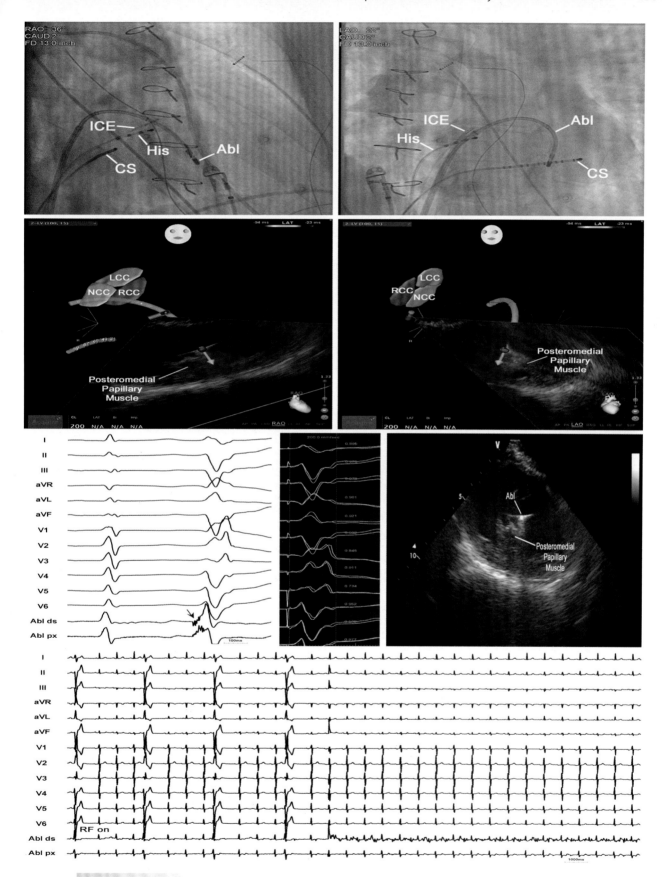

FIGURE 19-23 Posteromedial papillary muscle (PMP) PVC. At the successful ablation site (*red tag*), the bipolar electrogram is highly fractionated and precedes PVC onset × 26 ms. The pacemap score is 93%. Application of RF energy causes disappearance of the PVCs.

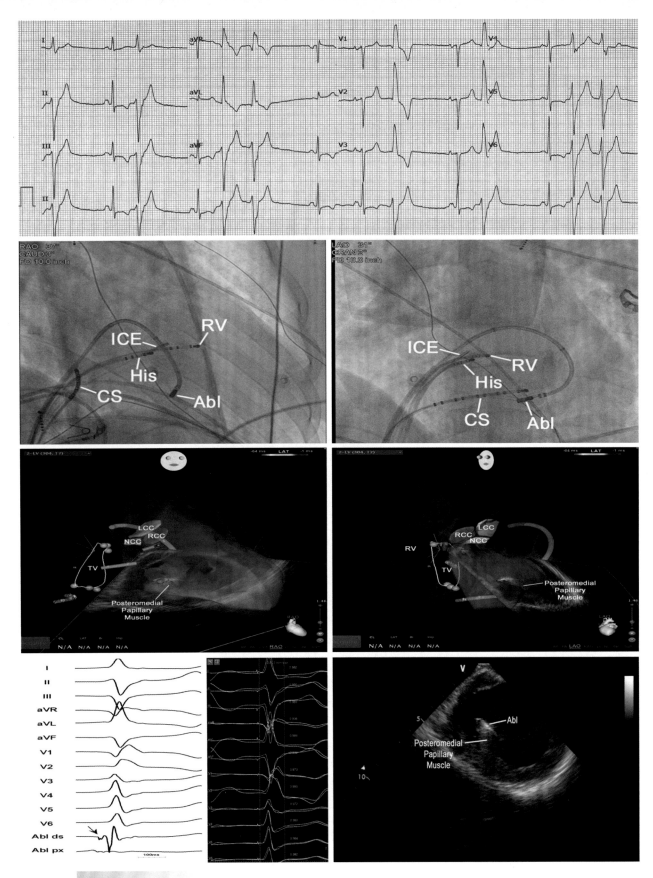

FIGURE 19-24 Posteromedial papillary muscle (PMP) PVC. The PVCs show an RBBB (V1 qR)/left superior axis. At the successful ablation site, the bipolar electrogram shows a small presystolic potential preceding PVC onset by 24 ms (*arrow*). The pacemap score is 97%.

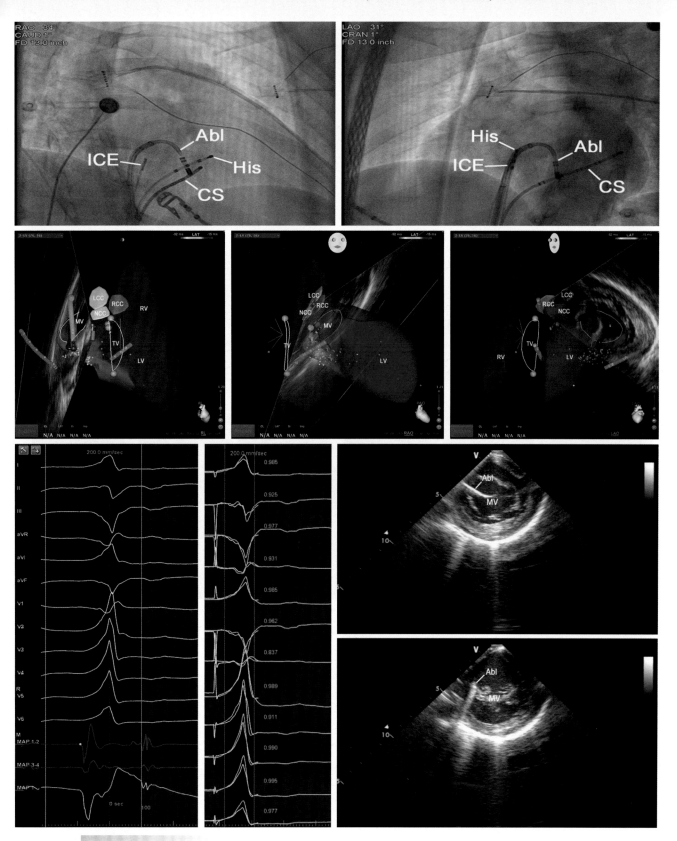

FIGURE 19-25 Mitral valve PVC. At the successful ablation site (*red tags*) along the posteroseptal mitral valve, the bipolar electrogram precedes PVC onset by 15 ms, the unipolar electrogram is "QS," and the pacemap score is 96%.

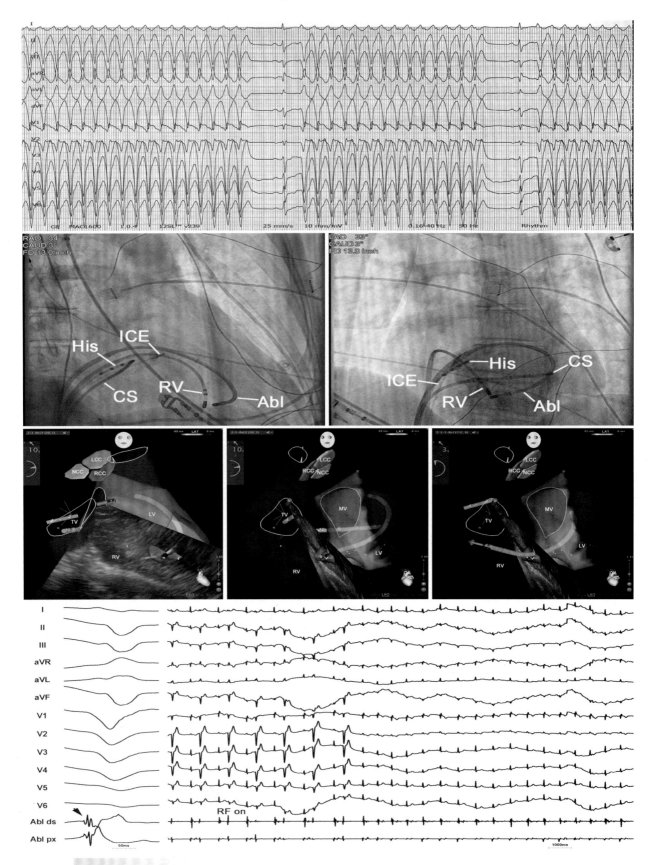

FIGURE 19-26 LV apical VT from a ventricular septal defect (VSD). Long salvos of rapid VT show negative precordial concordance and left superior axis. The successful ablation site (*red tags*) was at the mouth of the VSD on the LV side where bipolar electrograms precedes VT onset by 15 ms (*arrow*). Application of RF energy causes disappearance of identical focal PVCs in 4.9 sec. Further advancement pushes the ablation catheter across the VSD into the RV.

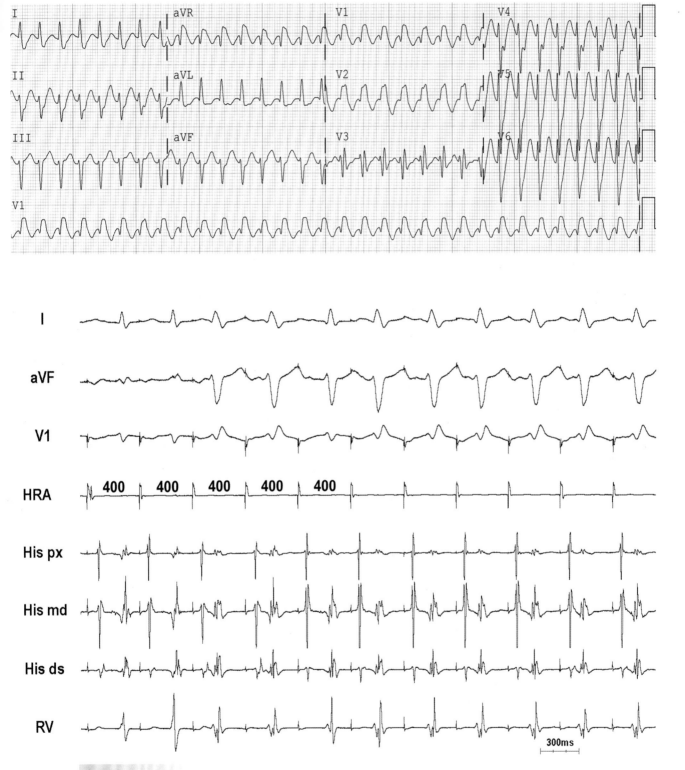

FIGURE 19-27 Idiopathic LV VT (Belhassen VT). VT shows a RBBB/left superior axis mimicking supraventricular tachycardia (SVT) with RBBB/LAFB. Induction by rapid atrial pacing is unique to this type of VT because of origin from/near the left posterior fascicle.

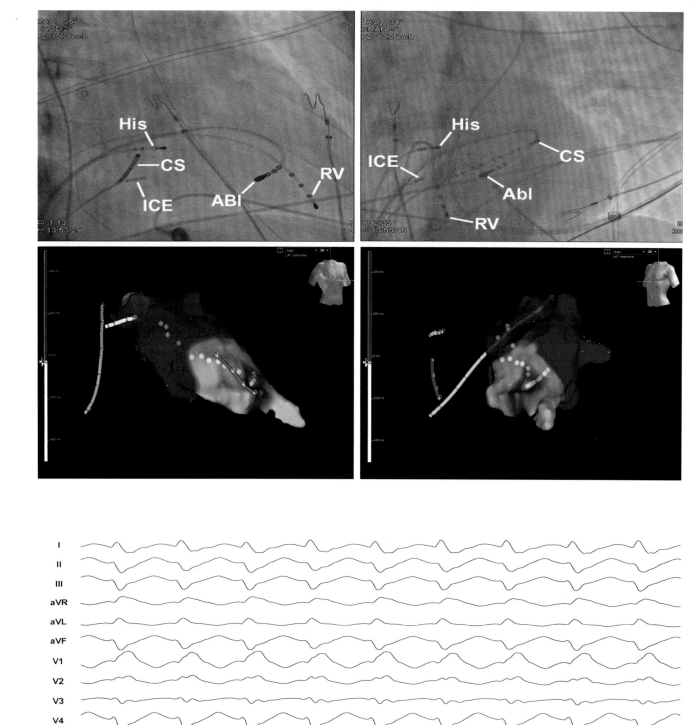

FIGURE 19-28 Idiopathic LV VT. At the successful ablation site along the inferior septum close to the apex (*white*), Purkinje potentials (*arrows*) are recorded during VT. Yellow tags denote Purkinje potentials.

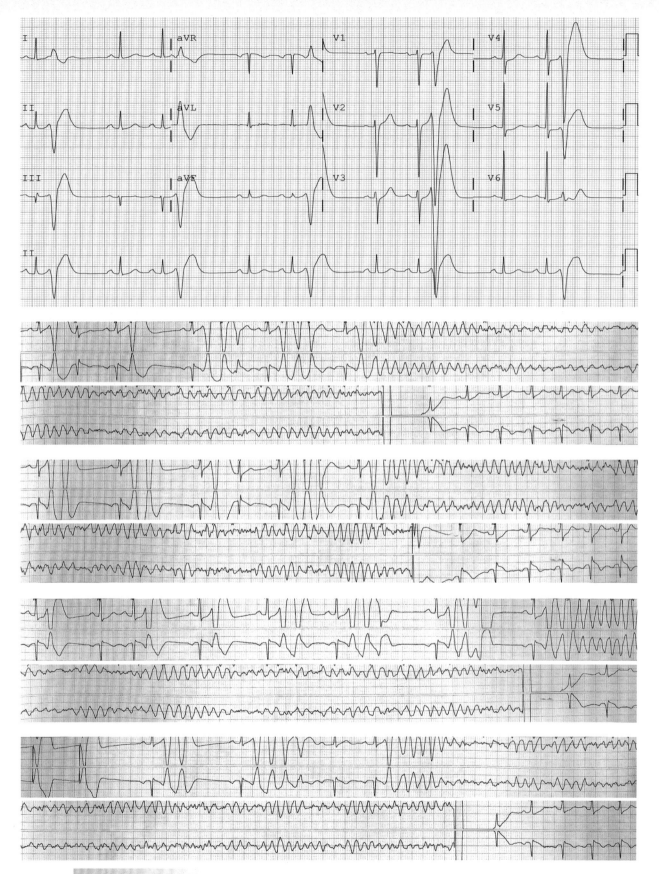

FIGURE 19-29 Idiopathic VF (moderator band PVCs). Frequent, short-coupled (260 ms) PVCs show LBBB/left superior axis and V5–V6 precordial transition. Multiple episodes of VF are triggered by these short-coupled PVCs requiring external defibrillation.

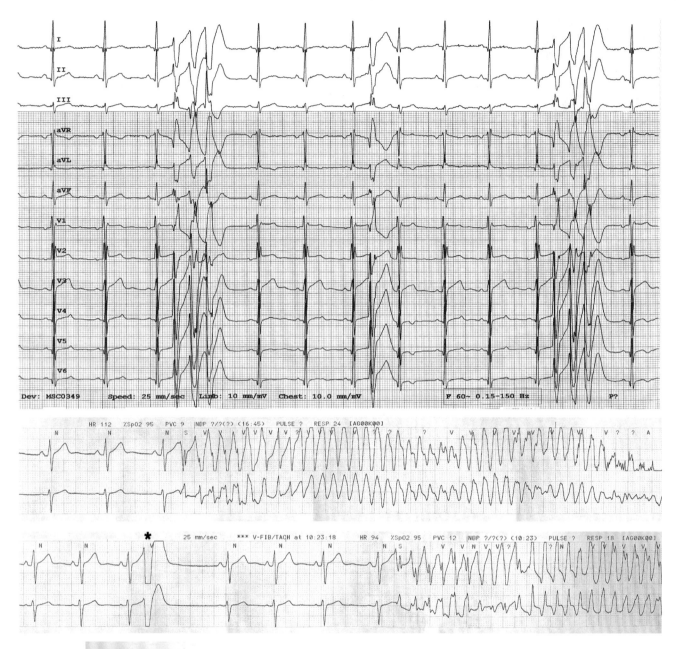

FIGURE 19-30 Idiopathic VF (left fascicular PVCs). Frequent, short-coupled (280 ms) PVCs are relatively narrow and show RBBB/RS axis. Multiple episodes of VF are triggered by these short-coupled PVCs. Note that short-coupled LBBB/left superior axis PVCs (*asterisk*) are also present.

muscles (particularly the RV moderator band), and RVOT. VT arising from the RV moderator band shows 1) LBBB morphology, 2) late precordial transition (>V4), and 3) left superior axis.[45] These trigger sources can be mapped and ablated by identifying the earliest electrogram relative to onset of the initiating PVC (**Figs. 19-31 to 19-33**). Purkinje potentials preceding ventricular activation during triggering PVCs indicate origin from the Purkinje system. During sinus rhythm, Purkinje potentials preceding the local ventricular electrogram >15 ms and <15 ms

indicate activation of proximal and distal Purkinje fascicles, respectively. Both short-coupled Purkinje foci falling into the vulnerable period and Purkinje-muscle reentry with wave breakup (putative mechanisms of VF initiation) are treated by targeted ablation of the Purkinje network. Absence of Purkinje potentials at the site of earliest ventricular activation during initiating PVCs suggests origin from ventricular muscle.[59–61] Delivery of RF energy to Purkinje triggers can result in transient exacerbation of the arrhythmia.[60]

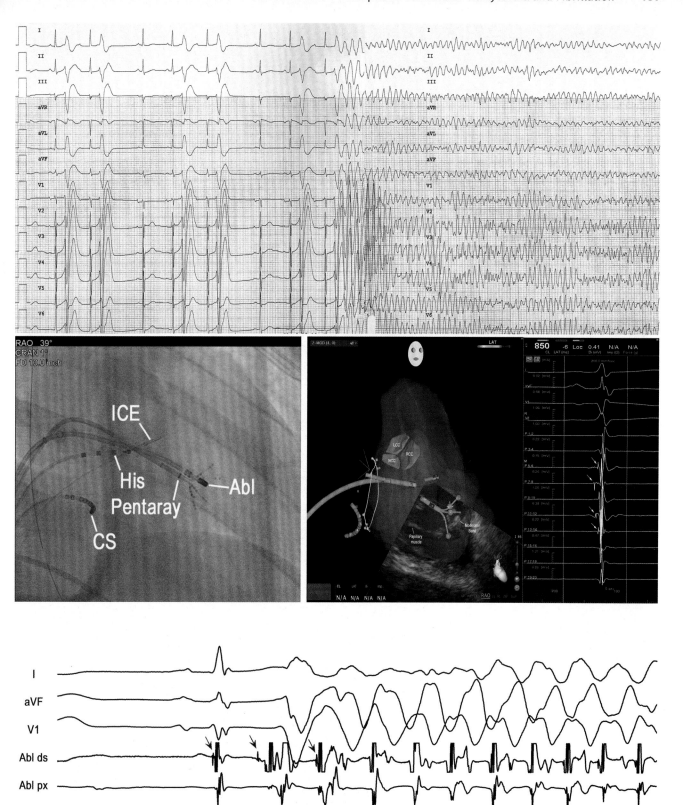

FIGURE 19-31 Idiopathic VF (not VT) (moderator band PVCs). Frequent, short-coupled (240 ms) PVCs with LBBB/ left superior axis and >V6 transition trigger VF. Successful ablation targeted Purkinje potentials (*yellow tags, white arrows*) along the moderator band–anterior papillary muscle complex—one of which was seen during sinus rhythm that preceded triggering PVCs by 103 ms (*black arrows*). Ablation caused RBBB but abolished all VF episodes.

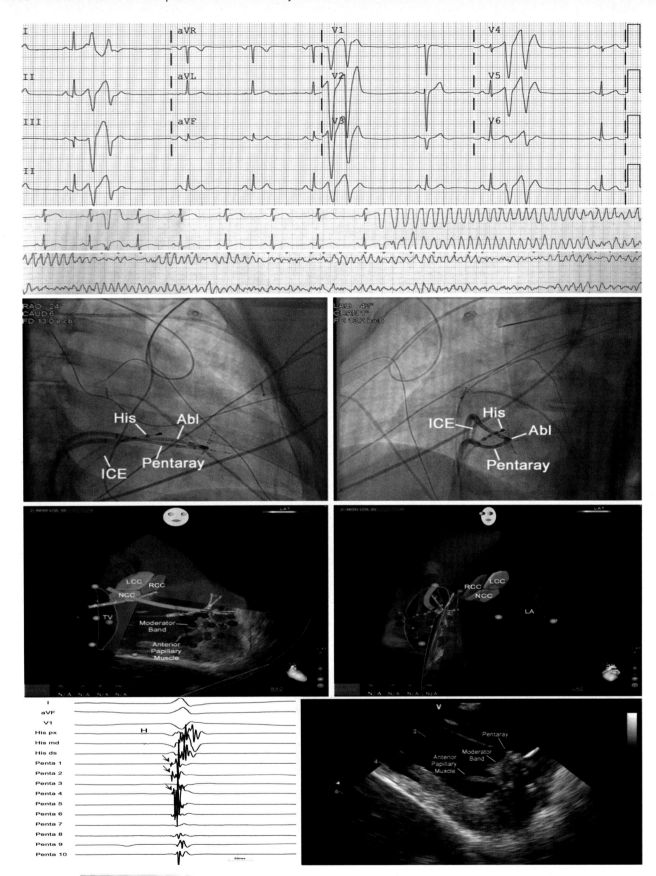

FIGURE 19-32 Idiopathic VF (moderator band PVCs). Frequent short-coupled (270 ms) PVCs with a LBBB/left superior axis and V6 transition trigger VF. Successful ablation (*red tags*) targeted Purkinje potentials (*yellow tags, black arrows*) along the moderator band–anterior papillary muscle complex.

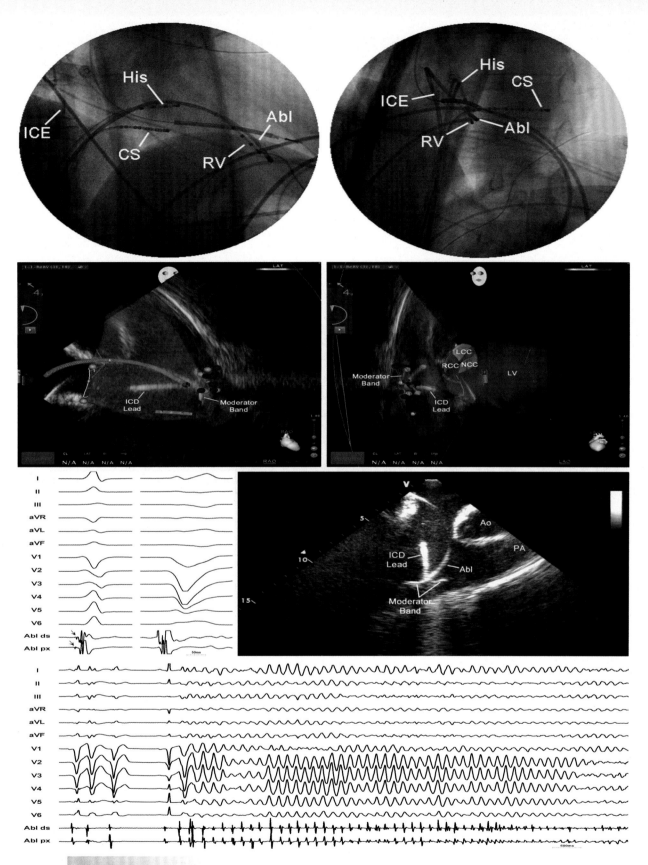

FIGURE 19-33 Idiopathic VF (moderator band PVCs). Short-coupled triggering PVCs have a LBBB/left superior axis and V5 transition. Successful ablation (*red tags*) targeted Purkinje potentials (*yellow tags*) along the moderator band–anterior papillary muscle complex. Purkinje potentials are recorded during sinus rhythm (*arrows*) where local ventricular activation precedes PVC onset by 28 ms.

REFERENCES

1. Lerman BB, Belardinelli L, West GA, Berne RM, DiMarco JP. Adenosine-sensitive ventricular tachycardia: evidence suggesting cyclic AMP-mediated triggered activity. Circulation 1986;74:270–280.
2. Lerman BB. Mechanism of outflow tract tachycardia. Heart Rhythm 2007; 4:973–976.
3. Gami AS, Noheria A, Lachman N, et al. Anatomical correlates relevant to ablation above the semilunar valves for the cardiac electrophysiologist: a study of 603 hearts. J Interv Card Electrophysiol 2011;30:5–15.
4. Yamada T, Litovsky SH, Kay GN. The left ventricular ostium: an anatomic concept relevant to idiopathic ventricular arrhythmias. Circ Arrhythm Electrophysiol 2008;1:396–404.
5. Enriquez A, Malavassi F, Saenz LC, et al. How to map and ablate left ventricular summit arrhythmias. Heart Rhythm 2017;14:141–148.
6. Kim RJ, Iwai S, Markowitz SM, Shah BK, Stein KM, Lerman BB. Clinical and electrophysiological spectrum of idiopathic ventricular outflow tract arrhythmias. J Am Coll Cardiol 2007;49:2035–2043.
7. Dixit S, Gerstenfeld EP, Callans DJ, Marchlinski FE. Electrocardiographic patterns of superior right ventricular outflow tract tachycardias: distinguishing septal and free wall sites of origin. J Cardiovasc Electrophysiol 2003;14:1–7.
8. Rodriquez LM, Smeets JLRM, Weide A, et al. 12 lead ECG for localizing origin of idiopathic ventricular tachycardia [abstract]. Circulation 1998;88:643.
9. Joshi S, Wilber DJ. Ablation of idiopathic right ventricular outflow tract tachycardia: current perspectives. J Cardiovasc Electrophysiol 2005;16: S52–S58.
10. Stevenson WG, Nademanee K, Weiss JN, Wiener I. Treatment of catecholamine-sensitive right ventricular tachycardia by endocardial catheter ablation. J Am Coll Cardiol 1990;16:752–755.
11. Klein LS, Shih H, Hackett FK, Zipes DP, Miles WM. Radiofrequency catheter ablation of ventricular tachycardia in patients without structural heart disease. Circulation 1992;85:1666–1674.
12. Coggins DL, Lee RJ, Sweeney J, et al. Radiofrequency catheter ablation as a cure for idiopathic tachycardia of both left and right ventricular origin. J Am Coll Cardiol 1994;23:1333–1341.
13. Liao Z, Zhan X, Wu S, et al. Idiopathic ventricular arrhythmias originating from the pulmonary sinus cusp: prevalence, electrocardiographic/electrophysiological characteristics, and catheter ablation. J Am Coll Cardiol 2015;66:2633–2644.
14. Zhang J, Tang C, Zhang Y, Su X. Pulmonary sinus cusp mapping and ablation: a new concept and approach for idiopathic right ventricular outflow tract arrhythmias. Heart Rhythm 2018;15:38–45.
15. Sekiguchi Y, Aonuma K, Takahashi A, et al. Electrocardiographic and electrophysiologic characteristics of ventricular tachycardia originating within the pulmonary artery. J Am Coll Cardiol 2005;45:887–895.
16. Srivathsan KS, Bunch TJ, Asirvatham SJ, et al. Mechanism and utility of discrete great arterial potentials in the ablation of outflow tract ventricular arrhythmias. Circ Arrhythmia Electrophysiol 2008;1:30–38.
17. Timmermans C, Rodriguez L, Crijns H, Moorman A, Wellens H. Idiopathic left bundle-branch-shaped ventricular tachycardia may originate above the pulmonary valve. Circulation 2003;108:1960–1967.
18. Betensky BP, Park RE, Marchlinski FE, et al. The V(2) transition ratio: a new electrocardiographic criterion for distinguishing left from right ventricular outflow tract tachycardia origin. J Am Coll Cardiol 2011;57:2255–2262.
19. Tanner H, Hindricks G, Schirdewahn P, et al. Outflow tract tachycardia with R/S transition in lead V3: six different anatomic approaches for successful ablation. J Am Coll Cardiol 2005;45:418–423.
20. Bala R, Marchlinski FE. Electrocardiographic recognition and ablation of outflow tract ventricular tachycardia. Heart Rhythm 2007;4:366–370.
21. Suleiman M, Asirvatham SJ. Ablation above the semilunar valves: when, why, and how? Part I. Heart Rhythm 2008;5:1485–1492.
22. Suleiman M, Asirvatham SJ. Ablation above the semilunar valves: when, why, and how? Part II. Heart Rhythm 2008;5:1625–1630.
23. Tabatabaei N, Asirvatham SJ. Supravalvular arrhythmia: identifying and ablating the substrate. Circ Arrhythm Electrophysiol 2009;2:316–326.
24. Hachiya H, Aonuma K, Yamauchi Y, Igawa M, Nogami A, Iesaka Y. How to diagnose, locate and ablate coronary cusp ventricular tachycardia. J Cardiovasc Electrophysiol 2002;13:551–556.
25. Lin D, Ilkhanoff L, Gerstenfeld E, et al. Twelve-lead electrocardiographic characteristics of the aortic cusp region guided by intracardiac echocardiography and electroanatomic mapping. Heart Rhythm 2008;5:663–669.
26. Wang Y, Liang Z, Wu S, Han Z, Ren X. Idiopathic ventricular arrhythmias originating from the right coronary sinus: prevalence, electrocardiographic and electrophysiological characteristics, and catheter ablation. Heart Rhythm 2018;15:81–89.
27. Bala R, Garcia FC, Hutchinson MD, et al. Electrocardiographic and electrophysiologic features of ventricular arrhythmias originating from the right/left coronary cusp commissure. Heart Rhythm 2010;7:312–322.
28. Callans DJ, Menz V, Schwartzman D, Gottlieb CD, Marchlinski FE. Repetitive monomorphic tachycardia from the left ventricular outflow tract: electrocardiographic patterns consistent with a left ventricular site of origin. J Am Coll Cardiol 1997;29:1023–1027.
29. Kanagaratnam L, Tomassoni G, Schweikert R, et al. Ventricular tachycardias arising from the aortic sinus of Valsalva: an under-recognized variant of left outflow tract ventricular tachycardia. J Am Coll Cardiol 2001;37:1408–1414.
30. Ouyang F, Fotuhi P, Ho SY, et al. Repetitive monomorphic ventricular tachycardia originating from the aortic sinus cusp: electrocardiographic characterization for guiding catheter ablation. J Am Coll Cardiol 2002;39:500–508.
31. Yamada T, Murakami Y, Yoshida N, et al. Preferential conduction across the ventricular outflow septum in ventricular arrhythmias originating from the aortic sinus cusp. J Am Coll Cardiol 2007;50:884–891.
32. Yamada T, Yoshida N, Murakami Y, et al. Electrocardiographic characteristics of ventricular arrhythmias originating from the junction of the left and right coronary sinuses of Valsalva in the aorta: the activation pattern as a rationale for the electrocardiographic characteristics. Heart Rhythm 2008;5:184–192.
33. Yamada T, McElderry HT, Okada T, et al. Idiopathic left ventricular arrhythmias originating adjacent to the left aortic sinus of Valsalva: electrophysiological rationale for the surface electrocardiogram. J Cardiovasc Electrophysiol 2010;21:170–176.
34. Yamada T, McElderry T, Doppalapudi H, et al. Idiopathic ventricular arrhythmias originating from the aortic root prevalence, electrocardiographic and electrophysiologic characteristics, and results of radiofrequency catheter ablation. J Am Coll Cardiol 2008;52:139–147.
35. Chen J, Hoff PI, Rossvoll O, et al. Ventricular arrhythmias originating from the aortomitral continuity: an uncommon variant of left ventricular outflow tract tachycardia. Europace 2012;14:388–395.
36. Yamada T, Lau YR, Litovsky SH, et al. Prevalence and clinical, electrocardiographic, and electrophysiologic characteristics of ventricular arrhythmias originating from the noncoronary sinus of Valsalva. Heart Rhythm 2013;10:1605–1612.
37. Daniels DV, Lu YY, Morton JB, et al. Idiopathic epicardial left ventricular tachycardia originating remote from the sinus of Valsalva: electrophysiological characteristics, catheter ablation, and identification from the 12-lead electrocardiogram. Circulation 2006;113:1659–1666.
38. Berruezo A, Mont L, Nava S, Chueca E, Bartholomay E, Brugada J. Electrocardiographic recognition of the epicardial origin of ventricular tachycardias. Circulation 2004;109:1842–1847.
39. Efimova E, Dinov B, Acou WJ, et al. Differentiating the origin of outflow tract ventricular tachycardia arrhythmia using a simple, novel approach. Heart Rhythm 2015;12:1534–1540.
40. Yamada T, Doppalapudi H, McElderry HT, et al. Idiopathic ventricular arrhythmias originating from the papillary muscles in the left ventricle: prevalence, electrocardiographic and electrophysiological characteristics, and results of the radiofrequency catheter ablation. J Cardiovasc Electrophysiol 2010;21:62–69.
41. Yamada T, Doppalapudi H, McElderry T, et al. Electrocardiographic and electrophysiological characteristics in idiopathic ventricular arrhythmias originating from the papillary muscles in the left ventricle: relevance for catheter ablation. Circ Arrhythm Electrophysiol 2010;3:324–331.
42. Doppalapudi H, Yamada T, McElderry T, Plumb VJ, Ebstein AE, Kay GN. Ventricular tachycardia originating from the posterior papillary muscle in the left ventricle: a distinct clinical syndrome. Circ Arrhythm Electrophysiol 2008;1:23–29.
43. Santoro F, Di Biase L, Hranitzky P, et al. Ventricular tachycardia originating from the septal papillary muscle of the right ventricle: electrocardiographic and electrophysiological characteristics. J Cardiovasc Electrophysiology 2015;26:145–150.
44. Enriquez A, Supple GE, Marchlinski FE, Garcia FC. How to map and ablate papillary muscle ventricular arrhythmias. Heart Rhythm 2017;14:1721–1728.
45. Sadek MM, Benhayon D, Sureddi R, et al. Idiopathic ventricular arrhythmias originating from the moderator band: electrocardiographic characteristics and treatment by catheter ablation. Heart Rhythm 2015;12:67–75.
46. Wasmer K, Köbe J, Dechering DG, et al. Ventricular arrhythmias from the mitral annulus: patient characteristics, electrophysiological findings, ablation, and prognosis. Heart Rhythm 2013;10:783–788.
47. Zipes, DP, Foster PR, Troup PJ, Pedersen DH. Atrial induction of ventricular tachycardia: reentry versus triggered automaticity. Am J Cardiol 1979;44:1–8.
48. Belhassen B, Rotmensch HH, Laniado S. Response of recurrent sustained ventricular tachycardia to verapamil. Br Heart J 1981;46:679–682.
49. Okumura K, Matsuyama K, Miyagi H, Tsuchiya T, Yasue H. Entrainment of idiopathic ventricular tachycardia of left ventricular origin with evidence for reentry with an area of slow conduction and effect of verapamil. Am J Cardiol 1988;62:727–732.
50. Okumura K, Yamabe H, Tsuchiya T, Tabuchi T, Iwasa A, Yasue H. Characteristics of slow conduction zone demonstrated during entrainment of idiopathic ventricular tachycardia of left ventricular origin. Am J Cardiol 1996;77:379–383.
51. Talib AK, Nogami A, Nishiuchi S, et al. Verapamil-sensitive upper septal idiopathic left ventricular tachycardia: prevalence, mechanism, and electrophysiological characteristics. JACC Clin Electrophysiol 2015;1:369–380.
52. Nakagawa H, Beckman K, McClelland JH, et al. Radiofrequency catheter ablation of idiopathic left ventricular tachycardia guided by a Purkinje potential. Circulation 1993;88:2607–2617.
53. Wen M, Yeh S, Wang C, Lin F, Chen I, Wu D. Radiofrequency ablation therapy in idiopathic left ventricular tachycardia with no obvious structural heart disease. Circulation 1994;89:1690–1696.

54. Tsuchiya T, Okumura K, Honda T, et al. Significance of late diastolic potential preceding Purkinje potential in verapamil-sensitive idiopathic left ventricular tachycardia. Circulation 1999;99:2408–2413.

55. Zhan H, Liang Y, Xue Y, et al. A new electrophysiologic observation in patients with idiopathic left ventricular tachycardia. Heart Rhythm 2016;13:1460–1467.

56. Zhan XZ, Liang YH, Xue YM, et al. A new electrophysiologic observation in patients with idiopathic left ventricular tachycardia. Heart Rhythm 2016;13:1460–1467.

57. Leenhardt A, Glaser E, Burguera M, Nürnberg M, Maison-Blanche P, Coumel P. Short-coupled variant of torsade de pointes. A new electrocardiographic entity in the spectrum of idiopathic ventricular tachyarrhythmias. Circulation 1994;898:206–215.

58. Haïssaguerre M, Shah DC, Jaïs P, et al. Role of Purkinje conducting system in triggering of idiopathic ventricular fibrillation. Lancet 2002;359:677–678.

59. Noda T, Shimizu W, Taguchi A, et al. Malignant entity of idiopathic ventricular fibrillation and polymorphic ventricular tachycardia initiated by premature extrasystoles originating from the right ventricular outflow tract. J Am Coll Cardiol 2005;46:1288–1294.

60. Haissaguerre M, Shoda M, Jaïs P, et al. Mapping and ablation of idiopathic ventricular fibrillation. Circulation 2002;106:962–967.

61. Nogami A, Sugiyasu A, Kubota S, Kato K. Mapping and ablation of idiopathic ventricular fibrillation from the Purkinje system. Heart Rhythm 2005;2:646–649.

62. Santoro F, Di Biase L, Hranitzky P, et al. Ventricular fibrillation triggered by PVCs from papillary muscles: clinical features and ablation. J Cardiovasc Electrophysiol 2014;35:1158–1164.

63. Ho RT, Frisch DR, Greenspon AJ. Idiopathic ventricular fibrillation ablation facilitated by PENTARAY mapping of the moderator band. JACC Clin Electrophysiol 2017;3:313–314.

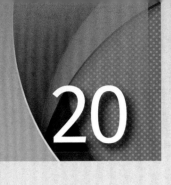

20 Ablation of Scar-Related Ventricular Tachycardia

Introduction

In addition to the implantable cardioverter-defibrillator, catheter ablation plays an important role in the treatment of patients with scar-related ventricular tachycardia (VT).

The purpose of this chapter is to:

1. Describe the macroreentrant circuit for scar-related VT.
2. Locate the VT exit site by the 12-lead ECG.
3. Discuss mapping techniques and target site criteria for ablation.

VT CIRCUIT

The primary mechanism underlying scar-related VT is macroreentry. Ventricles scarred by disease (e.g., infarction) or surgery (e.g., repaired tetralogy of Fallot) contain islands of surviving myocyte bundles interspersed among electrically unexcitable scar (EUS) creating isthmuses or zones of slow conduction that facilitate reentrant excitation.[1-4] Integral to the VT reentrant circuit is this critical isthmus of slow conduction protected by anatomical and/or functional barriers and is the primary target site for ablation.[1]

CIRCUIT MODEL

A two-dimensional model provides a working framework to guide ablation that centers around the critical isthmus (Fig. 20-1).[2,4] At the proximal end of the isthmus is an excitable point of entry called the entrance site. At its distal end, the exit site provides continuity between the circuit and the rest of the ventricle. The circuit is completed by dominant inner or outer loops connecting both ends of the isthmus allowing reentry—one type of which is figure of 8 reentry (Fig. 20-2). The difference between inner and outer loops is that outer loops connect entrance and exit sites around the periphery of scar, while inner loops travel within the scar and are, therefore, electrically isolated. During VT, the isthmus is activated from entrance to exit after which the wavefront leaves the circuit to activate the ventricle. The VT morphology, therefore, reflects the location of the isthmus exit site. Adjacent bystander sites are blind channels or alleys within scar that are passively activated during tachycardia and not essential to the reentrant circuit. Remote bystanders are noncritical sites located outside the circuit. The isthmus is a critical component of the circuit and, therefore, the target site

for ablation. Each circuit site is identified by specific entrainment mapping criteria.

In contrast to a simple two-dimensional working construct, actual VT circuits are complex, three-dimensional structures that can involve endocardial, mid-myocardial, and epicardial layers. The circuit for certain diseases (e.g., myocardial infarction) shows a predilection for the endocardium, while others (e.g., nonischemic cardiomyopathy, arrhythmogenic right ventricular [RV] cardiomyopathy, sarcoidosis) show a predilection for the mid-myocardium and epicardium.[5] For infarct VT, the macroreentrant circuit can span several centimeters with the length of isthmuses averaging approximately 3 cm. Exit sites tend to be located at the infarct border zone (defined by voltages = 0.5 mV − 1.5 mV), while central isthmus and entrance sites are located within dense scar (<0.5 mV).[6,7]

12-LEAD ECG DURING VT

The 12-lead ECG provides the approximate location of the VT exit site.[8] Because VT arises from the border zone of an infarct, Q waves are preserved during tachycardia and reflect both infarct location and exit site. The terminal QRS forces in lead V1 determine VT bundle branch block (BBB) morphology. Left bundle branch block (LBBB) VT (negative terminal forces in V1) identifies either a left septal or RV tachycardia. Right bundle branch block (RBBB) VT (positive terminal forces in V1) indicates a left ventricular (LV) tachycardia. VT with a superior axis arises from the inferior wall of the ventricle, while an inferior axis identifies an anterior or outflow tract origin. VT associated with inferior infarctions shows predilection for the LV base between the infarct border and the mitral annulus (submitral VT) with a zone of slow conduction running parallel to the mitral

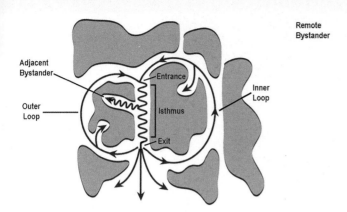

FIGURE 20-1 Figure of 8 (double loop) reentry. The protected isthmus is a region of slow conduction critical to the circuit. Proximal and distal isthmus sites are the entrance and exit, respectively. The exit site is the point where the activation wavefront leaves the circuit to depolarize the ventricles and, therefore, determines the VT morphology. Bystander sites are passively activated and not integral to tachycardia.

annulus and showing two characteristic morphologies: LBBB/LS axis (septal exit) and RBBB/RS axis (lateral exit).[9] Positive precordial concordance (all positive QRS complexes across the precordium) indicates a basal VT near the mitral valve. Negative precordial concordance (all negative QRS complexes across the precordium) identifies an apical VT (**Figs. 20-3 and 20-4**).

MAPPING AND ABLATION

Ventricular mapping can be performed either during VT (entrainment mapping) or sinus/paced rhythm (substrate-based ablation). Because the mechanism of scar-mediated VT is macroreentry, discrete electrograms can be recorded during the entire VT cycle length. The target of ablation is the critical isthmus: proximal (entrance), mid (central), and distal (exit) isthmus sites, which generate low-amplitude/fractionated early, mid-, and late diastolic potentials, respectively, during VT. While mid-diastolic potentials representing the central isthmus

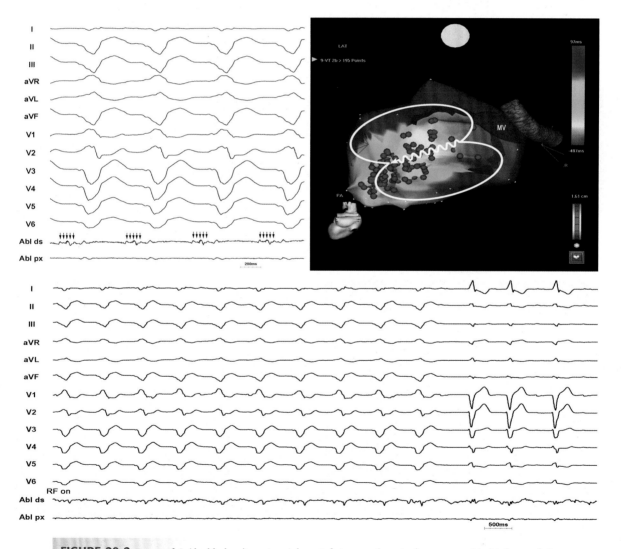

FIGURE 20-2 Figure of 8 (double loop) reentry. A large inferior scar (*gray tags*) creates a critical isthmus of slow conduction allowing figure of 8 reentry. Early (*red*) meets late (*purple*) on the lateral and septal sides of the mitral annulus. Long, fragmented mid-diastolic potential (*arrows*) representing slow asynchronous activation is recorded from the isthmus (*zigzag line*) where radiofrequency (RF) energy terminated VT.

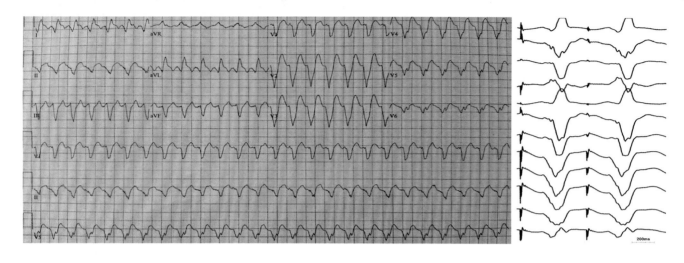

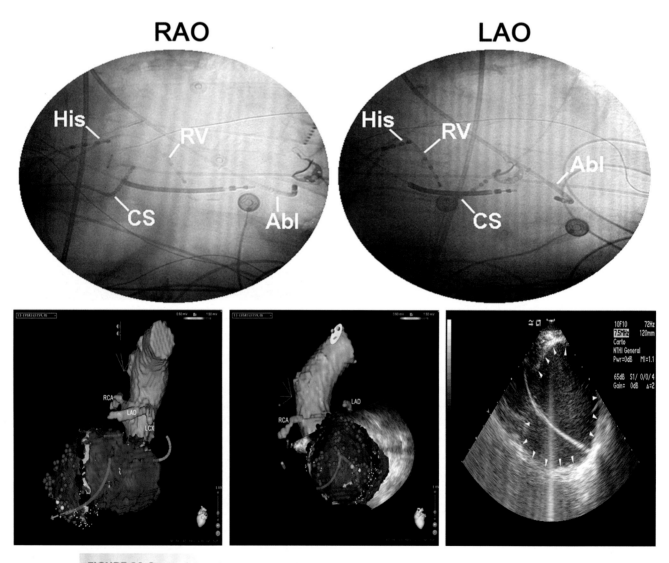

FIGURE 20-3 LV apical VT (negative precordial concordance). Electro-anatomic LV voltage map shows a large apical aneurysm with apical ballooning (*arrowheads*). Pacemapping within the aneurysm generates a long St-QRS interval and 12-lead ECG match to VT. Ablation lesions (*red tags*) are delivered to these sites and circumferentially around the border zone of the aneurysm. Gray tags denote EUS.

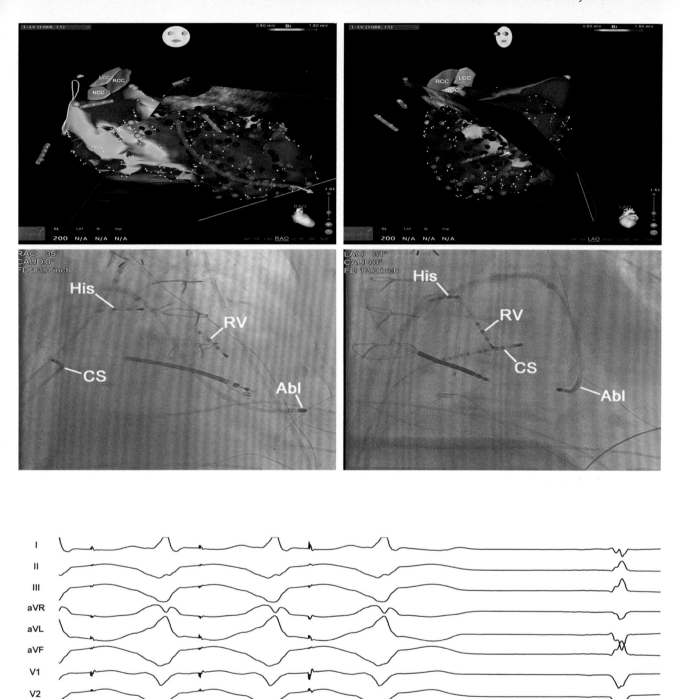

FIGURE 20-4 LV apical VT (negative precordial concordance). Electro-anatomic LV voltage map shows a large apical aneurysm. Pacemapping from the LV apex generates a long St-QRS interval with negative precordial concordance despite lack of a visible electrogram during sinus rhythm. Ablation lesions (*red tags*) are delivered to this site and throughout the aneurysm. Gray tags denote EUS, and black tags denote late potentials (LPs).

are important to identify, they are not specific for the critical isthmus and can be recorded from adjacent bystander sites. Therefore, entrainment mapping coupled with activation mapping should be performed to determine the value of the recording site to the reentrant circuit.

ENTRAINMENT MAPPING

Entrainment mapping is a valuable pacing maneuver that identifies functional components of the tachycardia circuit and differentiates them from bystander sites (Fig. 20-5).[10-13] During VT, pacing stimuli are delivered at a cycle length 10–20 ms shorter than the VT cycle length. It is imperative to confirm that pacing stimuli truly capture the ventricle and accelerate VT to the pacing cycle length (Fig. 20-6). Stimuli penetrating the circuit and entraining tachycardia give rise to orthodromic and antidromic wavefronts. The antidromic wavefront of the first stimulus collides with tachycardia, while its orthodromic counterpart advances the circuit. With continuation of pacing, the orthodromic wavefront of each pacing stimulus (n) advances the tachycardia and collides with the antidromic wavefront of

the subsequent ($n + 1$) stimulus (continuous resetting). When pacing stops, the last orthodromic wavefront has no antidromic wavefront with which to collide and completes one revolution around the circuit, and tachycardia continues.

Entrainment Criteria

Three criteria define each mapped site relative to the circuit: 1) paced QRS relative to tachycardia QRS morphology, 2) stimulus (St)-QRS relative to electrogram (egm)-QRS interval, and 3) post-pacing interval (PPI) relative to tachycardia cycle length (TCL). The St-QRS − egm-QRS and PPI–TCL are complementary to each other.

Concealed versus Manifest Fusion

Entrainment from isthmus (entrance, central, and exit), inner loop, and adjacent bystander sites activates the ventricle from the isthmus exit site so that paced QRS morphologies are identical to tachycardia (entrainment with concealed fusion) (Figs. 20-7 to 20-16). Collision between orthodromic and antidromic wavefronts occurs "upstream" to the pacing site within the circuit resulting in local fusion that is undetectable on the

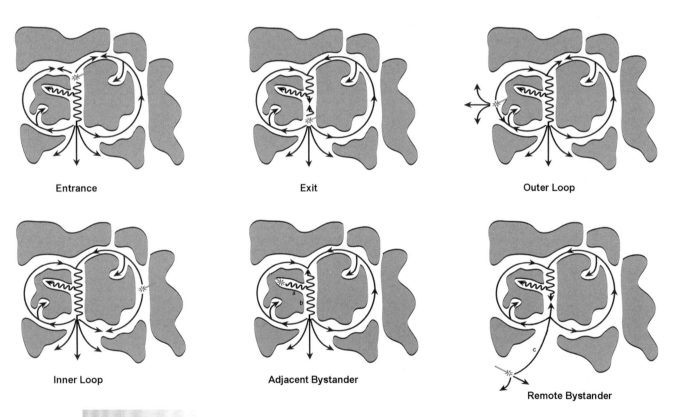

Entrance

Exit

Outer Loop

Inner Loop

Adjacent Bystander

Remote Bystander

FIGURE 20-5 Diagram illustrating the six different entrainment sites. Entrance site stimulation shows concealed fusion, long St-QRS = egm-QRS, and PPI = TCL. Exit site stimulation produces concealed fusion, short St-QRS = egm-QRS, and PPI = TCL. Outer loop site stimulation causes manifest fusion but PPI = TCL. Inner loop site stimulation shows concealed fusion, very long St-QRS = egm-QRS, and PPI = TCL. Adjacent bystander site stimulation generates concealed fusion, long St-QRS ≠ egm-QRS, and PPI ≠ TCL. (The St-QRS [a + b] > egm-QRS intervals [b − a] and the PPI = TCL + 2a provided that the conduction times in and out of the bystander pathway are equal. The letter a denotes bystander pathway conduction time, and b denotes conduction time from junction between bystander and isthmus to exit site.) Remote bystander site stimulation shows manifest fusion and PPI ≠ TCL. (The PPI = VTCL + 2c provided that the conduction times to and from the circuit are equal. The letter c denotes conduction time between pacing site and circuit.)

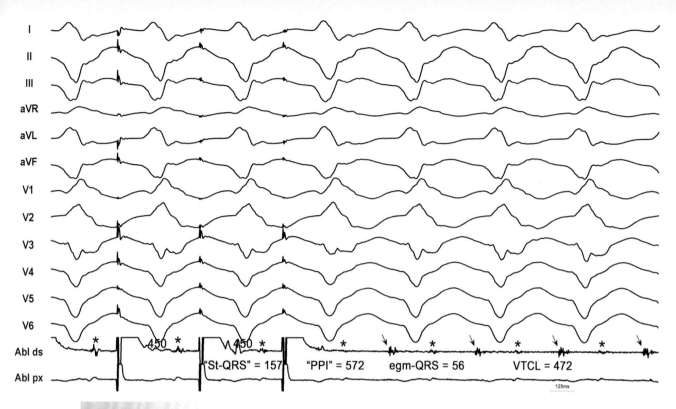

FIGURE 20-6 Pseudo-entrainment (noncapture). At first glance, it appears that the ventricle is entrained with concealed fusion, St-QRS (33% TCL) − egm-QRS = 101 ms, and PPI − TCL = 100 ms suggesting an adjacent bystander site. Close inspection, however, reveals that pacing stimuli fail to capture the ventricle (prolonging St-QRS intervals). Asterisks denote far-field electrograms. Arrows denote the putative near-field electrograms.

12-lead ECG (hence, the term "concealed"). Entrainment from outer loop and remote bystander sites produces paced QRS morphologies different from tachycardia (entrainment with manifest fusion) (**Figs. 20-17 to 20-20**).

St-QRS versus egm-QRS Interval

The St-QRS interval is measured from the pacing artifact to onset of the QRS complex. Entrance, central, and exit site stimulation produce long (51–70% VTCL), intermediate (31–50% VTCL), and short (≤30% VTCL) St-QRS intervals, respectively (**Figs. 20-7 to 20-13**). Because the inner loop is within scar proximal to the critical isthmus, stimulation from this site generates very long St-QRS intervals (>70% VTCL) (**Fig. 20-14**). The St-QRS intervals for outer loop and remote bystander sites are generally short because myocardial tissue outside the circuit is directly depolarized by the pacing stimulus unless stimulation occurs within remote scar (**Figs. 20-17 to 20-20**). In contrast, the St-QRS intervals for adjacent bystander sites are typically long and equals the conduction time over the bystander pathway plus the conduction time from its junction with the isthmus to the exit site (**Figs. 20-15 and 20-16**).

The egm-QRS interval represents the activation time from the mapping site to onset of the QRS complex. It is very long for inner loop sites and becomes progressively shorter as the mapping catheter heads toward entrance, central, and exit sites. Electrograms from the isthmus are typically low amplitude; fractionated; and occur during early (entrance), mid (central), or late ("presystolic") (exit) diastole.[14] Diastolic electrograms are not isthmus specific and can be recorded from bystander sites. Therefore, the egm-QRS relative to St-QRS intervals differentiates isthmus from bystander sites. Isthmus (entrance to exit) and dominant inner loop sites demonstrate matching St-QRS and egm-QRS intervals (≤20 ms) because they are participants in the reentrant circuit, while bystander sites (adjacent, remote) do not (>20 ms). The St-QRS interval for an adjacent bystander site is the conduction time out of the bystander pathway plus the conduction time from its junction with the isthmus to the exit site, while the egm-QRS interval is the difference between them. The St-QRS interval for a remote bystander site is generally 0 (unless in noncircuit scar) and does not match the corresponding egm-QRS interval, which is the conduction time from the exit to the remote bystander site. The St-QRS and egm-QRS intervals for outer loop sites depend on pacing location relative to the exit site and also generally do not match unless near the exit ("exit zone").

Post-pacing Interval–Tachycardia Cycle Length

The PPI is measured from the last pacing stimulus to the onset of the first spontaneous near-field electrogram recorded on

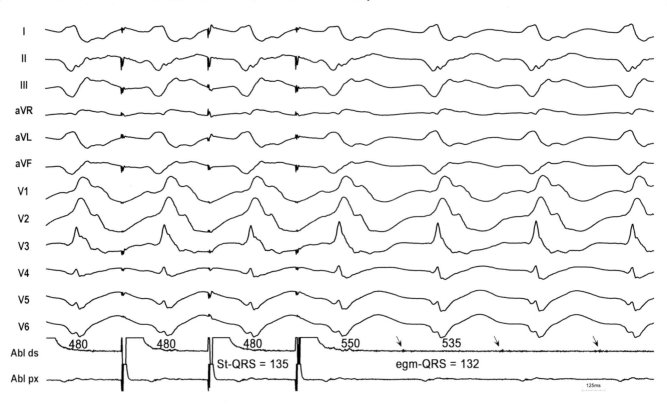

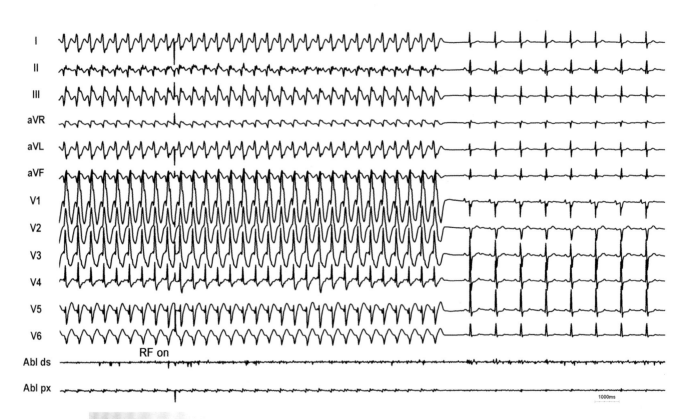

FIGURE 20-7 Exit site. Paced and VT complexes are identical (concealed fusion). The St-QRS (25% TCL) − egm-QRS = 3 ms. The PPI − TCL = 15 ms. Radiofrequency (RF) delivery terminates tachycardia in 11.1 sec.

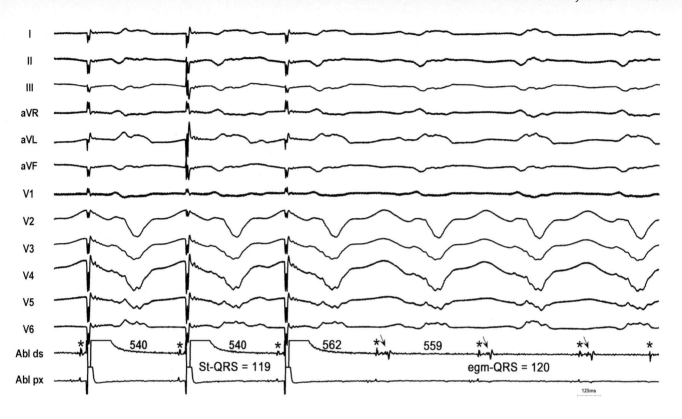

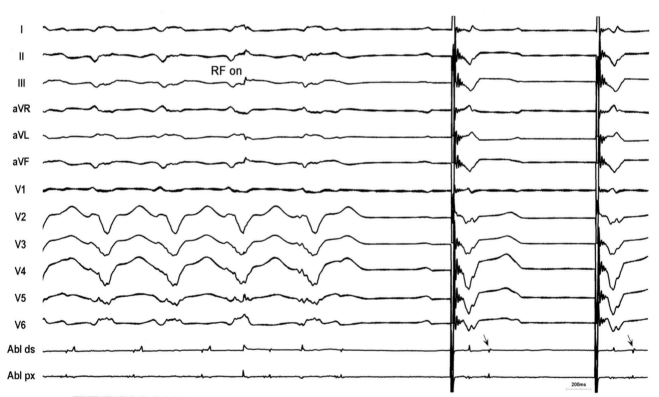

FIGURE 20-8 Exit site. Paced and VT complexes are identical (concealed fusion). The St-QRS (21% TCL) − egm-QRS = 1 ms. The PPI − TCL = 3 ms. Radiofrequency (RF) delivery terminates tachycardia in 0.8 sec. The ablation catheter records a split potential—the first component (*asterisks*) of which is not captured by pacing stimuli and, therefore, not used for PPI measurement. The second component (*arrows*) is the near-field electrogram of interest and also seen as a LP during ventricular paced rhythm.

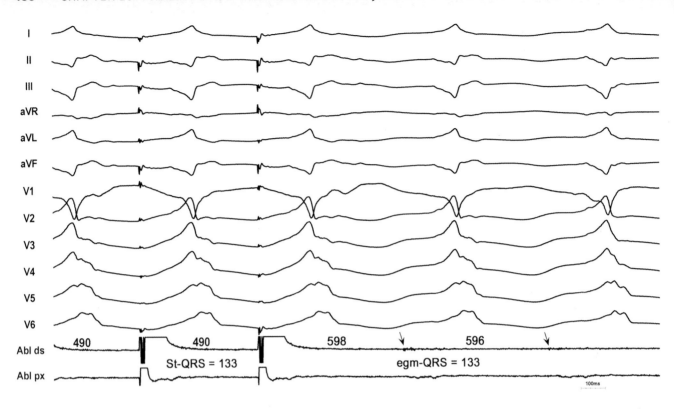

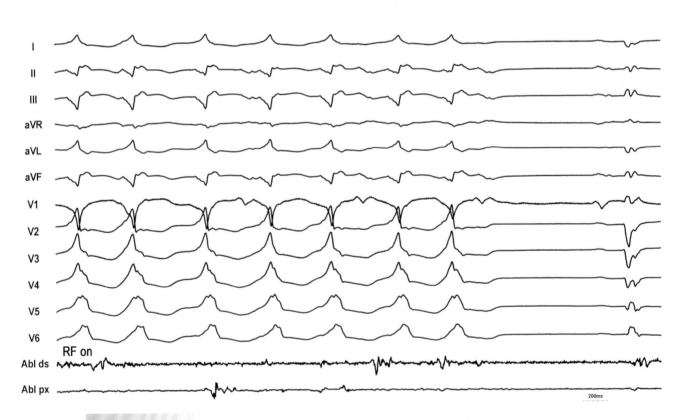

FIGURE 20-9 Exit site. Paced and VT complexes are identical (concealed fusion). The St-QRS (22% TCL) − egm-QRS = 0 ms. The PPI − TCL = 2 ms. Radiofrequency (RF) delivery terminates tachycardia.

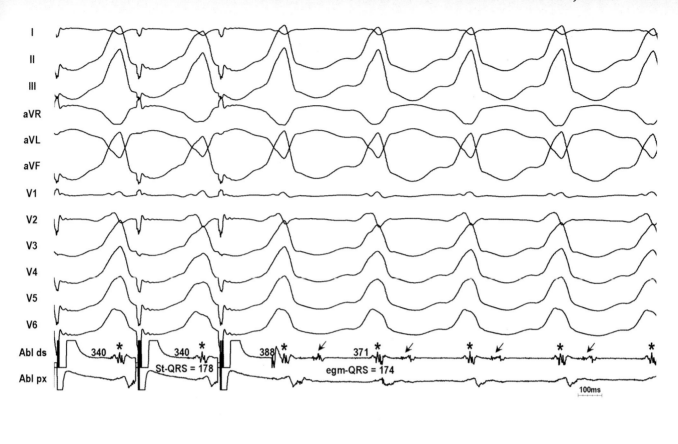

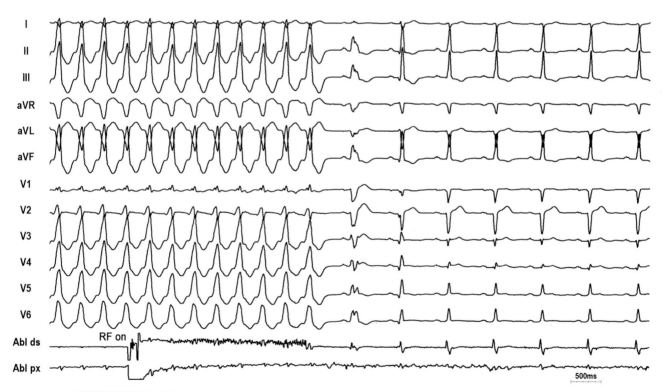

FIGURE 20-10 Central isthmus site. Paced and VT complexes are identical (concealed fusion) with subtle beat-to-beat alternation in QRS morphology (a form of multiple exit site (MES) stimulation (see below)). The St-QRS interval (48% TCL) − egm-QRS interval = 4 ms. The PPI − TCL = 17 ms. Application of radiofrequency (RF) energy terminates tachycardia in 3.1 sec. Asterisks denote far-field ventricular potentials not captured by pacing. Arrows denote the near-field electrograms of interest.

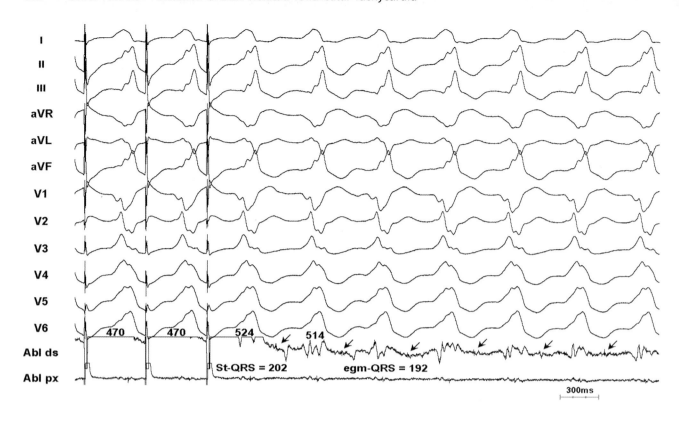

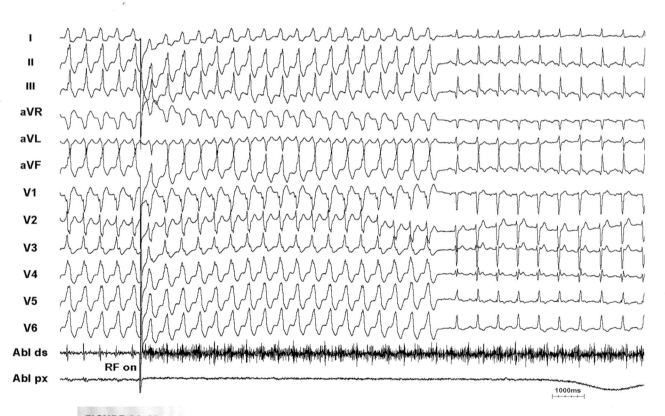

FIGURE 20-11 Central isthmus site. Paced and VT complexes are identical (concealed fusion). The St-QRS interval (39% TCL) − egm-QRS interval = 10 ms. The PPI − TCL = 10 ms. Application of radiofrequency (RF) energy terminates tachycardia in 9.2 sec.

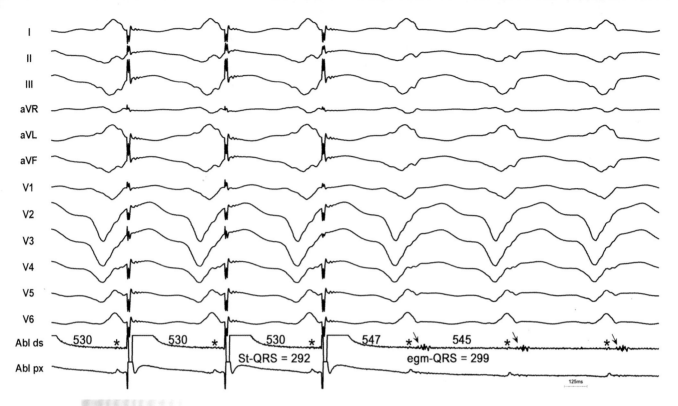

FIGURE 20-12 Entrance site. Paced and VT complexes are identical (concealed fusion). The St-QRS interval (54% TCL) − egm-QRS interval = 7 ms. The PPI − TCL = 2 ms. Asterisks denote far-field ventricular potentials not captured by pacing. Arrows denote the near-field electrograms of interest.

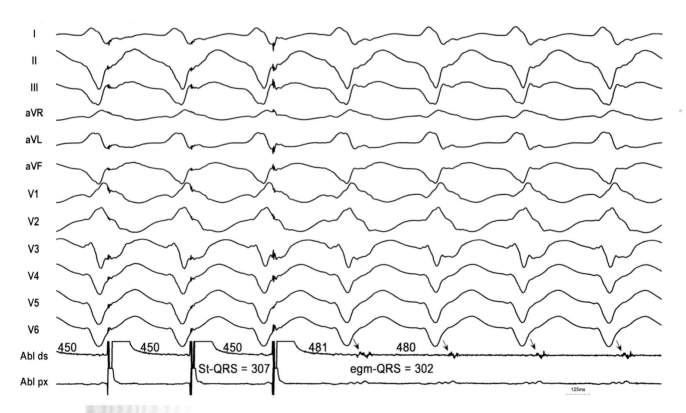

FIGURE 20-13 Entrance site. Paced and VT complexes are identical (concealed fusion). The St-QRS interval (64% TCL) − egm-QRS interval = 5 ms. The PPI − TCL = 1 ms.

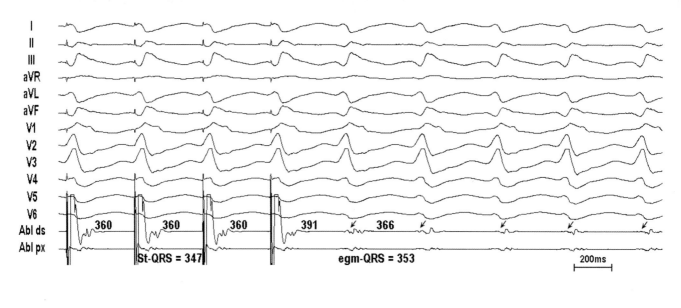

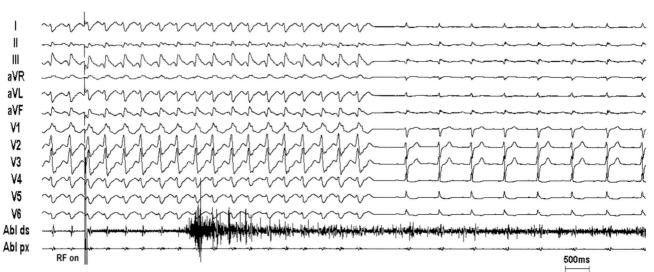

FIGURE 20-14 Inner loop site. Paced and VT complexes are identical (concealed fusion). The St-QRS interval (95% TCL) − egm-QRS interval = 6 ms. The PPI − TCL = 25 ms. Application of radiofrequency (RF) energy terminates tachycardia in 5.9 sec.

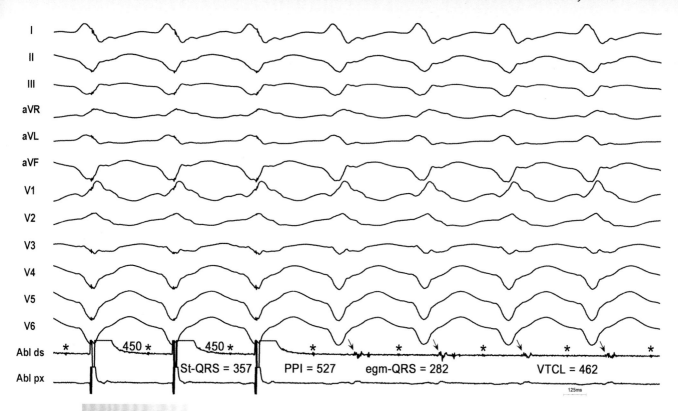

FIGURE 20-15 Adjacent bystander site. Paced and VT complexes are identical (concealed fusion). The St-QRS (77% TCL) − egm-QRS = 75 ms. The PPI − TCL = 65 ms. Asterisks denote far-field potentials not captured by pacing stimuli. Arrows denote the near-field electrograms of interest.

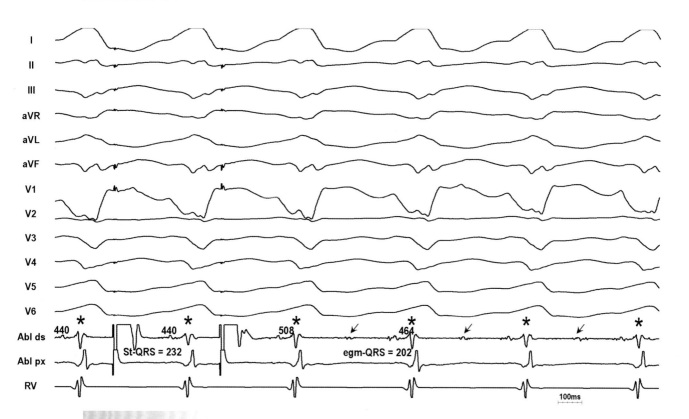

FIGURE 20-16 Adjacent bystander site. Paced and VT complexes are identical (concealed fusion). The St-QRS interval (50% TCL) − egm-QRS = 30 ms. The PPI − TCL = 44 ms. Asterisks denote far-field electrograms not captured by pacing stimuli. Arrows denote the near-field electrograms of interest.

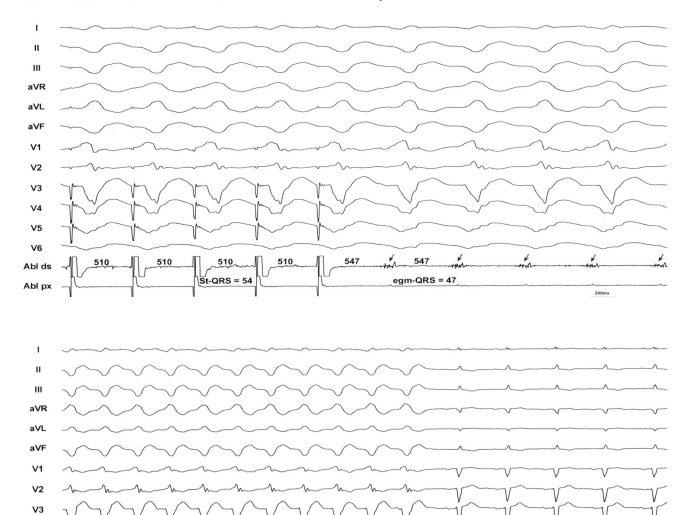

FIGURE 20-17 Outer loop site near exit (exit zone). Paced and VT complexes are subtly different (evident in lead V1) (manifest fusion). The St-QRS − egm-QRS = 7 ms. The PPI − TCL = 0 ms. Radiofrequency (RF) delivery terminates tachycardia in 5.2 sec.

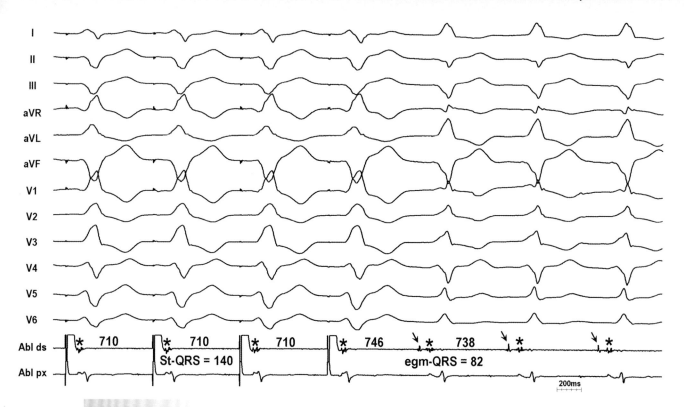

FIGURE 20-18 Outer loop site. Paced and VT complexes are different (manifest fusion). The PPI − TCL = 8 ms. Asterisks denote far-field potentials not captured by pacing. Arrows denote the near-field electrograms of interest.

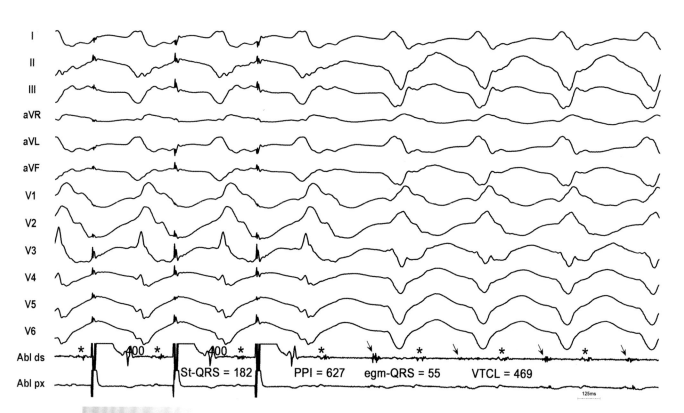

FIGURE 20-19 Remote bystander site. Paced and VT complexes are different (manifest fusion). The PPI − TCL = 158 ms. The St-QRS is long (182 ms) because of pacing within scar. Asterisks denote far-field electrograms not captured by pacing stimuli. Arrows denote near-field electrograms of interest.

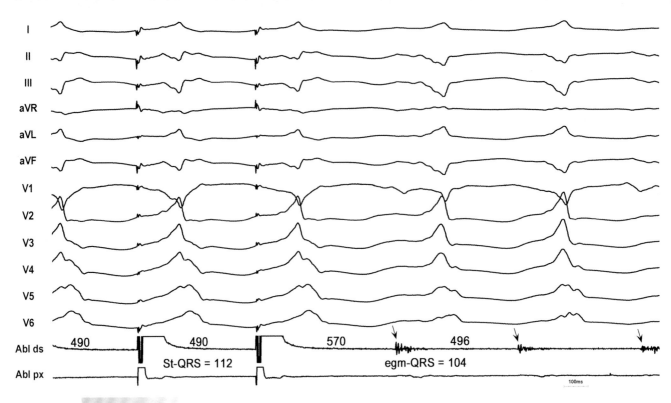

FIGURE 20-20 Remote bystander site. Paced and VT complexes are similar but not identical (manifest fusion). The PPI − TCL = 74 ms.

the mapping catheter. This near-field electrogram of interest is differentiated from far-field electrograms by its disappearance during pacing due to direct local capture at the stimulation site.[13] Far-field electrograms remain visible during entrainment and separate from the pacing stimulus. Analysis of orthodromically captured electrograms from neighboring dipoles (e.g., Abl px) can provide additional confirmation. Because the revolution time around the circuit equals the TCL, entrainment from a site within the circuit (isthmus, dominant inner and outer loop) results in PPI − TCL ≤30 ms. Entrainment from bystander sites (adjacent, remote) produces PPI − TCL >30 ms. The PPI for an adjacent bystander site is the conduction time out of the bystander pathway, once around the circuit, and back to the bystander pathway. Assuming that conduction times in and out of the pathway are equal, the PPI = TCL + 2 (bystander pathway conduction time). The PPI for a remote bystander site is the conduction time from pacing site to the circuit, once around the circuit, and back again to the pacing site. Assuming that the conduction times to and from the circuit are equal, the PPI = TCL + 2 (conduction time between pacing site and circuit). The PPI can be unexpectedly short if 1) high pacing output captures distant tissue (large virtual electrode), 2) entrainment momentarily accelerates VT, 3) pacing "short circuits" the actual circuit (e.g., transient conduction around a smaller nondominant inner loop), or 4) the near-field electrogram is orthodromically (not directly) captured (far-field

ventricular capture outside the circuit penetrates and orthodromically entrains the near-field electrogram inside the circuit in which case it occurs at the pacing cycle length).[15]

When the first return near-field electrogram on the mapping catheter cannot be measured because of pacing-induced saturation artifact, a complementary measurement is the n + 1 difference.[16] The interval between the last stimulus entraining tachycardia and a timing reference during the second beat after the stimulus (n + 1 beat) (e.g., St-QRS$_{n+1}$ or St-RV$_{n+1}$) is subtracted from the comparative interval involving the electrogram at the stimulation site in any following beat (e.g., egm$_{n+2}$ − QRS$_{n+3}$ or egm$_{n+2}$ − RV$_{n+3}$). The n + 1 difference correlates with the PPI–TCL.

Entrainment Sites

The characteristics of the different VT circuit sites identified by entrainment mapping and success with ablation are presented in Table 20-1. Termination of VT by radiofrequency application is most successful when targeting the isthmus (entrance to exit), although a focal lesion to an isthmus site might not terminate VT if the isthmus is too broad for a single lesion.

SUBSTRATE-BASED ABLATION

By evaluating its response to pacing, entrainment mapping allows identification of the exact isthmus responsible for a given VT, but its major limitations are the inability to induce VT, induction of

TABLE 20-1 Characteristics of macroreentrant VT circuit sites

Circuit site	Fusion type	St-QRS – egm-QRS	PPI – TCL	Ablation success[†]
Exit	Concealed	≤20 ms (St-QRS ≤30% TCL)	≤30 ms	37%
Central	Concealed	≤20 ms (St-QRS 31–50% TCL)	≤30 ms	23%
Entrance	Concealed	≤20 ms (St-QRS 51–70% TCL)	≤30 ms	25%
Inner loop	Concealed	≤20 ms (St-QRS >70% TCL)	≤30 ms	9%
Outer loop	Manifest	>20 ms (except near exit)	≤30 ms	10%
Adjacent bystander	Concealed	>20 ms	>30 ms	11%
Remote bystander	Manifest	>20 ms	>30 ms	3%

nonclinical VT, and hemodynamic instability during VT. While intravenous vasopressors or mechanical circulatory assist devices (e.g., Impella, TandemHeart) can provide hemodynamic support and allow entrainment mapping, substrate-based ablation is an alternative and complementary ablation strategy that does not require VT induction. While identifying the exact VT isthmus is less precise, substrate-based ablation targets putative circuits and shared common pathways based on the electrical content of the electrograms during sinus rhythm (or RV pacing) and response to direct stimulation (pacemapping).[17]

Sinus Rhythm Ventricular Electrograms

Myocardial scar contains strands of surviving myocyte bundles intermixed among fibrosis causing nonuniform anisotropic conduction and, therefore, slow, delayed, and asynchronous ("zigzag") activation.[18] Characteristic scarred ventricular electrograms show low voltage, long duration, and late onset. Other features include fragmentation or fractionation (continuous or multicomponent (multiple electrograms each separated by isoelectric intervals)). Characteristic target site electrograms include 1) low voltage, 2) late potentials (LPs), and 3) local abnormal ventricular activities (LAVAs). During sinus rhythm and ventricular pacing, it is important to differentiate far-field electrograms (lower dV/dt, not captured locally by pacing [seen before/after the pacing stimulus artifact]) from true near-field electrograms (higher dV/dt, captured locally by pacing [obscured by pacing stimulus artifact]).

Voltage Maps

Using an electro-anatomic mapping system, a sinus rhythm voltage map can be created to delineate scar. Standard endocardial bipolar voltage settings are normal myocardium (>1.5 mV), border zone of scar (0.5–1.5 mV), and dense scar (<0.5 mV).[19] A cutoff of 0.5 mV, however, does not differentiate excitable from inexcitable tissue (EUS). A lower setting (<0.1 mV) could be used to delineate complete scar.[20] Different anatomically deployed lesion sets can be scar-based: 1) linear spokes (guided by pacemapping) radiating from dense scar into either healthy myocardium or fixed anatomical boundaries, 2) circumferentially along the border zone of scar, and 3) completely covering the scar (homogenization) endo-/epicardially or isthmus-based (defined by entrainment or pacemapping): 1) short (4–5 cm) ablation lines transecting an isthmus and running parallel to the border zone and 2) circumferentially around an isthmus until exit block is achieved (core isolation) (**Fig. 20-3 and Figs. 20-21 to 20-23**).[19–23] A submitral VT after a remote inferior myocardial infarction can be treated by deploying an anatomic ablation line of block across the corridor between the infarct and mitral annulus.[9] Incisional VT (e.g., repaired tetralogy of Fallot) revolves around surgical incision lines manifesting double potentials along the incision that represents activation on both sides of the line. Four discrete anatomic isthmus sites after surgical repair of tetralogy of Fallot are located between 1) RV outflow tract (RVOT) free wall patch/scar–tricuspid annulus (most common), 2) RVOT free wall patch/scar–pulmonary annulus, 3) ventricular septal defect (VSD) patch—tricuspid annulus, and 4) VSD patch—pulmonary annulus.[24] Although ablation can target the critical isthmus, incisional VT can also be treated by an ablation line connecting the scar to a fixed anatomic barrier (e.g., right ventriculotomy scar to pulmonary annulus) (**Fig. 20-24**).[24–26]

With voltage mapping, upper and lower voltage thresholds can be adjusted to identify putative conducting voltage channels (corridor of "higher" border zone voltages among dense scar) that can be targeted for ablation, particularly when coupled with additional electrical information (e.g., LPs) from that site (**Fig. 20-25**).[27,28] The location and degree of scar transmurality based on late gadolinium enhancement on cardiac MRI can supplement electro-anatomic voltage maps and guide ablation.[29–31]

Late Potentials

Another ablation target are LPs (LP abolition), which reflect diseased sites with delayed activation due to slow conduction typically within dense scar (voltage <0.5 mV).[20,32–34] Because slow conduction is a prerequisite for reentry, ablation of LPs might interrupt a critical isthmus. LPs, however, do not differentiate isthmus from adjacent bystander sites.[32] LPs are generally low-amplitude, high-frequency, discrete, or fractionated potentials, which by definition occur late (after the QRS complex or >40–50 ms after the larger local ventricular electrogram) with different LP definitions varying on the degree of

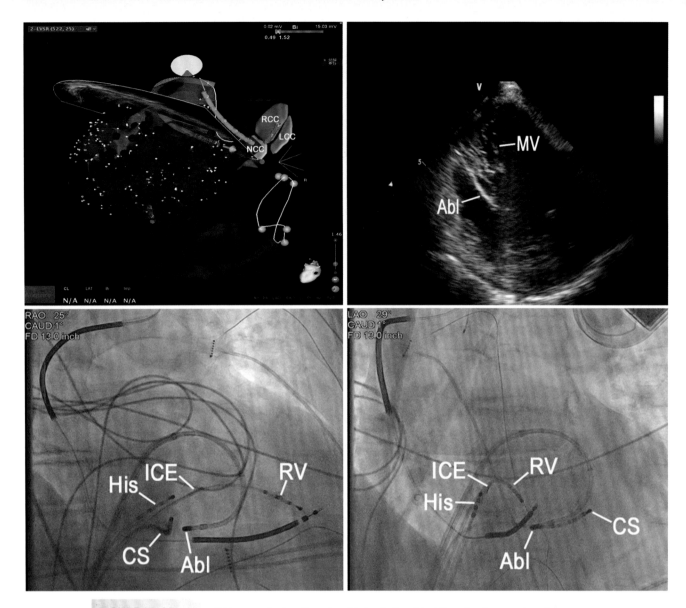

FIGURE 20-21 Endocardial homogenization. Extensive ablation (*red tags*) is delivered to homogenize a large postero-inferior infarct with the ablation catheter located beneath the septal mitral valve.

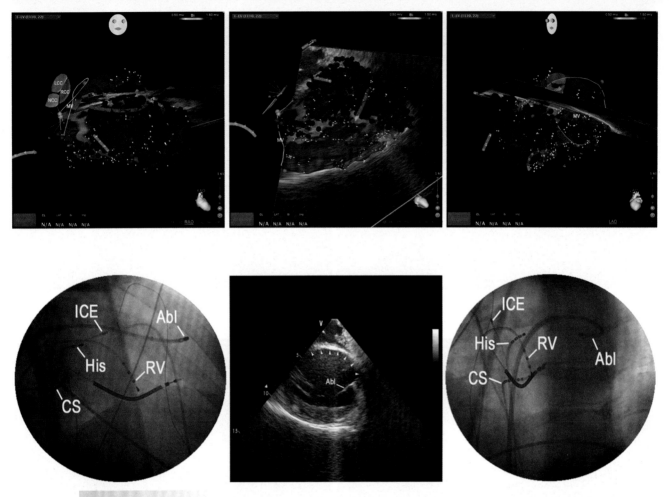

FIGURE 20-22 Endocardial homogenization. Extensive ablation (*red tags*) is delivered to homogenize a large LV anteroseptal aneurysm (*arrows*) with the ablation catheter located at the anterior border of the aneurysm. An ablation line is also created from the inferoseptal portion of the aneurysm to the mitral valve.

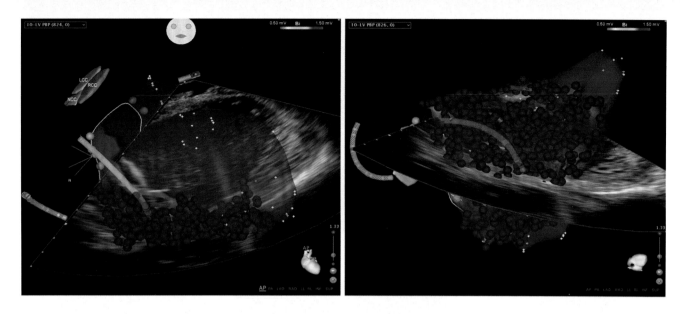

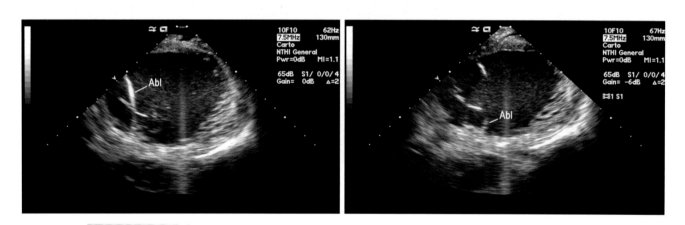

FIGURE 20-23 Endocardial homogenization. Extensive ablation (*red tags*) is delivered to homogenize a large inferior scar. The ablation catheter is positioned on the scar (patchy echogenic areas on intracardiac echocardiography [ICE]).

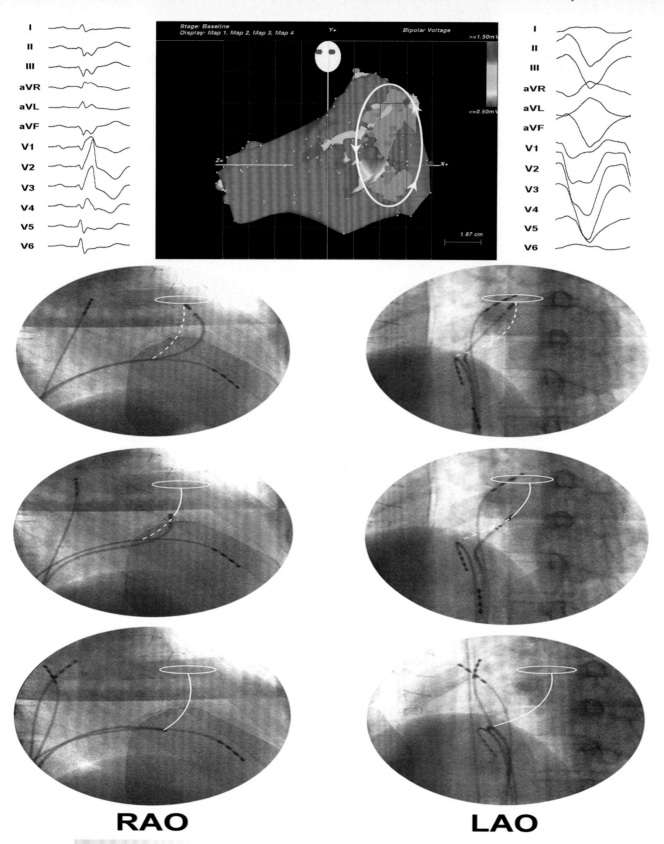

FIGURE 20-24 VT ablation following repaired tetralogy of Fallot. QRS complexes show RBBB during sinus rhythm and LBBB morphology during VT. Electro-anatomic RV bipolar voltage map delineating the ventriculotomy (*gray scar*) around which tachycardia revolves. An ablation line is deployed to create a "line of block" from the pulmonary annulus to the ventriculotomy and ventriculotomy to tricuspid annulus.

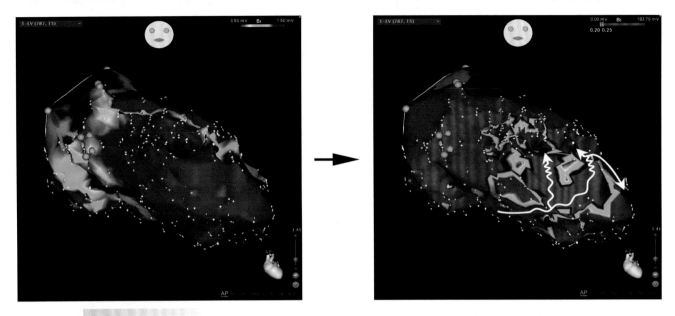

FIGURE 20-25 Voltage channels. *Left*: Electro-anatomic LV bipolar voltage map with standard voltage settings (<0.5 mV: dense scar; 0.5–1.5 mV: border zone; >1.5 mV: normal) showing a large dense anteroseptal scar. *Right*: Voltage threshold adjustment (0.2 mV/0.25 mV) identifies putative conducting channels within the scar with LPs (*black tags*) occurring at the entrance and dead ends.

LP lateness (**Figs. 20-26 to 20-28**). Isolated delayed components are a variant of LP not seen during sinus rhythm and unmasked by RV pacing.[20] One ablation strategy involves complete LP elimination within the scar (**Fig. 20-29**).[33,34] A more selective approach is scar dechanneling (conducting channel electrogram elimination based on the precocity of the LP relative to the local ventricular electrogram) (**Fig. 20-30**).[35,36] Scar dechanneling initially targets the conducting channel entrance (earliest LP) followed by the inner portion of the conducting channel (later LPs) if necessary. Targeting the conducting channel entrance site (which is not necessarily the critical isthmus entrance site) might close the channel as well as other interconnected channels and avoid the need for further ablation of those channels. Rather than a voltage map, a three-dimensional color-coded electro-anatomic map could be created to display the timing of LP and the degree of lateness within scar or isochronal late activation maps displaying regions of slow conduction propagating into the latest zone of activation (deceleration zones).[34,36,37]

Local Abnormal Ventricular Activities

One limitation of targeting LPs is their site dependency. During sinus rhythm, activation of the LV septum precedes the free wall. Late activation of septal scar might occur during ventricular activation and not produce a LP after the QRS complex. Furthermore, simultaneous activation around both sides of the scar can cause overlapping electrograms. While RV pacing could be used to expose LPs by changing the wavefront of activation and unmasking lines of block, LAVAs are a different electrogram target.[38,39] LAVAs are sharp, high-frequency potentials distinct

from the far-field ventricular electrogram that precede, overlap, or follow the far-field ventricular electrogram during sinus rhythm or precede it during VT (**Fig. 20-31**). They are further characterized by ventricular pacing techniques (e.g., extrastimulation) to dissociate them from the far-field ventricular electrogram. Pacing-induced delay between the LAVA and far-field ventricular electrogram indicates poor coupling between LAVA generating muscle bundles and the rest of the myocardium.

Pacemapping

Pacemapping provides complementary information to electrogram analysis during sinus rhythm (or RV pacing) to further guide substrate-based ablation.[40] Characteristic target site pacemaps include 1) perfect pacemaps, 2) long St-QRS intervals (≥40 ms), 3) multiple exit sites (MES), and 4) pacemapping induction (PMI) of VT.[41–46]

Paced QRS Morphology

Because VT morphology reflects the isthmus exit site, direct isthmus stimulation can produce a QRS morphology identical to tachycardia (perfect 12-lead ECG pacemap) (**Figs. 20-3 and 20-32**).[41,42] A short St-QRS interval and perfect (12/12 lead) pacemap indicate exit site stimulation, while a long St-QRS interval and perfect pacemap suggest stimulation from a protected region of slow conduction involving the isthmus (e.g., central isthmus, adjacent bystander). Similar to LPs, pacemapping does not differentiate isthmus from adjacent bystander sites. Imperfect pacemaps might occur with exit site stimulation because radial spread of ventricular activation from a point source during sinus rhythm might not mimic the

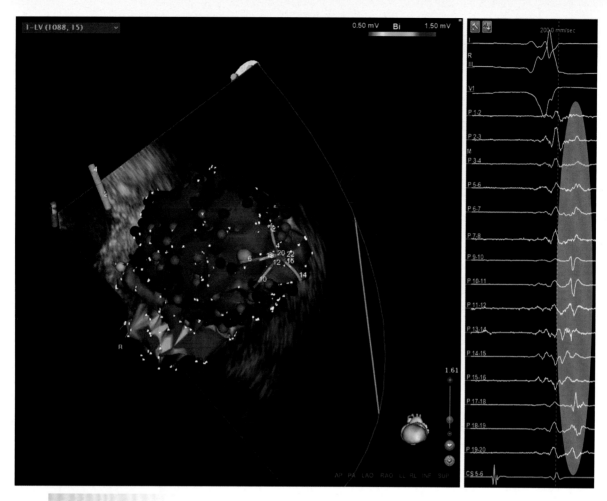

FIGURE 20-26 Late potentials (*encircled*) recorded from the Pentaray catheter positioned at the apex of a large antero-apical aneurysm.

activation wavefront and functional lines of block occurring during VT (eikonal relationship). Additionally, entrance site stimulation more often generate imperfect pacemaps because of antidromic capture of more proximal portions of the circuit.[7] In the absence of an available reference 12-lead ECG of VT for pacemapping, the morphology of stored defibrillator electrograms can be used as a substitute.[47]

Long St-QRS Intervals (≥40 ms)

Pacemapping with long St-QRS intervals (≥40 ms) indicates stimulation of slowly conducting tissue within scar—a prerequisite for reentry and potential isthmus or shared common pathway for VT. Targeting sites with long St-QRS intervals despite imperfect pacemaps could still be helpful during VT ablation.[43,44] Within scar, a relative correlation exists between presence of LP and long St-QRS intervals but is not absolute (which may reflect differences in bidirectional conduction in and out of the channel) (Fig. 20-33).[48] Rather than a voltage map, a three-dimensional color-coded electro-anatomic map could be created to display the degree of stimulus latency within scar.[40]

Multiple Exit Sites

Single site stimulation that produces multiple St-QRS intervals and paced QRS morphologies indicates a common conducting channel with multiple exits (shared common pathway) and is a target site for ablation (Fig. 20-34).[45,46]

Pacemapping Induction

Another functional pacemapping response is induction of VT with pacemapping (pacing cycle lengths = 400–600 ms) in a region of slow conduction (Fig. 20-35).[45] In particular, PMI of the targeted VT with a perfect pacemap predicts an acutely successful ablation site.

ENDPOINTS

The most common procedural endpoint is VT noninducibility. However, with substrate-based ablation, alternative endpoints depend on the strategy employed and include 1) complete LP elimination, 2) complete LAVA elimination (abolition or dissociation of all LAVAs from the far-field ventricular electrogram),

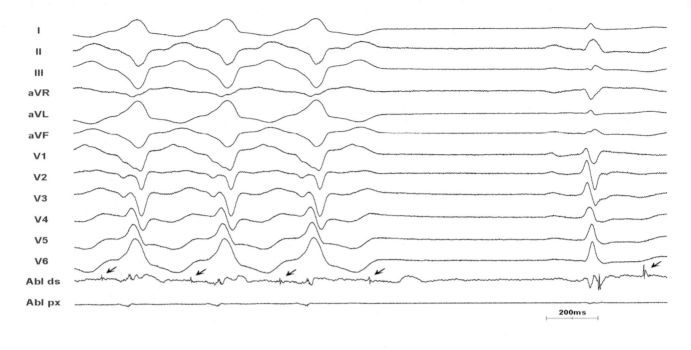

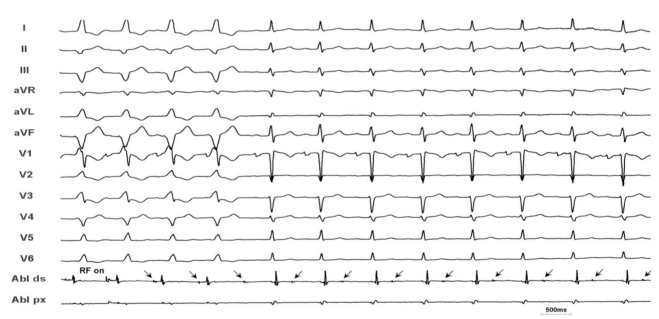

FIGURE 20-27 Late potentials. In both cases, mid-diastolic potentials are recorded during VT with very LPs during sinus rhythm (*arrows*). VT terminates spontaneously (*top*) and during radiofrequency (RF) delivery (*bottom*).

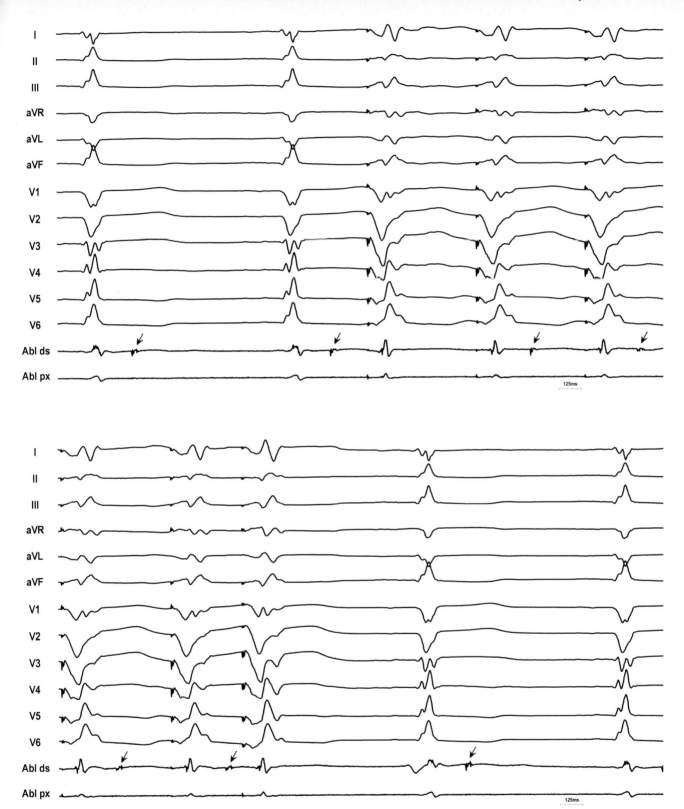

FIGURE 20-28 Late potentials. LPs (*arrows*) are recorded during sinus rhythm and ventricular pacing except following the first and last (extrastimulus) paced complex (tight coupling intervals encroach upon conducting channel refractoriness resulting in entrance block).

Pre RF

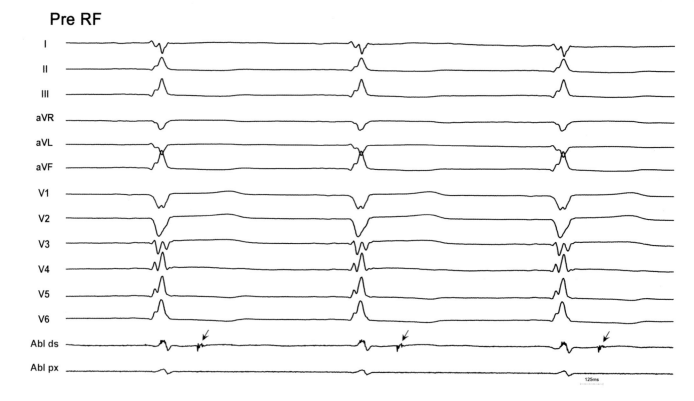

Post RF

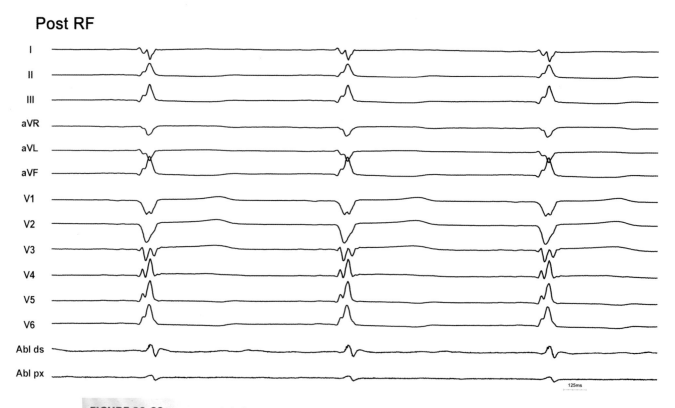

FIGURE 20-29 Late potential abolition. Discrete LPs (*arrows*) are recorded prior to radiofrequency (RF) delivery with their disappearance after ablation. Note that the far-field ventricular electrogram is unchanged (except for loss of high-frequency content).

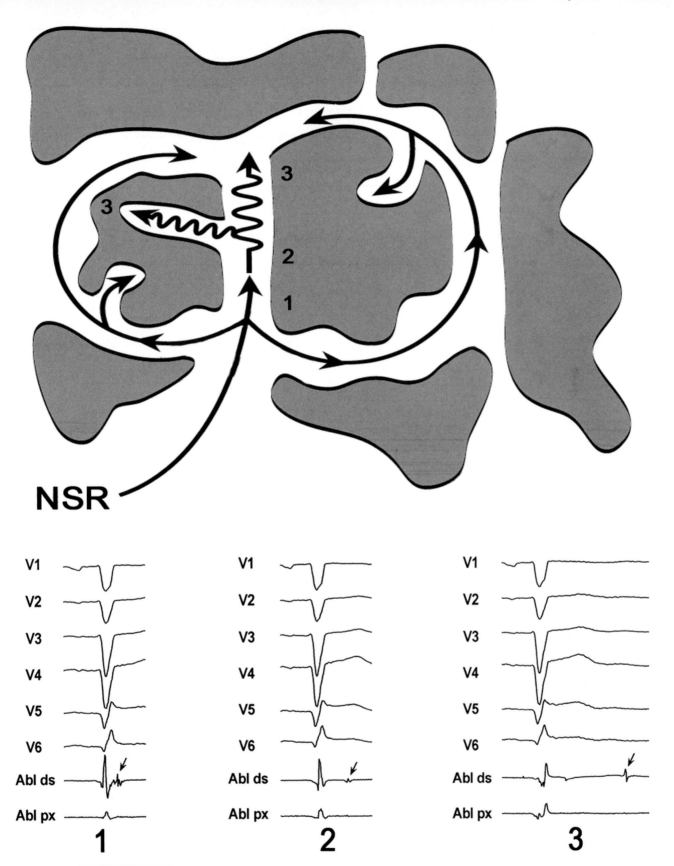

FIGURE 20-30 Scar dechanneling. The earliest and latest LP is recorded at the entrance (site 1) and end (site 3) of a conducting channel. Targeting the most precocious LP (entrance) might close the conducting channel responsible for VT.

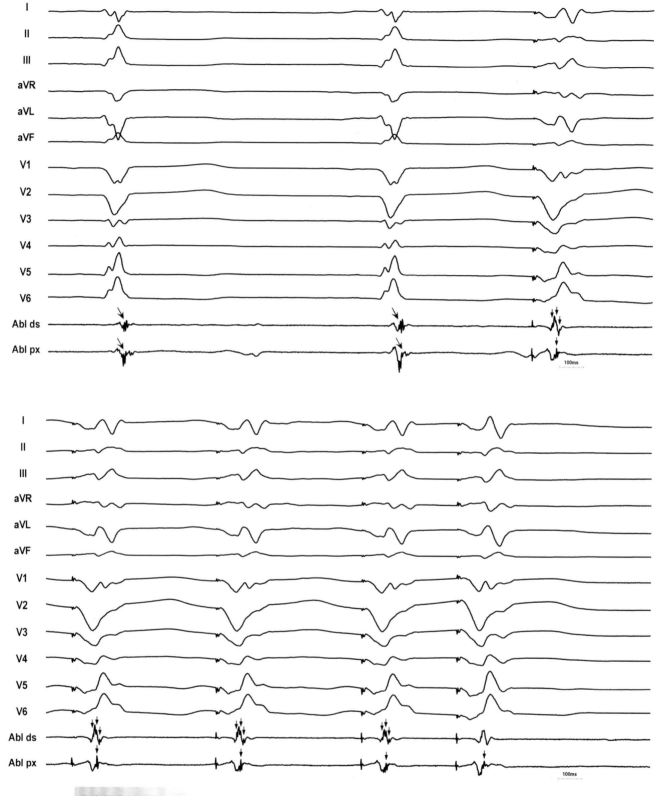

FIGURE 20-31 Local abnormal ventricular activities. Sharp, high-frequency potentials from the infarct border zone are recorded during sinus rhythm (*slanted arrows*) and RV pacing (*smaller, vertical arrows*); are distinct from the overlapping lower frequency, far-field ventricular electrogram; and disappear (Abl ds) after a ventricular extrastimulus (poor coupling between LAVA generating muscle bundles and the rest of the myocardium). Note that these LAVA potentials occur within the QRS complex during sinus rhythm and are therefore not LPs.

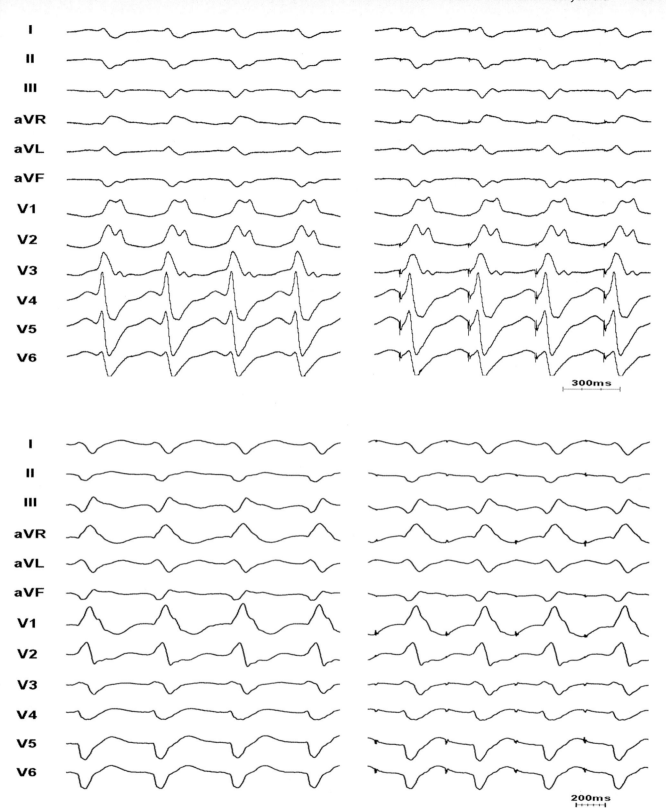

FIGURE 20-32 Pacemapping. VT (*left*) and perfect pacemaps (*right*). *Top*: The short St-QRS interval indicates exit site stimulation. *Bottom*: The long St-QRS interval indicates stimulation from a protected region of slow conduction within the circuit (e.g., central isthmus, adjacent bystander).

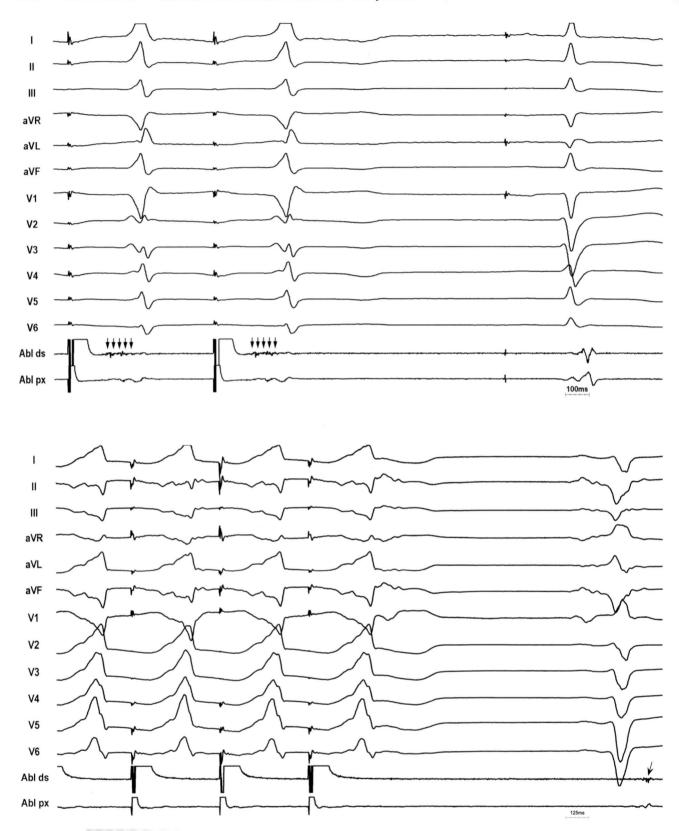

FIGURE 20-33 Long St-QRS intervals. *Top*: Pacing causes a very long St-QRS interval (219 ms) within which continuous, low-amplitude, fractionated potentials (*vertical arrows*) are recorded. *Bottom*: Pacing causes a long St-QRS interval (107 ms) at a site recording an LP (*slanted arrow*) during sinus rhythm.

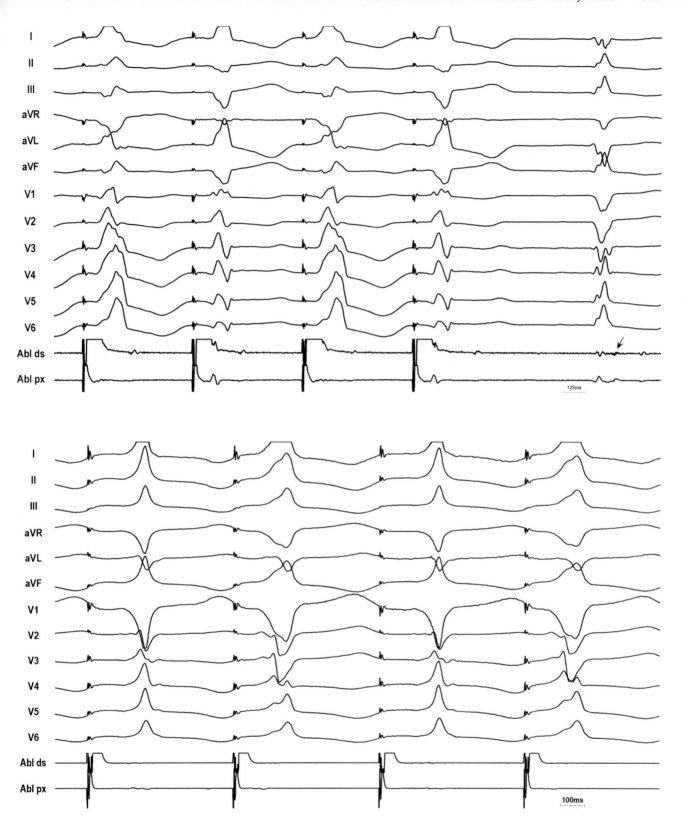

FIGURE 20-34 Multiple exit sites (MES). In both cases, pacing induces alternating stimulus latencies (St-QRS intervals) and QRS morphologies. A LP (*arrow*) is recorded in the top tracing.

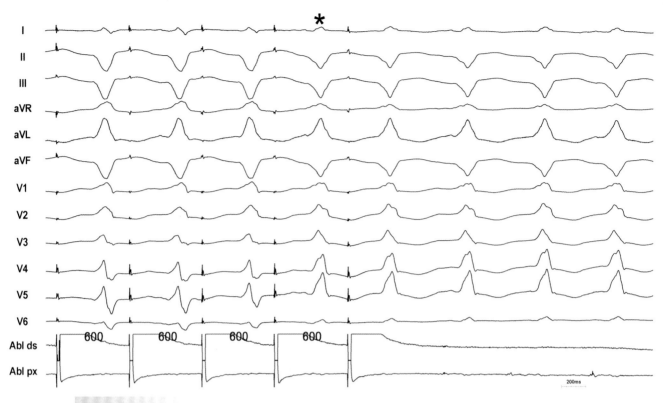

FIGURE 20-35 Pacemapping induction (PMI). Pacing generates long St-QRS intervals (305 ms) followed by VT onset of similar morphology (*asterisk*). Note the absence of electrical activity on the pacing channel.

and 3) rendering the entire scar (or the part containing VT circuit elements [core isolation]) electrically unexcitable (no capture despite high-output pacing [10 mA, 2 ms]) (with high-output stimulation, the virtual electrode generates a pacing field that is larger than the spacing between the true bipolar electrodes, and lack of capture indicates a larger amount of EUS than what is directly beneath the pacing electrodes).[49]

UNUSUAL ELECTROPHYSIOLOGIC PHENOMENA

NONGLOBAL CAPTURE

A pacing stimulus that fails to capture the ventricle but terminates tachycardia (nonglobal capture with or without local capture) is specific for a critical component of the reentrant circuit and should be targeted for ablation.[50–52] Such a nonpropagated stimulus either locally depolarizes or prolongs refractoriness of a critical isthmus rendering it refractory and terminating VT. Mechanisms include subthreshold stimulation of poorly coupled surviving myocytes within scar having both diminished excitability and complex anisotropy as well as postrepolarization refractoriness.[51] Another target for ablation are sites where mechanical trauma from catheter manipulation interrupts VT without inducing a PVC.[53]

SCAR CHANNEL ENTRANCE/EXIT BLOCK

Manifestations of entrance block into a scar channel are LPs during sinus rhythm demonstrating 2:1 or Wenckebach conduction or diastolic potentials during VT with 2:1 conduction. Manifestations of exit block from a scar channel include stimulation with 2:1 or Wenckebach conduction (**Fig. 20-36**).

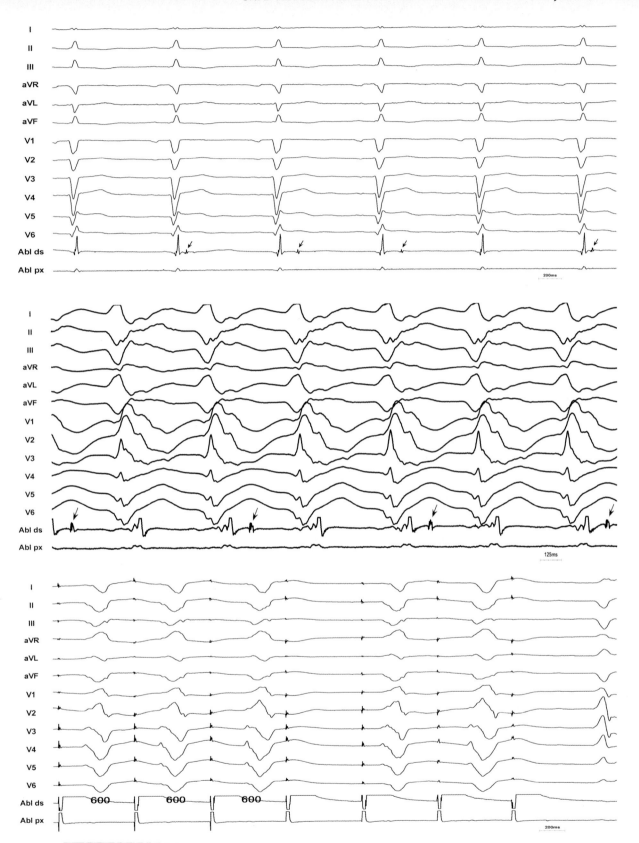

FIGURE 20-36 Scar channel entrance/exit block. *Top*: Entrance Wenckebach. During sinus rhythm, the degree of LP lateness (*arrows*) increases until block. *Middle*: Entrance 2:1 block. During VT, diastolic potentials (*arrows*) are seen on alternate beats. *Bottom*: Exit Wenckebach. Pacing causes increasing stimulus latencies (prolonging St-QRS intervals) and QRS widening prior to block ("noncapture").

REFERENCES

1. Morady F, Frank R, Kou WH, et al. Identification and catheter ablation of a zone of slow conduction in the reentrant circuit of ventricular tachycardia in humans. J Am Coll Cardiol 1988;11:775–782.
2. Stevenson WG, Khan H, Sager P, et al. Identification of reentry circuit sites during catheter mapping and radiofrequency ablation of ventricular tachycardia late after myocardial infarction. Circulation 1993;88(4, pt 1):1647–1670.
3. Morady F, Harvey M, Kalbfleisch SJ, El-Atassi R, Calkins H, Langberg JJ. Radiofrequency catheter ablation of ventricular tachycardia in patients with coronary artery disease. Circulation 1993;87:363–372.
4. Stevenson WG, Friedman PL, Sager PT, et al. Exploring postinfarction reentrant ventricular tachycardia with entrainment mapping. J Am Coll Cardiol 1997;29:1180–1189.
5. Sacher F, Roberts-Thomson K, Maury P, et al. Epicardial ventricular tachycardia ablation a multicenter safety study. J Am Coll Cardiol 2010;55:2366–2372.
6. Hsia HH, Lin D, Sauer WH, Callans DJ, Marchlinski FE. Anatomic characterization of endocardial substrate for hemodynamically stable reentrant ventricular tachycardia: identification of endocardial conducting channels. Heart Rhythm 2006;3:503–512.
7. de Chillou C, Groben L, Magnin-Poull I, et al. Localizing the critical isthmus of postinfarct ventricular tachycardia: the value of pace-mapping during sinus rhythm. Heart Rhythm 2014;11:175–181.
8. Miller JM, Marchlinski FE, Buxton AE, Josephson ME. Relationship between the 12-lead electrocardiogram during ventricular tachycardia and endocardial site of origin in patients with coronary artery disease. Circulation 1988;77:759–766.
9. Wilber DJ, Kopp DE, Glascock DN, Kinder CA, Kall JG. Catheter ablation of the mitral isthmus for ventricular tachycardia associated with inferior infarction. Circulation 1995;92:3481–3489.
10. Ellison KE, Friedman PL, Ganz LI, Stevenson WG. Entrainment mapping and radiofrequency catheter ablation of ventricular tachycardia in right ventricular dysplasia. J Am Coll Cardiol 1998;32:724–728.
11. Kocovic DZ, Harada T, Friedman PL, Stevenson WG. Characteristics of electrograms recorded at reentry circuit sites and bystanders during ventricular tachycardia after myocardial infarction. J Am Coll Cardiol 1999;34:381–388.
12. Delacretaz E, Stevenson WG. Catheter ablation of ventricular tachycardia in patients with coronary heart disease: part I: mapping. Pacing Clin Electrophysiol 2001;24:1261–1277.
13. Zeppenfeld K, Stevenson WG. Ablation of ventricular tachycardia in patients with structural heart disease. Pacing Clin Electrophysiol 2008;31:358–374.
14. Fitzgerald DM, Friday KJ, Wah JA, Lazzara R, Jackman WM. Electrogram patterns predicting successful catheter ablation of ventricular tachycardia. Circulation 1988;77:806–814.
15. Beaser AD, Chua KC, Upadhyay GA, Tung R. Entrainment of ventricular tachycardia: is the pacing site in or out? Heart Rhythm 2016;13:2399–2400.
16. Soejima K, Stevenson WG, Maisel WH, et al. The N + 1 difference: a new measure for entrainment mapping. J Am Coll Cardiol 2001;37:1386–1394.
17. Santangeli P, Marchlinski FE. Substrate mapping for unstable ventricular tachycardia. Heart Rhythm 2016;13:569–583.
18. de Bakker JM, van Capelle FJ, Janse MJ, et al. Slow conduction in the infarcted human heart. 'Zigzag' course of activation. Circulation 1993;88:915–926.
19. Marchlinski FE, Callans DJ, Gottlieb CD, Zado E. Linear ablation lesions for control of unmappable ventricular tachycardia in patients with ischemic and nonischemic cardiomyopathy. Circulation 2000;101:1288–1296.
20. Arenal A, Glez-Torrecilla E, Ortiz M, et al. Ablation of electrograms with an isolated, delayed component as treatment of unmappable monomorphic ventricular tachycardias in patients with structural heart disease. J Am Coll Cardiol 2003;41:81–92.
21. Soejima K, Suzuki M, Maisel WH, et al. Catheter ablation in patients with multiple and unstable ventricular tachycardias after myocardial infarction: short ablation lines guided by reentry circuit isthmuses and sinus rhythm mapping. Circulation 2001;104:664–669.
22. Tzou WS, Frankel DS, Hegeman T, et al. Core isolation of critical arrhythmia elements for treatment of multiple scar-based ventricular tachycardias. Circ Arrhythm Electrophysiol 2015;8:353–361.
23. Di Biase L, Santangeli P, Burkhardt DJ, et al. Endo-epicardial homogenization of the scar versus limited substrate ablation for the treatment of electrical storms in patients with ischemic cardiomyopathy. J Am Coll Cardiol 2012;60:132–141.
24. Zeppenfeld K, Schalij MJ, Bartelings MM, et al. Catheter ablation of ventricular tachycardia after repair of congenital heart disease: electroanatomic identification of the critical right ventricular isthmus. Circulation 2007;116:2241–2252.
25. Khairy P, Stevenson WG. Catheter ablation in tetralogy of Fallot. Heart Rhythm 2009;6:1069–1074.
26. Harrison DA, Harris L, Siu SC, et al. Sustained ventricular tachycardia in adult patients late after repair of tetralogy of Fallot. J Am Coll Cardiol 1997;30:1368–1373.
27. Arenal A, del Castillo S, Gonzalez-Torrecilla E, et al. Tachycardia-related channel in the scar tissue in patients with sustained monomorphic ventricular tachycardia: influence of the voltage scar definition. Circulation 2004;110:2568–2574.
28. Mountantonakis SE, Park RE, Frankel DS, et al. Relationship between voltage map "channels" and the location of critical isthmus sites in patients with post-infarction cardiomyopathy and ventricular tachycardia. J Am Coll Cardiol 2013;61:2088–2095.
29. Dickfeld T, Tian J, Ahmad G, et al. MRI-guided ventricular tachycardia ablation: integration of late gadolinium-enhanced 3D scar in patients with implantable cardioverter-defibrillators. Circ Arrhythm Electrophysiol 2011;4:172–184.
30. Perez-David E, Arenal A, Rubio-Guivernau JL, et al. Noninvasive identification of ventricular tachycardia-related conducting channels using contrast-enhanced magnetic resonance imaging in patients with chronic myocardial infarction: comparison of signal intensity scar mapping and endocardial voltage mapping. J Am Coll Cardiol 2011;57:184–194.
31. Sasaki T, Miller CF, Hansford R, et al. Myocardial structural associations with local electrograms: a study of postinfarct ventricular tachycardia pathophysiology and magnetic resonance-based noninvasive mapping. Circ Arrhythm Electrophysiol 2012;5:1081–1090.
32. Harada T, Stevenson WG, Kocovic DZ, Friedman PL. Catheter ablation of ventricular tachycardia after myocardial infarction: relation of endocardial sinus rhythm late potentials to the reentry circuit. J Am Coll Cardiol 1997;30:1015–1023.
33. Nogami A, Sugiyasu A, Tada H, et al. Changes in the isolated delayed component as an endpoint of catheter ablation in arrhythmogenic right ventricular cardiomyopathy: predictor for long-term success. J Cardiovasc Electrophysiol 2008;19:681–688.
34. Vergara P, Trevisi N, Ricco A, et al. Late potentials abolition as an additional technique for reduction of arrhythmia recurrence in scar related ventricular tachycardia ablation. J Cardiovasc Electrophysiol 2012;23:621–627.
35. Berruezo A, Fernández-Armenta J, Andreu D, et al. Scar dechanneling: new method for scar-related left ventricular tachycardia substrate ablation. Circ Arrhythm Electrophysiol 2015;8:326–336.
36. Tung R, Mathuria NS, Nagel R, et al. Impact of local ablation on interconnected channels within ventricular scar: mechanistic implications for substrate modification. Circ Arrhythm Electrophysiol 2013;6:1131–1138.
37. Irie T, Yu R, Bradfield JS, et al. Relationship between sinus rhythm late activation zones and critical sites for scar-related ventricular tachycardia: systematic analysis of isochronal late activation mapping. Circ Arrhythm Electrophysiol 2015;8:390–399.
38. Jais P, Maury P, Khairy P, et al. Elimination of local abnormal ventricular activities: a new end point for substrate modification in patients with scar-related ventricular tachycardia. Circulation 2012;125:2184–2196.
39. Sacher F, Lim HS, Derval N, et al. Substrate mapping and ablation for ventricular tachycardia: the LAVA approach. J Cardiovasc Electrophysiol 2015;26:464–471.
40. Baldinger SH, Nagashima K, Kumar S, et al. Electrogram analysis and pacing are complimentary for recognition of abnormal conduction and far-field potentials during substrate mapping of infarct-related ventricular tachycardia. Circ Arrhythm Electrophysiol 2015;8:874–881.
41. Josephson ME, Waxman HL, Cain ME, Gardner MJ, Buxton AE. Ventricular activation during ventricular endocardial pacing. II. Role of pace-mapping to localize origin of ventricular tachycardia. Am J Cardiol 1982;50:11–22.
42. Brunckhorst CB, Delacretaz E, Soejima K, Maisel WH, Friedman PL, Stevenson WG. Identification of the ventricular tachycardia isthmus after infarction by pace mapping. Circulation 2004;110:652–659.
43. Stevenson WG, Sager PT, Natterson PD, Saxon LA, Middlekauff HR, Wiener I. Relation of pace mapping QRS configuration and conduction delay to ventricular tachycardia reentry circuits in human infarct scars. J Am Coll Cardiol 1995;26:481–488.
44. Brunckhorst CB, Stevenson WG, Soejima K, et al. Relationship of slow conduction detected by pace-mapping to ventricular tachycardia re-entry circuit sites after infarction. J Am Coll Cardiol 2003;41:802–809.
45. Tung R, Mathuria N, Michowitz Y, et al. Functional pace-mapping responses for identification of targets for catheter ablation of scar-mediated ventricular tachycardia. Circ Arrhythm Electrophysiol 2012;5:264–272.
46. Tung R, Shivkumar K. Unusual response to entrainment of ventricular tachycardia: in or out? Heart Rhythm 2014;11:725–727.
47. Yoshida K, Liu T, Scott C, et al. The value of defibrillator electrograms for recognition of clinical ventricular tachycardias and for pace mapping of post-infarction ventricular tachycardia. J Am Coll Cardiol 2010;56:969–979.
48. Bogun F, Good E, Reich S, et al. Isolated potentials during sinus rhythm and pace-mapping within scars as guides for ablation of post-infarction ventricular tachycardia. J Am Coll Cardiol 2006;47:2013–2019.
49. Soejima K, Stevenson WG, Maisel WH, Sapp JL, Epstein LM. Electrically unexcitable scar mapping based on pacing threshold for identification of the reentry circuit isthmus: feasibility for guiding ventricular tachycardia ablation. Circulation 2002;106:1678–1683.
50. Garan H, Ruskin JN. Reproducible termination of ventricular tachycardia by a single extrastimulus within the reentry circuit during the ventricular effective refractory period. Am Heart J 1988;116:546–550.
51. Bogun F, Krishnan SC, Marine JE, et al. Catheter ablation guided by termination of postinfarction ventricular tachycardia by pacing with nonglobal capture. Heart Rhythm 2004;1:422–426.
52. Altemose GT, Miller JM. Termination of ventricular tachycardia by a non-propagated extrastimulus. J Cardiovasc Electrophysiol 2000;11:125.
53. Bogun F, Good E, Han J, et al. Mechanical interruption of postinfarction ventricular tachycardia as a guide for catheter ablation. Heart Rhythm 2005;2:687–691.

Bundle Branch Reentrant Tachycardia

21

Introduction

Bundle branch reentrant tachycardia (BBRT) ("bundle to bundle" tachycardia) is a macroreentrant ventricular tachycardia (VT) that utilizes both right bundle (RB) and left bundle (LB) branches as integral components of the reentry circuit.[1] Classically, BBRT occurs in patients with severe His-Purkinje disease with a clinical triad of 1) prolonged HV interval, 2) left bundle branch block (LBBB) (or IVCD), and 3) dilated cardiomyopathy. However, it can also occur in patients with isolated (fixed or functional) His-Purkinje system disease without cardiomyopathy (e.g., myotonic dystrophy, prior aortic valve replacement).[2–5] BBRT presents as syncope or cardiac arrest in 75% of patients.[6]

The purpose of this chapter is to:

1. Define the circuit and electrophysiologic features of BBRT.
2. Discuss mapping and ablation of the RB and LB branches.
3. Discuss the circuit and electrophysiologic features of interfascicular reentrant tachycardia (IFRT).

CIRCUIT

During typical BBRT, the antegrade and retrograde limbs of the circuit are the RB and LB branches, respectively, resulting in counterclockwise activation of the bundle branches (Fig. 21-1). Onset of ventricular activation occurs at the terminal branches of the RB resulting in typical LBBB QRS complexes that can appear identical to baseline LBBB (Fig. 21-2). After activating the RB, the depolarizing wavefront crosses the lower interventricular septum to retrogradely activate the LB. Following activation of the LB, the wavefront crosses the upper interventricular septum to again depolarize the RB. Sustained tachycardia requires that conduction times over each bundle exceed the refractory period of its counterpart. During atypical BBRT, the circuit is reversed and the bundle branches are activated in clockwise fashion.

ELECTROPHYSIOLOGIC FEATURES

The characteristic electrophysiologic features of typical BBRT are 1) typical LBBB QRS complexes, 2) His bundle potentials preceding QRS complexes, 3) $HV_{(BBRT)} \geq HV_{(NSR)}$, and 4) H-RB-LB activation sequence (Figs. 21-3 to 21-6).[6] Onset of ventricular activation from the RB produces QRS complexes showing typical LBBB. His bundle potentials precede each QRS complex. Although the HV interval is a pseudo-interval (simultaneous activation of the His bundle retrogradely and RB-V antegradely), anisotropic conduction across the His-Purkinje system produces HV intervals that exceed or equal those during sinus rhythm.[7] Close proximity between the upper turnaround site and the His bundle results in oscillations of the HH interval preceding and predicting oscillations in the tachycardia cycle length (TCL).[8,9] However, the His bundle itself is not truly an integral part of the circuit and can rarely be dissociated from BBRT.[10] In contrast to BBRT, septal VT with retrograde activation of the His bundle demonstrates shorter HV intervals during tachycardia compared to sinus rhythm ($HV_{[VT]} < HV_{[NSR]}$). Counterclockwise activation of the bundle branches produces H-RB-LB activation sequence. Atypical (reverse) BBRT manifests right bundle branch block (RBBB) QRS complexes and H-LB-RB activation sequences.

During sinus rhythm, QRS complexes often show typical LBBB resulting from antegrade His-LB conduction delay rather than failure. A rare finding is the occurrence of a second His bundle potential after conducted LBBB QRS complexes due to late retrograde activation of the LB and His bundle that can mimic a dual antegrade His bundle response (see Fig. 1-40).[3,11]

ZONES OF TRANSITION

INITIATION

Induction of typical BBRT by right ventricular (RV) extrastimulation requires that an impulse fall into the tachycardia window (defined as the difference in retrograde refractory periods between the RB and LB branches). A critically timed impulse 1) fails to conduct over the RB (unidirectional block) and 2) crosses the septum to retrogradely activate the LB and His

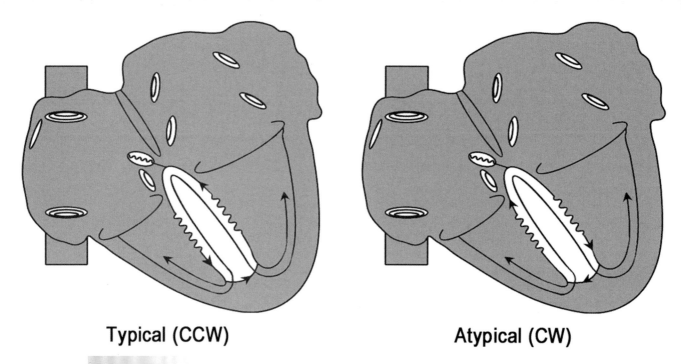

Typical (CCW)   **Atypical (CW)**

FIGURE 21-1 Diagram illustrating the circuits for typical (counterclockwise [CCW]) and atypical (clockwise [CW] or reverse) BBRT.

bundle resulting in a "VH jump" (slow conduction) (**Figs. 21-7 and 21-8**).[12] Sufficient VH delay allows the RB to recover excitability, conduct antegradely, and initiate tachycardia. The length of the VH jump is inversely related to the subsequent HV interval (VH/HV reciprocity). While induction of single BBR complexes by programmed ventricular extrastimulation is a common finding in normal individuals, development of sustained BBRT only occurs in patients with diseased His-Purkinje tissue. Induction of BBRT can be facilitated by procainamide (which further slows His-Purkinje conduction) or short-long-short sequences (pause protocol—which widens the tachycardia window by increasing the dispersion of refractoriness between the bundle branches) (**Fig. 21-9**).[13,14] Induction of BBRT can be abolished by simultaneous RV and left ventricular (LV) stimulation, which prevents transeptal conduction and the "VH jump." BBRT can also be induced from the atrium by pacing-induced functional block in the His-Purkinje system (e.g., abrupt HV prolongation with development of phase 3 LBBB).[4]

TERMINATION

Block in the RB or LB branch causes termination of BBRT. Spontaneous termination before the next His bundle potential or immediately after it during typical BBRT indicates block in the LB or RB, respectively (**Fig. 21-10**).

PACING MANEUVERS

ENTRAINMENT FROM THE ATRIUM

Reentry within the His-Purkinje system allows BBRT to be entrained from the atrium provided that the atrio-ventricular (AV)

node can accommodate rapid atrial pacing rates (which might require atropine/isoproterenol). Atrial pacing accelerates both the His bundle and ventricle to the pacing rate producing QRS complexes identical to those during tachycardia (orthodromically concealed QRS fusion), a feature not characteristic of myocardial VT.[15]

ENTRAINMENT FROM THE VENTRICLE

Reentry within the His-Purkinje system allows BBRT to be entrained from the RV apex near the terminal branches of the RB with constant manifest fusion (although concealed entrainment is possible if the collision point between orthodromic [*n*] and antidromic [*n* + 1] wavefronts is within the His-Purkinje system) (**Fig. 21-11**).[15] Because of the close proximity between the RV pacing catheter and BBRT circuit, post-pacing intervals (PPIs) are similar to the TCL (PPI − TCL <30 ms).[16] In contrast, atrio-ventricular nodal reentrant tachycardia (AVNRT) with LBBB and AV dissociation can mimic BBRT, but entrainment from the ventricle is only concealed and PPI − TCL >115 ms.[17]

MAPPING AND ABLATION OF BBRT

The bundle branches are integral components of the BBRT circuit and targets for ablation. While ablation of the RB is technically easier than the LB, it carries a risk of inducing AV block when LBBB (due to LB antegrade conduction failure) is present.

RIGHT BUNDLE ABLATION

The ablation catheter is advanced across the tricuspid valve into the RV and positioned along the anteroseptum slightly distal to the His bundle with clockwise torque. Target site criteria

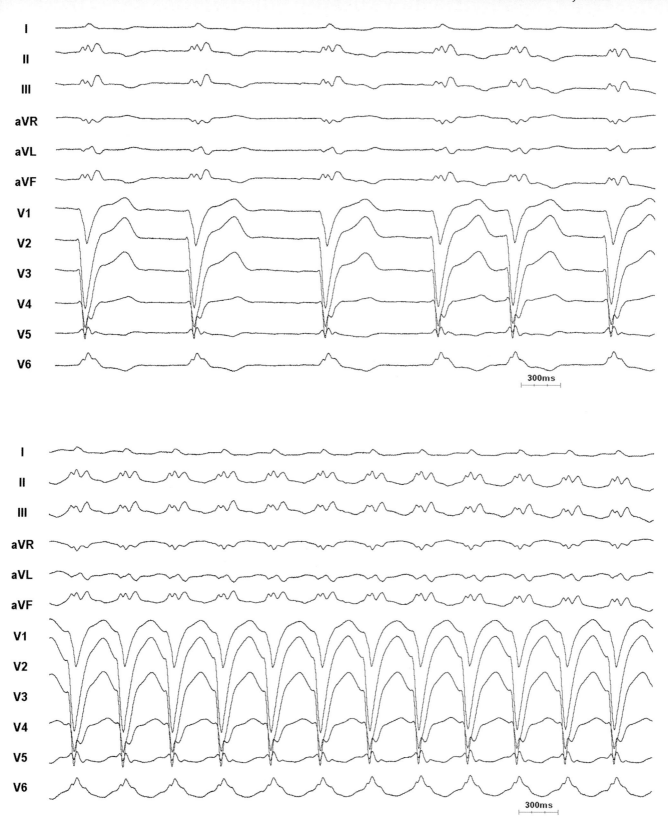

FIGURE 21-2 Atrial fibrillation with typical LBBB (*top*) and typical BBRT (*bottom*). QRS complexes are identical.

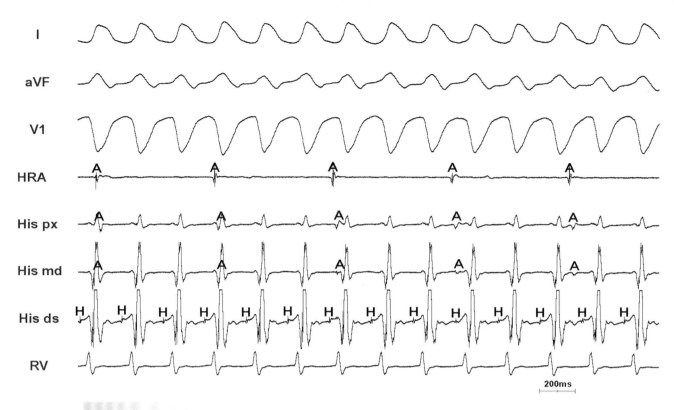

FIGURE 21-3 Typical BBRT. His bundle potentials precede typical LBBB QRS complexes (HV = 58 ms). AV dissociation is present.

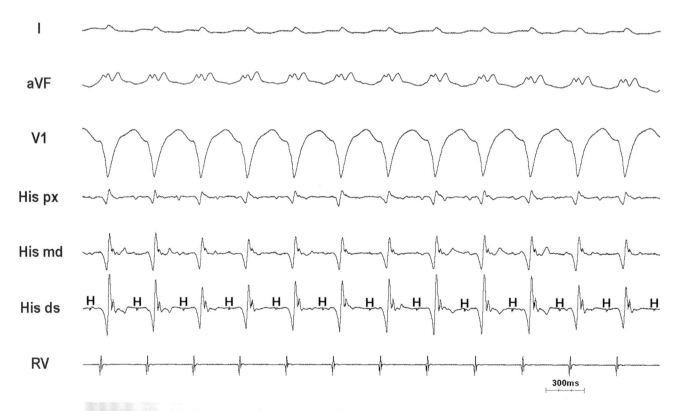

FIGURE 21-4 Typical BBRT. His bundle potentials precede typical LBBB QRS complexes (HV = 81 ms).

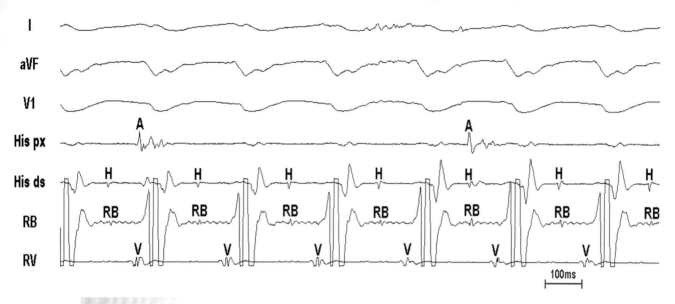

FIGURE 21-5 Typical BBRT. A His-RB activation sequence precedes LBBB QRS complexes. (HV = 82 ms). AV dissociation is present.

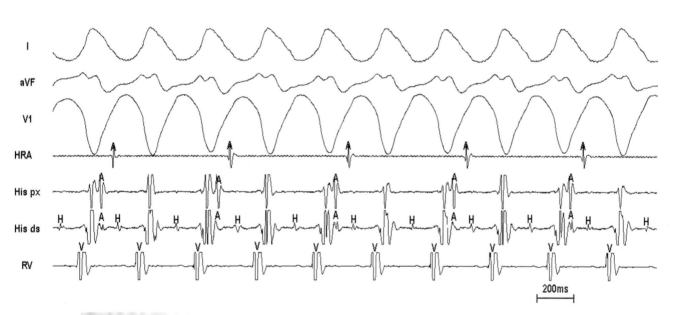

FIGURE 21-6 Typical BBRT. His bundle potentials precede LBBB QRS complexes (HV = 75 ms). 2:1 retrograde conduction occurs over the AV node.

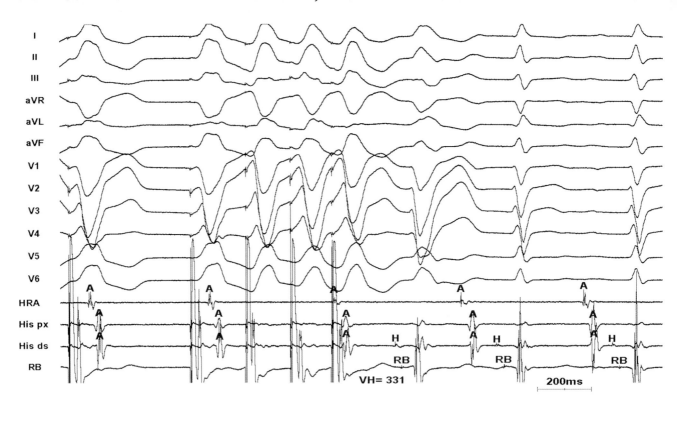

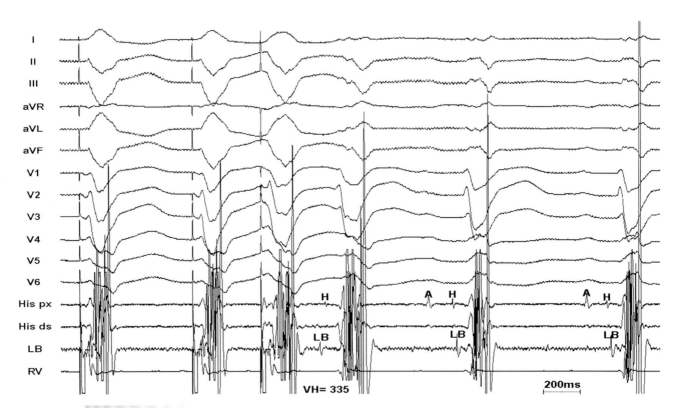

FIGURE 21-7 His/RB/LB activation patterns during typical BBR complexes. Single BBR complexes are induced by ventricular extrastimuli. *Top*: Following the "VH jump" (331 ms), RB follows His bundle potentials. *Bottom*: Preceding the "VH jump" (335 ms), LB precedes His bundle potentials.

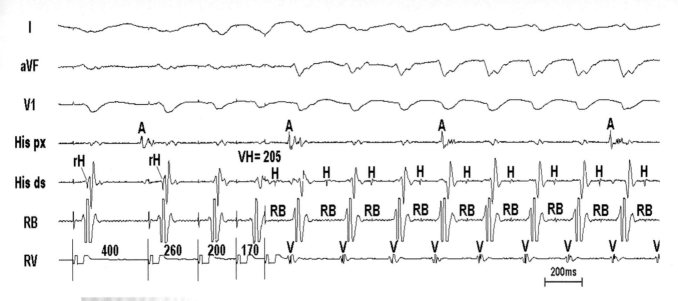

FIGURE 21-8 Induction of typical BBRT. During the drive train (400 ms), retrograde His bundle potentials (rH) precede local ventricular electrograms due to retrograde RB conduction. The second extrastimulus captures the ventricle, encounters RB refractoriness, crosses the septum, and retrogradely activates the LB and His bundle ("VH jump" = 205 ms). Sufficient LB delay allows the RB to recover excitability, conduct antegradely, and initiate tachycardia. The His bundle and RB are sequentially activated, and AV dissociation is present.

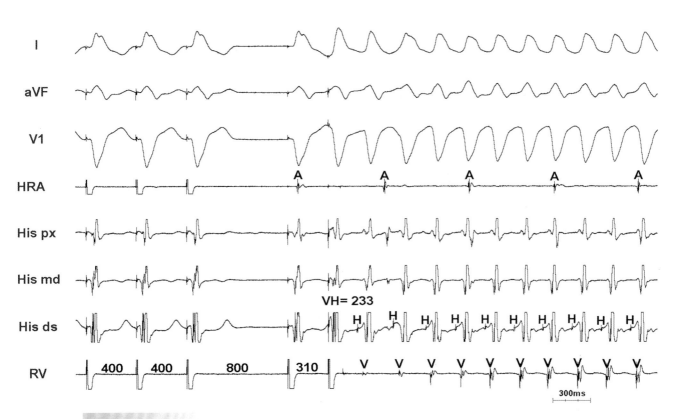

FIGURE 21-9 Induction of typical BBRT (pause protocol). The pause (800 ms) increases dispersion of bundle branch refractoriness so that the extrastimulus (310 ms) causes a "VH jump" (233 ms) and induces tachycardia. His bundle potentials precede QRS complexes (HV = 58 ms), and oscillations in the HH interval precede and predict VV intervals. AV dissociation is present.

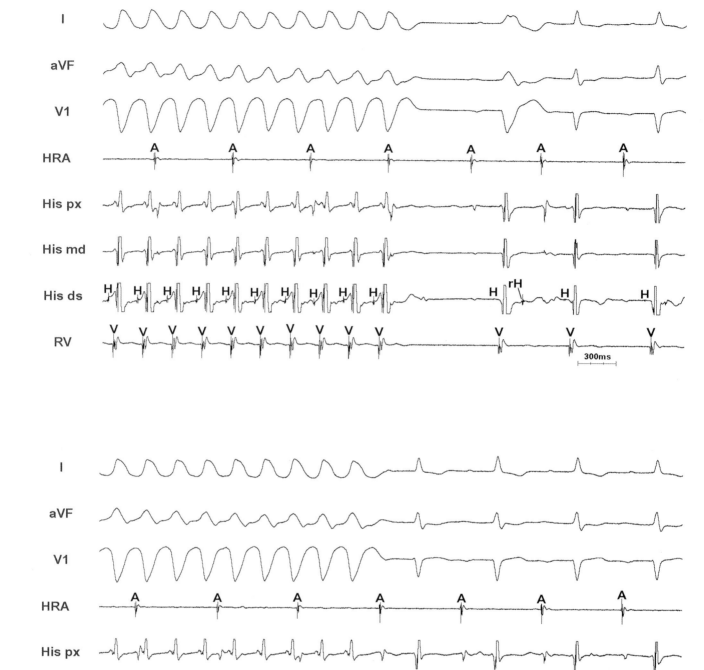

FIGURE 21-10 Termination of typical BBRT. Abrupt termination results from retrograde block in the LB. *Top*: Late timing of the first conducted sinus complex exposes the LB to a pause, which induces phase 4 LBBB. Phase 4 LBBB is followed by a retrograde His bundle potential (rH), but BBRT is not reinitiated because the pause prolongs RB refractoriness that prevents subsequent antegrade RB conduction. *Bottom*: Early timing of the first conducted sinus complex upon tachycardia termination prevents phase 4 LBBB.

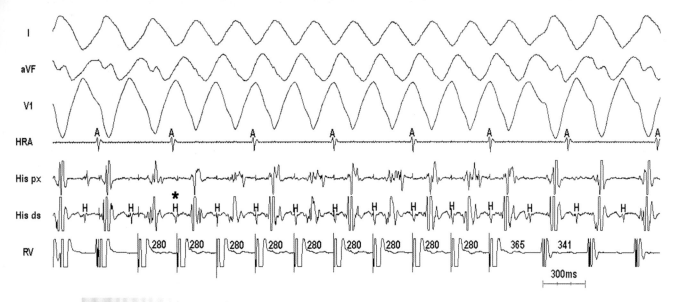

FIGURE 21-11 Entrainment of typical BBRT from the RV apex. The His bundle is orthodromically activated and accelerated to the pacing cycle length. Note that the His bundle is advanced (*asterisk*) by a fused ventricular paced complex (an indication of macroreentry). The PPI exceeds the TCL by only 24 ms.

are 1) absent or small atrial electrogram, 2) RB potential, and 3) large ventricular electrogram (**Figs. 21-12 and 21-13**).[18–22] Absence of an atrial electrogram differentiates a His bundle from RB potential when the RB-V interval is long (>35 ms) due to underlying RB disease. Ablation of the RB during preexisting LBBB often causes marked HV interval prolongation accompanied by a change to RBBB indicating that LBBB itself was due to antegrade conduction delay rather than failure.

LEFT BUNDLE ABLATION

With a transaortic approach, the ablation catheter is advanced retrogradely across the aortic valve into the LV and positioned along the septum. A right-sided His bundle catheter serves as a useful reference landmark of the His bundle region. Target site criteria are 1) absent or small atrial electrogram, 2) LB potential, and 3) large ventricular electrogram (**Fig. 21-14**). Ablation of the LB during preexisting LBBB causes further aberration of the QRS complex as delayed conduction over the LB fails.[21,22]

INTERFASCICULAR REENTRANT TACHYCARDIA

IFRT is a rare, unique form of His-Purkinje reentry that utilizes the left-sided fascicles as critical limbs of the reentrant circuit. In its common form, antegrade and retrograde conduction occur over the left anterior fascicle (LAF) and left posterior fascicle (LPF), respectively, resulting in 1) RBBB-RAD QRS complexes, 2) His bundle potentials preceding QRS complexes, and 3) $HV_{(IFRT)} < HV_{(NSR)}$ (**Fig. 21-15**).[23] Because His bundle potentials precede QRS complexes, HH oscillations precede and predict VV oscillations. The HV interval is a pseudo-interval that reflects simultaneous activation of the

truncal LB–His bundle axis retrogradely and LAF–LV antegradely after the reentrant wavefront reaches the upper turn-around point at the LPF–LAF junction. In contrast to BBRT, IFRT more commonly shows baseline RBBB and easier induction from the atrium.[23] The unusual observation that many cases of IFRT occur after catheter ablation of the RB for BBRT suggests that RB conduction is protective against IFRT. With RB conduction, transeptal conduction and retrograde activation of the LB system collides with antegrade LAF conduction preventing development of IFRT from the atrium. With RBBB, loss of RB conduction and retrograde concealment into the LAF allow a conducting impulse from the atrium to block antegradely in the LPF (unidirectional block), conduct slowly over the LAF (conduction delay), reenter the LPF retrogradely, and initiate IFRT. IFRT can be successfully treated by ablation of the LAF or LPF.

In contrast to scar-related VT, insulated conducting fascicles are the essential circuit components for His-Purkinje tachycardias (BBRT, IFRT). Entrainment mapping therefore requires determination of whether the fascicles (fascicular potentials "in" the circuit), adjacent ventricular myocardium ("out" of the circuit), or both are captured during pacing. Analogous to pure and parahisian entrainment, pure fascicular (selective) entrainment of the antegradely conducting fascicle would produce an "isthmus" site (St-QRS latency, concealed QRS fusion, PPI = TCL). (However, antidromic capture from the retrogradely conducting fascicle near the entrance might produce manifest fusion.) Para-fascicular (nonselective) entrainment would generate an "outer" loop site (manifest QRS fusion [due to surrounding myocardial capture], PPI = TCL). Entrainment with pure myocardial capture would produce a "remote bystander" site (manifest fusion, PPI > TCL), and the fascicular potential would be orthodromically (not directly) captured.

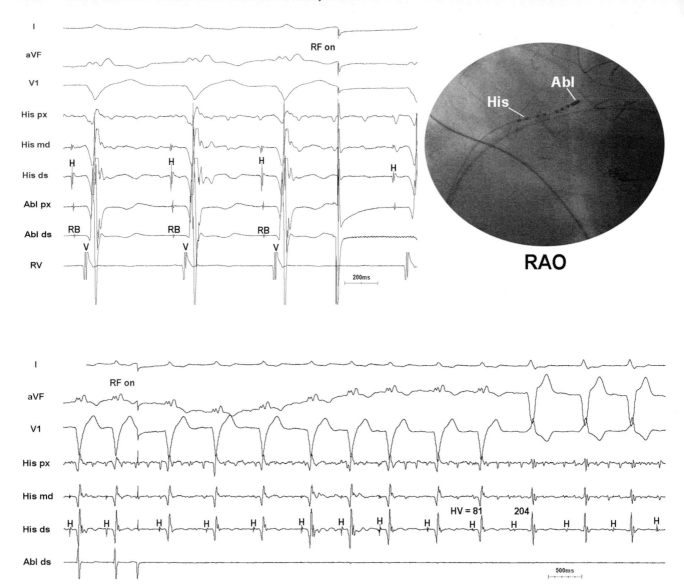

FIGURE 21-12 Ablation of the RB. The ablation catheter is positioned at the proximal RB distal to the His bundle where it records a RB potential and large ventricular electrogram (RB-V = 66 ms). Radiofrequency (RF) delivery changes the QRS morphology from LBBB to RBBB accompanied by 123 ms prolongation of the HV interval.

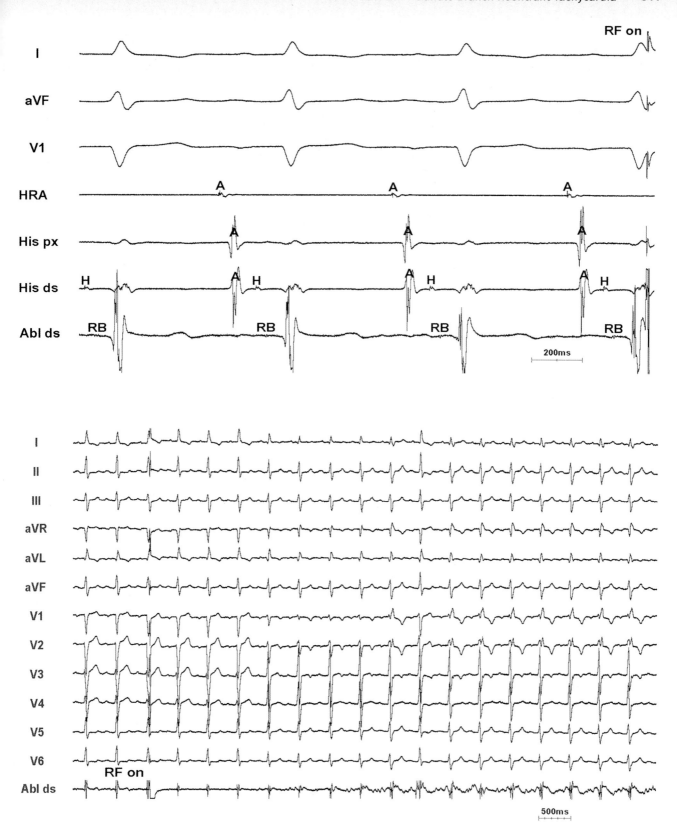

FIGURE 21-13 Ablation of the RB. The ablation catheter is positioned at the proximal RB distal to the His bundle where it records a small RB potential and large ventricular electrogram. Application of radiofrequency (RF) energy causes transient narrowing of the left IVCD (simultaneous and equal delay in both bundles) followed by complete RBBB.

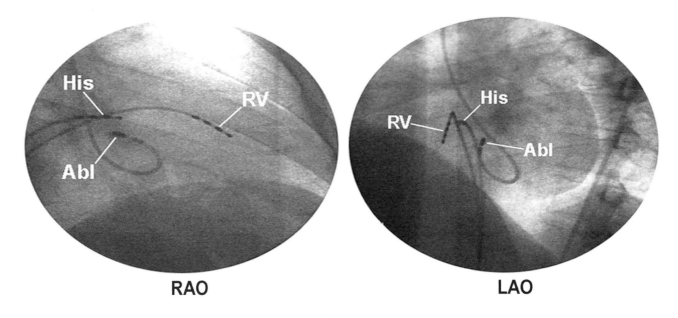

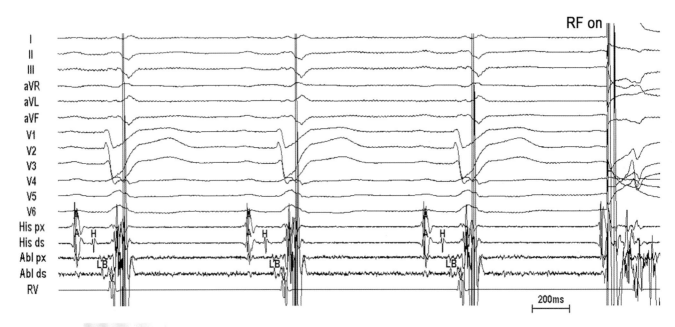

FIGURE 21-14 Ablation of the LB. The ablation catheter is advanced retrogradely across the aortic valve and positioned along the interventricular septum below the level of the right-sided His bundle catheter where it records a small far-field atrial signal, a LB potential, and a large ventricular electrogram. LB follows His bundle activation.

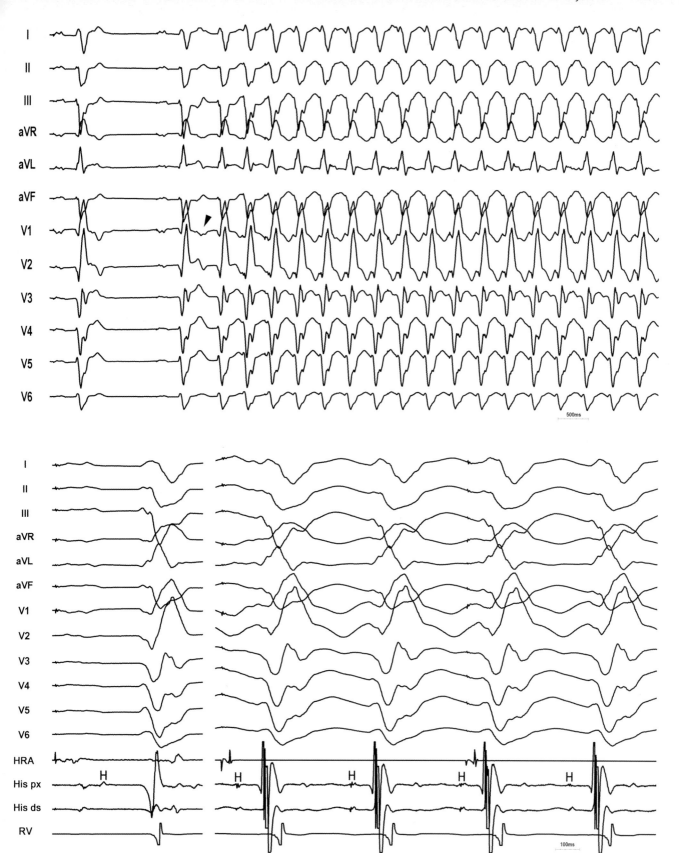

FIGURE 21-15 IFRT. *Top:* A single atrial premature depolarization (APD) (*arrowhead*) induces IFRT. *Bottom:* His bundle potentials precede each QRS complex (HV$_{[IFRT]}$ < HV$_{[NSR]}$). AV dissociation (atrial paced rhythm) is present. Note that RBBB/RS axis QRS complexes are identical during sinus rhythm and IFRT.

REFERENCES

1. Akhtar M, Gilbert C, Wolf FG, Schmidt DH. Reentry within the His-Purkinje system: elucidation of reentrant circuit using right bundle branch and His bundle recordings. Circulation 1978;58:295–304.

2. Narasimhan C, Jazayeri MR, Sra J, et al. Ventricular tachycardia in valvular heart disease: facilitation of sustained bundle-branch reentry by valve surgery. Circulation 1997;96:4307–4314.

3. Fedgchin B, Pavri BB, Greenspon AJ, Ho RT. Unique self-perpetuating cycle of atrioventricular block and phase IV bundle branch block in a patient with bundle branch reentrant tachycardia. Heart Rhythm 2004;1:493–496.

4. Li YG, Grönefeld G, Israel C, Bogun F, Hohnloser SH. Bundle branch reentrant tachycardia in patients with apparent normal His-Purkinje conduction: the role of functional conduction impairment. J Cardiovasc Electrophysiol 2002;13:1233–1239.

5. Kusa S, Taniguchi H, Hachiya H, et al. Bundle branch reentrant ventricular tachycardia with wide and narrow QRS morphology. Circ Arrhythm Electrophysiol 2013;6:e87–e91.

6. Blanck Z, Sra J, Dhala A, Deshpande S, Jazayeri M, Akhtar M. Bundle branch reentry: mechanisms, diagnosis, and treatment. In: Zipes DP, Jalife J, eds. Cardiac Electrophysiology: From Cell to Bedside. 3rd ed. Philadelphia, PA: W.B. Saunders, 2000:656–661.

7. Fisher JD. Bundle branch reentry tachycardia: why is the HV interval often longer than in sinus rhythm? The critical role of anisotropic conduction. J Interv Card Electrophysiol 2001;5:173–176.

8. Caceres J, Tchou P, Jazayeri M, McKinnie J, Avitall B, Akhtar M. New criterion for diagnosis of sustained bundle branch reentry tachycardia [abstract]. J Am Coll Cardiol 1989;13:21A.

9. Caceres J, Jazayeri M, McKinnie J, et al. Sustained bundle branch reentry as a mechanism of clinical tachycardia. Circulation 1989;79:256–270.

10. Nageh MF, Schwartz J, Mokabberi R, Dabiesingh D, Kalamkarian N. Bundle branch reentry ventricular tachycardia with His dissociation—the His bundle: bystander or participant? HeartRhythm Case Rep 2018;4:378–381.

11. Sarkozy A, Boussy T, Chierchia GB, Geelen P, Brugada P. An unusual form of bundle branch reentrant tachycardia. J Cardiovasc Electrophysiol 2006;17:902–906.

12. Akhtar M, Damato AN, Batsford WP, Ruskin JN, Ogunkelu B, Vargas G. Demonstration of re-entry within the His-Purkinje system in man. Circulation 1974;50:1150–1162.

13. Reddy CP, Damato AN, Akhtar M, Dhatt MS, Gomes JC, Calon AH. Effect of procainamide on reentry within the His-Purkinje system. Am J Cardiol 1977;40:957–964.

14. Denker S, Lehmann MH, Mahmud R, Gilbert C, Akhtar M. Facilitation of macroreentry within the His-Purkinje system with abrupt changes in cycle length. Circulation 1984;69:26–32.

15. Merino JL, Peinado R, Fernández-Lozano I, Sobrino N, Sobrino J. Transient entrainment of bundle-branch reentry by atrial and ventricular stimulation: elucidation of the tachycardia mechanism through analysis of the surface ECG. Circulation 1999;100:1784–1790.

16. Merino JL, Peinado R, Fernandez-Lozano I, et al. Bundle-branch reentry and the postpacing interval after entrainment by right ventricular stimulation: a new approach to elucidate the mechanism of wide-QRS-complex tachycardia with atrioventricular dissociation. Circulation 2001;103:1102–1108.

17. Michaud GF, Tada H, Chough S, et al. Differentiation of atypical atrioventricular node re-entrant from orthodromic reciprocating tachycardia using a septal accessory pathway by the response to ventricular pacing. J Am Coll Cardiol 2001;38:1163–1167.

18. Tchou P, Jazayeri M, Denker S, Dongas J, Caceres J, Akhtar M. Transcatheter electrical ablation of right bundle branch. A method of treating macroreentrant ventricular tachycardia attributed to bundle branch reentry. Circulation 1988;78:246–257.

19. Touboul P, Kirkorian G, Atallah G, et al. Bundle branch reentrant tachycardia treated by electrical ablation of the right bundle branch. J Am Coll Cardiol 1986;7:1404–1409.

20. Cohen TJ, Chien WW, Lurie KG, et al. Radiofrequency catheter ablation for treatment of bundle branch reentrant ventricular tachycardia: results and long-term follow-up. J Am Coll Cardiol 1991;18:1767–1773.

21. Balasundaram R, Rao HB, Kalavakolanu S, Narasimhan C. Catheter ablation of bundle branch reentrant ventricular tachycardia. Heart Rhythm 2008;5:S68–S72.

22. Schmidt B, Tang M, Chun KR. Left bundle branch-Purkinje system in patients with bundle branch reentrant tachycardia: lessons from catheter ablation and electroanatomic mapping. Heart Rhythm 2008;6:51–58.

23. Blanck Z, Sra J, Akhtar M. Incessant interfascicular reentrant ventricular tachycardia as a result of catheter ablation of the right bundle branch: case report and review of the literature. J Cardiovasc Electrophysiol 2009;20:1279–1283.

Unusual Electrophysiologic Phenomena

22

Introduction

Electrophysiology has many peculiar arrhythmias and patterns of conduction. One of them is the unexpected conduction of a premature impulse. This is manifested as either the unexpected narrowing of a QRS complex during bundle branch block (BBB) or the momentary resumption of atrioventricular (AV) conduction during AV block. Normally, closely coupled premature impulses fall into the relative (RRP) or effective refractory period (ERP) of a tissue (phase 3 of the action potential) and therefore conduct with delay or fail to conduct, respectively (phase 3 block (functional refractory period (FRP) of tissue proximally less than RRP/ERP of tissue distally)). Conduction of a more premature impulse is, therefore, paradoxical. Mechanism for the unexpected narrowing of BBB QRS by a premature impulse include 1) supernormality (**Figs. 22-1 and 22-2**), 2) gap phenomenon (**Figs. 22-3 and 22-4**), 3) resolution of phase 4 BBB (**Figs. 22-5 and 22-6; see also Fig. 1-40**), 4) bilateral bundle branch delay (**Fig. 22-7**), and 5) PVCs ipsilateral to the BBB (this latter mechanism is not the result of alterations in His-Purkinje conduction per se but early activation of the ipsilateral ventricle by the PVC cancelling the late unopposed ventricular forces from BBB).

The purpose of this chapter is to:

1. Discuss supernormality, gap phenomenon, and phase 4 block.
2. Discuss the concept of concealed conduction.
3. Discuss mechanisms for grouped beating: Wenckebach, exit block, and longitudinal dissociation.

SUPERNORMALITY

The supernormal period is a short window at the end of repolarization during which an impulse finds otherwise refractory tissue capable of conduction and/or excitability.[1,2] Because it occurs during repolarization, it behaves similarly to other repolarization phenomena showing cycle length dependency (restitution).[3,4] It is, therefore, not a static but rather a dynamic time window widening and shifting rightward with longer cycle lengths (analogous to the QT interval and QT dispersion). Its timing corresponds to the end or shortly after the T wave (the ECG marker of global ventricular myocardial repolarization), but it is repolarization of the tissue in question that determines the true supernormal period. Supernormality has been described in "all or none" (fast response) tissues with prolonged refractoriness (His-Purkinje, ventricular myocardium, accessory pathways [APs]) and not the AV node. Its most common manifestation is momentary resolution of BBB or AV block following a premature impulse (supernormal period of His-Purkinje conduction) (**Figs. 22-1, 22-2, and 22-8**).[5–9] While episodes of supernormality during AV block result in "better

than expected" conduction, sometimes "faster than expected" conduction occurs with paradoxical shortening of the PR interval (**see Fig. 1-35**). Spontaneous episodes of supernormality in APs are rare and require the unusual combination of AV block and a poorly conducting AP (**Fig. 22-9; see also Fig. 9-20**).[3,4,10–12] Supernormality in the ventricle occurs when otherwise subthreshold pacing stimuli capture the ventricle only during a critical period at the end of ventricular repolarization (supernormal period of ventricular excitability) (**Fig. 22-10**).[13] Supernormality might be due to a transient window of increased voltage in the transmembrane action potential at the end of repolarization.[2] However, the cellular basis of supernormality is unknown, and alternative mechanisms can also explain the phenomenon of unexpected conduction with prematurity.[14,15]

GAP PHENOMENA

During premature beats, the gap phenomenon refers to temporary loss of conduction over a structure at intermediate coupling intervals when longer and shorter coupling intervals are

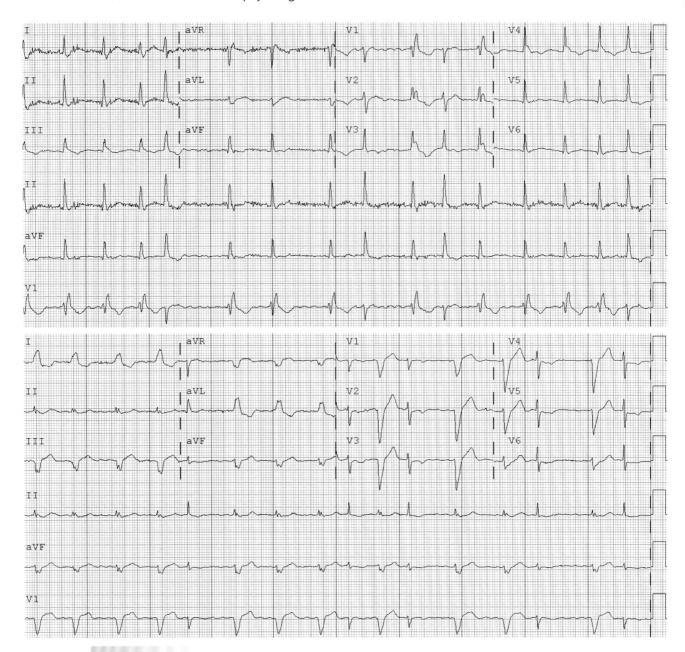

FIGURE 22-1 Supernormality in the right (*top*) and left (*bottom*) bundle. In both cases, the underlying rhythm is atrial fibrillation. QRS complexes normalize only during a short window at the end of repolarization when impulses fall into the supernormal period of the right and left bundle branch. Supernormality occurring later after the T wave results from concealed transeptal retrograde conduction from "unblocked" into "blocked" bundle—the late retrograde concealment into the "blocked" bundle shifts its supernormal period rightward.

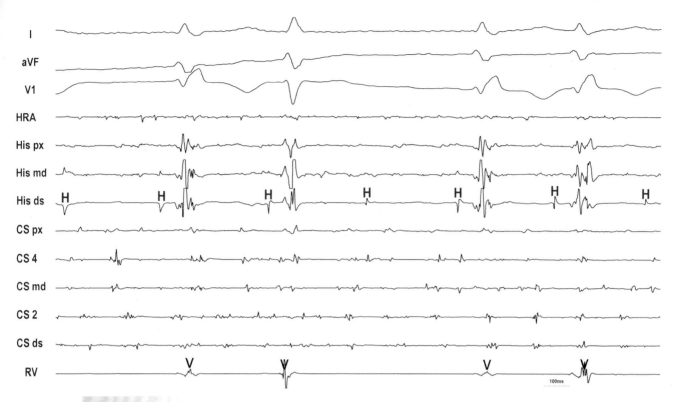

FIGURE 22-2 Supernormality in the right bundle. The underlying rhythm is atrial fibrillation with right bundle branch block (RBBB). Loss of RBBB occurs at a critical time at the end of repolarization during the supernormal period of the right bundle. Lack of HV prolongation indicates that QRS normalization is not due to simultaneous delay in the left bundle (equal bilateral bundle branch delay).

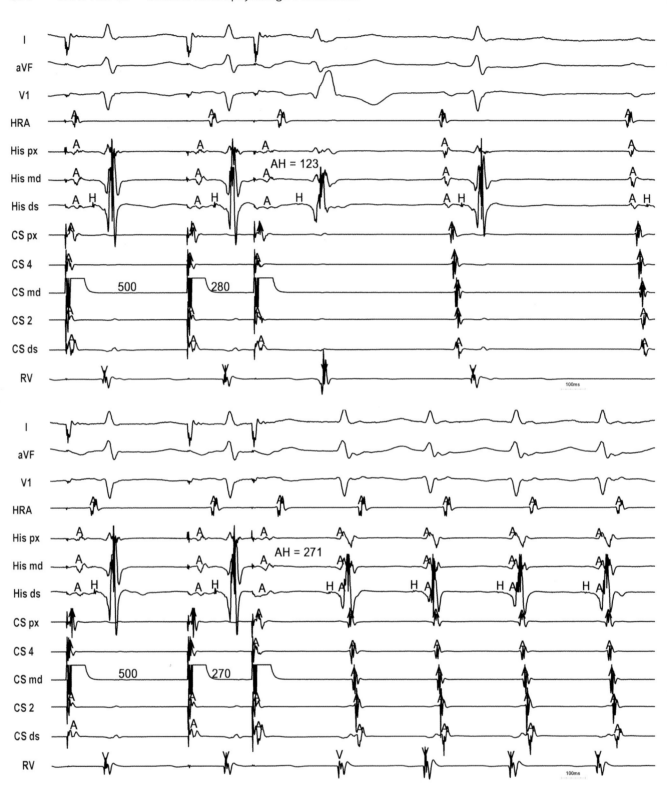

FIGURE 22-3 Gap phenomenon in the right bundle. During atrial extrastimulation at a coupling interval of 280 ms, conduction occurs over the FP (AH = 123), which encroaches on right bundle refractoriness causing right bundle branch block (RBBB). At 270 ms (FP ERP), conduction occurs over the SP (AH = 273 ms), allowing complete recovery of the right bundle, normalization of the QRS complex, and initiation of typical AVNRT.

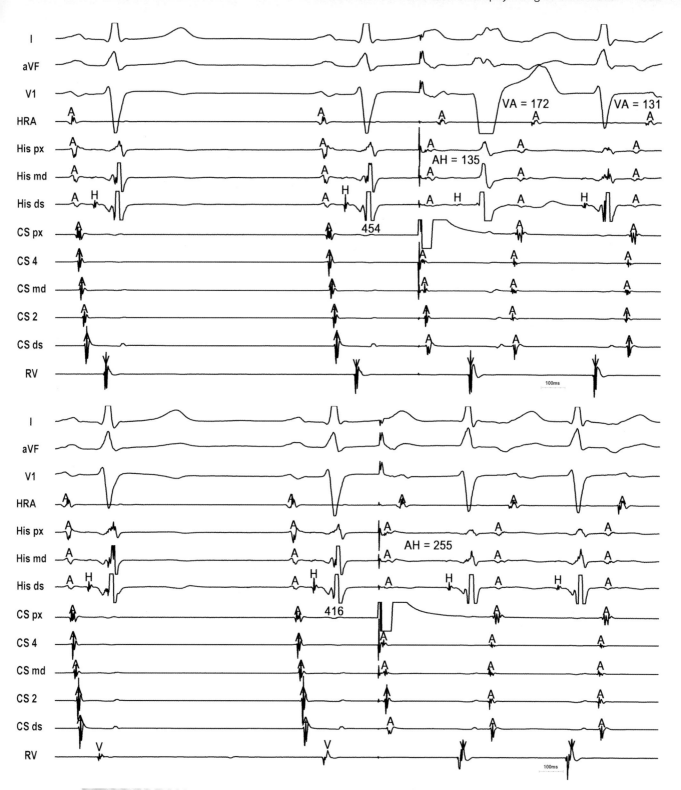

FIGURE 22-4 Gap phenomenon in the left bundle. A single atrial extrastimulus (coupling interval = 454 ms) conducts over the FP (AH = 135 ms) and encroaches on left bundle refractoriness causing left bundle branch block (LBBB). LBBB facilitates induction of orthodromic reciprocating tachycardia (ORT) using a left posterolateral AP. Note that the VA interval shortens by 41 ms with loss of LBBB. A shorter coupled extrastimulus (coupling interval = 416 ms) encounters FP refractoriness and conducts over the SP (AH = 255 ms) allowing complete recovery of the left bundle and normalization of the QRS complex. SP conduction facilitates induction of ORT.

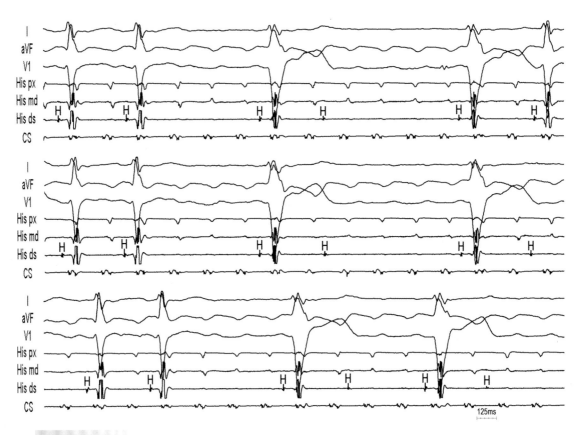

FIGURE 22-5 Phase 4 left bundle branch block (LBBB). The underlying rhythm is counterclockwise (CCW) cavo-tricuspid isthmus–dependent atrial flutter with phase 4 LBBB and infrahisian AV block. LBBB only occurs after long His-His intervals with paradoxical QRS normalization following short His-His intervals. Exposure of the His-Purkinje system to long–short sequences also causes phase 3 block in both bundle branches resulting in infrahisian AV block.

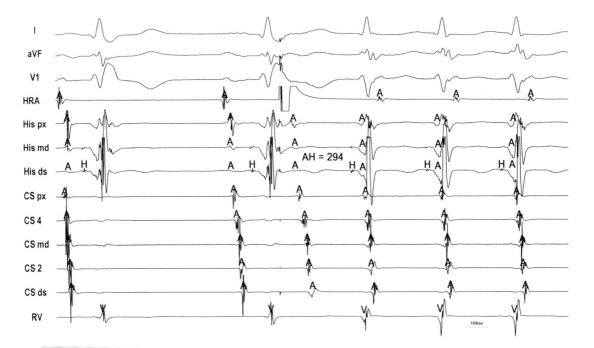

FIGURE 22-6 Phase 4 right bundle branch block (RBBB). A single atrial extrastimulus delivered during sinus rhythm encounters FP refractoriness, conducts over the SP (AH = 294 ms), and induces typical AVNRT. Phase 4 RBBB during sinus rhythm paradoxically disappears during AVNRT.

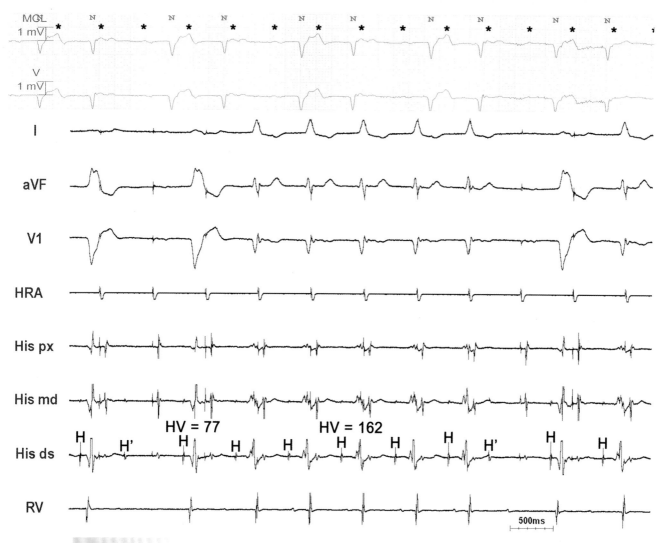

FIGURE 22-7 Bilateral bundle branch delay. The telemetry strip shows sinus rhythm (*asterisk*) with 3:2 Wenckebach AV block. Paradoxically, the first QRS complex shows left bundle branch block (LBBB), while the second QRS narrows. During HRA pacing, His bundle recordings show that QRS narrowing is preceded by an 85 ms prolongation of the HV interval, which in the setting of LBBB indicates simultaneous delay over the right bundle. Two His bundle extrasystoles (H′) cause pseudo AV block.

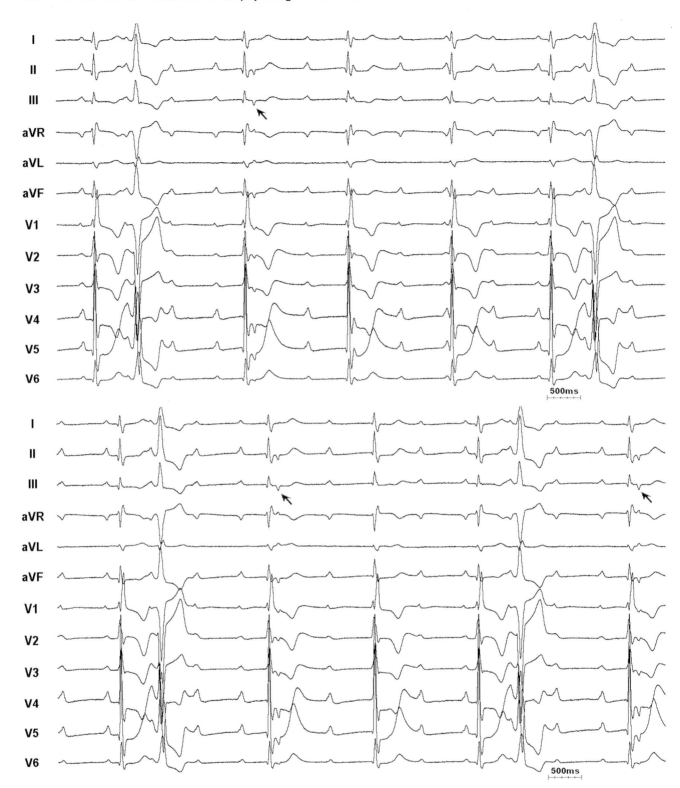

FIGURE 22-8 Supernormality in the right bundle. The underlying rhythm is sinus with complete AV block and a left ventricular escape rhythm. Critically timed P waves falling into the supernormal period of the right bundle (downslope of the T wave of escape complexes) conduct with left bundle branch block (LBBB). Note retrograde P waves (*arrows*) only follow escape complexes occurring in mid-diastole of the atrium.

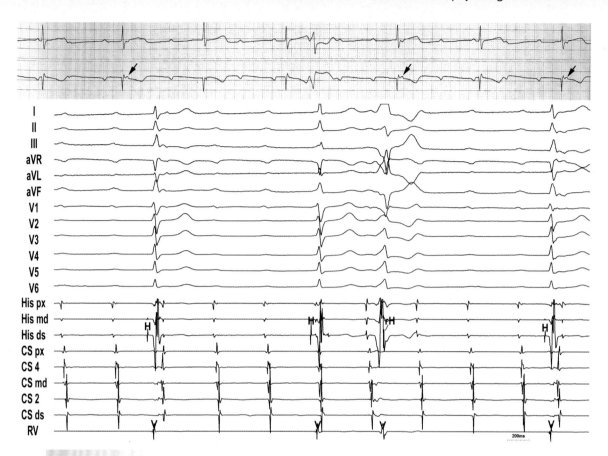

FIGURE 22-9 Supernormality in an AP. The underlying rhythm is sinus with complete AV block and a junctional escape rhythm. Only critically timed P waves falling into the supernormal period of the AP (end of the T wave of escape complexes) conduct with preexcitation. Junctional escape complexes occurring in mid-diastole of the atrium conduct retrogradely over the AP (*arrows*). The earliest site of atrial and ventricular activation during retrograde and antegrade AP conduction, respectively, is at the left posterior mitral annulus (CS md).

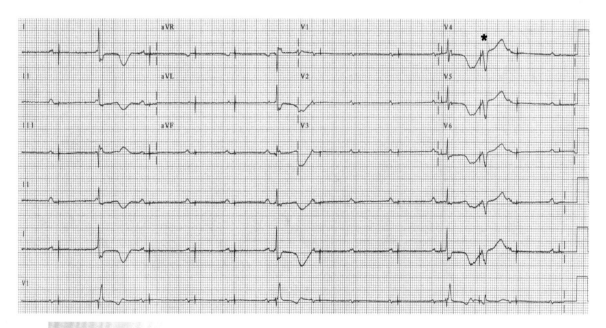

FIGURE 22-10 Supernormal period of ventricular excitability. The underlying rhythm is sinus with complete AV block and slow left ventricular escape rhythm. Atrial sensed-ventricular pacing stimuli are delivered—all of which fail to capture except for a single stimulus (*asterisk*) that falls into the supernormal period of ventricular excitability (end of the prolonged QT interval/T wave of the escape complex).

able to conduct (i.e., "gap" in conduction).[16,17] A premature impulse reaching a site in its absolute refractory period will fail to conduct (phase 3 block). A more premature impulse, however, might encounter relative refractoriness in tissue proximal to this site resulting in conduction delay. Enough delay proximally allows the previously blocked site sufficient time to recover excitability and conduct distally ("proximal delay allowing distal conduction"). Gap phenomena have been described both antegradely (six types) and retrogradely (two types) along the conduction system, particularly in the setting of dual AV node physiology (the slow pathway [SP] providing delay proximal to the His-Purkinje system) (**Figs. 22-3, 22-4, and 22-11 to 22-13**).[18–21]

PHASE 4 BLOCK

Phase 3 of the His-Purkinje action potential is the end of repolarization during which tissue is partially excitable or completely inexcitable. Impulses encroaching on refractoriness at this time conduct with delay or block (phase 3, acceleration-dependent, or tachycardia-dependent block). Phase 4 of the His-Purkinje action potential is during electrical diastole following complete repolarization during which tissue is fully excitable and capable of propagation. Diseased His-Purkinje tissue, however, can show spontaneous diastolic depolarizations of its transmembrane potential due to inward Na current. The longer the diastolic period, the more Na channels that are activated and the less Na channels available to elicit excitation and subsequent propagation (reduced Na channel reserve). In contrast to phase 3 block, phase 4 block (deceleration-dependent or bradycardia-dependent block) occurs after long diastolic intervals. Phase 4 BBB results in BBB at slower heart rates with resolution at faster rates (narrowing with prematurity) (**Figs. 22-5, 22-6, 22-14, and 22-15**).[22–24] Phase 4 AV block is one mechanism of paroxysmal AV block triggered by momentary slowing of the heart rate, particularly following the pause caused by premature beats (**see Figs. 1-22 to 1-26**).[25,26] Phase 4 AP block results in the paradoxical loss of preexcitation after long diastolic intervals (**see Figs. 9-17 and 9-18**).[27–29]

BILATERAL, EQUAL DELAY

The morphologic pattern of BBB results from conduction differences between the right and left bundle (conduction delay or failure of one bundle relative to the other). If BBB results from conduction delay and a premature impulse finds the contralateral bundle in its RRP, equal (or nearly equal) delay will cause simultaneous (or nearly simultaneous) activation of the ventricles from both bundles and narrowing of the QRS complex (narrowing with prematurity) (**Fig. 22-7**). During BBB, the HV interval reflects the conduction time over the faster or "unblocked" bundle. The hallmark of bilateral, equal delay therefore is prolongation of the HV (and PR) interval.

CONCEPT OF CONCEALED CONDUCTION

Concealed conduction explains many electrophysiologic phenomena, particularly unusual disturbances in AV conduction caused by retrograde concealment.[30,31] Concealed conduction itself is invisible with no direct expression on the ECG (hence, the term "concealed"), but its presence is inferred by the effect is has on subsequent events on the ECG. One of the most common manifestation of concealed conduction is retrograde penetration of a PVC into the AV node–His-Purkinje axis causing post-ectopic PR prolongation, post-ectopic AV block (and the subsequent compensatory pause), and post-ectopic BBB (**Fig. 22-16**). In normal His-Purkinje tissues, other manifestations of concealed conduction include 1) unmasking of dual AV node physiology during sinus rhythm by a PVC (retrograde concealed conduction into the SP and fast pathway [FP]) (**see Fig. 7-1**), 2) induction and termination of lower common final pathway (LCFP) block during atrio-ventricular nodal reentrant tachycardia (AVNRT) by ventricular pacing (retrograde concealed conduction into the distal AV node–His bundle) (**see Figs. 7-16 to 7-19 and 7-24**), and 3) resolution of functional BBB during supraventricular tachycardia (SVT) by a PVC (retrograde concealed conduction into the Purkinje system breaking the "transeptal link") (**see Figs. 5-3, 7-23, and 10-6**). In these cases, premature retrograde concealment into the nonconducting structure causes a leftward shift in depolarization (and therefore repolarization ("peeling back of refractoriness")), allowing a previously blocked impulse of the same timing to conduct. Conduction of this impulse then alters the timing and pattern of refractoriness interrupting the mechanisms perpetuating block (long-short sequences, transeptal linking), thereby facilitating conduction of subsequent impulses. In diseased His-Purkinje tissue, manifestations of concealed conduction include initiation of 1) phase 4 AV block by a PVC (**see Figs. 1-25 and 1-26**) and 2) transient complete AV block by rapid ventricular pacing/repetitive ventricular ectopy (fatigue phenomena) (**Fig. 22-17**; **see also Fig. 1-36**). Abrupt loss of preexcitation following a PVC results from retrograde concealment into the AP (**Fig. 22-18**). Following each normal QRS complex, repetitive retrograde concealment from His-Purkinje conduction into the AP renders the AP persistently refractory and maintains loss of preexcitation.

GROUPED BEATING

The phenomena of grouped beating has several different mechanisms including 1) Wenckebach periodicity, 2) exit block, and 3) longitudinal dissociation.

WENCKEBACH PERIODICITY

Mobitz type I or Wenckebach conduction is characterized by conduction delay followed by block.[32] It is the hallmark of decrementally conducting tissue, the classic structure being the AV node. Wenckebach periodicity can be typical or atypical—the latter being more common at higher (e.g., 5:4) conduction ratios.

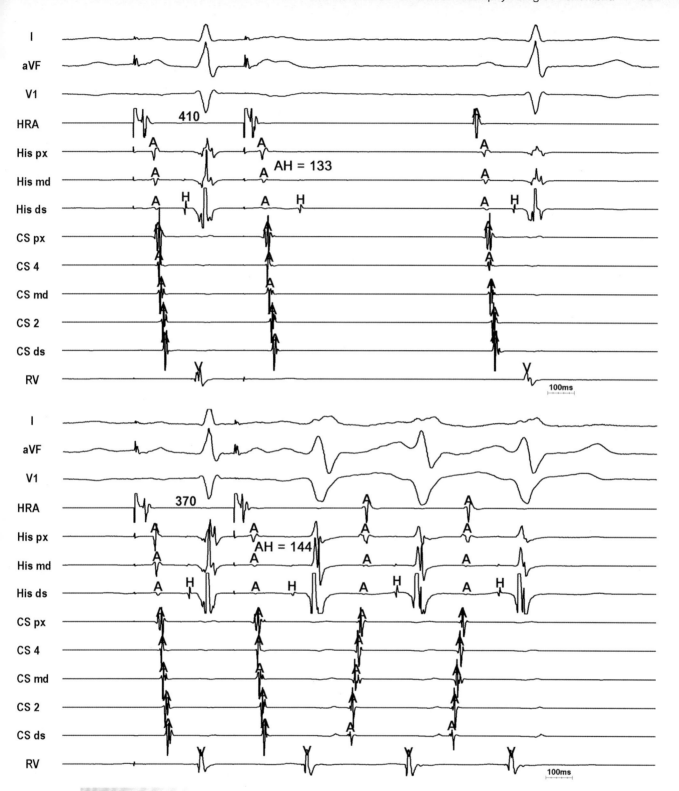

FIGURE 22-11 Gap phenomenon in the right bundle. During atrial extrastimulation at a coupling interval of 410 ms, conduction occurs over the AV node/His bundle (AH = 133 ms) but encounters physiologic refractoriness in the bundle branches (because of the long–short sequence inherent in programmed extrastimulation). At 370 ms, conduction delay over the AV node (AH = 144 ms) allows recovery of right bundle refractoriness resulting in left bundle branch block (LBBB) QRS complexes and induction of two orthodromic reentrant beats using a left free wall AP.

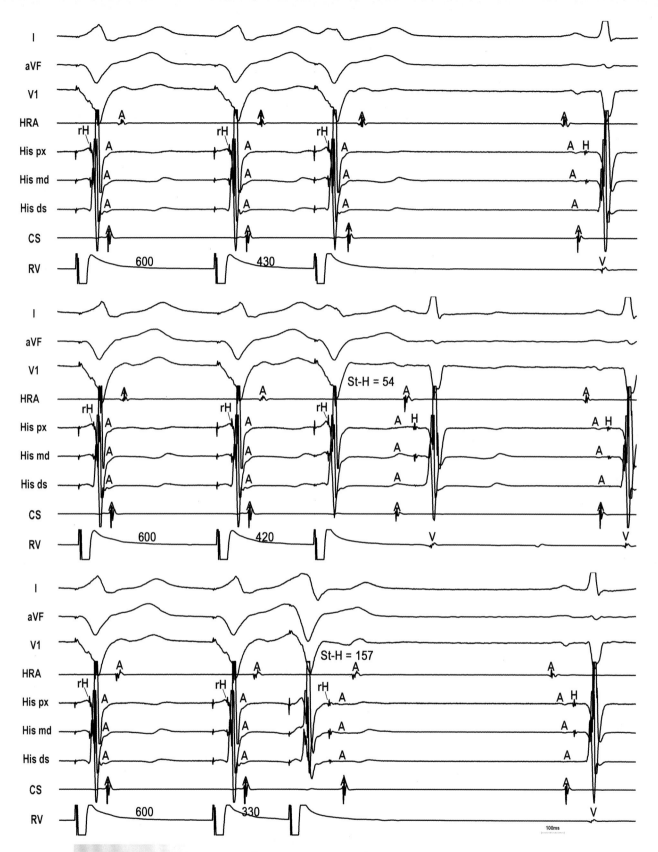

FIGURE 22-12 Gap phenomenon in the FP. During programmed ventricular extrastimulation at a coupling interval of 430 ms, retrograde conduction occurs over the FP (short HA, earliest atrial activation at His bundle region). At 420 ms (FP ERP), retrograde conduction occurs over the SP (long HA, earliest atrial activation at CS os). At 320 ms, retrograde block in the right bundle causes a "VH jump" (103 ms increase in St-H interval) allowing resumption of FP conduction.

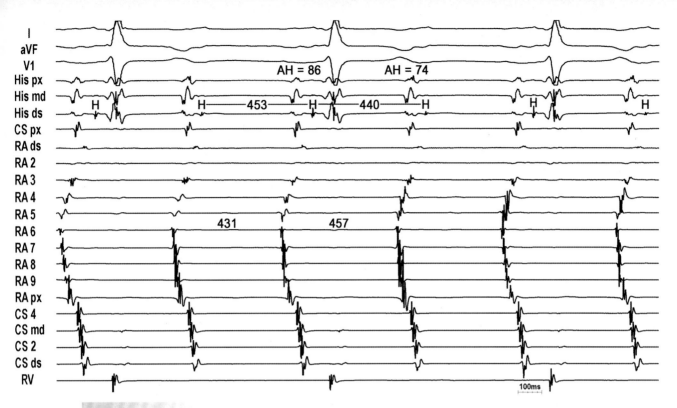

FIGURE 22-13 Gap phenomenon in the His-Purkinje system. The underlying rhythm is a right atrial tachycardia with cycle length alternans and 2:1 AV block below the His bundle. Paradoxically, longer AA intervals are followed by infrahisian block because they are followed by shorter AH (74 ms) and, therefore, HH (440 ms) intervals that encroach upon His-Purkinje refractoriness. In contrast, shorter AA cycles encroach upon AV nodal refractoriness producing longer AH (86 ms) and, therefore, HH (453 ms) intervals that allow His-Purkinje conduction.

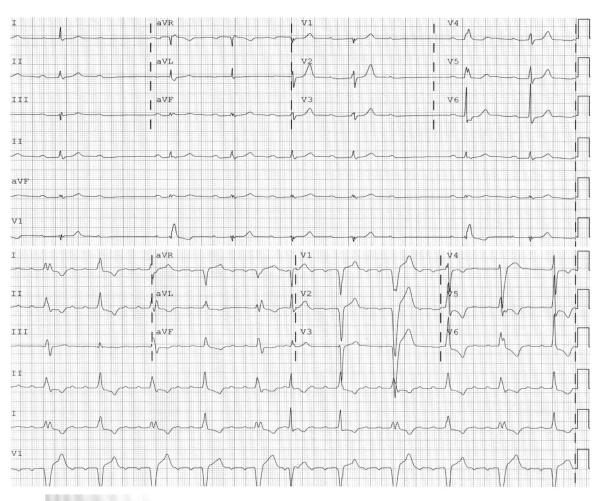

FIGURE 22-14 Phase 4 block in the right (*top*) and left (*bottom*) bundle. *Top*: The underlying rhythm is sinus with 5:4 Wenckebach AV block. Right bundle branch block (RBBB) follows each pause because of phase 4 block in the right bundle. *Bottom*: The underlying rhythm is a right atrial tachycardia/flutter with variable AV conduction and different degrees of left bundle aberration. Note that the degree of left bundle branch block (LBBB) correlates directly with the length of the preceding RR interval. (More left bundle fibers are exposed to phase 4 block at longer cycle lengths.)

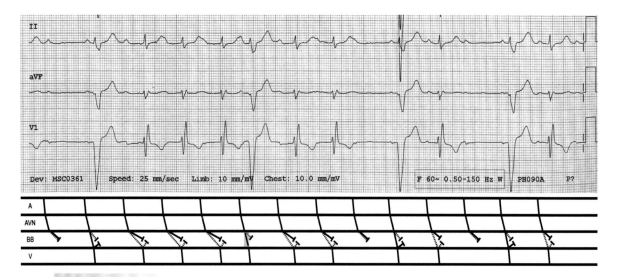

FIGURE 22-15 Phase 4 block in the left bundle. The underlying rhythm is sinus with alternating BBB and AV block. Left bundle branch block (LBBB) follows the longest and shortest RR intervals due to phase 4 block in the left bundle and supernormality in the right bundle, respectively. In the ladder diagram, solid lines denote right bundle (RB) conduction and dotted lines denote left bundle (LB) conduction. Shaded window denotes RB supernormal period.

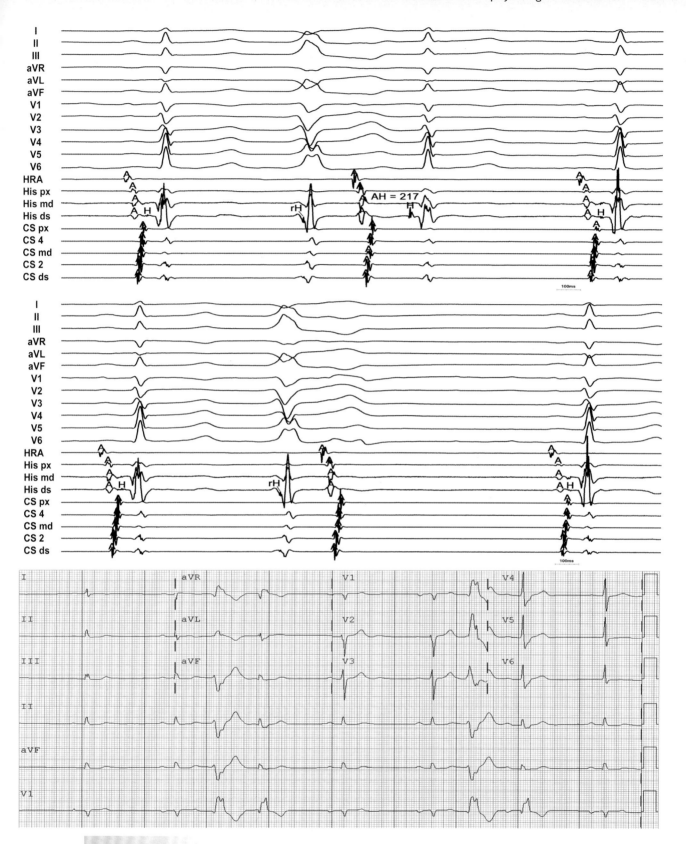

FIGURE 22-16 Concealed conduction into the AV node–His-Purkinje system. A right ventricle (RV) ventricular premature depolarization (VPD) retrogradely penetrates the right bundle (RB)-His bundle (rH) and conceals into the AV node. Subsequent longer and shorter coupled sinus beats encounter relative (*top*) and absolute (*middle*) AV nodal refractoriness resulting in post-ectopic PR prolongation and AV block, respectively. A left ventricle VPD retrogradely penetrates the His-Purkinje system. Later penetration of the RB than left bundle (LB) causes RB refractoriness with the subsequent sinus beat resulting in post-ectopic right bundle branch block (RBBB).

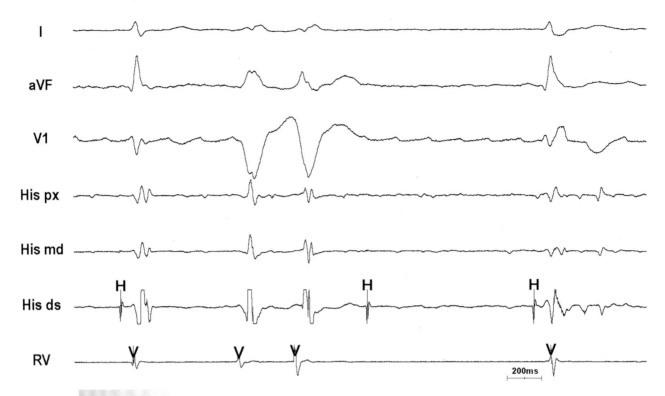

FIGURE 22-17 Concealed conduction into the His-Purkinje system. The underlying rhythm is atrial fibrillation. A ventricular couplet conceals retrogradely into the His-Purkinje system, rendering it refractory and causing one beat of infrahisian block. Note that the subsequent QRS complex manifests right bundle branch block (RBBB) due to persistent refractoriness in the right bundle.

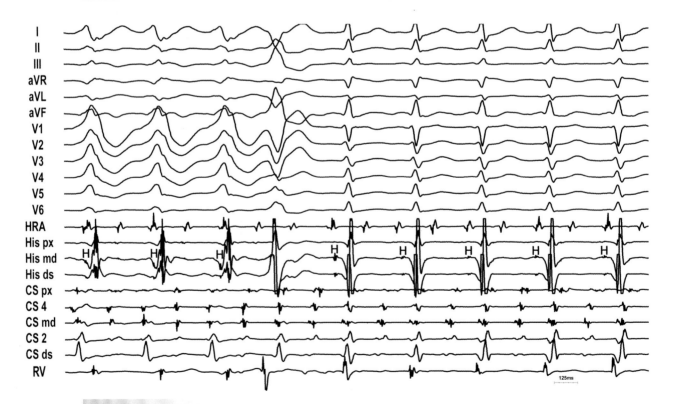

FIGURE 22-18 Concealed conduction into a left free wall AP. The underlying rhythm is preexcited atrial flutter. A spontaneous early-coupled ventricular premature depolarization (VPD) from the right ventricle conceals retrogradely into the AP rendering it refractory causing abrupt loss of preexcitation. Repetitive retrograde concealment from the His-Purkinje system into the AP maintains persistent loss of preexcitation.

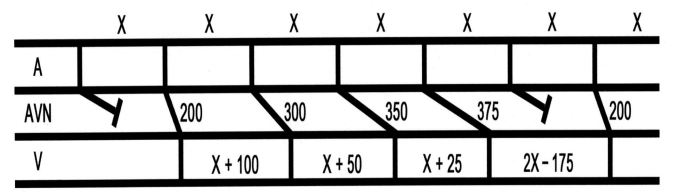

FIGURE 22-19 Diagram of typical AV node (AVN) Wenckebach periodicity. While PR intervals prolong, the increment in PR prolongation decreases causing progressive shortening of the RR interval. The length of each pause = 2 (sinus cycle length) – total increment in PR prolongation.

During typical AV node Wenckebach, PR intervals progressively prolong but the increment in PR prolongation shortens, resulting in successive shortening of the RR interval (Fig. 22-19).[32] The largest increment in PR prolongation, therefore, follows the second P wave of each Wenckebach cycle. The length of each pause equals 2(basic cycle length) – total increment in PR prolongation. During atypical Wenckebach, the increment in PR prolongation within each cycle can lengthen, shorten, or remain the same so that RR intervals lengthen, shorten, or remain the same. In addition to the AV node, however, diseased "all or none" tissue including the His-Purkinje system and myocardium can show Wenckebach phenomena (Fig. 22-20; see also Figs. 1-13, 1-15, and 1-16).

EXIT BLOCK

Exit block refers to failure of impulse propagation beyond an automatically discharging focus when the surrounding tissue is not refractory.[33] Perifocal conduction and block can show 2:1, Mobitz type I (Wenckebach) or Mobitz type II behavior. Mobitz type I and II blocks result in a pause that is less than (Mobitz type I) or equal to (Mobitz type II) twice the basic cycle length

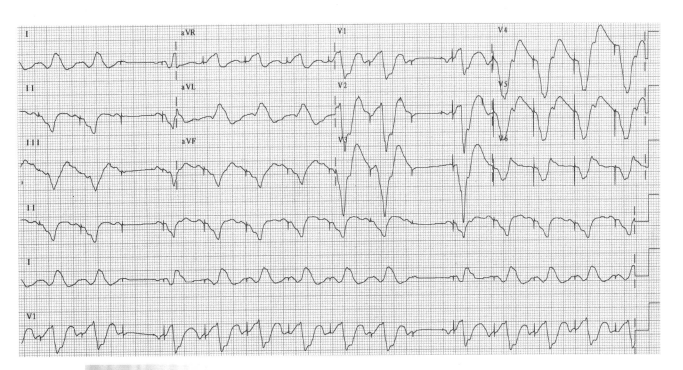

FIGURE 22-20 Wenckebach in ventricular muscle. The underlying rhythm is AV sequential pacing with complete AV block and periodic ventricular noncapture. Paced ventricular complexes progressively widen until noncapture (myocardial Wenckebach with either true noncapture or local capture and ventricular propagation failure (global block)).

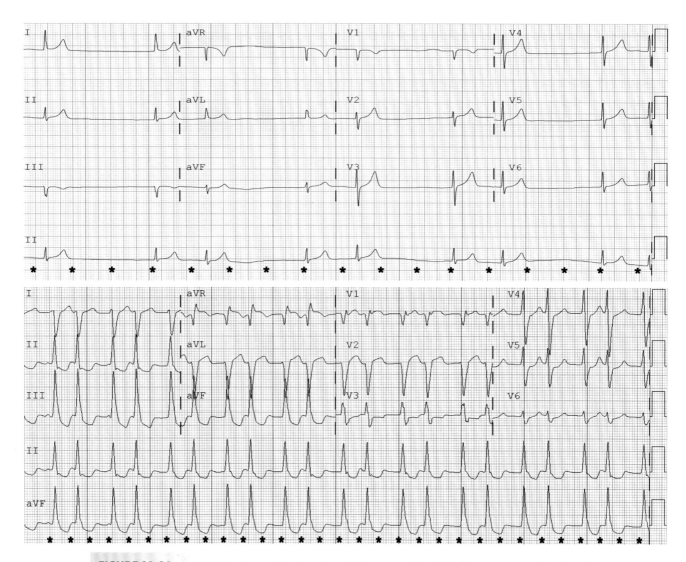

FIGURE 22-21 Exit block. *Top:* Junctional tachycardia with 4:2 exit Wenckebach block. *Bottom:* Ventricular tachycardia with 3:2 exit Wenckebach block. The asterisk denotes the discharging focus.

of the discharging focus. Exit block has been observed for the sino-atrial (SA) node, AV junction, ventricular tachycardia, and paced rhythms (**Fig. 22-21; see also Fig. 1-2**). One intriguing automatically discharging focus showing exit block is parasystole. A parasystolic focus has entrance block (not reset by sinus rhythm) and exit block. The ECG manifestations of parasystole are therefore 1) variable coupling intervals (entrance block), 2) fusion complexes, and 3) interectopic parasystolic intervals that are a multiple of a basic parasystolic interval (exit block) (**Fig. 22-22**).[34] Incomplete entrance block, however, allows re-setting of the parasystolic focus (modulated parasystole) allowing for fixed coupling intervals and grouped beating.

LONGITUDINAL DISSOCIATION

A structure with longitudinal dissociation has two functional and/or anatomical parallel pathways—one with slower conduction/shorter refractoriness and the other with faster conduction/longer refractoriness. Alternate conduction over each pathway gives rises to long–short cycles and grouped beating. The classic structure with longitudinal dissociation is the AV node (**see Figs. 7-45, 10-30, and 10-31**).[35] Rarely, an AP can manifest longitudinal dissociation resulting in grouped beating during orthodromic and antidromic reciprocating tachycardia.[36] Longitudinal dissociation has also been described for the His bundle (committed fibers destined for the right or left bundle) and the cavo-tricuspid isthmus.[37,38]

Other mechanisms of grouped beating include 1) escape-capture bigeminy and 2) supernormality. Escape complexes followed by fortuitously-timed sinus captures or reciprocating echoes cause bigeminal beating (**Fig. 22-23**). In the setting of AV block, isolated or repetitive episode of supernormal AV conduction causes grouped beating (**see Figs. 1-34, 1-35, and 9-20**).[39,40]

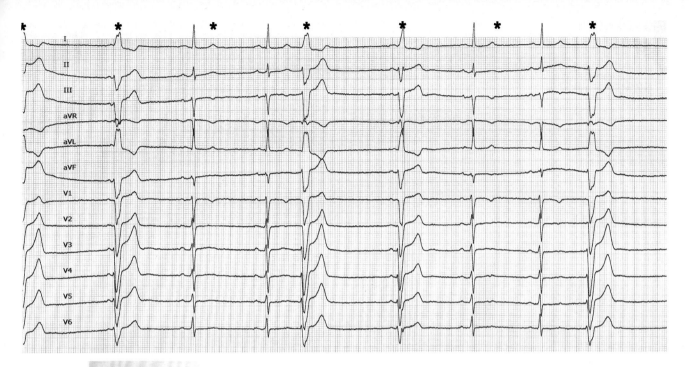

FIGURE 22-22 Parasystole. The underlying rhythm is sinus with frequent, unifocal ventricular ectopy. Ectopic beats exhibit left bundle branch block (LBBB) morphology, greater than V6 transition, and left superior axis suggesting origin from the moderator band. They show variable coupling intervals (entrance block), fusion, and interectopic intervals that are twice the basic parasystolic interval (exit block). The asterisk denotes the discharging focus.

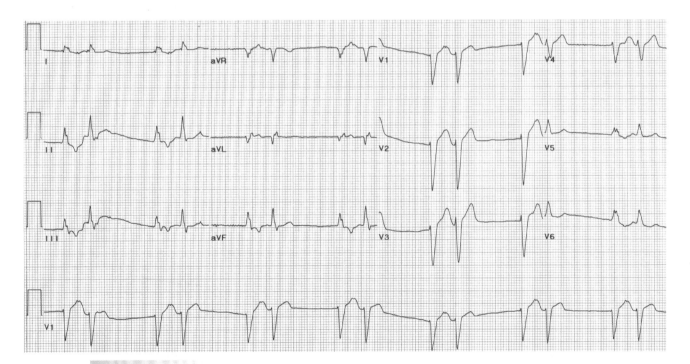

FIGURE 22-23 Escape-capture bigeminy. Junctional escape complexes are followed by atypical AV nodal echoes causing grouped beating with underlying left bundle branch block (LBBB).

REFERENCES

1. Adrian ED, Lucas K. On the summation of propagated disturbances in nerve and muscle. J Physiol 1912;44:68–124.
2. Massumi RA, Amsterdam EA, Mason DT. Phenomenon of supernormality in the human heart. Circulation 1972;46:264–275.
3. Lum JJ, Ho RT. Dynamic effects of exercise and different escape rhythms on the supernormal period of an accessory pathway. J Cardiovasc Electrophysiol 2007;18:672–675.
4. Przybylski J, Chiale A, Sánchez RA, et al. Supernormal conduction in the accessory pathway of patients with overt or concealed ventricular pre-excitation. J Am Coll Cardiol 1987;9:1269–1278.
5. Ho RT, Stopper M, Koka A. Alternating bundle branch block. Pacing Clin Electrophysiol 2012;35:223–226.
6. Ho RT. An uncommon manifestation of atrio-ventricular block: what is the mechanism? Pacing Clin Electrophysiol 2014;37:900–903.
7. Ho RT, Rhim ES, Pavri BB, Greenspon AJ. An unusual pattern of atrioventricular block. J Cardiovasc Electrophysiol 2007;18:1000–1002.
8. Lewis T, Master AM. Supernormal recovery phase, illustrated by two clinical cases of heart block. Heart 1924;11:371.
9. Kline EM, Conn JW, Rosenbaum FF. Variations in A-V and V-A conduction dependent upon the time relations of auricular and ventricular systole: the supernormal phase. Am Heart J 1939;17:524–535.
10. McHenry PL, Knoebel SB, Fisch C. The Wolff-Parkinson-White (WPW) syndrome with supernormal conduction through the anomalous bypass. Circulation 1966;34:734–739.
11. Calabrò MP, Saporito F, Carerj S, Oreto G. "Early" capture beats in advanced A-V block: by which mechanism? J Cardiovasc Electrophysiol 2005;16:1108–1109.
12. Chang M, Miles WM, Prystowsky EN. Supernormal conduction in accessory atrioventricular connections. Am J Cardiol 1987;59:852–856.
13. Soloff LA, Fewell JW. The supernormal phase of ventricular excitation in man. Its bearing on the genesis of ventricular premature systoles, and a note on atrioventricular conduction. Am Heart J 1960;59:869–874.
14. Gallagher JJ, Damato AN, Varghese PJ, Caracta AR, Josephson ME, Lau SH. Alternative mechanisms of apparent supernormal atrioventricular conduction. Am J Cardiol 1973;31:362–371.
15. Moe GK, Childers RW, Merideth J. An appraisal of "supernormal" A-V conduction. Circulation 1968;38:5–28.
16. Wit AL, Damato AN, Weiss MB, Steiner C. Phenomenon of the gap in atrioventricular conduction in the human heart. Circ Res 1970;27:679–689.
17. Wu D, Denes P, Dhingra R, Rosen KM. Nature of the gap phenomenon in man. Circ Res 1974;34:682–692.
18. Brodine WN, Lyons C, Han J. Dual atrioventricular nodal pathways associated with a gap phenomenon in atrioventricular nodal conduction. J Am Coll Cardiol 1983;2:582–584.
19. Mirvis DM, Bandura JP. Atrioventricular nodal gap conduction as a manifestation of dual nodal pathways. Am J Cardiol 1978;41:1115–1118.
20. Bonow RO, Josephson ME. Spontaneous gap phenomenon in atrioventricular conduction produced by His bundle extrasystoles. J Electrocardiol 1977;10:283–286.
21. Akhtar M, Damato AN, Caracta AR, Batsford WP, Lau SH. The gap phenomena during retrograde conduction in man. Circulation 1974;49:811–817.
22. Massumi R. Bradycardia-dependent bundle-branch block. A critique and proposed criteria. Circulation 1968;38:1066–1073.
23. Fisch C, Miles W. Deceleration-dependent left bundle branch block: a spectrum of bundle branch conduction delay. Circulation 1982;65:1029–1032.
24. Schamroth L, Lewis CM. Normalisation of a bundle branch block pattern in early beats. The "supernormal" phase of intraventricular conduction, intraventricular block due to phase 4 diastolic depolarisation. J Electrocardiol 1971;4:199–203.
25. Mallya R, Pavri BB, Greenspon AJ, Ho RT. Recurrent paroxysmal atrioventricular block triggered paradoxically by a pacemaker. Heart Rhythm 2005;2:185–187.
26. El-Sherif N, Jalife J. Paroxysmal atrioventricular block: are phase 3 and phase 4 block mechanisms or misnomers? Heart Rhythm 2009;6:1514–1521.
27. Przybylski J, Chiale PA, Quinteiro RA, Elizari MV, Rosenbaum MB. The occurrence of phase-4 block in the anomalous bundle of patients with Wolff-Parkinson-White syndrome. Eur J Cardiol 1975;3:267–280.
28. Lerman BB, Josephson ME. Automaticity of the Kent bundle: confirmation by phase 3 and phase 4 block. J Am Coll Cardiol 1985;5:996–998.
29. Fujiki A, Tani M, Mizumaki K, Yoshida S, Sasayama S. Rate-dependent accessory pathway conduction due to phase 3 and phase 4 block. Antegrade and retrograde conduction properties. J Electrocardiol 1992;25:25–31.
30. Langendorf R. Concealed A-V conduction: the effect of blocked impulses on the formation and conduction of subsequent impulses. Am Heart J 1948;35:542–552.
31. Langendorf R, Pick A. Artificial pacing of the human heart: its contribution to the understanding of the arrhythmias. Am J Cardiol 1971;28:516–525.
32. Friedman HS, Gomes JA, Haft JI. An analysis of Wenckebach periodicity. J Electrocardiol 1975;8:307–315.
33. Fisch C, Greenspan K, Anderson GJ. Exit block. Am J Cardiol 1971;28:402–405.
34. Moe GK, Jalife J, Mueller WJ, Moe B. A mathematical model of parasystole and its application to clinical arrhythmias. Circulation 1977;56:968–979.
35. Moe GK, Preston JB, Burlington H. Physiologic evidence for a dual A-V transmission system. Circ Res 1956;4:357–375.
36. Atié J, Brugada P, Brugada J, et al. Longitudinal dissociation of atrioventricular accessory pathways. J Am Coll Cardiol 1991;17:161–166.
37. Narula OS. Longitudinal dissociation in the His bundle. Bundle branch block due to asynchronous conduction within the His bundle in man. Circulation 1977;56:996–1006.
38. Shen MJ, Knight BP, Kim SS. Fusion during entrainment at the cavotricuspid isthmus: what is the mechanism? Heart Rhythm 2018;15:787–789.
39. Satullo G, Donato A, Busà G, Grassi R. 4:2 Atrioventricular block: what is the mechanism? J Cardiovasc Electrophysiol 2003;14:1252–1253.
40. Trohman RG, Pinski SL. Supernormality with cycle length-dependent intra-His alternans: a new cause of group beating. Pacing Clin Electrophysiol 1997;20:2496–2499.

Index

Page numbers followed by *f* or *t* refer to figures or tables, respectively.